PSYCHOLOGY LIBRARY EDITIONS: NEUROPSYCHOLOGY

Volume 9

NEUROPSYCHOLOGY AFTER LASHLEY

NEUROPSYCHOLOGY AFTER LASHLEY

Fifty Years Since the Publication of *Brain Mechanisms and Intelligence*

Edited by
JACK ORBACH

Routledge
Taylor & Francis Group
LONDON AND NEW YORK

First published in 1982 by Lawrence Erlbaum Associates, Inc.

This edition first published in 2019
by Routledge
2 Park Square, Milton Park, Abingdon, Oxon OX14 4RN

and by Routledge
711 Third Avenue, New York, NY 10017

Routledge is an imprint of the Taylor & Francis Group, an informa business

British Library Cataloguing in Publication Data
A catalogue record for this book is available from the British Library

ISBN: 978-1-138-48894-6 (Set)
ISBN: 978-0-429-45935-1 (Set) (ebk)
ISBN: 978-1-138-59245-2 (Volume 9) (hbk)
ISBN: 978-1-138-59332-9 (Volume 9) (pbk)
ISBN: 978-0-429-49003-3 (Volume 9) (ebk)

Publisher's Note
The publisher has gone to great lengths to ensure the quality of this reprint but points out that some imperfections in the original copies may be apparent.

NEUROPSYCHOLOGY AFTER LASHLEY

Fifty Years Since the Publication of *Brain Mechanisms and Intelligence*

Edited by

JACK ORBACH

Queens College

City University of New York

LAWRENCE ERLBAUM ASSOCIATES, PUBLISHERS

1982 Hillsdale, New Jersey London

Lawrence Erlbaum Associates, Inc., Publishers
365 Broadway
Hillsdale, New Jersey 07642

Library of Congress Cataloging in Publication Data
Neuropsychology after Lashley.

Originally presented as a series of lectures at Queens College of the City University of New York.
Includes bibliographies and index.
1. Neuropsychology—Addresses, essays, lectures.
2. Lashley, Karl Spencer, 1890-1958. Brain mechanisms and intelligence. I. Orbach, Jack, 1927–
II. Beach, Frank Ambrose, 1911– . [DNLM:
1. Psychophysiology. WL 103 N4935]
QP360.N494 612.8 80-28787
ISBN 0-89859-088-4
Printed in the United States of America
10 9 8 7 6 5 4 3 2 1

Contents

Preface

These lectures grew out of a graduate seminar in contemporary neuropsychology that I planned for the fall semester in 1979 at Queens College of the City University of New York. In preparation, I began with the following notation, "1979—50 years after the publication of Lashley's *Brain Mechanisms and Intelligence*. The aim is to review Lashley's major contributions and to trace the development of physiological psychology through the experimental work of Lashley's students and colleagues (e.g., Beach, Chow, Evarts, Hebb, Pribram, Riesen, Sperry) and those influenced by Lashley's writings (e.g., Diamond, Doty, John, Lindsley, the Pasiks, Riopelle, Robert Thompson, Weiskrantz)." Though the task seemed formidable, the occasion was appropriate, and I began toying with the idea of a lecture series to celebrate the semicentennial of publication of Lashley's monograph. Titled "Neuropsychology After Lashley: 50 Years Since the Publication of *Brain Mechanisms and Intelligence*," the lectures would be sponsored by the Neuropsychology Program at Queens College of the City University of New York and delivered at Queens College during the fall semester, 1979–1980. Why not invite these individuals to review their own experimental work in a lecture, one per week during the semester, and to indicate how Lashley's seminal contributions might have exerted an influence in shaping or directing their thinking? Our students would benefit by having firsthand contact with eminent neuroscientists at the formal lectures and after, at a cocktail party and reception. And I would help reawaken an interest in Lashley's contributions and focus attention on those of his students. I saw my own role as convener of the lectures, as reviewer of Lashley's work a generation after his retirement, and as editor of the resulting volume.

Before I could proceed, I had to determine whether prospective participants would in fact respond positively to my invitations. Most did. Those who could not participate in the lecture series, for one reason or another, responded positively to my request for a chapter to be included in the volume, either an original manuscript or a recent reprint. Those individuals were Beach, Hebb, and Sperry, as well as A. J. Berman, E. R. John, and Robert Thompson. Regretfully absent as appropriate participants and obviously missed were Klüver, Krech (Krechevsky), and Teuber.

In all, some 18 noted neuroscientists who were students and colleagues of Lashley or who were strongly influenced by him participated in the series. Each participant was asked to describe how his work had been influenced by the contributions of Lashley. Enclosed with the letter of invitation was a list of areas in which, the editor felt, Lashley had made major and lasting contributions. (This list is reproduced below.) The participant was asked to select from this list one or more areas to illustrate the influence that Lashley exerted on him through his research, writings, and personal contacts. Each lecture was meant to be an in-depth account of the participant's own research and thinking and not merely an appreciation of Lashley as a man or a review of his work. The editor encouraged each participant to include original data in the course of the lecture.

LASHLEY'S MAJOR CONTRIBUTIONS TO NEUROPSYCHOLOGY (LISTED UNDER CATEGORIES CONTAINING OVERLAPPING TOPICS)

Methodology
- Animal testing—maze, latch box, jumping stand, discrimination
- Systematic testing of cortical function—capacities at birth, innate behavior, instincts, intelligence, learning, and memory
- Plot of lesions, brain reconstructions, degeneration methods

Ablation Method
- Use and logic of
- Diaschisis, degeneration, recovery of function

Sensory Systems
- Thalamocortical projection, sensory cortex
- Vision

Attention
- Noncontinuity in learning
- Presetting and the semiautonomous central process
- Conditions for association

Equipotentiality
- Vicarious function
- Sensory and motor equivalence
- Generalization and transfer of training

Mass Action
- Cortical reflexology, synaptic resistance
- Localization of function, search for the engram
- Electrochemical fields, reduplicated traces, resonances
- Cortical cytoarchitecture

Serial Order in Behavior
- Language, thought, emotion

Students
- Graduate and postdoctoral fellows

To translate the plan into a practical endeavor, I needed funds. It quickly became clear to me that no one source at the university would furnish sufficient sums to cover all the expenses (travel, honoraria, promotion, etc.), and I began to visit the various administrative offices at Queens College and the City University of New York in an attempt to assemble the necessary funds. With an initial commitment of seed money from Lawrence Erlbaum, publisher, each of the administrators came through: Presidents Saul Cohen of Queens College and Harold Proshansky of the Graduate School of CUNY; Deans Elie Hayon and Norman Goldman and Gad Hakerem, Chairman of Psychology at Queens College; and Florence Denmark, Executive Officer of Psychology at CUNY. Finally, The Commonwealth Fund awarded a subvention for publication of the resulting volume. To all these individuals and to The Commonwealth Fund, I am greatly indebted.

My own research into Lashley's career and contributions was greatly assisted by a number of individuals. I met with the participants of the lecture series prior to their lecture, and each one helped me place him or her in the context of Lashley's career and contributions. Before the series began, I visited on separate occasions with K.-L. Chow, Austin H. Riesen, and Murray E. Jarvik in their laboratories in California, and they shared with me many of their experiences at the Yerkes Laboratories of Primate Biology in Orange Park, Florida.

I spent a delightful morning in February 1979 at the Faculty Club, McGill University, chatting and reminiscing with Don Hebb, the man who introduced me to Lashley in the course of his graduate seminar, 1949–1950, and whose book, *Organization of Behavior*, I studied in page proof. It wasn't until 1952 that I finally met Lashley in person and became his last student, but I knew him quite well by then through the medium of Hebb's seminar and book.

The present director of the Yerkes Primate Research Center in Atlanta, Fred King, kindly opened to me the Archives of the Orange Park Laboratories dating back to the days when Yerkes was still director. Among other things, I found in the archives the day-to-day log of the laboratories, Lashley's correspondence, his *Annual Reports* submitted to the Board of Scientific Directors, his grant applications and research reports. It seems that very little was discarded when Lashley retired in 1955 and when the laboratories were moved to Atlanta in 1962. King and I agreed that there is a veritable treasure in the archives, and that a definitive history of the Yale/Yerkes Laboratories from their inception in 1930 will one day have to be written.

Along with the invitations to prospective participants went an invitation to Claire S. Lashley to be present at the inaugural lecture and to share in the semicentennial celebration honoring her late husband. Because of her commitments in Jacksonville, Florida, she was unable to join us that day. Mrs. Lashley lives at Fiddler's Cove and teaches foreign and classic languages at the Bartram School. We finally persuaded her to fly to New York for the eighth lecture, but her plane was many hours late. Though she missed the lecture, she arrived before the reception ended and had a chance to visit with us and with an old friend, Marianna Teuber. That night was long and memorable. Mrs. Lashley is a bundle of energy. We sat up many hours into the night listening to her anecdotes of Lashley. She described her entry to the United States with Paul Schiller and their ultimate reception in Orange Park, and she brought with her a bound volume of birthday letters that was presented to her husband on his 60th birthday in 1950. These letters reveal aspects of Lashley's relationships with people that cannot be inferred from any other source. Excerpts of many letters are brought together in Chapter 4.

During the course of his lecture, Don Lindsley showed a film of eminent psychologists photographed over the years at various professional meetings. In it, we saw sequences of Lashley taken in the early 1950's in animated discussion with Henry Nissen, Frank Beach, and Wolfgang Köhler (see Chapter 15). This film is a remarkable historical document, and I am indebted to Dr. Lindsley for showing it. Perhaps with a little nudging, he could be persuaded to prepare the appropriate sound track (which he delivered live at his lecture, with wit and affection for his colleagues in the film) and deposit a copy in the Archives of the American Psychological Association.

In drawing the portrait of Lashley in the first three chapters of the book, I returned to some of the arguments and debates that Lashley generated in the 1930s. As I prepared this section, I became aware that I was stoking old embers, and I began to suspect that my discussions may appear anachronistic to the modern student of neuropsychology, more suitable for students of that earlier era. Yet Lashley's problems do have a modern ring to them when framed in contemporary terminology. Whatever the case, students should be exposed to neuropsychological problems in historical perspective, and that is what I have tried to do through the medium of Lashley's contributions. The reader is urged to approach this section as a historical account of the development of Lashley's brand of neuropsychology. The anecdotal material is meant to add a lighter side (which Lashley cultivated in himself) and to give the portrait some color.

I want to thank those who helped me assemble the materials for this book. Karen Orbach spent considerable time on the problem of compiling the list of students and colleagues of Lashley. Gloria Kopp did a magnificent job of typing and retyping the manuscript and got to know Lashley and his students very well in the process. Though I enjoy editing the work of others, writing does not come easily to me. Harold Schuckman reminded me of my need to revise and improve my material, and Doreen Berman's examination of the legacy and portrait of Lashley prompted a revision of the manuscript. It was my wife, Louise, who urged me to take advantage of the semicentennial of publication of Lashley's monograph to begin the story of Orange Park that I had been saving for so many years, and it was she who hit on the idea of rendering the cellist in Figure 2.1.

I am chiefly indebted to Karl Lashley. Though he would disclaim teaching anyone anything, I learned the most difficult lessons from him as a graduate student: that "facts" are opinions; that seeing is disbelieving; and that the brain is not a bowl of cherries.

Introduction

The lectures upon which this volume is based were each preceded by a short introduction consisting for the most part of vignettes of Lashley during his Orange Park, Florida, years. Before introducing the first lecturer, the editor had this to say:

> Today we inaugurate a series of lectures at Queens College titled *Neuropsychology After Lashley* to celebrate the semicentennial of publication of *Brain Mechanisms and Intelligence*. In doing so, we honor the author, Karl Spencer Lashley, a man of many skills, who is perhaps the most important of the founders of modern neuropsychology. Brilliant as a researcher and theoretician, he was the archcritic of establishment neuroscience. As iconoclast, Lashley enjoyed repeating that he had disproved all neuropsychological theories including his own. An eccentric in appearance, a nonconformist in dress and behavior, Lashley designed and maintained his own sailboat, he made his own candy and sewed his own drapes. A nonbeliever, he delighted in being irreverent and uttering outrageous opinions. Impatient with pat answers and simplistic positions, Lashley might lean back in his chair to draw a book off a shelf and proceed to feign reading in the middle of a professional talk. Always out to elicit reactions of disbelief, Lashley could be dramatic, mocking, puckish, and whimsical, all at the same time. Never fastidious as a technician, he could fashion a surgical instrument in the workshop from a kitchen spoon just before scrubbing for sterile surgery, and he could repair his own cello and a fellow musician's violin with clamps and a bit of glue at a moment's notice. A careful observer, Lashley might call excitedly to his histological assistant to share the experience of identifying obscure microorganisms in a drop of brackish

water he picked up on his way to the laboratory. Lashley was a neurosurgeon who could miss his mark as often as he hit it, but would persevere until he assembled adequate numbers of hits to permit interpretation of the data. What a singular man!

In the spring of 1945, Lashley received a letter from T. G. Andrews at the University of Chicago requesting some information about his life. Andrews explained that he planned to offer a seminar on Lashley's work and, in preparation, could find no biographical material in the literature. Indeed, there was none. Lashley had earlier turned down a request from Murchison for a contribution to his series *A History of Psychology in Autobiography*.

Lashley obliged Andrews. In the archives of the Yerkes Primate Center in Atlanta, Georgia, the editor found the autobiographical letter dated June 13, 1945, addressed to Andrews. In staccato style, Lashley recorded some personal and professional milestones. Between the lines, can be heard his impish voice, his outrageous opinions, and his lack of conformity. Here are some excerpts.

On his roots. "Of ancestry I know little. Lashley is an English name; those that I know have been farmers or unambitious merchants. Descent through maternal grandmother is from New England Edwards family, which may have genetic significance." To understand that cryptic remark, note the following statement I found elsewhere: "It is clear that the intellectual curiosity and drive descended through the maternal line."

Early years. "Born in lumber town of 2,000; started school at 4; during next 5 years lived in various towns of West Virginia, Los Angeles, Seattle, and . . . Klondike gold rush. . . . Returned to Davis and school in '99 [at nine years of age]. Was pushed ahead with older children in school, worked in father's store with lessons at night so had little contact with other children; [developed] asocial attitude. . . . High school under Latin disciplinarian; no interest except in animal pets."

On sailing. "Went through Klondike gold rush with parents. Got permanent liking for small boats from 1,000 mile trip down the Yukon in an open boat . . . Pittsburgh, in 1911 . . . bought me a sixty-foot seine and turned me loose in November. Caught one catfish in three months. . . . Harvard 1935; chief attraction, ocean sailing; sailing not so hot, climate abominable."

On undergraduate studies. "Prep school . . . 1905. As freshman, 1906, discovered zoology under J. B. Johnston as the one interesting thing in college and thereafter took no course voluntarily except in biological sciences. Freshman grades: Zoology 96, Military Science 96, Latin 75, English 23." (A mischievous Lashleyan hyperbole. His actual Freshman grades were: Latin 75, 70, 83; English 94, 80, 88; Chemistry and Physics 82, 89; Algebra 73; History 86; Military Science 96. He did receive a grade of 23, but it was in his sophomore year and not in English but in rhetoric, which he hated with a passion. Whether his gentle distortion of the facts made a better story is debatable.) "Laboratory assistant in zoology with A. M. Reese 1907–10 with varied experience ranging from boiling out human skeletons to teaching classes. Undergraduate thesis on histology of intestine of chimeroid fish."

On master's program. "Teaching fellowship in biology, Pittsburgh, 1911. Department was all bacteriology; chairman suggested as master's thesis study of effects of water pollution on distribution of fishes in rivers at Pittsburgh . . . master's thesis on bacteriology of rotten eggs; three courses in psychology including Wundt's theory of apperception . . . don't know yet what it was about."

On pre- and postdoctoral studies. "Hopkins 1911-17. Few courses, thesis with Jennings and volunteer assistant to Watson during whole time. Thesis, a reply to criticisms of Jennings. . . . Spring 1913, with Watson on Tortugas [Bird Key, where the two studied homing, nesting, and reproductive behavior of sooty and noddy terns]. Spent one year after doctorate trying to develop further pure work with rotifers, desmids, Difflugia, and bacteria but could see no future in work. Meantime increased interest in conditioned reflex and decided to shift to that field."

On Shepherd Ivory Franz. "Met S. I. Franz in 1915 and proposed study of amount of practice necessary to reduce habits to subcortical level; volunteered to train rats if he would operate. Weekly trips to Washington with rats."

On John B. Watson. "Started infant work with Watson but disliked the little bastards and quit. . . . [In 1918] with Watson on study of motion pictures for sex education [a subject that generated many a tale later on]. . . . Interest in sex leading to work of Stone, Ball and Beach."

On the Minnesota years, 1917-18; 1920-26. "Escaped draft, bad vision; heavy teaching schedule but flu epidemic closed school and gave me chance to get big experiment started; thereafter teaching suffered. 1920-26 interesting department, Elliot (Harvard), Woodrow (Columbia), Fernald (Chicago), Foster (Cornell), representing all schools and encouraging more catholic point of view. Taught comparative, abnormal, physiological, learning. Experiments planned from conditioned reflex theory; results never consistent with theory; increasing scepticism toward Pavlovian behaviorism. Good students, Stone, Landis, Ball, Jacobsen; Klüver came in 1924 and profoundly influenced my point of view."

On the Chicago years, 1925-1935. "Three ideal years at the Behavior Research Fund on full time research. Debates and friendship with Koffka. With Herrick got funds to bring Poljak, learned some neurology from him. Problems getting narrower and more exacting; increasing doubt of the value of psychological theory based on few facts. [University of] Chicago, 1929, when Behavior Research Fund seemed likely to go under. Six good years with excellent support and interesting students: Maier, Schneirla, Krechevsky, Ingebritsen, Tsang, Hebb, Beach. Lectures London, Berlin, Moscow, 1932. Visited Pavlov; more impressed with the man than with his work.[1] Methods of testing rat vision opened possibilities of study of visual system and further restricted program."

On Harvard and directorship of the Yerkes Laboratories of Primate Biology. "Harvard, 1935; Orange Park and the chance to develop a research program on the primate brain under ideal working conditions.'' [Not so ideal, to judge from complaints embodied in the *Annual Reports*.]

On life's themes. ''Read Ingersol and Paine at 10 and developed active antagonism to religion which holds over in mechanistic philosophy and distrust of majority opinion. . . . Under influence of Darwin, Huxley, Haeckel; interest in the brain as a machine with psychology only a tool for study of the brain; . . . Attempt to validate asocial attitude and rejection of accepted standards.''

The letter ended as follows:

> This is my first and, I hope, last attempt at autobiography. Murray has pointed out, apparently with surprise, that a great many psychologists are not interesting people. I am one of that sort and would be a lot more interesting to myself if I could develop a good visual agnosia or other trait related to my problems. But then I should probably object to an immediate autopsy and so be as useless as other human subjects.
>
> You will find numerous contradictions in my work. I make no apology for them; interpretations were based on facts available and later experiments changed the picture. Recent on lack of effect of transcortical connections...may knock all. my theories cockeyed. That may mean some progress.
>
> Mixed wishes for your course.

[1]In response to an inquiry by B. P. Babkin at McGill University, Lashley prepared a statement evaluating Pavlov's influence on behaviorism in America. This statement is included in Chapter 1 *On Pavlov: An Exchange and Evaluation*.

1 The Legacy of *Brain Mechanisms and Intelligence*[1]

Jack Orbach
Queens College,
City University of New York

The period of modern experimental physiological psychology may be dated from the publication of *Brain Mechanisms and Intelligence* in 1929. In this volume, Karl Spencer Lashley formulated neuropsychological problems which he attacked with the new methods that he developed in the laboratory; he set exacting standards of analysis which themselves became the standards of contemporary brain ablation research; and he summarized the results of his now-famous brain ablation experiments on rats which he conducted in Chicago in the 1920s. Introduced by his teachers to a Sherringtonian and Pavlovian reflexology and a Watsonian empiricism, his early data and his inclinations toward genetics led him away from these positions. Instead he boldly borrowed ''mass function'' from embryology and ''action commune'' from Flourens, and embodied them in his concepts of equipotentiality and mass action in cortical function. Little more than summary statements of his data, these concepts were used to mean that a part of a defined area of cerebral cortex surviving after damage can function for the whole and that maze performance of rats deteriorates in direct proportion to the total mass of cortex destroyed and not as a function of the locus of the lesion. Theoretical refinements of these concepts came later (in 1942b, 1951, and 1958, especially), but the attack on the strict connectionism of the day had begun. The monograph created a stir in the neuroscientific community, it stimulated considerable research that continues to this day, and it generated a number of significant debates.

[1]Treated along with his monograph (1929) is Lashley's address titled *Basic Neural Mechanisms in Behavior*, delivered in 1929 at the Ninth International Congress of Psychology (Lashley, 1930).

Lamentably, over the years, Lashley's positions have been exaggerated and distorted by well-meaning interpreters of his views and caricatured by his critics. And today, in the climate of modern neo-connectionism, his assault on cortical reflexology is all but forgotten. Contemporary students are not exposed to Lashley's conceptual contributions. Few psychologists still remember that the dicontinuity position in learning was first enunciated in 1929. This volume is meant to reawaken interest in Lashley's experimental and theoretical work through the contemporary contributions of his students, colleagues, and those strongly influenced by him.

THEME AND VARIATIONS

Fifty years after the publication of *Brain Mechanisms and Intelligence,* rereading the volume reminds one of the principal theme that Lashley proclaimed in 1929 and to which he returned over and over again. The theme is an argument against reflex conduction as a model of behavioral and cortical function. Lashley played the theme in many variations:

The search for the engram and localization of function
Cortical field theory and connectionism
Sensory and motor equivalence
Noncontinuity and orderliness in learning
Mass action and equipotentiality

Though they may appear to be independent of each other, all are essentially variations on the principal theme. Lashley performed them in various guises and combinations in this volume and in subsequent publications, and the critique grew into a grand assault. The whole piece was executed in a style that captured the attention of the community of psychologists, and with solo virtuosity, Lashley turned the course of neuropsychological theory away from Pavlovian reflexology. The assault culminated, just 20 years later, in Hebb's acknowledgment of the cogency of Lashley's argument and his proposed rapprochement (1949).

A subsidiary theme, perhaps as important as the principal one, appeared early in the volume. This merits a few preliminary observations.

Methodology

Lashley's emphasis on standard procedures of testing was important because it permitted verification of data and replication of experiments. Each procedure had already found its place in the laboratory prior to Lashley's descriptions, but the consistent rigor in experimentation and the relentless review and reanalysis of data had not. Lashley insisted on the following:

Strict criteria of learning.
Multiple measures of learning—time, trials, and errors to meet the criterion of learning.
Reliability of measurements.
Distinction between postoperative retention and postoperative initial learning.
Standard postoperative recovery period. In Lashley's experiments with rats, 10 days was chosen because it appeared to be ample time for recovery from operative shock.
Histological verification of site and size of lesions. This is amplified later.

The rat was selected as the subject of investigation over, say, the monkey not only because it was cheaper and more convenient to use but also because of certain of its anatomical and behavioral features. For one thing, it has a smooth brain which simplified the characterization and quantification of experimentally produced cortical lesions. The problem was to produce a circumscribed lesion and to communicate to the reader in a precise way its site and size. Without verification of the lesion after autopsy, Lashley insisted, the results would have limited significance because replication of the experiment could never be completely successful.

Lashley's early diagrams of brain lesions did not prove to be satisfactory; these were based on camera lucida drawings of the fixed brain, prepared in 1917 with Franz. Then, in 1921, Lashley described a method of reconstructing the lesion from histological material.

> Serial frontal sections of the brain were prepared, stained in iron hematoxylin, and mounted in balsam. Sections at intervals of 0.25 mm were outlined under the camera lucida at a magnification of ten diameters. The extent of the lesions in each section was determined under higher power and indicated on the outline. The level of the section was next determined and the dimensions of the lesions were transferred to the diagram of the brain by means of proportional dividers. The points so determined were connected by lines and the resultant areas inked in. Only obvious lesions, absorption of tissue or complete degeneration of the cortex were recorded, so the diagrams represent the minimal extent of the lesions. The diagrams are probably accurate to within 0.5 mm when reduced to the dimensions of the brain [p. 458; a sample diagram is shown in Fig. 1.1].

This method resulted in a diagram that showed the size and location of the lesion but not the serial sections on which the diagram was based or their position on the diagram. Lashley added this information on drawings published in 1924 showing reconstructions of a monkey brain. Using the method already described, he reconstructed the brain and the lesion from serial coronal sections, but this time he included drawings of representative sections through the lesion on which he based the reconstruction, and he located each section on the reconstructions. These drawings of sections were included to indicate the depth of the lesion and perhaps to encourage the community of psychologists to read and use the anatom-

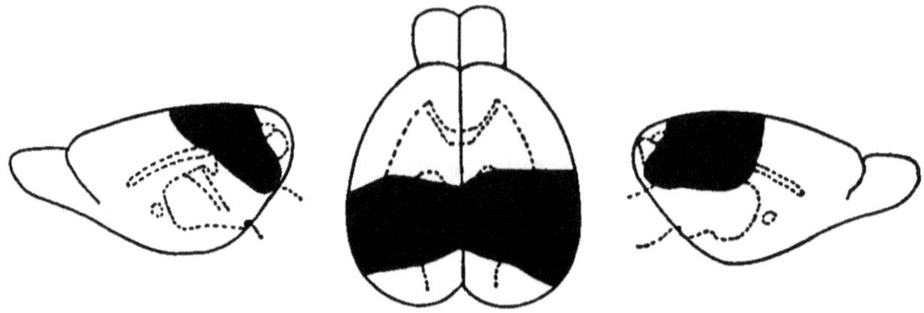

FIG. 1.1. Anatomical reconstruction of a rat brain showing surface lesion (from Lashley, 1921).

ical material. A sample reconstruction together with the serial sections is shown in Fig. 1.2.

For the rat brain, the procedure could be simplified by starting with a standard diagram of the dorsal and lateral surfaces of the brain on which were superimposed the positions of serial coronal sections .25 mm apart. The appropriate sections would be selected for study, and the dimensions of the lesion would be transferred to the standard diagram. This was the method Lashley used in his 1929 monograph, and Fig. 1.3 shows an example. Still missing was a record of retrograde degeneration in the thalamus. This was rectified beginning in the early 1930s when drawings of representative sections through the thalamus were added. This method was widely adopted by students of Lashley and others in the 1940s and 1950s.

How the Rat Solves the Maze Problem

Following the work of Thorndike on cats, it was generally assumed that animals engage in trial-and-error learning, and in random exploration, in the puzzle box. The solution, when it comes, can therefore be termed "accidental." If the problem is a complex one, in the sense that it requires serial solutions or a sequence of acts, such as an alley maze, then a chaining of specific responses is required for ultimate solution of the problem. Lashley's monograph contains an extended argument against this position. His critique can be divided into two parts—the argument against random, continuous learning; and the agrument against the acquisition and utilization of specific movements in maze performance. Recast in positive terms, Lashley argued that learning is orderly and discontinuous and that, instead of specific movements, the rat acquires and retains a general orientation in the maze.

On orderliness of learning, Lashley noted that the rat approaches the problem in a systematic way. If the rat tripped the release mechanism of the puzzle box door by falling, for example, it might climb and fall many times before abandoning this *attempted* (but unsuccessful) solution. A record of the rat's responses on

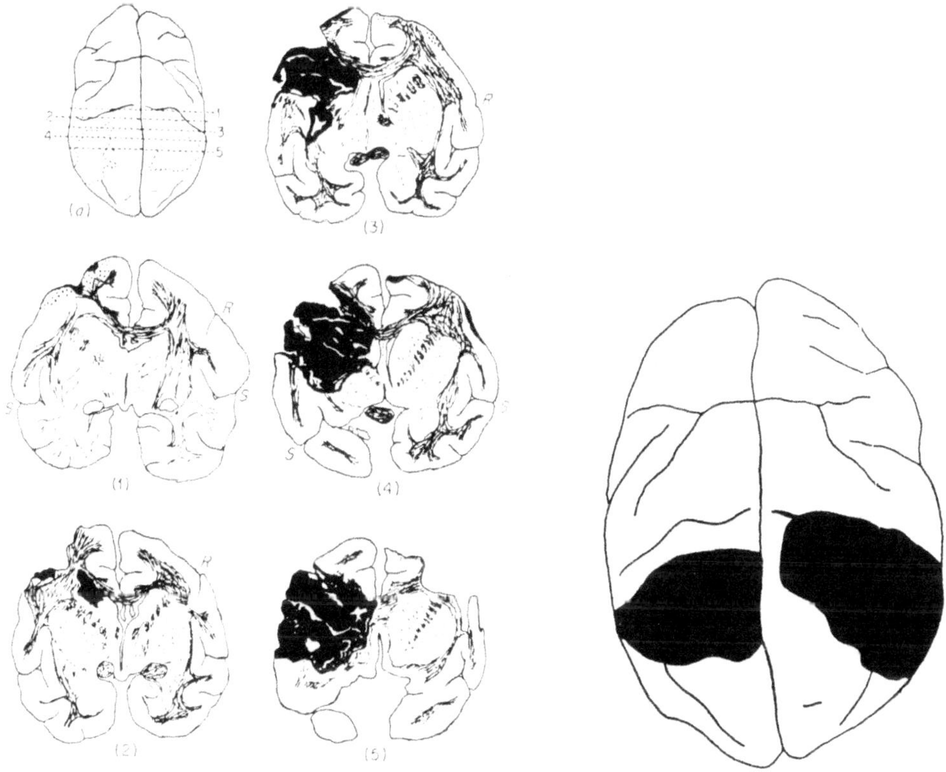

FIG. 1.2. Anatomical reconstruction of a monkey brain showing surface lesion and representative coronal sections through the lesion (from Lashley, 1924).

successive trials reveals that it tried responding to position, for example, or alternating between positions, or responding to the experimenter's movements, etc.—all incorrect solutions but all systematic attempts, not random responses. Lashley pointed out (1929):

> One does not recognize the meaning of "random" behavior until he has compared a normal animal with one having extensive cerebral destruction. The normal animal almost never re-enters a cul-de-sac without intervening explorations of other parts of the maze. An animal with severe lesions may repeat a single error as many as two hundred times before passing to other parts of the maze [p. 138].

A scientific determinism demanded an analysis of random behavior, and it is remarkable that none was offered prior to Lashley's.

As the animal solved the problem box and acquired discrimination habits, Lashley noted that the typical learning curve is one with a sudden drop in errors

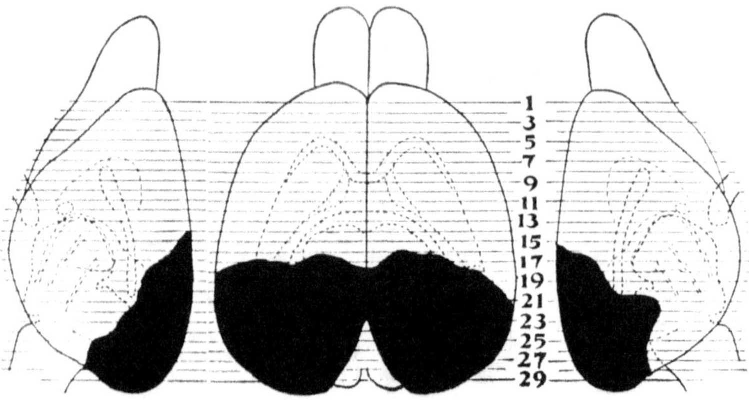

FIG. 1.3. Anatomical reconstruction showing surface lesion on a standard diagram of the rat brain (from Lashley, 1929).

after a period of little or no change.[2] This form of the learning curve suggests that the actual association is formed very quickly and that the practice preceding, and the errors following, are irrelevant to the actual formation of the association. In short, a simple association is acquired only after a number of more familiar responses have been tried unsuccessfully.

''There are many indications,'' Lashley wrote (1929), ''that animals . . . experiment with many solutions. . . . Responses to position, to alternation, or to cues from the experimenter's movements usually precede the reactions [to the relevant cue] and represent attempted solutions which are within the rat's customary range of activity [p. 135].'' The ''attempted solution'' during the presolution period was later called a ''hypothesis'' by Krechevsky, and the idea that ''attention'' is a factor in discrimination learning was largely instrumental in generating the continuity-noncontinuity controversy of the 1930s and 1940s.

In 1942, Lashley recalled that, some 6 years earlier, Spence had proposed a theory of the nature of discrimination learning using Hullian principles which contrasted with his (Lashley's) view that such learning involved a series of ''attempted solutions.'' In offering an experimental critique of noncontinuity, Spence referred to this position as ''Lashley's theory.'' Lashley accepted the christening and remarked (1942a) on Spence's rough handling of the theory: ''Since Spence's treatment of the foundling seems less than just, I am willing to accept the responsibilities of paternity, though from a certain purposive cast in the infant's features I suspect that I am cuckold'' [p. 241].''

[2]A gradual decrease does occasionally appear, but this is likely to occur after the animal has made more than a chance number of errors and, hence, depends upon factors other than discrimination. For example, many rats tend to explore the entire box on every trial until they become thoroughly adapted to the routine of training, and the gradual improvement is due to the reduction in exploration.

Confronted earlier with the evidence of noncontinuity, Spence (1940) had backed down: "The mere presence of the cue stimulus somewhere in the experimental situation does not guarantee its impingement on the animal's sensorium [p. 276]." This was a concession; Spence seemed to require that the rat look at (fixate) a particular aspect of the situation. The sensorium was thus identified with the "focus of attention." Indeed, Spence acknowledged that his statement referred to "attention." Recast, Spence seemed to say that *all stimuli in the focus of attention* at the time of response became associated with that response. This statement was certainly acceptable to Lashley, and the controversy with Spence was at an end.

On the role of proprioception and movement sequences in the solution of the maze problem, Lashley (1929) had this to say:

> Habits like the maze . . . have most frequently been interpreted as series of chain reflexes. Washburn (1916) calls these "movement systems" and defines them as "*a combination of movements so linked together that the stimulus furnished by the actual performance of certain movements is required to bring about other movements.*" There is no direct evidence . . . of the correctness of this analysis. . . . The demonstration that the habit is not dependent upon stimulation of exteroceptors (Watson, 1907) and observations upon the effects of changing the length of alleys (Carr and Watson, 1908) have shown that the execution of the habit is internally conditioned. . . . The observation on spinal lesions . . . (Lashley and Ball, 1929), seems to reduce the kinesthetic and motor patterns to the same status as the exteroceptors in the performance of the maze habit. They may be utilized as cues to orientation but are not essential to the correct performance of the habit.
>
> Observations on the behavior of animals with pronounced motor disturbances following spinal or cerebellar injuries emphasize the relative unimportance of the movement system. Animals which have learned the maze before the development of the motor inco-ordination continue to traverse it, although the manner of progression may be almost completely altered. One drags himself through with his forepaws; another falls at every step but gets through by a series of lunges; a third rolls over completely in making each turn, yet manages to avoid rolling into a cul-de-sac and makes an errorless run. . . . If the customary sequence of movements employed in reaching the food is rendered impossible, another set, not previously used in the habit, and constituting an entirely different motor pattern, may be directly and efficiently substituted without any random activity [pp. 136–137]. . . .
>
> An animal was . . . placed in the starting compartment [of a maze without its wire mesh cover and the entrance blocked] and kept under observation. Of 20 so tested, 5 pursued the most direct course across the tops of the partitions to the food with practically no random exploration . . . they were perfectly oriented with respect to its direction, although they had never before reached it save by the indirect path of the maze. . . . [This suggests] that the rat forms, from the indirect path of the maze, some generalization as to the relative positions of the starting and food boxes. . . .
>
> The available evidence seems to justify the conclusion that the most important features of the maze habit are a generalization of direction from the specific turns of

> the maze and the development of some central organization by which the sense of general direction can be maintained in spite of great variations of posture and specific direction of running [pp. 137–138].

How reminiscent of modern cognitive theory! The student of Tolman may find this 1929 statement quite familiar and may even hear *sotto voce* the suggestion that the rat develops a map of the maze in its mind. In a direct line of descent is Hebb's spatial hypothesis (1949) and his attempt to assess rat intelligence via the Hebb–Williams maze (1946).

The Logic of the Ablation Method

In the course of interpreting the effects of cortical lesions, Lashley presented a logic for the ablation method that had not been offered earlier. Let us assume, Lashley argued, that specific symptoms follow circumscribed cortical lesions. In order to attribute the symptoms to the damage of particular cortical cells, it is necessary to rule out a number of factors that may influence the result.

1. *Individual variation in localization.* The results may be obscured by this factor. Lashley considered both anatomical variation and functional variation over time.
2. *Specific shock and/or diaschisis.* Cortical damage might cause a lowered efficiency of nervous tissue not involved in the primary lesion via the toxic products of cell degeneration; changes in circulation with resultant trophic disturbances; mechanical distortion and pressure and withdrawal of necessary facilitation to an intact area (diaschisis).
3. *Vicarious functioning.* Though the initial symptoms are due to a specific lesion, reeducation induces uninjured cortex to take over the function that was lost by the lesion. Hence, improvements in performance after cerebral injury complicate the conclusions regarding localization of function.
4. *Disturbances in equilibrium within functional systems.* Some symptoms may result from disturbances in the functional equilibrium between centers, although no tissue essential to the performance of the disturbed activities is directly involved in the lesion. For example, unilateral lesions to the extrapyramidal system may produce a marked incoordination though bilaterally symmetrical lesions do not.
5. *Equipotentiality and mass function.* According to Lashley (1929):

> The term equipotentiality [was] used to designate the apparent capacity of any intact part of the functional area to carry out, with or without reduction in efficiency, the functions which are lost be destruction of the whole. *This capacity varies from one area to another and with the character of the functions involved. It probably holds only for the association areas and for functions more complex than simple sensitivity or motor co-ordination. . . .*

> *Equipotentiality is not absolute but is subject to a law of mass action* whereby the efficiency of performance of an entire complex function may be reduced in proportion to the extent of brain injury within an area whose parts are not more specialized for one component of the function than for another [p. 25; italics mine].

Thus, the underlying assumption that the site of the lesion is always responsible for the specific behavioral disturbances is questioned on a number of grounds, and equipotentiality and mass function are offered among several alternative interpretations. Lashley's use of these concepts and their limits are carefully spelled out.

Unfortunately, Lashley's monograph is remembered simply as rejecting localization of function in rat cortex, period. It is plain, however, that this does not reflect the breadth of Lashley's research. Consider the following examples. For solution of the double latch box, anterior lesions produced a loss of retention;

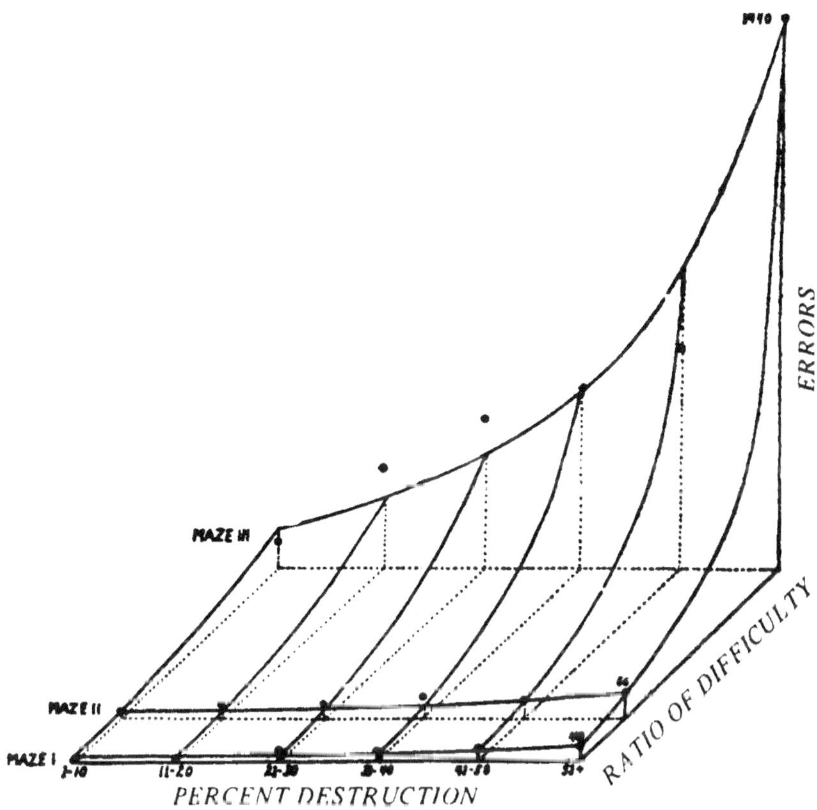

FIG. 1.4. The original diagram upon which mass action was based, showing the relation between extent of cortical lesion, difficulty of the mazes, and errors to meet criterion of learning (adapted from Lashley, 1929, p. 74).

posterior lesions did not. Conversely, posterior lesions disrupted brightness discrimination; anterior lesions did not (Lashley, 1935). Following Teuber's scheme, we would regard this as an application of the double dissociation paradigm, the paradigm of choice to demonstrate the validity of localization of function.

Cortical versus Peripheral Blinding

Lashley *did* conclude that equipotentiality and mass action were the most reasonable statements summarizing the relation between disturbances in performance of the alley maze and the size of the cortical lesions, not their site. However, it is easy to reify these concepts. The postoperative impairment that Lashley observed was of acquisition and retention of the alley maze habit, and he concluded that learning ability and memory were governed by equipotentiality and mass action of cortical function. Lashley himself recognized the pitfalls in such an argument, and this led him to consider an alternative interpretation. Suppose that the progressively larger cortical lesions interfere with more and more sensory processes. Suppose, too, that the alley maze is a multimodality task. Did it not follow that the larger lesion, the lesion that would more likely deprive the rat of more sensory input, should have a more deleterious effect on maze performance? A comparison of the effects of cortical and peripheral blinding on maze performance provided the answer.

Lashley found empirically that at least 10% of the entire cortical mass had to be eliminated before maze performance was affected by the lesion. One region of cerebral cortex that was known to be highly specialized was striate cortex, the so-called visual area. Coincidentally, striate cortex in the rat amounts to approximately 10% of the entire cortex. Lashley had already determined that destruction of striate cortex interfered with maze performance, a result to be expected from the "10% rule." Was the impaired maze performance due to a visual impairment? If so, Lashley reasoned that rats blinded by enucleation should be equally impaired (or even more impaired) compared to the cortically blinded rats.

In one experiment, rats were blinded by enucleation and then trained on the maze. The resulting habit was thus formed without visual cues. Though blind, these rats lost the maze habit after striatectomy! As in sighted rats, the loss was roughly proportional to the extent of the lesion. Control data showed that peripheral blinding did not interfere appreciably with the maze habit. "It can scarcely be maintained," Lashley wrote (1929) triumphantly, "that a partial loss of vision through central scotomata can have any greater effect than a total loss by enucleation [p. 111]." It is thus impossible to ascribe the loss of the maze habit in animals with normal eyes and occipital lesions to any simple disturbance of visual function. In what way the occipital lesions interfere with the maze habit cannot be determined, but it is certainly not through the production of cortical blindness. It must be concluded that visual cortex has some general function ("action commune") in addition to a specific sensory one ("action propre").

Hunter reopened the issue of multisensory loss following progressively larger cortical lesions in his critique of mass action in 1930, and he put students on the problem to check the relative effects of peripheral and cortical blinding on maze performance. After the challenge by Finley (1941), Lashley settled the matter to his own satisfaction in a paper published in 1943. And in 1959, Orbach described similar nonvisual disturbances following striate cortex lesions in monkeys.

Cortical Field Theory

Lashley's involvement in the dispute over the functional significance of cortical fields can only be understood if a distinction is made between the law of mass action (1929)—called here the mass action correlation, derived from empirical data—and the theory of mass action—variously called the reduplicated trace theory and the interference patterns theory (1942b).

No one seriously disputes the mass action correlation for maze performance of rats. The experiments have been replicated many times, and none of Lashley's critics (e.g., Hunter and Hebb) have ever challenged the data. Nor does anyone seriously dispute Lashley's argument regarding equivalence of stimuli and responses. Modern neuropsychologists acknowledge the challenge of these data (e.g., Hebb, 1949; John, 1972; Miller, Galanter, & Pribram, 1960; the one exception was Pavlov in 1932/1955, but Pavlov never recognized the cogency of Lashley's argument, and his position was never made clear on this issue). Thus, Lashley's case for cortical fields is solid as far as behavior is concerned. The dispute is not even whether recognition and recall require the excitation of specific neural cells or not, as Hebb alleged, since Lashley subscribed explicitly to a connectionism based on the anatomic arrangements proposed by Lorente de No. This is an important point, as I show later.

Then what is the dispute about? Part of the dispute revolves around the mechanism of generation of cortical fields, and here Lashley's dispute is with Köhler and with nobody else. To characterize Lashley's theory of cortical function as a field theory and to treat equipotentiality together with Köhler's field theory is to obscure the fundamental differences between the two positions. Unfortunately, Hebb's critique of cortical field theory in Chapter 3 of his 1949 monograph, though brilliant at the time, tended to close this debate. The issue is a bit passé and belongs in the history of neuropsychology. But the weight of evidence is with Lashley, as his argument (1942b) that follows attests:

> The anatomic studies of Lorente de Nó (1934) have revealed a system of cross connections in the cortex which will permit the spread of excitation in any direction along the surface . . . the whole system is organized as a network, with loops of

> various lengths and complexity, capable of transmitting impulses from cell to cell across the cortex, or of re-exciting initial points of stimulation by the action of return circuits [pp. 312–313].

Here Lashley draws on the then-current concepts of neuro-anatomy and -physiology to sketch his theory of irradiating waves and interfering patterns (1942b):

> From such a structural organization, functional properties may be inferred. . . . Excitation started at any point must spread from that point throughout the system. . . . If the system is uniform . . . a series of radiating waves should be produced. . . . The timing of the waves should be uniform, *since it is dependent upon the speed of conduction and the refractory periods of the elements in the system* [italics mine; this is hardly to be confused with a conception of the cerebral cortex as a quasi-homogenous medium through which direct currents flow] With . . . many points of excitation, interference patterns will be formed . . . the action should be somewhat analogous to the transmission of waves on the surface of a fluid medium. Interference of waves in such a system produces a pattern of crests and troughs which is characteristic for each spatial distribution . . . and which is reduplicated roughly over the entire surface. . . . Spatially distributed impulses reaching the cortex from the retina . . . will give rise to a different and characteristic pattern of standing waves, reduplicated throughout the extent of the functional area [pp. 313–314].

This conception cannot be given the status of a theory, and Lashley (1942b) acknowledged this:

> The analogy with wave motion in a homogenous liquid cannot be applied seriously . . . since the cortical tissues have inherent characteristics as a transmitting mechanism quite different from those of a fluid. The analogy is presented only to give a conceptual picture of a reduplicated system which may serve as a starting point for a more adequate conception of the structure of the memory trace [p. 314].

If you remain unconvinced that Lashley has sketched a connectionist's conception of cortical function, consider his summary statement (1942b):

> The scheme of nervous organization . . . makes no assumptions concerning elementary nervous activities beyond those established in studies of reflex conduction. It suggests a mechanism for action of the system as a whole which is also subject to analytic treatment in terms of nerve transmission. *In this respect, it is a substitute for field theory and, if of lesser immediate predictive value, is more consistent with elementary nerve physiology, and is more open to experimental examination* [pp. 320–321; italics mine].

In his treatment of equipotentiality in 1949, Hebb saw the problem generated by cortical field theory quite differently. His clarification of the concept, equipotentiality, is noteworthy. Lashley's nativistic predilection led him to the view that cortical cells, when challenged by ablation of neighboring cells, for example, necessarily acquire the functions of the ablated cells. Though Hebb conceded that cortical cells are indeed able to acquire the functions of neighboring cells, he noted that they do not always do so, and even when they do, an empiricistic explanation can quite reasonably account for the data.

Hebb cited the following hypothetical "transfer" experiment and applied Lashley's nativistic interpretation (Fig. 1.5). Suppose that a circle is positioned to excite particular cells in the right hemiretinas and that a response is required of

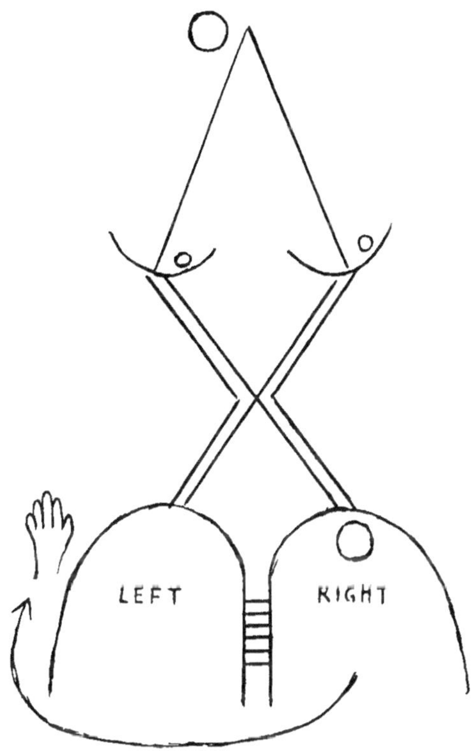

FIG. 1.5. Hebb's illustration of equipotentiality. The animal is taught to respond with a movement of the left extremity to a circular pattern that always excites the same retinal cells in the right hemiretinas. Although stimulation has been confined to the right hemisphere via the geniculostriate system and the response has been determined by motor systems also in the right hemisphere, equipotentiality implies that the *left* hemisphere will mediate recognition of the pattern and will mediate the response (adapted from Hebb, 1949, p. 40).

the left hand. It might be said that it is the right hemisphere primarily that is active in this habit. According to Hebb, Lashley's equipotentiality implies that (1) other retinal cells excited in a circular pattern, even in the left hemiretinas, will elicit a similar response, with the right as well as left hands ("sensory and motor equivalence"); (2) the right hemisphere may be ablated, and the left would continue to mediate the habit; and (3) this transfer of learning from one set of cells to another depends on the innate properties of cortical cells (and not on earlier experiences that set up connections between them, as Hebb believed). Thus, a particular habit does not depend upon the excitation of any particular cortical cells, because ablation of these cells will not abolish the habit.

Hebb conceded the implications of points 1 and 2 but disputed point 3. Later, in his analysis, Hebb showed that it is possible to endorse a behavioral equipotentiality, and in his 1949 monograph, he proceeded to develop a neural mechanism of the origin of sensory and motor equivalence involving specific neural connections influenced by past experience.

Here rests the matter on cortical fields. What was the tempest about? The problem was to account for the mass action correlation and for the equivalence of stimuli and responses (generalization, transfer of training, relative choice, etc.) in terms that require the excitation of specific neural cells in cortex. Having overpowered Köhler and Pavlov by the weight of argument (Lashley, 1942b; Lashley & Wade, 1946) and experimental data (Lashley, Chow & Semmes, 1951; Sperry, 1947), Lashley was in the uncomfortable position of having no one to tilt with. And the problem remains unresolved despite the cries of success from the neo-connectionists.

ON PAVLOV: AN EXCHANGE AND EVALUATION

According to Lashley (1930), the Pavlovian theory of reflex conduction was extended to cerebral function by adding

> localized areas as relay points or centers along the course of the reflex arc and . . . seemed to explain the functional relations of the areas. However, the theory has not worked well in application to the details of behavior. To understand the difficulties we should have clearly in mind the form and limitations of the theory. It states that the mechanism of cerebral function is essentially the same as that of the spinal reflexes, involving the conduction of nerve impulses from the sense organs over definite, restricted paths to the effectors. The performance of a habit, whether of speech or of manipulative movement, is determined by the existence of definite connections between a limited number of nerve cells, which are always functional in that habit . . . the essential feature of the reflex theory is the assumption that individual neurons are specialized for particular functions. The explanatory value of the theory rests upon this point alone, and no amount of hypothetical elaboration of connections alters the basic assumption [p. 3].

So spoke the president of the American Psychological Association before the Ninth International Congress of Psychology in 1929. As he proceeded, Lashley turned the address into a sweeping indictment of reflex and conditioned reflex theory. Citing the evidence of sensory and motor equivalence and the plasticity in central organization, Lashley concluded that there is no constant anatomical localization at any point from receptors to effectors. Without referring directly to Pavlov, he concluded the indictment with the following statement (Lashley, 1930): "In the study of cerebral functions we seem to have reached a point where the reflex theory is no longer profitable either for the formulation of problems or for an understanding of the phenomena of integration. . . . It is now becoming an obstacle rather than a help to progress [p. 12]."

Accustomed to respect and praise, Pavlov was deeply hurt by the attack. In "A Reply of a Physiologist to Psychologists," which he published in 1932, Pavlov selected Lashley (as well as Guthrie and Köhler) as the objects of his scorn. What particularly rankled him was Lashley's opinion, expressed so candidly, that reflex theory was becoming an obstacle to the understanding of cerebral function. How could anyone take such a position, wrote the affronted Pavlov, after 30 years of his work and that of his collaborators? "No one has the right to say that" (Pavlov, 1932/1955; p. 425).

After redefining the reflex, Pavlov (1932/1955) reviewed the evidence in support of cortical localization of function (chiefly his own) and ended his exposition with this statement of cortical mechanism: "The basic processes of cortical activity are excitation and inhibition, their spread in the cortex in the form of irradiation and concentration and their reciprocal induction [p. 434]." Though Lashley might challenge the use of Pavlov's concepts of irradiation and induction, nothing in Pavlov's defense of the reflex would have disturbed him greatly—certainly not the principle of determinism as embodied in Pavlov's concept of the reflex and which Pavlov believed Lashley had abandoned.

When Pavlov turned to Lashley's ablation results, the argument became acrimonious. Mass action was ridiculed. First Pavlov chided Lashley for ignoring the obvious fact that the maze is a multimodality task. Was Pavlov unaware of Watson's studies of the sensory control of the maze and Lashley's reference to them? "Neither the author [Lashley] nor anyone else has ever performed such experiments" (Pavlov, 1932/1955; p. 439). Then he offered the alternative interpretation that the larger cortical lesions necessarily encroached on more and more sensory tissue. Hunter had already offered this interpretation in 1930, and Lashley himself had raised this possibility in his 1929 monograph, though he rejected it on the grounds that cortical blinding had deleterious effects on maze performance even in enucleated rats. Was Pavlov unaware of the psychological literature? The author [Lashley] pays no attention to such possibilities, was Pavlov's unjustified complaint. Lashley's suggestion that the rat develops a sense of direction in the maze rather than a series of specific movements was also derided as "some kind of bodiless reaction" (Pavlov, 1932/1955; p. 439).

Most important to note here is Pavlov's handling of the main thrust of Lashley's critique of reflexology: the problems raised by sensory and motor equivalence and cerebral plasticity. Here Pavlov faltered. Not able to give an inch on the issue of specificity, he accused Lashley of deluding himself if he believed that equivalence and plasticity weakened the theory of reflex conduction. His defense was based principally on an anatomical argument: that the details of central projection and of peripheral connections were not yet known, and that the experimental interruption of connections could not be guaranteed with the technology then available.

Lashley: Assuming specificity of cortical function, how is it that some lesions seem to have no effect on behavior?

Pavlov (1932/1955):

> Isolated destruction can hardly ever be obtained mechanically or chemically. . . . If . . . we sometimes do not observe any change in the animal's behavior (after surgical destruction), this is due to the self-evident fact that we have not yet decomposed the animal's behavior into all its elements, the number of which must be enormous. And for this reason, the disappearance of some of them naturally escapes our attention [p. 436].

By the same token, incisions meant to section association and projection tracts in the hemisphere are rarely effective (Pavlov, 1932/1955):

> Let us recall . . . the case of recurrent sensibility in the spinal roots and the innervation of a single muscle by fibers from different roots. How much more diverse and delicate . . . must this be in the central nervous system with its immense connections. . . . Since at present we cannot claim complete knowledge of all the connections . . . our experiments with incisions, sections, etc., . . . do not accomplish our aim of disjunction since the apparatus proves to be more complicated . . . than we anticipated. It is . . . risky to draw definite . . . conclusions on the basis of such experiments [p. 440].

Referring to Lashley's failure to observe disturbances of a motor habit after destruction of the cortical motor area, Pavlov suggested (1932/1955) that Lashley did not extirpate the motor region fully; "the remaining parts are still sufficient for a mechanical habit [p. 443]." Is it possible that Pavlov was inadvertently describing something akin to equipotentiality?

How did Pavlov respond to Lashley's claim that the same retinal cells are not always reexcited every time the organism responds to a particular visual pattern? He denied it (Pavlov, 1932/1955): "Usually each part of the retina serves for a corresponding reaction to the given object [p. 444]." In his discussion, Pavlov neglected the phenomenon of interocular transfer as described by Lashley in 1924.

How did Pavlov respond to Lashley's claim that the trained rat proceeds in the right direction in the maze after damage to the cerebellum in spite of the fact that it circles its way through; or that the trained rat swims its way through the maze filled with water without making an error? Where, in these instances, are the specific connections between stimulus and response? Pavlov insisted (1932/1955) that the specific connections are there: "The rat constantly moves forward and makes turns to the right and to the left with the help of the same muscles in all the cases mentioned here, the rest are additional movements determined by other additional stimuli [p. 445]." Curiously, Pavlov seemed to concede (1932/1955) Lashley's point invoking, at the same time, his principles of summation and irradiation. "Have we not known for a long time that a decapitated frog, [removes] acid placed on the thigh of one of its extremities by using the foot of the same extremity, [but] if unable to do so because of amputation of that foot, will use the other foot after a few unsuccessful attempts with the disabled extremity [p. 446]." (In his last publication, in 1958, Lashley cited the example of the spinal frog removing acid from its rump to illustrate the features of *voluntary* action!)

How did Pavlov handle the absence of stereotypy in instinctive behavior as in the building of nests by birds? His solution (1932/1955) to the apparent absence of specific connections was cryptic: "The phenomenon of individual adaptation exists throughout the animal world. And this is precisely the conditioned reflex . . . which is effected on the principle of simultaneity [p. 446]."

Shortly after this exchange, Lashley and Pavlov met. In a letter written to T. G. Andrews in 1946, Lashley noted that he was more impressed with the man than with his work. It is interesting that Lashley rarely referred to Pavlov by name in his later publications except in his foray into, and critique of, *The Pavlovian Theory of Generalization* (Lashley & Wade, 1946).

In the course of writing a biography of the great physiologist, a student of his, B. P. Babkin, put to Lashley the following question: "How does Pavlov's work on conditioned reflexes influence the development of psychology?" The question aroused Lashley's interest and made him wonder just what influence Pavlov really had on American psychology. Representing himself as one of the early behaviorists in America, Lashley sent to Babkin a thoughtful evaluation of Pavlov's work in relation to the development of psychology. The letter, dated February 8, 1946, is here reproduced in full (except for some personal notes). It needs no further comment.

> I have been fairly close to the development of objective psychology in this country since its beginning. . . . Pavlov's work came to the serious attention of American psychologists between 1910 and 1915. At that time subjective psychology, represented by the structuralism of Titchener and the functionalism of Angell was dominant, but a trend toward objectivism was developing in the work of students of animal behavior, of learning, and of the testing methods of Cattell and Binet. This trend was without coherent expression and did not yet constitute a systematic position opposed to subjectivism. Watson's "Psychology as the Behaviorist Views It," was the first attempt here to formulate an objective program. It

was written in 1912 before Watson had been significantly influenced by Pavlov's work. Only in the following year did we begin a study of the writings of Pavlov and Bechterev. The ground was then already prepared for acceptance of an objective and physiological point of view. The conception of the reflex basis of behavior, sketched by John Dewey about 1906, was exemplified in the work of the Russian investigators. They provided not only theory but an experimental method and concrete results in support of their views. Bechterev was actually more influential than Pavlov in the early days. He appeared to have a more conprehensive grasp of psychological problems than did Pavlov and the French edition of his objective psychology provided a more complete account of his position than was available for that of Pavlov. The early experimental work, presented in Watson's presidential address, was based on Bechterev's accounts and designed to test his interpretations. However, Bechterev held to a psychophysical parallelism which did not fit with the anti-introspection movement which characterized behaviorism and his terminology was rejected in favor of Pavlov's more rigorously physiological one.

Without the earlier growth of the movement toward objectivism, Pavlov's work would probably have aroused little interest in America, as was the case in Germany and France. Without his work, behaviorism would have developed, though perhaps in a different way. Few details of Pavlov's experiments were available to English readers until the translation of his book in 1927. (In 1913 I compiled a bibliography of more than 300 Russian titles on the conditioned reflex of which only 7 were available in the major libraries of America.) In consequence, there was little understanding of physiological theories and the earlier books of Watson, Weiss, Holt and other behaviorists used the conditioned reflexes merely as a substitute for association, translating the psychology of Mills and later associationists into terms of connection between stimulus and response instead of association between ideas.

Pavlov's early influence derives from three chief sources, I believe. 1. He formulated learning in terms of association between stimulus and response, thus avoiding the association of images or of ideas, which had offered difficulties to objective psychology; he insisted that all learning could be reduced to that formula and he provided evidence which would be cited in support of such an interpretation. 2. The conditioned reflex offered a potential method for study of psychological processes which could be opposed to introspection and so gave ammunition to the objective movement. 3. He emphasized the possibility of a psychology without mentalistic elements with some evidence of progress toward such a goal.

In actual practice his work provided a set of slogans for the objective movement rather than an influence on the direction of development of that movement. Pavlov believed, I am sure, that an understanding of behavior could be gained only by study of the physiology of the brain, and that such studies should be as direct as possible. He was primarily an experimenter and had little use for the construction of conceptual systems, except as they could be supported step by step by direct experimental evidence. But the history of the conditioned reflex in America has been diametrically opposed to what was, I believe, his philosophy of science. He pointed the way to fundamental investigation of the physiology of the brain. No one in America has ever systematically followed that way or added significant factual information to the fund that Pavlov provided; a few experiments to extend his findings to striped muscle conditioning or to man, but no progress in analysis of brain physiology by his methods. Rather, his tentative experimental conclusions were imported as ultimate universal laws upon which to build elaborate speculative systems. From the weight of the super structures, they have acquired the rigidity of all fixed ideas whose change would involve the collapse of a philosophical system of values. Even the experimental study of neuroses, which is the most direct development of Pavlov's work, looks more like the exploitation of his ideas by a school, the environmentalists, than an open-minded attempt to investigate the problems which he formulated (why, otherwise, the neglect of his work on neurotic types?).

As details of his work have become better known, more of his conceptions have become embodied in speculative systems culminating in that of Hull. Such systems, from Watson to the present have exercised a tremendous influence on the direction of psychological thought, as does every comprehensive systematization but they have in them nothing of Pavlov's experimental attitude.

All of this is no fault of Pavlov's. He was one of the great pioneers in experimenting and inductive reasoning. But it seems to me that these characteristics of his work which give him greatest claim to genius have been least influential in American psychology. It has been his misfortune to fall into the hands of the philosophers. His influence has been rather that of a Descartes than of a Pasteur.

As to my personal attitude: what has been my life work was initiated by the hope of tracing conditioned reflexes through the brain and understanding the mechanism of their establishment. I worked for several years with the conditioning technique but came to the conclusion that the conditioned reflex presented complexities far beyond that implied in its American interpretations. In particular, I became involved in problems which Pavlov had dismissed (or set aside for future investigation) as the work of the analyzers, and increasingly felt the need for more fundamental research in this field before the conditioned reflex could be used as a genuinely physiological and explanatory concept. My statement that the conditioned reflex was becoming an obstacle to progress[3] was based on the extent to which the concept was being used as a form of verbal magic to dismiss genuine problems instead of submitting them to analytic investigation. It was a protest not against the rightness of Pavlov's point of view and experimental methods, but against the perversion of his work from physiological fact to psychological mumbo-jumbo (e.g., Hull's irradiation of conditioning along the physical dimensions of a stimulus series).

REFERENCES

Finley, C. B. Equivalent losses in accuracy of response after central and after peripheral sense privation. *Journal of Comparative Neurology*, 1941, *74*, 203–237.

Franz, S. I., & Lashley, K. S. The retention of habits by the rat after destruction of the frontal portion of the cerebrum. *Psychobiology*, 1917, *1*, 3–18.

Hebb, D. O. *The organization of behavior*. New York: Wiley, 1949.

[3]Reference to Lashley's 1929 address, published in 1930 (Editor).

Hebb, D. O., & Williams, K. A method of rating animal intelligence. *Journal of General Psychology*, 1946, *34*, 59-65.

Hunter, W. S. A consideration of Lashley's theory of the equipotentiality of cerebral action. *Journal of General Psychology*, 1930, *3*, 455-468.

John, E. R. Switchboard versus statistical theories of learning and memory. *Science*, 1972, *177*, 850-864.

Lashley, K. S. Studies of cerebral function in learning II. The effects of long continued practice upon cerebral localization. *Journal of Comparative Psychology*, 1921, *1*, 453-468.

Lashley, K. S. Studies of cerebral function in learning V. The retention of motor habits after destruction of the so-called motor areas in primates. *Archives of Neurology and Psychiatry*, 1924, *12*, 249-276.

Lashley, K. S. *Brain mechanisms and intelligence*. Chicago: University of Chicago Press, 1929.

Lashley, K. S. Basic neural mechanisms in behavior. *Psychological Review*, 1930, *37*, 1-24.

Lashley, K. S. The mechanism of vision. XII. Nervous structures concerned in the acquisition and retention of habits based on reactions to light. *Comparative Psychology Monographs*, 1935, *11*(52), 43-79.

Lashley, K. S. An examination of the "continuity theory" as applied to discriminative learning. *Journal of General Psychology*, 1942, *26*, 241-265. (a)

Lashley, K.S. The problem of cerebral organization in vision. *Biological Symposia*, 1942, *7*, 301-322. (b)

Lashley, K. S. Studies of cerebral function in learning XII. Loss of the maze habit after occipital lesions in blind rats. *Journal of Comparative Neurology*, 1943, *79*, 431-462.

Lashley, K. S., Chow, K. -L., & Semmes, J. An examination of the electrical field theory of cerebral integration. *Psychological Review*, 1951, *58*, 123-136.

Lashley, K. S., & Wade, M. The Pavlovian theory of generalization. *Psychological Review*, 1946, *53*, 72-87.

Lashley, K. S. Cerebral organization and behavior. In the Brain and Human Behavior. *Proceedings of the Association for Research in Nervous and Mental Diseases*. 1958, *36*, 1-18.

Miller, G. A., Galanter, E. & Pribram, K. H. *Plans and the structure of behavior*. New York: Holt, 1960.

Orbach, J. "Functions of striate cortex and the problem of mass action. *Psychology Bulletin*, 1959, *56*, 271-292.

Pavlov, I. P. A reply of a physiologist to psychologists. *Psychological Review*, 1932, *39*, 91-127. (Reprinted in Pavlov, I. P. *Selected Works*. Moscow: Foreign Languages Publishing House, 1955.)

Spence, K. W. Continuous versus non-continuous interpretations of discrimination learning. *Psychological Review*, 1940, *47*, 271-288.

Sperry, R. W. Cerebral regulation of motor coordination in monkeys following multiple transection of sensorimotor cortex. *Journal of Neurophysiology*, 1947, *10*, 275-294.

2 At the Yerkes Laboratories of Primate Biology, Orange Park, Florida

Jack Orbach
Queens College,
City University of New York

DIRECTOR, 1942–1955

The student of neuropsychology who was interested in nonhuman primate, brain–behavior relationships had few laboratory options in the 1930s, 1940s and early 1950s. As far as chimpanzees were concerned, the only laboratory in America offering opportunities for their study was the primate station in Orange Park, Florida. Established by Robert M. Yerkes in 1930, the laboratory came to be known as the southern station of the Yale Laboratories of Primate Biology. An eminent primatologist, Yerkes selected the site in Orange Park for its favorable semitropical climate and its isolation from worldly distractions. Though the choice of location turned out to be unfortunate, the laboratory was to contain a chimpanzee breeding colony and a behavioral research center of international renown.

Fronting the highway on part of a 200-acre tract and surrounded by a high, woven steel fence topped with electrified wire, the laboratories occupied a cluster of small buildings which contained modest offices and laboratory rooms. Nearby were the living quarters for some 60 chimpanzees. Over the years, many were born on the premises and were reared and studied with elaborate care. The living quarters for each chimpanzee or pair of chimpanzees consisted of an indoor "bedroom" with a concrete slab for a bed and an interconnecting outdoor exercise cage or solarium. There were also two or three large group-enclosures, a nursery for human-reared youngsters, and a small infirmary for the sick. The grounds were lush, planted here and there with exotic flora, and nurtured by the semitropical downpours. Between the entrance gate and the main building, a set of lawn furniture was set out in a circle. Here, in the open, staff members would meet regularly for lunch, to chat, and to engage in lively debates. Ada Yerkes, a botanist and Robert's wife, called the southern station, in an idyllic prose portrait, "Yale in Florida."

When Yerkes retired in 1942, the station was renamed the Yerkes Laboratories of Primate Biology, and its new director, Lashley, was selected by Yerkes and the Board of Scientific Directors that included one psychologist, Leonard Carmichael. Financial support came primarily from the Rockefeller Foundation, but also from the Carnegie Corporation and from Harvard (Lashley's salary) and Yale (Assistant Director Henry Nissen's salary). The budget to conduct the laboratories for the 1st year was something under $68,000. On that budget, there were some 50 chimpanzees and 18 humans to support.

In 1943, Yerkes published a summary of studies of chimpanzees conducted at Yale Laboratories that revealed a knowledge of the life history, physiology, and behavior of these primates, more extensive than that available for any other species with the possible exception of the laboratory rat. Among the more important publications issued prior to Lashley's appointment as director were the determination of the time of ovulation (Yerkes & Elder, 1936); the study of morphine addiction (Spragg, 1940); the functions of the frontal lobes (Jacobsen, 1935; Jacobsen's discoveries were to contribute to the development of prefrontal lobotomy in the treatment of "insanity," to use Lashley's term); and Spence's contributions to learning theory during the years 1935–1940 (e.g., Spence, 1940).

Lashley reviewed the state of knowledge and resources when he became director in 1942 and decided to concentrate on four major areas of research: growth and development; physiology and psychology of sex; comparative individual psychology (intelligence and emotion); and cerebral functions in behavior. He promptly expanded the colony to include monkeys and began to recruit research personnel. He proposed to appoint a senior and junior investigator with special competence in each of the four fields. From the earlier administration, he had Nissen and Riesen in growth and development and Young in the physiology of sex. Hebb was appointed to head the area of comparative individual psychology. Then, in quick succession, two postdoctoral fellows arrived, Sperry and George Clark. Among the students, Birch was an early arrival. Lashley reserved the studies of cortical structure and function for himself and his students. As the work expanded, the expertise of individuals overlapped, and specific responsibilities were obscured. A second generation of personnel began to arrive in 1947. These included Hayes, Schiller, Chow, the Blums, and Evarts. By 1952, a third generation began to appear (e.g., Jarvik, Hutt, and Orbach), but Lashley's retirement was approaching and his illness, beginning in 1953, restricted his activities.

From the beginning of his tenure, Lashley complained in his *Annual Reports* that he was unable to recruit suitable personnel to fill the available research positions. There were a number of reasons for this. First, during the war years, 1942–1945, all able-bodied young men were in the armed forces. Not only was recruitment difficult, but the laboratories lost one member of the staff to the armed forces (Riesen). Second, the location of the laboratories, away from urban centers and unaffiliated with a nearby university, did not help matters. And then, to top it off, a Naval Air Station was located close by, reducing the availability of housing for laboratory personnel. As a result of all these factors, Lashley never succeeded in developing a pool of candidates from which to draw. There was no neighboring university that might supply graduate students (Jacksonville had the dubious distinction of being the largest city in the United States without a university), and the two sponsoring universities, Harvard and Yale, were too distant for a regular exchange of personnel. In the last analysis, graduate students were simply not attracted to Orange Park to conduct their thesis research, despite the renown of Lashley and the laboratories. Those who were attracted, by Lashley or for some other reason, found the laboratories a lonely and isolated place where there was nothing to do but work. North Florida was a cultural wasteland; and Orange Park itself was in the middle of nowhere. In this setting, marital relationships were frequently strained, sometimes broken, and otherwise rearranged. In struggling to survive, it helped to have strong personal resources, some talent, and practical skills. Hopefully, one day, a definitive history of the laboratories, from their inception in 1930 until they were moved in 1962, will be told.

Despite the recruitment problems, the roster of personnel, though limited in length, turned out to be very impressive (see Chapter 5). An air of excitement pervaded the laboratories. There was always something to be learned from colleagues, chiefly about their successes and failures in the laboratory and their methodological expertise, but also about their extracurricular activities and even about their domestic problems. Those who witnessed the routine of the staff remember the luncheon group, sitting in the open in a large circle on lawn furniture amid lush, semitropical flora in lively debates about every issue of the day—from McCarthyism to the markings of venomous snakes and the permeability of the eggshell. Every issue appeared to be in Lashley's area of expertise.

Now and then, Lashley's flair for the dramatic was displayed in this setting. Frequently the subject was insects, a subject that seemed to preoccupy Northerners, to Lashley's great amusement. Opening his lunch box one noontime, Lashley extracted an apple that had a large hole in it. Noting that many of the staff were curiously eying the apple, he held it up for all to see and, pointing to the hole, pronounced, "See that? My roach ate that." Smacking his lips, he proceeded to eat the apple with relish.

On another occasion at lunch, he cautioned a staff member not to move. "There's a scorpion on your shoe," he whispered. The group watched apprehensively as the scorpion finally crawled off the shoe. Slowly, the staff member raised his foot and poised it, ready to stamp down. With a great flourish, Lashley grabbed his arm and demanded, "What are you doing? Did the scorpion sting you?"

In the *Annual Report* of 1950, Lashley remarked on the morale in the laboratory. "In the past two years, there has been a marked increase in the proportion of collaborative work among members of the staff so that it is becoming difficult to say who is responsible for a given study. In many of the experiments, three, four or more people are involved in entirely voluntary cooperation. That is, I think, an indication of excellent morale." Lashley was referring to the Blums, Chow and Pribram, and, to a lesser degree, to Nissen and Riesen. This group began to fragment around 1949 with the departure of Riesen and Pribram and Robert Blum's death. No other collaborative group during Lashley's tenure as director matched that one.

As an administrator, Lashley left much to be desired. He practiced laissez faire on himself as he did on others. Maintenance chores were left mainly for Nissen, perhaps because Lashley himself avoided working with chimpanzees; perhaps because he had no interest in housekeeping detail and was not particularly good at it. Hebb saw (1980):

> no sign of any control of research by Lashley. Having assembled a staff, he left it to them to get to work; . . . He argued vigorously for his own theoretical views but he did not force them on the rest of us. It was not necessary to agree with him, and in fact I never did persuade him that I was not still a Pavlovian. . . . He had curious lapses of memory in some respects. Very flexible in discussion, he would admit the force of contrary argument on some point—but if one came back to the same point a month or two later, one would find him back at the old stand, ready to persuade again, and forget again [pp. 297–298].

Hebb recounted an occasion that revealed another side of Lashley. While waiting for Lashley one day at Harvard, his old friend, Taliaferro, asked Hebb what experiments Karl was engaged in. Hebb recalled (1980):

> I had to say I didn't know . . . Taliaferro, with a sort of grin, then asked if he had said anything about being all washed up experimentally and thinking about going to the medical school to make cell counts in human brains. As a matter of fact, he had, and Taliaferro told me that Lashley's repeated pattern was one of furious work for eight or ten or twelve months, followed by a longer period of no ideas, feeling all washed up, and thinking of falling back on the cell-counting project (which he never did) [p. 298].

Lashley's interests in research and theory did not vary much over the years. Judging by the titles of his early bibliography, his initial research interests centered chiefly around heredity, instinct, and discrimination. These topics continued to preoccupy him while he broadened the spectrum of his research activities. His own listing of interests in successive volumes of *American Men of Science* is revealing. In the 1933 edition, he listed the following interests: heredity, color vision, instincts of birds and primates, learning, cerebral localization, reeducation, and sex behaviors of animals. In the 1938 edition, the list was substantially the same; a minor change was the substitution of neural anatomy and physiology for cerebral localization and reeducation. In the 1944 edition, two items were added: meningitis and human parasitology; nothing related specifically to chimpanzees. In 1949, the list read: genetics of protozoan and coelenterate, conditioned reflexes, learning in animals, and functions of the cerebral cortex.

A careful examination of his bibliography reveals that Lashley did not return to heredity and color vision as subjects of laboratory investigation once he left for the University of Minnesota in 1917 and the initial research period was over. He did, however, return to instinct repeatedly in his speculative and review papers, most notably in 1937, 1938, 1947, and 1956; and his students, Stone, Russell, Beach, and others, made substantial laboratory contributions in this area. But it is the titles, "Studies of Cerebral Function in Learning" (13 papers so titled) and "The Mechanism of Vision" (18 papers so titled), that best characterize his later interests. In these papers and in others bearing related titles, the topics discrimination, cerebral localization, reeducation, and sexual behavior appear repeatedly.

The output of the Yerkes Laboratories of Primate Biology is a matter of public record and is not reviewed here. A complete list of publications was issued by the Yerkes Primate Research Center in Atlanta to commemorate 50 years of publications, 1925–1974. Most of the items numbered 217–451 (something over 200 of them) belong to the period of 13 years during which Lashley was director. Only 21 of these (about 10%) bear Lashley's name as an author. Granting that Lashley's name did not appear gratuitously on others' publications, this was not a large output by any standards.

As is the practice in most laboratories, not all the experiments were published. Some were never completed; others were simply aborted and never written up in the form of a publishable paper. Nor were Lashley's opinions of the work of his staff published. However, a running record of the activities of members of the staff, together with brief evaluations and comments by Lashley, can be found in the *Annual Reports* that were prepared for the Board of Scientific Directors and the granting agencies. A perusal of these *Annual Reports,* which are deposited in the Archives of the Yerkes Primate Research Center in Atlanta, reveals that they contain much fascinating information on research, personnel, budget, and opinions not available anywhere else. For this section, I selected those items that illustrate Lashley's opinions and biases and have not appeared elsewhere.

Contracts under the Office of Scientific Research and Development (OSRD)

During the second world war, the laboratories received a number of requests from OSRD to provide materials and facilities for various studies of importance to the military. One was a project on the selection and training of oscilloscope operators, a project directed by Donald B. Lindsley (who was really not connected with the Yerkes Laboratories in any way). Nissen served as technical representative. Lashley had no role except to provide material, facilities, and personnel, if necessary. In addition to an investigation of methods of selecting and training operators, a number of variables were studied, including optimal illumination of radar scopes, learning of radar code, length of training, and effects of fatigue. The reports were classified at that time (e.g., Lindsley, 1945), and the material reached the public domain only years later. In the early 1950s, a former student of Lashley undertook to investigate the effects of fatigue and boredom on radar operators at the request of the Canadian Defense Research Board. For this, college students were restricted in an unvarying laboratory environment for days on end, and the effects on learning, memory, perception, imagery, and motivation were noted. These reports were made public. One account was published in the *Scientific American* (Heron, 1957), but the experiments achieved notoriety earlier in relation to so-called brainwashing during and after the Korean war. The site of the laboratory was McGill University, and the student was D. O. Hebb.

In 1944, a Committee on Sensory Devices was set up under an OSRD contract to develop mechanical aids for the blind and the partially sighted. Lashley was a member of the committee. Reports of the work were published in a volume titled *Blindness,* edited by Paul A. Zahl (Lashley, 1950b). In his paper, Lashley pointed out that the development of guidance devices for the blind raised problems of scanning that led him to reformulate some basic concepts of cerebral function in the combining of successive stimuli into a percept and to examine temporal sequences of action. These ideas were elaborated in the celebrated paper delivered in 1949, "The Problem of Serial Order in Behavior" (See Beach, Hebb, Morgan, & Nissen, 1960; Lashley, 1951).

A third project under an OSRD contract was conducted under the direction of Paul Weiss at the University of Chicago. He assigned a graduate student of his in Orange Park to work on problems of nerve grafting. This young embryologist severed nerves and resutured them in order to study the course of growth and regeneration. During these investigations, a tantalum sleeve was developed to promote and guide peripheral nerve regrowth. Studies of regeneration and behavioral recovery that were even more imaginative and daring involved crossing nerves and inverting the eye. The student's name was Roger Sperry.

Despite the favorable outcomes of some of these investigations, Lashley never became enthusiastic about supporting studies dictated by military considerations or about applying for contracts, though he lent the facilities and personnel and otherwise cooperated and even contributed to the efforts. Some of the proposed animal studies were obviously impractical, failing to recognize basic structural differences between chimpanzee and human (see "The Problem of Instinct"). Other studies were described by Lashley as "lying mostly outside the main objectives of the Laboratories but participation in them was nevertheless of value in formulating some basic problems." And in spite of interruptions caused by the war and the pressures to contribute to the war effort, many basic problems to which Lashley was dedicated were focused upon and studied in the laboratory. One was the problem of instinct.

The Problem of Instinct

As a trained geneticist, Lashley showed an enduring interest in innate patterns of behavior. The subject of his doctoral thesis was the inheritance of asexual reproduction in hydra. Though his association with Watson and Franz led him to a lifelong study of learning in rats and monkeys, learning ability, for Lashley, was also a product of inheritance. That the memory trace could not be located in any circumscribed portion of the cerebrum did not vitiate his argument in favor of genetic determination. Throughout his career, Lashley referred repeatedly to unlearned or instinctive behavior, even in the human.

In his recruitment of personnel, Lashley seemed to favor individuals who shared his point of view or who could be proselytized. Hebb is an interesting example. An avowed Pavlovian to begin with, Hebb interpreted his thesis data (on the effect on vision of dark-rearing rats from birth) along the lines of his sponsor's nativistic position (1937). It was not until 1946 that Hebb reanalyzed and reinterpreted his rat data to match those of Riesen's chimpanzees (Hebb, 1980). Lashley could not have foreseen Hebb's theoretical about-face.

With Paul Schiller, Lashley experienced a community of interests. The last contribution that Lashley made to psychology was in an introduction to Schiller's book *Instinctive Behavior*, which was translated and edited by Schiller's widow, Claire, later to become Lashley's second wife. Citing some important observations on insightful behavior in primates, Lashley (1957) wrote: "The insight is the immediate one-trial learning to use the innate manipulative acts in the manner discovered by chance, and the generalization of the acts to other, similar situations . . . ; an extension of the same concepts to the manipulation of ideas may well lead to the conclusion that man has failed to identify his own instincts because he calls them intelligence [p. xii]."

In 1943, shortly after Lashley assumed the directorship, L. H. Snyder, one of the foremost students of human genetics, was invited to visit the laboratories and advise on a program of breeding chimpanzees that might be fruitful and that would reveal genetic factors in physical and behavioral traits. He spent 2 weeks at Orange Park, studying individual differences among chimpanzees and analyzing records of matings. To initiate studies of inheritance, he recommended that a selective breeding program be considered in order to develop distinct races, differing in measurable physical and behavioral traits, which might then be crossed for study of genetic patterns. The physical data accumulated on pigmentation and body proportions, plus some behavioral data, would provide material for genetic analysis, especially when combined with a study of wild racial types. This program would justify appointing an investigator with training in population methods.

Lashley had to face the fact that a selective breeding program was a protracted undertaking that must extend over many generations. Obviously, the slow sexual maturation of the chimpanzee, with 7 or more years to menarche, rendered the plan unsuitable for most studies of genetics. On the other hand, hybridization between two or more known species could be considered if the various specimens could be obtained. In this way, the selective breeding part of the experiment on inheritance could be eliminated, and fewer generations would be required. However, attempts to identify differenct species of chimpanzees failed. Except for the dwarf chimpanzee, there seems to be a continuous range of variation.

Though the project was of considerable interest to him, Lashley was a realist, and the project never really materialized. In his penultimate report of 1953, Lashley reflected regretfully on the stillbirth of the project. His final notation raised the specter of eugenics and interspecies breeding: "Requests to use the colony for experiments on crossing with man have been declined, because the scientific value of any outcome seemed incommensurate with the social risks involved." Indeed, the townsfolk of Orange Park must have had something like that in mind when they asked laboratory personnel on more than one occasion, "What d'you all do there behind the fence?"

Lashley seemed to regret the disfavor to which "instinct" had fallen in the psychology of his time. In his eleventh *Annual Report,* dated June 1953, 2 years before his retirement, Lashley noted:

> Since 1900, the attitude of psychologists on the question of human instincts has twice shifted radically. At the beginning of the century, the views of James and MacDougall prevailed. They ascribed to man a great number and variety of instincts and sought to explain many social and cultural developments by them. A reaction against this view was started by Watson and Dunlap and, by 1920, it was rather generally denied that man has any instincts whatever. Since then, opinion has swung back from this extreme view but the nature and even the existence of instinctive behavior in man is still controversial.

This *Annual Report* is replete with accounts of experiments bearing on the constitutional–experiential debate to which most members of the laboratory contributed. To set the stage, Lashley wrote, "The relative importance of heredity and education in the development of general and special abilities has been a matter of controversy for many years. A majority of educational psychologists who use Binet or similar scales for measuring intelligence insist on the constancy of the I.Q.; that is, that the rate of growth of intelligence with age depends upon hereditary constitution and is not affected by education." The dissenting opinions led Lashley to suggest that animal experiments can solve the problem. Since the education of human children cannot be controlled or varied experimentally to a significant degree, the chimpanzee reared in a controlled environment should be used in more decisive studies of the role of education in the development of abilities. In these studies, Lashley advocated a longitudinal approach: "Almost all the data for human children have been obtained by measuring different children in each age group and plotting averages . . . to obtain a growth curve. There are serious defects in this method and 'longitudinal' curves based on the growth of the same individuals make it possible to correct some of the inaccuracies inherent in the more usual methods."

The developmental studies of behavior in Orange Park took two directions: first, rearing the chimpanzee with the increased advantages of a human home (represented by the Viki experiment); and second, great restriction of early experience by eliminating a sense modality (represented by the dark-rearing experiments). For the most part, the data did not support Lashley's nativistic point of view. At best, the data were ambiguous. In his comments, Lashley sometimes conceded the point; at other times, he was more guarded. One of the entries read: "Early observations on nest-building suggest that this is probably a social tradition. . . . The wild chimp builds a simple sleeping platform even in captivity, if captured young. The laboratory reared chimpanzees have never made any attempt at nest construction." This is a concession. The standard of comparison must have been nest building in the rat.

Nissen's study of growth and maturation of the chimpanzee lent itself to the systematic investigation and identification of unlearned patterns of behavior. One apparently innate pattern is copulation. This appears after sexual maturation, without tutoring, in all species that had already been studied. In this area, Lashley was in for a shock. Here is his report of June 1952:

> For several years before puberty the chimpanzees . . . were kept with males and females separated. When . . . they had reached sexual maturity, observations on sex behavior were begun with four males and four females. They were paired when the females were in maximal genital swelling and kept under constant observation for many hours. During two years, . . . with more than 100 hours of observation, no copulations have occurred. This systematic study . . . seems to establish the fact that, unlike all other animals which have thus far been studied, the chimpanzee lacks a definite instinctive pattern of sexual behavior. Opportunity to watch copulation by other animals did not facilitate mating behavior in the inexperienced animals. Some of the chimpanzees . . . have now been mated with older experienced animals and the acquisition of normal sexual behavior under tuition by experienced animals is being followed.

Lashley extended his report the following year:

> The use of sophisticated partners as "tutors" was a more successful method of inducing the mature pattern of mating, although even here progress was slow. . . . Although the component elements of the act of copulation are present in the repertoire of adolescent behavior, the integration of these into the proper se-

> quence involves "trial and error" or the chance patterning of acts in play. . . . In the chimpanzee the hormonal influences are reduced to a minimum and psychological factors largely replace them. We see here the beginning of a "traditional" culture. . . . Distinct preference in mating [partners] are evident, a phenomenon rarely observed in other species.

As far as cognition was concerned, the exasperatingly slow learning by chimpanzees puzzled Lashley. Shortly after he arrived in Orange Park, Hebb tried his hand at developing problems whose solutions would be immediately apparent to the chimpanzee. He found that the adult chimpanzee was astonishingly dense on these problems. Lashley found, too, that many chimpanzees required 100 or more repetitions to learn a simple discrimination, something a rat (or the occasional chimpanzee) might learn in a single trial. Lashley was constantly on the lookout for instances of one-trial learning in the hope that the instance would reveal the "unit" of behavior.

For an association to be formed quickly, the objects associated must have some sort of unity for the animal (e.g., physical contact; Jarvik, 1953, 1956). Years earlier, Thorndike made a somewhat different claim as far as humans are concerned: Names with intervening conjunctions are more likely to be associated than names without, even though the latter stand in closer contiguity to each other (*John* and *Henry; William* and *George; Tom* and *Peter,* etc.). The problem was to identify the analogue of *and* in animal learning. Neither Lashley nor his students succeeded in this regard.

The possibility that motivation for success on cognitive tasks is lagging in the chimpanzee was considered. Lashley attempted to speed up learning by modifying rewards and by adding punishment for errors, but again with little success. As an application of the longitudinal approach, Nissen and Gardner attempted to rear chimpanzee youngsters under conditions that demanded work for everything they got (working for a living, so to speak) in the hope of setting up "habits of industry," but this project had to be abandoned "because it required too large an investment of time."

Viki's Instincts and Intelligence

The results of the Viki project could only strengthen Lashley's conviction regarding the relative importance of inheritance in the shaping of behavior. A number of attempts had already been made to teach chimpanzees to communicate. Kellogg's was the first; the second was carried out by Finch at the Yale Laboratories over a 2½-year period. Finch's service in the military interrupted that work but not before he came to recognize the impossibility of maintaining comparable conditions in the rearing of ape and child. After these vain attempts came the Nissen–Gardner effort to force chimpanzees to communicate by gesture (sic!) to get food. Lashley claimed that their chimpanzees never developed a representational language nor showed any evidence of abstract thinking. As a matter of fact, their chimpanzees *did* respond to gestures but actually made few of them themselves. Then came the Viki project, which was initiated and carried out by Keith and Cathy Hayes. Viki was adopted after birth and was educated in the Hayes home much as a human child would be.

On Viki's failure to develop speech by age 6 years, Lashley wrote in 1953:

> Viki's training has been centered on methods of communication, since some form of transmission is essential for any sort of general education. Early and continued efforts to develop speech have been unsuccessful. Viki passed through a brief babbling stage as does the human infant but failed to develop the characteristic human interest in verbal play. With great labor, she was taught to enunciate some six words, but progress was so slight that this training was abandoned. Her understanding vocabulary may include a score of words. This is in contrast to the average vocabulary of 2,000 words of the six year old human child.

On the other hand, imitation was used effectively as a means of communicating.

> Viki was trained to imitate a number of acts and eventually generalized the training so that she will now imitate all sorts of new activities. This complicates living for the Hayes', as when Viki seasons their food with a can of household cleaner. Her own communication is chiefly by pointing or guiding the experimenter's hands to indicate what she wants done with objects. . . . To play Viki prefers manipulative tasks and the use of implements. She uses most household utensils effectively, opening cans and bottles, using hammer and pliers, lighting cigarettes, etc. She builds blocks, solves form-board puzzles and manipulates mechanical toys. In these activities, she is not markedly inferior to human children of her own age group.

A concession again, but what does Lashley conclude from this impressive repertoire?

> The mere fact that Viki has progressed beyond the performance of the wild or cage-reared animal is of limited significance, since we already have similar evidence of the efficacy of special training in the records of the "seeing-eye" dog and the like.

Finally, to strengthen further his case that innate patterns characterize the behavior of the chimp, Lashley suggested that many postural differences between human and chimp, including Viki, are attributable to morphology such as size of head and length of neck and to differences in innate behavior. The example he gave is the tendency of chimpanzee youngsters to explore their environment with lips and tongue rather than with hands. To this I can attest. At a dinner party at the Hayes' one evening, I found myself beside Viki, who was seated in a high chair. I watched with disbelief as she picked up her fork, poised it, and neatly impaled the raw vegetable on her plate, bringing it to her mouth with Victorian grace. But before I could comment on her table manners, I heard a sharp hoot as she pounced onto the dinner table and proceeded to lap the sauce from my beef bourguignon, all the while with her rump in my face. The pandemonium at the dinner table subsided when Cathy Hayes chastised Viki; at this point Viki leapt off the table hooting, caught the nearest drape, and swung back and forth.

By the time she was 6 years old, it became obvious that Viki could not be kept indefinitely in the wood frame house where she had, until then, lived intimately with a human family. A concrete blockhouse on laboratory grounds was therefore prepared as her home. Windows were protected with hardware cloth; plumbing was encased. Generous sleeping quarters and an outdoor play area were constructed, and plans were made to introduce her gradually to other members of her species. In April 1954, after a short time in her new home and brief contacts with other chimpanzees, Viki became seriously ill. Competent medical help was obtained, and heroic efforts were made to save her; but her condition deteriorated steadily, and on May 11 she died. Autopsy revealed that she had a virus encephalitis. Having been raised without contact with other members of her species, she probably never developed immunities necessary to survive contact with laboratory-raised chimpanzees.

Lashley's final report on Viki emphasized the cumulative effects of education, new knowledge, and skills, building on those previously acquired. Many of Viki's later performances went far beyond those shown by any laboratory chimpanzee of that era. For example, Viki demonstrated considerable skill in the use of tools such as files, crowbars, can openers, and even fire. Needing a long stick, she was able to construct one by using a kinfe to whittle the end of a short stick until it fit into the hole at the end of a thicker stick. But attempts to teach Viki to count ended in failure. Whether the difficulty was intellectual or motivational or whether training was inadequate was never determined. Pulling a number of levers in a certain order also proved difficult. And though vocal language seemed beyond her ken, Viki showed progress in devising various gestural and other nonverbal ways of communicating her desires. One of her last achievements was mastery of a conditional matching problem that required generalized responses to color and form indicating human-level conceptualizations. At the end, Lashley acknowledged the results of the Viki project as an important contribution to the field of comparative psychology. With the new generation of claims of success in teaching chimpanzees to communicate in a humanlike manner, and the notes of caution sounded by Terrace, Petitto, Sanders, and Bever (1979) and by Premack (1976), Lashley's opinions must be seen as remarkably prophetic.

Dark-rearing Studies

According to Riesen, the dark-rearing studies of chimpanzees were originally conceived in 1941 within the rubric of the Infant Studies Program under Nissen's direction. The first study involved one chimpanzee, Jent, who was blindfolded for 12 weeks. This animal developed a convergent squint, probably because of the effort involved in peeking from behind the blindfold toward the nasal field (see Riesen's chapter in this volume, Chapter 9). When Lashley entered the picture, he hoped that more information concerning the innate organization of vision could be gained from such studies of chimpanzees.

Lashley's first reference to the dark-rearing studies was in his *Annual Report* dated December 1945. Under the heading, "The Nature of the First Visual Impression," Lashley asked: "How much of visual perception is dependent upon visual experience and how much is innate?" After referring to his work with Russell (1934) and Hebb (1937)[1] and to the clinical protocols of Senden, Lashley reported that two chimpanzees, Snark and Alfalfa, were being reared in darkness. Though cared for in light, they were hooded whenever the room was lighted so that the regimen in darkness would never be broken. Since Riesen was on leave in the armed forces, Birch was designated to conduct this testing. However, circumstances changed once again 6 months later when the chimps had matured sufficiently and were ready for testing: Birch resigned and Riesen returned. Finally, Riesen and Hebb were scheduled to conduct the testing.

The early results certainly astounded Lashley. In June 1947, he wrote:

> The visual capacity of two chimpanzee infants, which were kept in darkness for the first eighteen months, is being measured. From earlier studies with birds and rats we expected to find a considerable development of visual organization independent of learning. On the contrary, although optic reflexes were normal, these infants gave no indication of the perception of objects. They were essentially blind except to differences in the intensity of light and to movement. During six months of training and testing they have learned to distinguish a few objects but the learning is extremely slow and includes recognition of simple objects only such as the feeding bottle and targets which are presented with electric shock. If such results prove to be general for sensory capacities, they will require extensive revision of psychological theories of development.

Unprepared for such a revision, Lashley's suspicions of the data nevertheless remained groundless until June 1949 when he had the ammunition.

> Five chimpanzees have been kept in darkness for periods ranging from 3 to 22 months, with subsequent studies of vision. The degree of visual defect is roughly proportional to the period of light deprivation [shades of mass action!]. It now seems likely that the defects are due to direct physiological change in the retina, rather than to lack of visual experience. To control this, animals are being reared under photic stimulation, but with eyes so screened as to prevent the formation of visual images [with the use of a translucent dome over the head].

---

[1]Hebb reported that rats reared to maturity in total darkness showed discrimination of visual distance, and recognition of differences between visual patterns, at their first exposure to light.

As far as the influence of experience is concerned, Lashley's concession was limited.

> A critical factor in such [visual] habits is the acquisition of eye-muscle coordinations which can be learned only when there are points and contours in the visual vield which permit the development of fixation and following. The experiment is closely related to the problem of suppression of vision in human cases of extreme squint. There is much disagreement among clinicians as to the nature and likelihood of success in treatment of this condition and the experiments with the chimpanzees should be of value in clarifying this problem [*Annual Report*, June 1950].

The diffuse-light-rearing experiments were reviewed by Lashley in June 1951. Were the visual defects due to the absence of light stimulation or of opportunity to learn the meaning of visual stimuli by combined vision and manipulation? During a 90-minute period each day for the first 8 months, one chimpanzee was exposed to homogeneous light while the second was allowed to see and handle objects. The first was indistinguishable visually from those kept continually in the dark, whereas the other behaved normally. A third infant was reared like the first, under conditions that permitted seeing objects but without the ability to move about or touch them (strapped down but without the translucent dome). This chimpanzee showed some defect in near adaptation but little else. Lashley's conclusion followed Riesen's: "It appears that the absence of *patterned* stimulation is the chief factor in producing the deficits." However, the results on a light-reared infant placed in the dark for 16 months at the age of 8 months led Lashley to modify his opinion. At 24 months, this chimpanzee behaved as though he never had vision, suggesting that the defect was due, not to failure of development, but rather to suppression of visual function, perhaps because of dominance of touch and other senses. The problem had become dismally complicated, particularly since one of the first dark-reared animals had become stone-blind during the 3 years in normal daylight, probably because of retinal degeneration. At this point, Lashley advocated studies of effects of light privation on the structural integrity of the retina and brain.

An interesting sidelight came up in the *Annual Report* of June 1952, when the question was raised of whether the fusion of images in binocular vision is the result of learning. To test this, a chimpanzee infant was raised for 6 months with vision restricted to one eye at a time; on alternate days the right and left eyes were blindfolded. At the end of this period, she was trained in habits of visual discrimination, using only one eye. She performed these habits correctly when the blindfold was transferred to the other eye. Lashley concluded that "although the nervous excitations from the two eyes are transmitted to the cerebral cortex by different pathways, their community of central connections is independent of any learning resulting from simultaneous stimulation of the two eyes." This statement by Lashley anticipates the later work of Sperry on the mechanisms of interocular transfer. It should be noted that Lashley was perhaps the first in

America to introduce the problem and methodology of interocular transfer (Lashley, 1924).

According to Riesen, an ophthalmologist was consulted some time around late 1948 in relation to the determination of visual acuity in chimpanzees. The question raised was whether the visual disturbances shown by the dark-reared chimps were due to acquired refractive errors that might by corrected. It was in the course of refracting the eyes that pallor of the optic discs was noted. Mindful of the clinical syndrome of "miner's" nystagmus, observed repeatedly in conjunction with pallor of the optic discs, Lashley was able to argue in June 1953 that prolonged absence of light leads to retinal degeneration, which in turn results in visual disturbances (amblyopia ex anopsia?). It was not until 1957 that Lashley's early suspicions were vindicated by anatomical studies of the retina of a dark-reared chimpanzee, which revealed degeneration of ganglion cells (Chow, Riesen, & Newell, 1957).

The dark-rearing studies had an enormous influence on contemporary psychological thought. References can be found in the literature of almost every division of psychology—sensory and perceptual, developmental and comparative, physiological and clinical—and textbook accounts are directed to students at every level. The data appeared at a propitious point in time in America, when interests were about to veer in the direction of the deprived human condition. The applications quickly became obvious. Among the spin-offs were studies of deprivation involving the nonvisual modalities—auditory, tactile, proprioceptive; the interocular transfer experiments; the multisensory deprivation experiments; the effects of social and parental restriction; receptive field properties; developmental studies of transmitter substances and dendritic spines; etc., etc.

Lashley's own influence on the course of this work has never been clarified. He must have served as a gadfly during the conduct of the research, and he must have contributed a share to the methodology used by Riesen. The large, painted plaque that approached the chimpanzee and delivered the milk bottle for a correct response and an electric shock to the nose for an error was probably designed with Lashley's assistance. And Lashley's suspicions of the emerging data must have goaded Riesen and others toward anatomical and biochemical considerations. But credit for popularizing the early light-deprivation work must be given to Hebb, who used Riesen's data skillfully to underpin his neuropsychological theory of perceptual development and later initiated an era of interest in multisensory deprivation.

Early Brain Damage and the Brain-Scarring Project

Lashley's first reference in his *Annual Reports* to age and brain-scarring as variables in the determination of behavioral disturbances after brain damage appeared in June 1947. Those references were made in relation to the operation of prefrontal leukotomy in the treatment of psychotic conditions. Developed as a result of the work of Jacobsen at the northern station of the Yale Laboratories, the operation seemed then to be most effective in the treatment of agitated depression. After expressing dissatisfaction with the mass of contradictory and poorly controlled observations, Lashley promised to undertake a systematic analysis of frontal lobe functions in monkeys and chimpanzees. Various considerations were cited as meriting attention: (1) structural variation within species; (2) species differences; (3) failure to understand the significance of the diagnostic tests; (4) crude and unreliable surgical procedures; (5) age of onset of cortical damage; and (6) differential effects of maximal and minimal scar formation.

It is interesting to note in this connection that Penfield was appointed to the Board of Scientific Directors just 1 year earlier and that Hebb, for whom these two factors were central, was about to leave. In a personal interview in 1979, Hebb reminisced regretfully that although age of onset of brain damage was the variable that originally drew him to Orange Park, the first infant was operated just months before he left.

That first reference to the age factor read as follows:

> The capacity for recovery from injuries seems more likely to produce generalized intellectual dificits; tumors or traumatic injuries in adults produce more limited and specific symptoms [no reference to Hebb's 1942 publication]. It is impossible to make anatomic comparisons of these conditions in man. The infantile injury may prevent development of general capacities or there may be important differences in character of the injuries. Experiments with rats and monkeys have indicated a quicker and more complete recovery of the infant than of the adult from similar injuries, but have dealt with very primitive capacities. A comparison of similar lesions in infant and adult chimpanzees has been undertaken. The prefrontal region has been removed from an 8 weeks infant and the parietal areas will be removed later. Development of the infant will be followed closely and his later capacities compared with those of adults with similar lesions. We plan to include additional infants in this study as they become available.

Following this up, in June 1951, Lashley wrote:

> Two of our chimpanzees had their prefrontal lobes removed at about six weeks of age and the parietal lobes were also removed from one of these animals at about twelve weeks. They have been tested in many ways during the four years since operation and, in every function tested, have come well within the range of normal animals of their age group . . . attention . . . discriminative learning and habit interference. . . . Publication of this material has been delayed, since the Director insists that the operations be confirmed by histological studies of the brains before conclusions are published.

As a matter of fact, the material was never published in the form of a research report.

The results of the brain-scarring project fared no better. The idea of scarring cortical tissue experimentally, rather than removing it, must have developed out of discussions with Hebb and Penfield no later than 1947, but the project did not get under way until some 5 years later, in 1952, when Lashley received a 3-year research grant from the Office of Naval Research.

Here is Lashley's rationale as stated in the 1953, 1954, and 1955 *Annual Reports:*

> Experimental ablation of the "associative areas" of the cerebrum in animals produces significant effects on behavior only when large areas are removed from both hemispheres. In monkeys these areas include frontal, temporal and parietal lobes. In contrast to this, severe behavioral disturbances in man are often ascribed to small traumatic lesions or localized tumors. There are several possible explanations of this apparent contradiction: the tests used with animals may not be sufficiently sensitive; the human functions may be more fragile than those of lower animals; the anatomic data used in delineating the lesions in many may be inadequate to reveal widespread damage; the damage in the human brain from trauma, hemorrhage or tumors produces irritative scars which are avoided in the clean surgical removal of tissue in the experimental laboratory. Nerve cells in such scars might fire in abnormal combinations and so produce disturbances in the activity of surrounding normal tissue.

The experiments were designed to test the last alternative—that experimentally produced irritative scars would have a more deleterious effect on behavior than clean removals of equal size and location. The underlying assumptions were that the scar contains neurons that remain functional but have abnormal connections, and that the abnormal firing of such cells would disorganize the activities of much larger cortical areas.

Some of the lesions were restricted to about 2 cm^2, centered in frontal or parietal areas, complete destruction of which is known to produce severe behavioral disturbances. More than 20 different methods of damaging the cortex were used, such as subpial hemorrhage, insertion of copper plates, devascularization, freezing, crushing, multiple stab wounds (in one case, some 700 over the entire exposed cortex), and cauterization with heat, electric current, and various chemicals. Other lesions were designed to produce increased intracranial pressure. Foreign bodies were inserted—in one case, a marble; in another case, bone splinters. Carcinogenic materials were also tried. Some 38 monkeys were tested on a variety of tasks that are known to reveal deterioration after extensive cortical removals.

In no case was it possible to demonstrate any disturbance of behavior after surgery, not even in those monkeys that showed marked abnormality in their EEG records. In general, *restricted* lesions of associative cortex, however produced, did not result in measurable symptoms in the monkey, whereas *extensive* cortical removals did. These results did not support the idea that abnormal activity of scar tissue in a circumscribed cortical areas is responsible for the behavioral disturbances in humans.

Although the experiments were restricted to the brain-scarring aspect of the problem, the results had a bearing on the other alternatives. The tests applied to monkeys did reveal agnosias, apraxias, and other defects comparable to the human symptoms when the lesions were extensive, so they could scarcely be regarded as insensitive. On the question of whether human cortical function is especially fragile, Lashley noted again that extensive lesions in the monkey produced symptoms comparable to those in the human. Was it possible that small lesions in humans produced severe symptoms by some mechanism of disorganization involving the abnormal firing of cells? This seemed to be ruled out by the successful performance of operated monkeys that had abnormal EEG records. The results of all these experiments raised the question of whether in human cases, the severe symptoms might be due to more widespread damage, vascular change or cell damage, which is not revealed by the customary methods of histological analysis. This remained a possibility, for Lashley's survey of the clinical literature revealed that anatomic verification of lesions had rarely been adequate, and the effects of edema with subsequent vascular and tissue damage had never been given adequate consideration.

At the end of the funding period, the unexpended funds were returned to the granting agency. A brief account was included in George W. Gray's (1955) very readable portrait, "The Yerkes Laboratories," in *Scientific American*, but a research report was never issued.

Temporal Integration

In his paper on serial order in behavior delivered in 1949 at the Hixon Symposium at the California Institute of Technology, Lashley offered some fascinating glimpses into the problem of temporal organization of behavioral elements. Focusing on the organization of words in meaningful sentences, Lashley illustrated the integrative functions of the cerebral cortex in human thought. However, temporal integration is not found exclusively in language. Behavioral instances to which Lashley would have liked to address himself include the coordination of leg movement in insects, the song of birds, and rat's running errorlessly through the maze. In the same way, human endeavors like the architect's designing a house and the carpenter's sawing a board present a problem of sequences of action that cannot be explained in terms of successions of external stimuli. In developing the TOTE model, Miller, Galanter, and Pribram (1960) seem to have been much influenced by Lashley's critique of the reflex and his analysis of temporal organization in behavior. Unfortunately, Lashley himself never pursued this line of thinking in systematic laboratory research. The following brief review of the 1951 paper illustrates how fresh and stimulating Lashley's serial order problem remains to this day.

Traditionally, behavioral integration has been ascribed to the spatial distribution of excitations in the nervous system. Using the principle of isomorphism, the Gestalt psychologists have provided examples of the relation between spatial distribution and perceptual integration. The Gestalt laws of organization, such as the law of proximity, relate the spatial features of the stimulus and isomorphic excitation in cerebral cortex. Temporal patterning has generally been neglected in neuropsychological theory. Though the concepts of "summation," "facilitation," "excitation," "inhibition," "after-discharge," and the like operate over time, little effort has been expended to translate the time factor into the neural activity that must account for behavioral integration.

Consider Lashley's (1951) illustrative sentence: "The mill-wright on my right thinks it right that some conventional rite should symbolize the right of every man to write as he pleases [p. 116]." The word arrangement is obviously not due to any direct associations of the word *right* with other words, but to meanings of words. The individual items of the series are not temporally polarized in their associative connections with other items. The order is imposed by some other agent. This is true not only of language but of all skilled movements or successions of movements. In the gaits of horses, trotting, pacing, and single footing involve essentially the same pattern of muscular contraction in the individual legs. However, the specific gait is imposed by some mechanism in addition to the direct relations of reciprocal innervation among the sensorimotor centers of the legs. Similarly, the order in which the fingers of the musician fall on the keys or fingerboard is determined by a set that is not inherent in the association of the individual movements.

What did Lashley mean by "set"? Prior to the enunciation of the sentence, an aggregate of word units is partially activated or readied. Lashley derived evidence in support of this idea from errors of speech and writing. The most frequent typing errors are those of anticipation: the inclusion in the word being typed of some part of a word or word structure that should properly occur later in the sentence. It may be only a letter. For example, Lashley wrote "*wrapid* writing," carrying the *w* from the second word to the first. Not infrequently words are introduced that should occur much later in the sentence, often five or six words in advance.

In oral speech, Spoonerisms illustrate similar transpositions of words. Spoonerisms are most frequently inversions of subject and object: "Let us always remember that waste makes haste." But they may also be only transpositions of parts of the words: "Our queer old dean" for "our dear old queen." "For real enjoyment, give me a well-boiled icycle," and "I have just received a blushing crow," etc. In some types of aphasia the tendency to disordered arrangment of words is greatly increased, and the attempt to speak results in a word hash with complete loss of grammatical organization. Lashley suggested that Spooner probably suffered from a mild form of aphasia. In these slips, it is as if the aggregate of words were in a state of partial excitation held in check by the requirements of the grammatical structure, but ready to activate the final common path if the effectiveness of this check is in any way interfered with. These slips provide further evidence for preexcitation of the elements and cannot be ascribed to differences in the relative strength of associative bonds between the elements of the act. The understanding and production of speech demand the postulation of an aftereffect or after-discharge of the sensory components for a significant time following stimulation.

The eye is alleged to be the only sense organ that gives simultaneous information concerning space in any detail. All the other senses are activated by a distribution of stimulation over time. The shape of an object impressed on the skin can scarcely be detected from simultaneous pressure, but the same shape can readily be distinguished by touch when traced on the skin with a stylus or when explored by tactile scanning. The temporal sequence is readily translated into a spatial concept. Even for vision it might be questioned whether simultaneous stimulation gives rise directly to space concepts. The visual object is generally surveyed by eye movements, and its form is a reconstruction from such a series of excitations.[2] Even with tachistoscopic exposures, the after-discharge permits a temporal survey, and with visual fixation, shifts of attention provide the possibility of a central "scanning." This reference to central scanning was extremely bothersome for it raised questions of the validity of tachistoscopic studies of visual recognition as a function of local retinal stimulation (e.g., Orbach, 1967).

Lashley's final topic was his favorite one—memory. Since memory traces are static and persist simultaneously, it must be assumed that they are spatially differentiated. Nevertheless, reproductive memory appears almost invariably as temporal sequence, either as a succession of words or of acts. Lashley wrote (1951):

> Even descriptions of visual imagery are generally descriptions of sequences, of temporal reconstructions from very fragmentary and questionable visual elements. Spatial and temporal order thus appear to be almost completely interchangeable in cerebral action. The translation from the spatial distribution of memory traces to temporal sequence seems to be a fundamental aspect of the problem of serial order [p. 128].

Though all behavior involves temporal integration (and certainly maze performance involves a series of responses in proper sequence), Lashley never conducted experiments directed specifically to the problem of understanding

---

[2]Shortly after this analysis, the method of stabilizing the image on the retina was devised, and Hebb quickly noted that the fading of parts of the stabilized image supported his conception of the cell assembly underlying the perceptual "unit." Lashley, however, never commented on the significance of the stabilized image evidence for perceptual theory, in general, or for temporal integration in vision, in particular.

serial order. After his marriage in 1957, Lashley and his wife Claire planned a program of studies of temporal organization in language. His death just 1 year later put an end to these plans.

A STUDENT OF HEBB WITH LASHLEY IN ORANGE PARK

In the spring of 1952, Lashley delivered the four Vanuxem Lectures at Princeton University. The audience was drawn not only from the faculty and student body at the university but also from the Institute for Advanced Study and neighboring institutions. After the series was over, a dinner party was arranged in Lashley's honor at the Nassau Inn. Though only a graduate student at the time, I was invited to join the group because I had studied with Lashley's student Hebb, and was preparing myself for a career in physiological psychology. At dinner, I found myself seated beside Lashley, and I remember him as quite animated and our conversation was exhilerating. When I finally screwed up my courage and told him that E. G. Wever had me placing recording electrodes on the round window of the guinea pig cochlea and that my heart was not in it, Lashley suggested that I prepare a proposal for research on primates, and he would see whether he could offer me a stipend at the Yerkes Laboratories of Primate Biology in Orange Park, Florida.

I quickly wrote up a proposal that involved rearing monkeys from birth in a visually distorted environment. The experiment took off from Sperry's eye rotation work on amphibians (1943) and from Hess' visual displacement work on chicks (1950). Designing with Hebb's theory of visual development in mind, and guessing Lashley's disapproval of Hebb's physiologizing, I mailed the proposal with some trepidation.

The offer in response to my proposal came in the form of a choice between an assistantship on the brain-scarring project supported by a Navy grant or an assistantship on general funds, both to start that fall. I hesitated because neither stipend amounted to a living wage, but then Lashley offered to accept my wife as a histological assistant and that clinched it. After consulting with Hebb on the choice, I took the assistantship on general funds. By that time, I had completed the academic requirements for the Ph.D degree at Princeton, and I was sent off with Wever's blessing to do my thesis *in absentia*. The assistantship on general funds would permit me to work out a research program of my own choosing.

When I arrived at the Yerkes Laboratories in 1952, Lashley spent the better part of the first day with me, beginning with a grand tour of the laboratories which involved leading me past each of the 60-odd adult chimpanzees then housed in Orange Park. The welcome I received from some of the chimpanzees was a rousing one. I was given a dazzling display of harp playing on the chain-linked fence by Don and a dousing with water as I turned to follow Lashley to the next cage. ''Look out,'' Lashley shouted, deliberately late, I would guess. It must have been a pint of water with which Don clandestinely filled his mouth. Swinging back and forth to gain momentum, his accuracy even from a distance of 10 feet was remarkable, and my shirt was drenched. Some caged chimpanzees have been described as spitters, but this description hardly does justice to Don's prowess. Near the end of the tour, Lashley was again late in warning me to keep my distance. This time it was a fecal missile that struck me hard on the left shoulder and knocked me off balance, a sight that Lashley must secretly have enjoyed. No hostility intended on Lashley's part, just good-natured humor.

After this initiation, Lashley sat down with me in the library room and proceeded to review the research that was then in progress. Included was the Infant Studies Program directed by Nissen and the ablation program in which he, Chow, the Blums, and others had recently been engaged. He described the daily distribution of cabbage-quarters throughout the colony, an activity that provided Nissen with the occasion to observe the physical condition of each and every chimpanzee (health, sex skin, etc.), and he urged me to join Nissen so that I could meet the chimpanzees and familiarize myself with their individual behaviors. "Don't get involved in the dark-rearing studies," he cautioned. Seeing my astonishment, he explained that the results were difficult to interpret, and he was convinced that the proper explanation had to await anatomical studies which would modify the conclusions drawn earlier by Riesen and popularized by Hebb. His reservations became clear to me later, when histological studies revealed degeneration in the retina resulting from disuse and I discovered the three papers by Walls, "The Problem of Visual Direction" (1951). Disregarding his injuction, I began to plan studies of pattern vision of chimpanzees and monkeys reared in intermittent illumination (Orbach & Miller, 1969). Lashley never approved, but I did get funds for the strobe equipment I needed.

Lashley as Teacher

In his supervision of student research, Lashley tended to be quite permissive and informal. At the Orange Park laboratories, students were given free reign to develop and execute experiments. Unless the student asked for it, Lashley himself imposed little guidance. This method worked well for postdoctoral fellows, not always for the shy and awed Ph.D. candidate who floundered without direction or reassurance. Lashley disliked teaching in the sense of giving formal lectures in the classroom, nor was he particularly good at it.[3] But as a supervisor of research, he could be extremely effective on a one-to-one basis or in small, informal discussion groups. In these settings he was animated, friendly, and helpful, though the relationship was almost always impersonal and distant with staff as well as with students. He addressed most everyone by their last names,

[3] "It's no use to teach people," he aphorized, "because those that need teaching can't learn and those that can learn don't need to be taught."

and most everyone reciprocated with the inevitable "Dr. Lashley." Exceptions included some members of the Board of Scientific Directors—Yerkes, Carmichael, and Taliaferro, who addressed him as "Karl." To his assistant director, Nissen, he was "Dr. Lashley."

If the student requested it, discussions involving progress in research might occur formally in Lashley's office or in the library room across the hall. Without a request, the discussion would more likely take place informally when the staff gathered for lunch outdoors. This laissez faire attitude seems to have been a studied one on the part of Lashley in order to foster resourcefulness and creativity.

Despite all the informality, however, students were expected to appear periodically with research plans and thereafter with data and publishable manuscripts. The one formal requirement of each member of the laboratory staff was an annual report in written form and orally before the Board of Scientific Directors.

When a research proposal was brought to him, Lashley would give it a sympathetic ear. That done, he would point to the inevitable conceptual and methodological shortcomings, sometimes dismissing the proposal as impractical or as downright impossible. As a critic he was a demolition expert. In 1952, I presented a plan to Lashley to plot the residual visual fields of monkeys following subtotal resections of striate cortex. The basic requirement, as I saw it, was a matrix of test points of light and a method to insure fixation. To trigger the test flash, I suggested a photoelectric system using a tiny mirror mounted on the eyeball. Point by point, Lashley proceeded to tear the plan apart. His parting shot at me was, "If you succeed in plotting the visual fields of the monkey, you will get the Nobel Prize." Though meant to inspire me, it did not. (Later, Cowey and Weiskrantz reported on just such an effort [1963].) After another occasion or two like that, Lashley began to identify me as the student with the impossible problems.

Although each proposal got the demolition treatment, I never heard Lashley forbid a proposal—quite the contrary. He frequently followed up by encouraging the student. "Try it," he would challenge. In the last analysis, however, he held the purse strings, and his approval could be measured by the funds he would release and by the reluctance he showed in releasing them. Two examples are worth noting. Lashley never seemed to approve the study of chimpanzees raised in darkness. As a consequence, the behavior of these chimpanzees was hardly ever recorded cinematographically. Movie film was rarely available in the lab, and one test sequence of the chimpanzees Snark and Alfalfa is all there is on film to show of this project. Later, one of the younger staff needed a large group of subjects to check a deduction from learning theory. His request for rodents in a primate laboratory seemed the height of indignity. Lashley was ill at the time and there was a long delay, but he finally did get his rats, though grudgingly.

Following is an example of Lashley's method with students drawn from an experience I had shortly after arriving in Orange Park. A paper of mine had just appeared in print in which I reported that English words were better recognized in the right visual field than in the left when projected tachistoscopically. The opposite seemed to be true for Yiddish words. The data suggested a limited intraocular transfer of learning to recognize words (and, hence, a limited equipotentiality of cortical tissue). In line with Hebb's critique of equipotentiality theory, I proposed that the limited transfer might be due to past reading experience and differential reading habits, not to the innate properties of cortical tissue (Orbach, 1952). With some trepidation, I left a reprint for Lashley, and the very next day he came looking for me.

First, Lashley complimented me on an interesting experiment. He would not have predicted my results, he admitted, but after reflection he was not surprised by them. I braced myself for the critique.

(*Question*): Did you realize that verbal material is polarized and not symmetrical?

(*Answer*): Yes, I did, and I said so in my paper. I even considered a vertical as well as a horizontal polarization. (What is this about? I wondered. Is he suggesting that the differential recognition was due to this polarization?)

(*Question*): Did you realize that tachistoscopic recognition requires a scanning of the word—not by the retina, to be sure—but by a central mechanism?

(*Answer, weakly*): Yes, I did, but how does this scanning influence my interpretation?

Gently, Lashley reviewed the argument in his "serial order" paper (1951), and he ended with the declaration that my test of equipotentiality left something to be desired.

This exchange, telegraphed above, lasted perhaps 10 minutes, but I was exhausted. When it was over, Lashley pulled a book off the shelf and opened it at random. Have you ever noticed, he asked animatedly, what happens to the recognizability of a word when it is rotated away from the horizontal? He began to read out loud, rotating the book slowly in his hands. As he passed the 90° point of rotation (reading upward with the words on their sides), he began to stumble over the words. Stopping triumphantly, he exclaimed, see what happens? You don't get a progressive drop in recognizability as you would predict if reading habits determined recognizability. Instead recognizability drops off sharply just beyond 90°. How do you explain it? he asked archly.

Confused, I repeated his question, how do *you* explain it? Ignoring the question, Lashley placed the book in my hands and urged me to try the little experiment myself, but I stumbled from the beginning. Seeing my discomfort, Lashley suggested that I check this casual observation in the laboratory. "Try it," he urged.

I remember going home depressed that evening. It had been a rather formidable encounter. Not only had I failed in the debate; I wasn't sure that I had followed Lashley's argument. That evening, I pulled out the "serial order" paper and studied it. The next day, when I tried Lashley's little experiment on my wife, the results were by no means obvious. I decided to try it in the laboratory as Lashley suggested.

Using tachistoscopic exposure of words in seven orientations (0° [normal horizontal], 30°, 60°, 90°, 120°, 150°, 180° [upside down, right-to-left], each produced by rotating the word counterclockwise from the horizontal, I tested laboratory personnel and plotted the data: percent recognition as a function of stimulus angle. To me, it appeared that recognizability dropped off continuously as the word was rotated from the horizontal until a low was reached at 150°; beyond, at 180°, recognizability rose slightly. I remember exulting despite the fact that I was not sure how to interpret the data.

It didn't take me long to complete the experiment; Lashley had the graphs in his hands within 3 weeks or so. He studied them silently. "That's interesting," he said finally, "but it's not the experiment I suggested. You presented the words tachistoscopically, requiring central scanning, a process we do not understand." I remember that we debated the matter and puzzled over the rise in recognizability at 180°. Finally, I proposed to repeat the experiment, this time studying reading rate as a function of stimulus angle, and Lashley concurred.

I selected seven paragraphs from Thoreau's *Walden* (I had just read *Walden Two*), equated more or less for textual difficulty, and presented each, in counterbalanced order, at one of the seven stimulus angles. The instructions were, "Read the paragraph aloud as fast as you can." The plotted data—reading rate as a function of stimulus angle—revealed the very same gradual drop-off, this time in reading rate, to a low at 150° followed again by a small rise at 180°. Though a little brusque, I thought, Lashley was genuinely puzzled. For relevant references, he promised to write to Beebe-Center at Harvard, who, he pronounced, was familiar with most of the international literature in psychology.

Sure enough, it took no more than a couple of weeks, and I had in my hands a reference in the German literature: "Aulhorn, O. Die lesegeschwindikeit als Function von buchstaben and zeilenlage *Pflüg. Arch. ges. Physiol.*, 1948, *250*, 12-25." Aulhorn had published the results of an experiment similar to mine but using German reading material. Imagine our astonishment when we found my graphs in Aulhorn's paper—the same gradual drop-off in recognizability to 150° and the small return at 180°. I marveled at the zeitgeist, but Lashley lost interest in the problem and I got involved in my thesis research.

A generation later, the problem and the proposed solutions have become much more complicated. Cerebral asymmetries have been implicated, and a central scanning process seems to be required to account for the results reported in the voluminous literature on recognition differentials in tachistoscopic perception.

Lashley expected a sudden drop in recognition when words were rotated beyond 90°. What really intrigued him, however, was the lack of a significant drop in recognizability of the rotated word over what he believed was a broad span of orientation ranging from −90° through 0° (normal horizontal orientation) to +90°. Left-to-right reading habits certainly could not be responsible for successful recognition of words exposed at orientations never used in normal reading. Instead, cortical cells that never mediated recognition in the past must have the potential to mediate successful recognition. However, the data simply did not conform to Lashley's expectations: A progressive drop in recognition took place before 90° was reached. In addition, the improvement in recognition of words at 180° suggested that a *horizontal* scanning, both ocular and central, is responsible. The data have transcended the original problem.

Early in 1953, I proposed as a thesis problem the effects on learning and retention of striate cortex removals in peripherally blinded monkeys. Though Lashley seemed to respond positively to my suggestion on this occasion, I got the usual demolition treatment on methodology once again. "Monkeys don't run mazes," he said when I outlined my plan, "certainly not horizontal ones. They climb. Why don't you try a vertical maze?"

Seeing myself clambering madly after monkeys to retrieve them, I abandoned the plan to use a locomotor maze and settled on a stylus maze. Lashley approved, and I went ahead to design a maze that the monkey could manipulate without vision. Though we chatted together almost every day and he assisted me with the enucleations and striate cortex removals (I saw the proverbial "spoon" used on one of these occasions), very little passed between us on my thesis problem. When I did come to him many months later, it was with preliminary data on four monkeys. My mood was gloomy, for the data were essentially negative: I had failed to pick up effects on learning and retention following the cortical blinding, and I feared a veto on the project. But I was in for a surprise. After carefully examining the data and noting some interesting side issues, Lashley congratulated me on a job well done. His earlier interpretation based on rats simply did not apply to monkeys, he concluded, and he was prepared to accept my work on the four preliminary monkeys as my thesis. No need to do it again. I was stunned but relieved, and later I determined not to abandon the problem until I could clarify the discrepancy between the data of rat and monkey.

Now, with my thesis out of the way, I disregarded Lashley's early advice and returned to the original plan that involved the use of the alley maze. Laboriously, I trained peripherally blinded monkeys to run errorlessly through a giant replica of Lashley's maze III. This time the striate cortex removals had a profound effect on maze performance, and Lashley was as astonished as I was. The results, together with an interpretation, were published in a review article (Orbach, 1959).

Lashley's Extracurricular Activities

Away from the laboratory, Lashley could drop the relaxed formality and take on the role of an erudite, though opinionated, conservative American. Hebb has noted (1959) that Lashley loved good plays and classical music except opera, which he ridiculed, and he also enjoyed burlesque and vaudeville. He told good stories with a mischievous humor, and he loved to puncture another's argument with a chuckle. Sometimes he played on his political conservatism to outrage his liberal students. On the night of the presidential election in November 1952, the laboratory personnel assembled at the home of one of the staff in Orange Park for a chess tournament. As they listened at the same time to the early returns on radio, it became clear that Eisenhower was winning by a wide margin. I remember that my wife was distressed that the brilliant, articulate, and charismatic Stevenson was headed for defeat. She commiserated with those around her until finally Lashley heard what was going on. "Why are you so upset?" he asked innocently. My wife stared incredulously at him. "You mean, you're for Eisenhower?" "No, no," Lashley answered with a twinkle in his eye. He waited for the puzzled look to broaden on her face, then added, "I'm for Taft."

Lashley himself was a sailing enthusiast. It was, for him, an important skill to compete at and a source of enjoyment. As in the case of many of his other skills, sailing was self-taught. Hebb, who was a fellow enthusiast, noted (1959) that Lashley mastered the art "by trial and error and sheer force of intellect [p. 147]." In the early 1930s, Lashley and Wiley would venture forth on Lake Michigan on a 30-foot yawl to return only by the grace of God, for in those days, Lashley could not swim. In a birthday felicitation in 1950, Wiley recalled the excitement of wind and water and the pranks they played on some of Lashley's guests.

Lashley's other great hobby was music. At 11, he was taught the piano but rebelled against the practice of scales. His real interest in music did not develop until much later. At 18, he picked up the violin and taught himself to play. Later he did the same with the cello, which became his instrument. Whether it was the music itself or the shop work involved in maintaining the instrument that fired the original interest is not clear—probably both.

His first wife, Edith, was a professionally trained pianist who could have concertized had her asthmatic condition permitted it. The two of them maintained their musical activities throughout their marriage. Lashley met many professional musicians through Edith, and he devoted at least one evening per week to playing chamber music selected from his personal library. In Jacksonville, he formed a string quartet with musicians from the Jacksonville Orchestra, and they gathered to rehearse at his home, "Fiddler's Cove," in which one of the rooms was air-conditioned. Together with occasional chess games and tournaments with laboratory personnel, these were Lashley's principal extracurricular activities.

Shortly after I arrived in Orange Park in 1952, Lashley discovered that I was a fiddler myself, and he suggested that I join him for the weekly rehearsals of the Jacksonville Orchestra. A bit shy, and awed by Lashley as a man of many talents, I tried to beg off each week with one excuse after another, but he persisted. Finding myself pinned without an excuse one afternoon, I was ready to succumb, then remembered with relief that my violin was in need of extensive repair. "It's open at the seams," I explained. "Bring it in tomorrow," Lashley

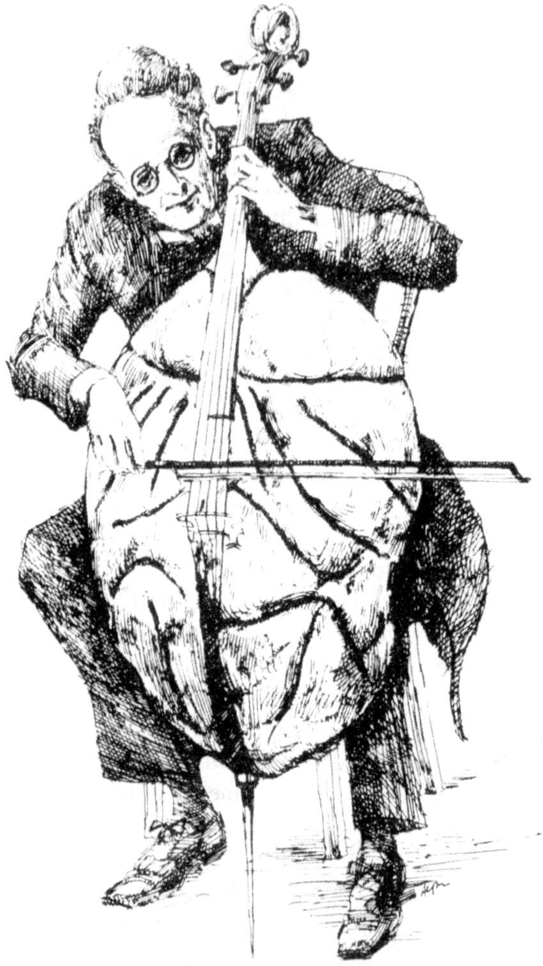

FIG. 2.1. Fiddling with the brain.

suggested. I was astonished to learn the next day that he had the tools, the material, the craft, and the inclination to do the repair himself. I remember wondering, as I watched him work, whether I should offer to pay him. The product was a messy one, but the violin was indeed repaired and my last excuse evaporated. The following week, I found myself with him at the rehearsal and regularly thereafter. But I breathed a sigh of relief when I first heard him play. He was certainly no Casals, as I was no Heifetz. Each week he insisted on driving, and the exchanges with him in his Hudson were memorable. But those rides! Lashley's misdeeds as a driver were legendary. He had a disdain for the vehicles around him that was not to be believed, and I had to endure some hair-raising experiences.

Early in his career, Lashley proclaimed himself a materialist, a position that he maintained steadfastly throughout his life. It was clear to him that human behavior is determined by the activity of the brain. He could speak of mind, but in doing so, he did not fall back on some animistic principle; he was referring to a manifestation of neural function. Lashley's materialism was uncompromising. The elements of his psychology were stimuli and responses, and the principle of combination was association. But the reflex was for him an oversimplification, and he was forced to introduce the concept of equivalence both in the sensory and motor realms to account for the data. He eschewed the Pavlovian mechanisms of conditioning, particularly that of generalization[4], and was branded an idealist by the Soviets. His response was to grin and thumb his nose in disdain. He certainly was no dialectical materialist, and on this matter, the Soviets were quite right.

Lashley would frequently raise questions that sounded mentalistic, such as, "How many items can you keep in mind at the same time?" but the question was asked in relation to neural function. The association of "ideas" interested him greatly, but the "idea" was a central process. Even the concept "intelligence" did not trouble him greatly. Whimsically he once assigned an IQ of 300 to a particular rat of his.

Lashley's scorn for religion was legendary, and he never passed up the occasion to heap ridicule on the church. After he became ill in 1954, I visited him a number of times at St. Vincent's Hospital in Jacksonville. When I arrived on the first occasion, he was in bed tossing and squirming uncomfortably. Every now and then he eyed a large crucifix which was mounted on the wall over his bed. We exchanged pleasantries, but he was obviously making a show of his discomfort. Finally he could contain himself no longer. "Do you know what that is on the wall?" Not realizing that he had prepared a witticism, I mumbled something about a crucifix. "Not at all," he pronounced triumphantly, "that's a Texan longhorn." After the chuckle, he told me that he had demanded that the crucifix be removed, and when the startled nurse demurred, he announced sacrilegiously that, though he was a pagan, he found a cow over his bed distasteful.

What, then, did Lashley have to say about the soul? To Sir Francis Walshe, the British neurologist who was a Roman Catholic, he delighted to repeat that psychologists had long ago buried the soul. Their debates on this subject were conducted in good humor. Years later, in his memoir of Lashley (Walshe, 1958), Sir Francis recollected his repartee at their last meeting in London. He suggested that Lashley had got it reversed: It was not the soul that had been buried, but the body! And he quoted an American anthem in support. Was it not John Brown's

[4]Note the letter of evaluation of Pavlov reproduced in Chapter 1.

body that lay a'mouldering in the grave and his soul that went marching on? "What loyal American," Walshe asked (1958), "could doubt the oracular quality of this pronouncement [p. 870]?"

Sir Francis had got in the last word.

REFERENCES

Beach, F. A., Hebb, D. O., Morgan, C. T., & Nissen, H. W. (Eds.). *Neuropsychology of Lashley*. New York: McGraw-Hill, 1960.

Chow, K.-L., Riesen, A. H., & Newell, F. Degeneration of retinal ganglion cells in infant chimpanzees reared in darkness. *Journal of Comparative Neurology*, 1957, *107*, 27-42.

Cowey, A., & Weiskrantz, L. A perimetric study of visual field defects in monkeys. *Quarterly Journal of Experimental Psychology*, 1963, *15*, 91-115.

Gray, G. W. The Yerkes Laboratories. *Scientific American*, 1955, *192*, 67-77.

Hebb, D. O. The innate organization of visual activity: I. Perception of figures by rats reared in total darkness. *Journal of Genetic Psychology*, 1937, *51*, 101-126.

Hebb, D. O. The effects of early and late brain injury upon test scores and the nature of normal adult intelligence. *Proceedings of the American Philosophical Society*, 1942, *85*, 275-292.

Hebb, D. O. Karl Spencer Lashley: 1890-1958. *American Journal of Psychology*, 1959, *72*, 142-149.

Hebb, D. O., D. O. Hebb. In G. Lindzey (Ed.), *A history of psychology in autobiography*, 1980, *7*, 273-303. San Francisco: W. H. Freeman.

Heron, W., Doane, B. K., and Scott, T. H. Visual disturbances after prolonged perceptual isolation. *Canadian Journal of Psychology*, 1956, *10*, 13-16.

Hess, E. H. Development of the chick's response to light and shade cues of depth. *Journal of Comparative and Physiological Psychology*, 1950, *43*, 112-122.

Jacobsen, C. F. Functions of frontal association area in primate. *Archives of Neurology and Psychiatry*, 1935, *33*, 558-569.

Jarvik, M. E. Discrimination of colored food and food signs by primates. *Journal of Comparative and Physiological Psychology*, 1953, *46*, 390-392.

Jarvik, M. E. Simple color discrimination in chimpanzees: Effect of varying contiguity between cue and incentive. *Journal of Comparative and Physiological Psychology*, 1956, *49*, 492-495.

Lashley, K. S. Studies of cerebral function in learning. VI. The theory that synaptic resistance is reduced by the passage of the nerve impulse. *Psychological Review*, 1924, *31*, 369-375.

Lashley, K. S. Psychological problems in the development of instrumental aids for the blind. In P. A. Zahl (Ed.), *Blindness*. Princeton, N. J.: Princeton University Press, 1950. (b)

Lashley, K. S. The problem of serial order in behavior. In L. A. Jeffress (Ed.), *Cerebral mechanisms in behavior*. New York: Wiley, 1951.

Lashley, K. S. Introduction. In Paul H. Schiller, [*Instinctive behavior: The development of a modern concept*] (Claire I. Schiller, Ed. and trans.). New York: International Universities Press, 1957.

Lashley, K. S., & Russell, J. T. The mechanism of vision. XI. A preliminary test of innate organization. *Journal of Genetic Psychology*, 1934, *45*, 136-144.

Lindsley, D. B. *Final report in summary of work on the selection and training of radar operators*. Office of Scientific Research and Development, 1945, Research Report No. 19.

Miller, G. A., Galanter, E., & Pribram, K. H. *Plans and the structure of behavior*. New York: Holt, 1960.

Orbach, J. Retinal locus as a factor in the recognition of visually perceived words. *American Journal of Psychology*, 1952, *65*, 555-562.

Orbach, J. "Functions" of striate cortex and the problem of mass action. *Psychological Bulletin*, 1959, *56*, 271-292.

Orbach, J. Differential recognition of Hebrew and English words in right and left visual fields as a function of cerebral dominance and reading habits. *Neuropsychologia*, 1967, *5*, 127-134.

Orbach, J., & Miller, M. H. Visual performance of infra-human primates reared in an intermittently illuminated room. *Vision Research*, 1969, *9*, 713-716.

Premack, D. *Intelligence in ape and man*. Hillsdale, N.J.: Lawrence Erlbaum Associates, 1976.

Spence, K. W. Continuous vs. non-continuous interpretations of discrimination learning. *Psychological Review*, 1940, *47*, 271-288.

Sperry, R. W. Effect of 180° rotation of the retinal field on visuomotor coordination. *Journal of Experimental Zoology*, 1943, *92*, 263-279.

Spragg, S. D. S. Morphine addiction in chimpanzees. *Comparative Psychology Monographs*, 1940, *15* (7), 1-132.

Terrace, H. S., Petitto, L. A., Sanders, R. J., & Bever, T. G. Can an ape create a sentence? *Science*, 1979, *206* (4421), 891-902.

Walls, G. L. The problem of visual direction. Parts I, II and III. *American Journal of Optometry*, 1951, *28*, 55-83; 115-146; 173-212.

Walshe, F. Karl Spencer Lashley. *Neurology*, 1958, *8*, 870.

Yerkes, R. M. *Chimpanzees: A laboratory colony*. New Haven, Conn.: Yale University Press, 1943.

Yerkes, R. M. & Elder, J. H. Oestrus, receptivity, and mating in chimpanzee. *Comparative Psychology Monographs*, 1936, *13*, (5), 1-39.

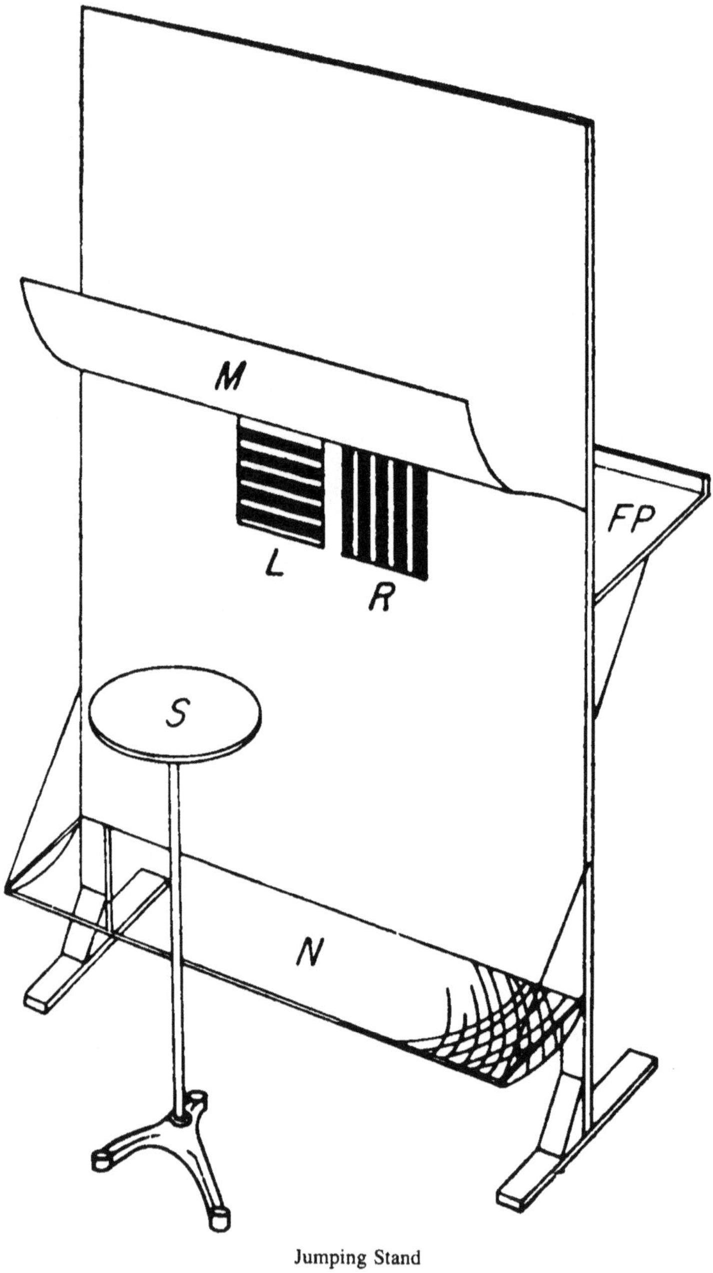

Jumping Stand

3 The Canadian Connection[1]

Jack Orbach
Queens College
City University of New York

D. O. Hebb is perhaps Lashley's most eminent student. Briefly at the University of Chicago as a Ph.D. candidate with Lashley, he transferred to Harvard when Lashley made the move in 1935. Hebb got the Harvard Ph.D. in 1936, remained another year in order to complete earlier work, and then left for postdoctoral studies at the Montreal Neurological Institute (1937-1939) and a faculty appointment at Queens University, Kingston, Ontario (1939-1942), in his native Canada.

It must have come as something of a shock to the faculty at Harvard that Lashley, though appointed there as "the best psychologist in the world" (Boring, 1952, p. 45), was unsystematic, nonconforming, and unorthodox—in short, a thorn in the side of the academy. Though there was genuine admiration and affection for the man, there must have been a collective sigh of relief in 1942, when he was appointed Director of the Yerkes Laboratories of Primate Biology in Orange Park, some 1200 miles away. The sum total of his duties at Harvard thereafter was to conduct a 2-week seminar each fall; otherwise he was rarely seen again in Cambridge.

Lashley invited Hebb to join his staff in Orange Park, and Hebb accepted, arriving shortly after Lashley did, in 1942. In his autobiography, Hebb (1980) mused ruefully that

> exposure to the chimpanzee was broadening indeed even though none of the work planned at first ever came to pass. Lashley's research program was that he and Henry Nissen . . . would study various aspects of learning and problem solving, and

[1]This section contains excerpts from three of D. O. Hebb's publications (1959, 1963 and 1980).

> that I would develop measures of temperamental variables. Then he would operate on the animals' brains, we would retest them, and thus we would see what sort of brain injury affected what behavior over a broad front. [In his first *Annual Report*, dated December 1, 1943, Lashley recorded that he and Hebb were working on a battery of tests to be used pre- and postoperatively in the measurement of the effects of cerebral lesions on intelligence.] However, the first step in this program was for Lashley to train a large group of adult chimpanzees in about thirty different habits which he expected would be easy to do given the high intelligence of the chimpanzee. When he found instead that it took about 300 trials to train a chimpanzee in a form discrimination that the rat would have mastered in sixty trials, the program was off. The first brain operation on an adult animal was made five years later, in the last month of my stay at the laboratories [p. 293].

Hebb went on to an analysis of chimpanzee temperament, emotion, and the recognition of chimpanzee emotion by human observers. At the same time, he began to work on the theory that prompted his celebrated *Organization of Behavior*. Hebb has conveyed some of the excitement he experienced in this venture. In 1946, when it became clear that there was something to the theory, he went to Lashley (Hebb, 1980):

> and proposed that we work it out and publish together. . . . Between us, a much better job was possible, in both theory and presentation; and with him as joint author, the book would get a hearing that I did not expect I alone would get. But Lashley was entirely uninterested and remained skeptical of the whole thing. . . . This led me for the first time to a realization of how completely Lashley's interest in theory was negative and critical [p. 296].

Recalling another incident, Hebb recorded (1980) that the only paper of his that Lashley praised wholeheartedly was one that was entirely devoted to criticizing the work of others (the data and methods of those who reported disturbances after frontal lobe damage in humans; Hebb, 1945).

> He [Lashley] told me he wished he had written it, which was praise indeed. . . . I once told Harry Harlow . . . that Lashley was so interested in criticizing others' theories and so little interested in developing one himself. Harry, I think, had the right diagnosis: "It's hard to get over having been a genius at twenty-five." That was not the right age . . . but his tremendous experimental success between 1921 and 1930 . . . was at a relatively early age and it was entirely destructive. . . . He made a career of finding things that were hard for others to explain [p. 297].

In his fifth *Annual Report*, dated June 30, 1947, Lashley noted: "Dr. Hebb has been engaged in development and elaboration of a theory of nervous integration which gives some promise of clarifying discrepancies between neurological and psychological theory. It will probably be published in book form." Apparently this was notice enough, for Hebb's book received no other mention in any of Lashley's publications. Although it is true that Lashley was not in the habit of citing his student's work, this could not have been mere oversight or benign neglect. Lashley seemed to avoid the subject of Hebb's theory. As a graduate student in 1952, I asked Lashley what he though of the theory. He feigned ignorance; "I don't understand it," was his loconic reply, all the while grinning innocently. In his last publication, in 1958, Lashley sketched a theory of cerebral organization that he "dreamed up in the course of years." In that sketch he referred to "trace systems," "partially activated systems," and the like—highly reminiscent of Hebb's concepts of cell assemblies and the semiautonomous central process. And in the Vanuxem Lectures, delivered at Princeton University in 1952, Lashley spoke of a cortical "presetting," again reminiscent of Hebb's neurologizing on "attention." On the other hand, Lashley's theoretical paper in *Biological Symposia* published in 1942 seems to have influenced Hebb's thinking. Moreover, the debates that took place between 1942 and 1947 in Orange Park must have resulted in considerable cross-fertilization, thus rendering unresolvable the question of priority. What seems clear is that the sharp disagreements drawn by Hebb in Chapter 3 of his 1949 monograph on the issue of cortical field theory, and tacitly accepted by Lashley, were not always evident in their respective writings. This point is elaborated in Chapter 1.

Hebb paid his filial and professional respects to Lashley in a warm and generous memoir published in 1959. Lashley's death a year earlier brought to an end a brilliant career, he wrote—

> perhaps the most brilliant in the psychology of this century. In particular, the sustained vigor of his studies on the mechanisms of learning from 1920 to 1929 seems to me to be without equal in recent experimental psychology. His career was also a controversial one, for the general tenor of his work was critical: first, in the series of experiments that destroyed the simple stimulus-response theories of the day; and, secondly, in his later theoretical papers, which addressed themselves with vigor to the shortcomings of current explanatory notions. The net effect, however, was more than a critique of theory, to be forgotten when the theory itself is outmoded. In support of his criticism he sought new phenomena and new analyses of behavior with which to confront the ideas he was opposing, and these additions to knowledge, together with his mastery of a widely scattered literature, make his work of continuing importance for psychology as well as for the neurological sciences.
>
> Because his work impinged on neurology and neurophysiology, psychologists have been known to assert that Lashley was "only a physiologist," with the implication that for "pure" psychology his papers are not required reading. Undoubtedly such an idea, especially since the recent development of positivistic ideas in psychology, has led to some neglect of his papers. No idea could be more wrong.
>
> Though his formal training was chiefly in biology, he was in his own eyes a psychologist. . . . He became an accomplished anatomist and histologist and made great use of surgical methods, but for him these skills were avenues to the all-

> important problem of behavior. Lashley regarded behavior as a biological phenomenon and saw no reason why he should not use every means at hand for analyzing it, including surgical operations; but he also contributed brilliant studies of the intact organism. Whatever else he may have been, he was in addition, by any definition and in the strict sense, an experimental psychologist of the first rank [p. 142].

Hebb has articulated, better than any of his other students, Lashley's impact on the neuropsychology of his day. In the memoir (1959) Hebb wrote:

> It is not an easy task to evaluate Lashley's contributions to science, and especially to psychology. He made important contributions to neurophysiology and neuroanatomy, in two early studies of the motor area and in studies of the anatomy of the visual system and of thalamo-cortical projection in the rat. An outstanding study was the critique of cortical architectonics with George Clark. In the first years of the present century, Brodmann, Campbell and others had described differences in the finer structure of the cortex, all of which, it came to be assumed, represented differences of function. Brodmann defined some 47 distinct areas in the human cortex. Others made a further subdivision into more than a hundred areas all told, each of which might be thought of as a separate "organ," with its distinctive role in psychological processes. Lashley and Clark put an abrupt end to such extravagances, showing that all but a half-dozen or so of the areas existed only in the eye of the beholder and provided no basis for localization of function. [See Diamond's discussion in Chapter 6 of this volume.]
>
> He kept constantly before him his question, from undergraduate days, of "how the frog worked"—the whole frog (or whole man). He was a dedicated materialist, to whom it was clear that what man does is determined by the brain and not by any animistic principle. To have recourse to animism . . . was, for him, to give up any attempt to solve the problem; and to approach it by way of intervening variables, without physiological definition, was simply to avoid or postpone it. . . .
>
> He clarified many problems, often by setting them in a new context that his own research or scholarship made possible, with corresponding implications for new research. He certainly had biases and fixed ideas, resulting from earlier controversies, biases which affected these formulations. On such points he was undogmatic and open to conviction in the course of a discussion, but he did not remain convinced: it seems, essentially, that he failed to realize how great the impact of his own work had been, even for those who opposed his views. In 1945, he still saw the issues of the innate vs. the acquired, of S–R connections, and of the law of effect, very much as he had seen them in the twenties. On the question of the innate, for example, he tended to regard his opponents as Watsonian empiricists still, who would deny all hereditary organization. But a remarkable feature of his earlier analysis is the extent to which it clarified the great continuing problems of psychology. Thus his thinking remains relevant today, even though it was tied to problems formulated earlier. . . .
>
> Within psychology today [1959] his work is not given the attention it had earlier, but this in a way was his own doing. In 1929 he demolished physiological

conceptions of learning so completely that physiologizing became slightly ridiculous. Having burnt its fingers, psychology turned away in the thirties to E. C. Tolman's intervening variables or B. F. Skinner's positivism. Neither Tolman nor Skinner adopted his own position because of Lashley; yet it seems clear that the appeal of such positions must have been greater in the negativistic climate created by Lashley's work. One extreme, the naive physiologizing of the twenties, was corrected by another, an antiphysiological one, in which Lashley's work inevitably came to be neglected [pp. 147–150].

The rather startling idea that Lashley stultified the development of physiological psychology by the sheer brilliance of his critiques was elaborated in the introduction that Hebb contributed to the Dover edition of *Brain Mechanisms and Intelligence* issued in 1963:

Is consciousness due to an impulse crossing high or low resistance at the synapse? In which cells do memories reside? Does conscious mean cortical and unconscious subcortical? Lashley's monograph put an end to this type of carefree neurologizing and after 1930 budding theoreticians avoided physiological problems. In the perspective of time one can see an extraordinary change of theoretical climate between, say, 1928 and 1938. From Wundt onward psychology had been predominantly physiological psychology, however fanciful. Now psychology became anti-physiological or a-physiological, a theme most effectively presented in the work of B. F. Skinner and E. C. Tolman. Both these men argued that talking about the nervous system is unnecessary, even a positive hindrance, in behavioral analysis. C. L. Hull seems to have taken a less extreme position, but the fact that his highly influential theorizing made no real use of neurological conceptions was a vote cast on the same side. . . .

Now the positivistic views of Skinner and Tolman are really extreme . . . it is astonishing that they could have been so successful in so short a period of time allowing for the conservativeness of scientific thought—except for one thing.

The traditionalist, the man who might have argued the opposing case, found himself at once without arguments. The stock-in-trade of physiological behavior theory had been synaptic resistances, detailed localizations of cortical function, and new paths from point to point in the cortex for new habits. Now, suddenly, it appeared from Lashley's work that such ideas were fantasy, not science. In these circumstances the positivistic *coup d'etat* becomes more intelligible. Neither . . . Tolman nor Skinner adopted his position because of Lashley, but one hardly doubts that their success in carrying others along with them owed much to work that made the ideas of physiological theory more than slightly ridiculous.

The literature of the day does not directly reveal the impact made by the book. . . . It can be seen however in what was *not* said after 1930, what people *stopped* writing . . . Tolman's *Purposive Behavior in Animals and Men* took over in 1932, to be followed by Skinner's *The Behavior of Organisms* in 1938, with hardly a murmur from the defenders of physiological psychology. The defenders had in fact become few in number [pp. v–vii].

Nor was the 20-year period beginning in 1930 or so an especially exciting time in the neuropsychological laboratory. Except for the development of electrophysiological techniques (to which Lashley did not contribute), culminating in the discovery of the reticular activating system, there was little to capture the imagination of the student of brain-behavior relationships. It was not until the appearance of Hebb's provocative monograph in 1949 that interest in neuropsychological theory reemerged among experimental psychologists. In a sense, Hebb's speculations filled a void, and from then on, neurologizing in psychology could be more firmly rooted in the data of the day.

REFERENCES

Boring, E. G. Edwin Garrigues Boring. In E. G. Boring, H. S. Langfeld, & R. M. Yerkes *A history of psychology in autobiography,* 1952, Worcester, Mass.: Clark University Press, 1952.

Hebb, D. O. Man's frontal lobes: A critical review. *Archives of Neurology and Psychiatry,* 1945, *54,* 10–24.

Hebb, D. O. *The organization of behavior.* New York: Wiley, 1949.

Hebb, D. O. Karl Spencer Lashley: 1890-1958. *American Journal of Psychology,* 1959, *72,* 142-149.

Hebb, D. O. Introduction to Dover Edition. In K. S. Lashley *Brain mechanisms and intelligence.* New York: Dover, 1963.

Hebb, D. O. D. O. Hebb. In G. Lindzey (Ed.), *A history of psychology in autobiography,* 1980, *7,* 273-303.

Lashley, K. S. The problem of cerebral organization in vision. *Biological Symposia,* 1942, *7,* 301-322.

Lashley, K. S. *Vanuxem lectures.* Delivered at Princeton University, 1952, unpublished.

Lashley, K. S. Cerebral organization and behavior. In "The brain and human behavior." *Proceedings of the Association for Research in Nervous and Mental Diseases,* 1958, *36,* 1-18.

4 Biography and Evaluations

Jack Orbach
Queens College
City University of New York

A VIEW FROM CAMBRIDGE[1]

In July 1949 the Society of Experimental Biology and the Institute of Animal Behavior together organized a Symposium for the discussion of a wide range of problems, neurological, physiological and psychological, in which the members of both groups were interested. The Symposium was held in the Zoological Laboratory of the University of Cambridge. K. S. Lashley came to England for this meeting, and no member of the large audience who heard him describe how he had set out ''In search of the engram'', and what its upshot had been, is likely ever to forget the tremendous impression that he made.

After the public discussions one morning, I walked with him back from the Zoological Department to Corpus Christi College, where he was staying. The sun shone with unclouded brilliance, and when we reached the College Lashley, who seemed, perhaps, a little tired, sat himself down on the stone steps leading to the main gate, one long leg stretched out towards the pavement, with not a single care for the curious, and slightly shocked glances of some of the passers-by. We were talking, not about any intricacies of animal behavior, but about sailing and the sea, which he loved. He told me something about his own boats, and journeys he had made in them; but more about longer and unconventional voyages in small tramp steamers which took a long time, wherever they were going, and called at ports little known to the big luxury vessels for which he had no use at all.

Here was Lashley, sitting where hardly anybody ever did sit, talking quietly and naturally about things that I suppose very few, if any, of the others who came to that conference could, or would, talk about. It was an occasion which I am glad that

[1]Excerpts of a memoir by F. C. Bartlett. Karl Spencer Lashley, 1890–1958. *Biographical Memoirs of Fellows of the Royal Society*, 1960, *5*, 106–118.

I can remember. For, as I see them, all Lashley's scientific explorations, most of them planned and carried out with infinite care, and all the exercise of his superb intelligence, were a prolonged and serious adventure. In his experimental and theoretical work, and in his life outside the laboratory as well, he would go where he wanted, he would say what he believed, not because he was insensitive to influences from other people, but because his only ultimate compulsion came from inside himself. . . .

Somewhere around 1915 Lashley definitely decided that he would make his career in psychology, and from this decision he never swerved. The psychology that attracted him, however, was not the rather prim and respectable laboratory exercises of the earlier Germans, which were being imitated in those American Universities that allowed psychology a place in the structure of their studies; and it certainly was not introspectionism run to extremes. He was now working fairly closely with J. B. Watson, and Watson was as much of an adventurer in the fields of animal and human behaviour as he was himself, though nowhere near as cautious. Lashley had had several years of training and research in zoology, together with a fair amount of anatomy and physiology, and some neurology. All of these, in their relation to the behaviour of animals, seemed to be impelling him towards an experimental examination of the directions, character and final upshot of conduction in the central nervous system. There have been plenty of psychologists who, having made a careful firsthand study of behavior, have been willing to speculate about its underlying physiological and neurological conditions, though of these they usually could claim no more than an inadequate and second-hand knowledge. It has perhaps been still commoner for people who have come from one or more of the other biological sciences, when they get to the level of behaviour itself, to suppose that no specially controlled observation and experiments are needed. In this field, they seem to assume, nothing is required beyond the exercise of common sense or the acceptance of established views. It was a part of Lashley's great strength and originality that he was, all his scientific life, prepared and able to take one side as seriously and as experimentally as the other.

For a few years still Lashley could, and did, allow free play to a lively curiosity that took him in many different directions. Students and colleagues who knew him well then have recorded that, though what he would say or do next was highly unpredictable, there was all the time a kind of "contagion of excitement" about him. . . .

At the end of his address on the engram Lashley rather wryly said, "This series of experiments has yielded a good bit of information about what and where the memory trace is not." But everybody who heard him knew that though the words may have been negative, he finished still full of the ardor of the research, still resolved that he, and others, must continue it, and that in spirit he was optimistic and positive. For anybody who looks there are, in this study as in very many others that he made, flashes of insight springing out of the level of scientific caution. "It is highly probable that immediate memory is maintained by some sort of after-discharge of the originally excited neurones. Such can scarcely be the basis of more permanent memory." No doubt others before him had made much the same suggestion but not with the same background or to the same purpose. Again, "The serial timing of actions is among the most important and least studied of behavioral patterns." And "Skilled acts involve a timed series of actions which cannot be accounted for as a simple chain of conditioned reflexes." We have to keep in mind that for him these suggestions, of memory, for example, as a skill, and of all skills as timed series of actions were not merely general notions gained by reflection. They were a summing up of a great mass of original, highly controlled observations; and since Lashley made them their definition and significance have increased.

Lashley possessed, indeed, extreme scientific honesty and carefulness, combined both with outstanding technological and manipulative skill, and with a capacity for brilliant intuition. The first two working in fields full of hastily framed hypotheses and theories, were bound to issue largely in destructive criticism. Scientific intuition, reaching forward towards discovery before the evidence... is known, is always preponderantly positive. It is beyond any possibility of dispute that in each of these ways Lashley's achievements will remain of permanent and outstanding significance. At the same time it is highly probable that many of his suggestions which could not at the time be fully substantiated, of the remarks which he seemed to make "by the way" and of his flashes of insight will be found to have contributed most of all towards the solution of his problems. . . .

In appearance Lashley wsa rather tall, and rather loosely built. He had a sensitive and expressive face, maybe a little sad in repose, but capable of lighting up into a most charming smile. Wherever he was present he could not be overlooked at the time, or soon forgotten. This was not, generally, because he talked a lot or pushed himself forward in any way; it was because he was one of those rare folks from whom a kind of excitement seems to spread out. Some found him shy, reserved and even stand-offish. Certainly he had little relish for the company of the unintelligent or the pretentious, and he did not love convention for convention's sake. But when he met a person, or faced an audience, whose intelligence and honesty could make some sort of a match with his own, he could be splendidly witty, gay and wise. No doubt there were ways in which rebels attracted him. At various stages he was much interested in J. B. Watson, in Pavlov, in Freud and in the Gestalt psychologists—all at odds against the respectable opinions of their day and clime. But he maintained his own integrity and was never swept away by any of them, for with a certain liking for intellectual risk and sweeping assertion he combined the scientist's loyalty to empirical observation and respect for experimental facts.

A BIOGRAPHICAL MEMOIR BY FRANK A. BEACH[2]

Eminent psychologist with no earned degree in psychology
Famous theorist who specialized in disproving theories, including his own
Inspiring teacher who described all teaching as useless

[2]Reprinted from *Biographical Memoirs of the National Academy of Sciences*, 1961, 35, 162–204 (courtesy National Academy of Sciences). Omitted are a photograph of Lashley; evaluations of mass action, equipotentiality, and other contributions; and some appreciative statements. Lashley's bibliography is also omitted since it has been reprinted a number of times

KARL SPENCER LASHLEY, one of the great psychologists of our time, was born on June 7, 1890, and died on August 7, 1958. His birth occurred in Davis, West Virginia; his death in Poitiers, France. Over a span of sixty-eight years Karl Lashley grew from a small-town boy with the heart of a naturalist to become an eminent neuropsychologist. He helped to shape the beginning of a new era in physiological psychology, and his research and theorizing concerning the brain and behavior had an important influence upon contemporaneous thought in psychology and neurology.

Ancestry. Lashley came from substantial, middle-class stock of English derivation. Henry Lashley, Karl's paternal great-grandfather, owned a tannery and a brickyard in the village of Gilpin, Maryland, which was located about twelve miles from Cumberland. He also owned, at various times, small stores in Flintstone, Cumberland, and Davis. Henry had little use for formal education, and as soon as his sons had completed their elementary schooling they became clerks in one of his merchandising establishments. Three sons eventually became managers of branch stores.

Karl's grandfather, Jacob Lashley, managed the store in Davis, and was succeeded by Charles Gilpin Lashley, Karl's father. Charles had at one time expressed an ambition to "read medicine" with a local physician, but Jacob persuaded him to follow the family tradition. In addition to managing the family store, Charles Lashley organized a small bank in Davis, and held a number of political posts. He served as mayor for several terms, and was appointed postmaster during the administrations of Harrison, Coolidge, and Hoover. Fragmentary notes left by Karl portray his father as a kindly man with a certain talent for local politics, some business acumen, and strong family ties and affections, but without any pow-

(e.g., in Bartlett [1960] and in Beach, et al. [1960]. However, for completeness, an abstract should be added to the published list:

Clark, G., & Lashley, K. S. Visual disturbances following frontal ablations in the monkey. *Anatomical Records*, 1947, 97, 326.

It should also be noted that Lashley's review, "Learning. III. Nervous Mechanisms in Learning," in Murchison's *Handbook* (1934) is a reprint verbatim of the review "Learning. I. Nervous Mechanisms in Learning" in Murchison's *Foundations* (1929).

erful ambition or drive—all in all not a likely sire to a famous scientist.

On the distaff side, Lashley's great-grandfather was Osa Spencer, also of English blood. By his second wife, Ann Mercer, Osa fathered seven children including David Hatton Spencer, grandfather to Karl. David married Maria Chalfonte who must have been a woman of great energy and strong character for she not only raised nine children, but, following her husband's death, successfully managed the family farm for thirty-six years until her death at the age of ninety. Karl's grandmother Maria was the daughter of William Chalfonte and Elizabeth Edwards. Elizabeth, in turn was descended from Jonathan Edwards, to whose judgment General George Washington often deferred with the statement, "We must consult Brother Jonathan." Although, as noted later, Karl steadfastly refused to prepare a formal autobiography, he did occasionally jot down casual notes and observations concerning his own history. At one time he wrote of his hereditary background, ". . . it is clear that the intellectual curiosity and drive descended through that maternal line."

The plausibility of this conclusion is increased by consideration of the talents and accomplishments of Karl's mother. Maggie Blanche Spencer, daughter of David and Maria, had a normal school education and began teaching country school at the age of sixteen. She was always an avid reader, and she amassed a personal library of more than 2,000 volumes.

Throughout her life she manifested great reverence for learning, and although she resigned her school position at the time of her marriage to Charles Lashley, Maggie never ceased teaching. The Lashley home in Davis became a center for what today would be called "adult education" where women came for instruction in a variety of subjects ranging from civics to Greek poetry and drama. Not content with caring for her family and acting as instructress to her neighbors, Maggie Lashley opened and operated a commercial photographic studio. As a hobby she learned the art of painting and firing chinaware, and became expert in the production of delicate, translucent cups, saucers, and other pieces.

Considering the accomplishments of Henry, Jacob, and Charles Lashley, and comparing these with the descriptions of Osa and Maggie Spencer, one is strongly inclined to agree with Karl's belief that the hereditary elements contributing to his own intellectual reach and thirst for knowledge are traceable chiefly to "Edwards genes."

The Early Years. The remarkable woman, Maggie Lashley, exerted a very powerful influence upon the early development of Karl, her only child. They were extremely close, and from his mother the boy acquired a love of nature and of learning. In later years he was wont to say that he was reared on a combination of Nestle's Food and Nietzsche, although later we shall have something to say concerning Lashley's love of the "low bow."

In any event, Lashley's mother encouraged him in intellectual pursuits, with the result that he could read at the age of four, and throughout his childhood made avid use of the extensive family library. But Karl was not destined to be merely a bookworm for he had the instincts of a naturalist, and from early childhood displayed a deep interest in plant life and in all kinds of animals, both wild and domestic. A favorite boyhood pastime was to wander through the woods and fields, observing and sometimes collecting various plants and animals. At different times he maintained collections of butterflies, snakes, frogs, and snails, not to mention pet mice and racoons.

Upon at least one occasion young Karl's interest in animal behavior took a practical turn. The family barn was infested by large numbers of rats, and his father offered to pay five cents for each rodent bagged. The first day of trapping yielded thirty-six rats; the second brought twenty-seven. At this point Lashley senior prudently terminated the contract.

An interest in animals persisted throughout his life, and Lashley was never without some kind of pet. At one time he owned a cat and a parrot, but the combination created certain unexpected problems when the voluble bird displayed a disconcerting tendency to adopt the cat's new-born kittens. The roster of pets included another cat (Gottlieb Teufel), a cockateel, a monkey, and several dogs, the last of which was Till Eulenspiegel, who developed, under her master's tutelage, an inordinate fondness for daiquiris and pink ladies.

It is of considerable significance that during his childhood, while he was exploring the countryside or browsing in his mother's library, Karl had very few playmates. Most of his time seems to have been spent in solitude or in the company of adults. It was a prophetic pattern, in a way, for many years later Lashley told the present writer that some of his happiest days were spent all alone on an island in the Dry Tortugas.

During his childhood Karl discharged the usual stint of chores expected of a boy living in a small town near the turn of the century. He was responsible for the care of a pair of fine carriage horses owned by his father, and at the close of each day he brought in the family cow. The latter was no mean feat since there was no fenced pasture, and the beast was free to roam the countryside at will. When he grew a bit older Karl was also expected to clerk in his father's general store.

Lashley's pronounced aptitude for mechanical achievement showed itself when he was quite young. He was fascinated by his mother's sewing machine, and learned to use it very efficiently,—an accomplishment which proved useful later when he made sails for the boats which he owned at different times. His preoccupation with sewing was so intense that Karl's father was afraid the machine would wear out, and as a substitute the boy was presented with a jigsaw outfit. This opportunity to construct things with his hands was welcome, and from his new workshop there issued a steady flow of expertly designed and finely executed articles ranging in size from spectacle cases to living room furniture. The pleasure derived from this form of creativity persisted throughout life, and even after his retirement Lashley continued with his cabinet making, and extended his efforts to include the remodeling of his house.

Most of Karl's childhood was spent in Davis, but there was a four year interlude during which the family moved several times. Between 1894 and 1898 they lived in Elk Garden, and Hartmansville,

West Virginia, Los Angeles, and Seattle. The move to Seattle in 1897 resulted in experiences which made a strong impression on the seven-year-old boy. In an informal account set down years later Lashley recalled the fever of the gold rush, and meetings with such swashbuckling characters as Swiftwater Bill and Klondike Pete who sported nugget jewelry and recounted tall tales about fabulous "strikes" and the dangers of encountering bird-sized Alaskan mosquitoes.

Like so many others, Charles and Maggie Lashley fell prey to gold fever and decided to go north to prospect. The decision brought with it one welcome release for Karl. Recalling the occasion he wrote, "The happy event for me was the cutting of my long blond curls, à la Fauntleroy, which had been my shame for two years."

Two of Charles' brothers were persuaded to leave the East and join the Lashley party. Because there was a near famine in Dawson in 1897, the Canadian Government required that prospectors bring with them provisions sufficient for two years. This amounted to one ton per person. Eventually an outfit was assembled and the four adults and one child took passage on the steamer *Queen,* sailing from Seattle to Skagway. Lashley's vivid recollections of the passage included the memory of colorful fellow passengers such as, "miners, cheechawkers, dance hall girls, and a deckload of dogs ranging from a ten-pound terrier to a huge mastiff,—few more suited to the trail than their masters."

At Skagway the party disembarked and then proceeded by dog sled for some distance. Eventually all supplies and equipment had to be transferred to hand sleds for the arduous climb over Chilkoot Pass. Lashley's written reminiscences of this experience are full of color and vitality. The primitive Chilkoot trail must have taxed a seven-year-old boy's endurance, but the memory was so rewarding that Lashley arranged to revisit the site of these childhood adventures in 1948 and again in 1957. The fragmentary account of the original trip was found in an album of snapshots which were taken when he retraced portions of the original route in 1948.

Following the Alaskan excursion the Lashley family returned to Davis and resettled there in 1899.

School and College. Karl was entered in a private school at the age of four. In 1895 he attended the public school in Elk Garden, and the next year the one in Hartmansville. There followed two interrupted terms at the Denny School in Seattle, and the remainder of Lashley's precollege education was received in the public system in Davis where he graduated from high school when he was fourteen years old.

Because Davis High School was not accredited Karl did not qualify as a freshman when he entered the University of West Virginia, but had to spend one year in the "Preparatory Department" of that institution. During the subsequent year as a freshman he was, as he later wrote, "thoroughly lost." He was "vaguely inclined to engineering"; his father wanted him to study medicine, but his mother insisted on his earning an A.B. degree, and this he did.

His first plan was to major in Latin, but the university registrar instructed him to make English his major.* To fill a vacant hour in his schedule Karl enrolled in a course in zoology. His professor was John Black Johnston, a neurologist and the only teacher of zoology in the university. The contact with Johnston and his subject matter had a profound influence upon the sixteen-year-old boy. Of the first course he later wrote, "Within a few weeks in his class I knew that I had found my life's work."

At the beginning of the next academic quarter Lashley rebelled against his faculty advisor's order that he drop the course in zoology and replace it with one in Old English. Instead of complying, the young freshman changed his major from English to zoology. Explaining this decision in retrospect he wrote as follows:

"Zoology attracted me because of my prior interest in animals, because it required much freehand drawing, which I enjoyed, and because it seemed to support the materialism which, even at 16, I was beginning to formulate vaguely."

During his freshman year Karl studied general zoology and comparative anatomy with Johnston, but Johnston left at the close of the spring term and was replaced by Albert M. Reese. Reese appointed

*(Editor's note) Enjoying the shock it produced in his audience, Lashley sometimes told students that his early training was in Latin.

Lashley departmental assistant, at a salary of twenty-five cents per hour. One of the new assistant's first tasks was to sort out various materials that Johnston had left behind. The result of this assignment can best be expressed in Lashley's own words:

"Among them I found a beautiful Golgi series of the frog brain. I took these to Reese and proposed that I draw all of the connections between the cells. Then we would know how the frog worked. It was a shock to learn that the Golgi method does not stain all cells, but I think almost ever since I have been trying to trace those connections."*

As a sophomore Karl took several courses in zoology including embryology, histology, animal behavior, and general technique. At the start of his junior year he wanted to register for an advanced course in zoology, but as the only zoologist on the faculty Reese was too busy to conduct a one-student seminar. Nevertheless Lashley learned a great deal in the course of his assistantship. Reese's instructions were such as to encourage, in fact to compel, the exercise of initiative, and to develop independence of thought and action, "You will find some bones in the basement. Go work up a course in comparative osteology." Another time Lashley was told, "Here is a copy of Burkholder. Get some sheep brains and work up the anatomy. I want you to take charge of the laboratory course in neurology next term." This experience had lasting effects upon Lashley's philosophy of education and influenced his treatment of his own students in later years.

Advanced Training. After earning his A.B. at West Virginia in 1910, Lashley applied for and was awarded a teaching fellowship in biology at the University of Pittsburgh. He taught several laboratory sections of the biology course, and carried out the research for his Master's thesis. Unquestionably the most important aspect of Lashley's year at Pittsburgh was his contact with another teaching fellow, Karl Dallenbach, a psychologist. Dallenbach's memory of their year together includes the following observation:

*(Editor's note) Only later did Lashley realize that functional variables rendered his original plan unrealistic, variables such as spatial and temporal summation, excitatory and inhibitory states, and *in vivo* micromovements of elements influencing synaptic contact.

"Lashley's laboratory was on the floor above mine. Though he had never taken a course in psychology, he was permitted, because he was a fellow, to elect my laboratory course in experimental psychology. The class was small and we worked intimately together upon the various experiments. Lashley was intensely interested and was the outstanding student in the class—as one might expect being a graduate student in an undergraduate class, but he was more than a run-of-the-mine graduate student. He showed in that course the promise that he later fulfilled."

Receiving his Master's degree in June, 1911, Lashley spent the summer at the Carnegie Laboratories at Cold Spring Harbor. There he studied the variability in the number of cirri in the ciliate, *Stylonychia.* This work attracted the attention of H. S. Jennings, professor of zoology at the Johns Hopkins University, and he offered Lashley a fellowship which was accepted.* At Hopkins Karl participated in Jennings' research on paramecia, and also worked with S. O. Mast on the behavior of various invertebrates. His thesis dealt with inheritance in the asexual reproduction of *Hydra,* and he received the Ph.D. degree in 1914.

The interest in psychology, first aroused by Dallenbach, continued while Lashley was at Hopkins. He was greatly stimulated by contact with Adolf Meyer, professor of psychiatry and director of the newly established Henry Phipps Clinic. While majoring in zoology, Karl took two minors. One was with Meyer, and the other was with a psychologist destined for fame, John B. Watson. The impact of Watson's behavioristic approach was so great that forty-four years later Lashley asserted, "anyone who knows American psychology today knows that its value derives from biology and from Watson."

During the year following the granting of the Ph.D. Lashley remained at Hopkins as a Bruce Fellow in zoology. In the summer of 1914 he and Watson carried on field experiments on the behavior of sea birds. They made their observations on Bird Key in the Dry

*(Editor's note) His first paper on form and size discrimination in the rat was published in 1912 in the second volume of the *Journal of Animal Behavior.* Later, when he was at the height of his career, in the 1930s and early 1940s, he returned with a long series of penetrating experimental studies of visual mechanisms.

Tortugas, studying chiefly the homing, nesting, and reproductive behavior of sooty and noddy terns. That same year Lashley carried on experiments on the acquisition of motor skills in human subjects, color vision in birds, and conditioning of the salivary reflex.

During the academic year of 1915–1916 Lashley continued at Hopkins with an appointment as Johnston Scholar. He occupied a basement laboratory adjacent to one which housed a beginning graduate student, W. H. Taliaferro, who became a life-long friend, and was for a while Lashley's colleague at the University of Chicago.

While he held the Johnston Scholarship, Lashley continued to work with Watson, studying, among other problems, the effects of strychnine and other drugs upon maze learning in rats. At this time Shepherd Ivory Franz was examining the behavior of brain-injured patients at Saint Elizabeth's Hospital in Washington, D. C. He was also carrying out experiments with animals to investigate the behavioral effects of surgically inflicted brain lesions. Lashley became greatly interested in Franz's program and journeyed frequently to Washington to observe the brain-operated monkeys.

Lashley was anxious to learn surgical techniques from Franz, but first he was required to participate in a study of body types which involved the photographing of nude women. Surviving this first assignment he was permitted to graduate to the study of neurological cases on the wards. Eventually he acquired the surgical and histological skills which permitted the inception of a major program of studies on the neural basis of learning. With the inauguration of this program, which eventually brought eminence and world-wide recognition, Lashley's research career was solidly launched, and this terminated his period of training.

Professional Posts. Lashley's first, full-time professional position was that of instructor in psychology at the University of Minnesota, where he took up his duties in the fall of 1917. The appointment was arranged by Robert M. Yerkes who was slated to assume the chairmanship of the psychology department. However, Yerkes became involved in the organization of the new National Research Council and was forced to remain in Washington instead of taking up his administrative duties at Minnesota. Because of this, or for other reasons, departmental morale was not high, and Lashley left at the end of his first year, taking a leave of absence.

From Minnesota he went to Baltimore, accepting a position with the United States International Hygiene Board. His vision was too poor to meet Army standards and the wartime program to which he was assigned was aimed primarily at educating the public with respect to the dangers of venereal disease. Working once more with Watson, Lashley participated in showing and discussing motion picture films designed to further the campaign against this particular affliction. In later years he enjoyed telling of one time when he and Watson went into a small town and distributed advertisements announcing a free motion picture show. The announcements included no mention of the subject matter, and, according to Lashley, he and Watson were fortunate to escape from the Sheriff and outraged citizenry with whole skins.*

In 1920, R. M. Elliott, who had become chairman of the department of psychology at the University of Minnesota, persuaded Lashley to return as an assistant professor. This promotion was made at Elliott's insistence. In his contribution to *A History of Psychology in Autobiography,* Elliott recalls Lashley's career at Minnesota in vivid terms.

When he had been back for just one year, Elliott insisted "violently" that Lashley be promoted to associate professor. In another two years he was advanced to full professorship, at which time he was thirty-four years old. John Black Johnston, under whom Lashley had studied at West Virginia, was then a dean at Minnesota.

Referring to Lashley's situation at Minnesota in the early twenties, Elliott has written as follows:

"Lashley's intellectual pre-eminence and the brilliant reports of study after study of brain function in rats and monkeys presented

*(Editor's note) This early interest in sex blossomed later on in the animal work of his students. Lashley himself rarely studied human subjects, but there is no doubt that he saw human sexual behavior as a fundamental problem for psychological study and he was a longstanding member of the National Research Council's Committee for Research on Problems of Sex and a good friend of Kinsey.

at our all-department seminar placed him in the prestige spot among us. I constituted myself guardian and protector outside his laboratory door, fending off official expectations of a usual teaching load and other threats to his research productivity, all the while shoving into him and his students (how the good ones do flock around a good man!) whatever supplies and equipment they needed. We think those six years were the most productive period of Lashley's career."[1]

In 1926 Lashley left Minnesota for Chicago to accept an appointment as a research psychologist associated with the Behavior Research Fund at the Institute for Juvenile Research. In 1929 he became professor of psychology at the University of Chicago. In this position he remained until 1935.

When James B. Conant succeeded Lowell as president of Harvard University one of his early acts, according to E. G. Boring, was to appoint his first ad hoc committee to find the "best psychologist in the world" to elect to a Chair at Harvard.[2] Lashley was chosen by the committee. He was first elected professor of psychology, and only then was he informed of this action and asked whether he would accept. He did so, and was given laboratory space in the new Biological Laboratories.

In 1937 Lashley was made research professor in neuropsychology. Retaining this title, he became, in 1942, Director of the Yerkes Laboratories of Primate Biology, and continued in this position until his retirement in 1955. During the thirteen-year period at the Yerkes Laboratories in Orange Park, Florida, Lashley journeyed to Cambridge once each year to give a two-week seminar for graduate students.

Research. Throughout his professional life Lashley persisted in his attempts to discover "how the frog works" by learning how the nervous system works. Despite the world-wide recognition accorded his research, Lashley did not feel that he or anyone else had made much progress toward a solution of the central problems involved.

---

[1] *A History of Psychology in Autobiography*, Vol. IV, edited by E. G. Boring, H. S. Langfeld, and R. M. Yerkes (Worcester, Mass.: Clark University Press, 1952), p. 88.

[2] *Ibid.*, p. 45.

Toward the close of his life he expressed his views in a letter to Sir Francis Walshe:

"Brain function presents the most difficult and elusive problems in science and I have little hope of seeing any of them solved . . . But if we have contributed something of orientation and scientific approach to the problems I think we may feel that we have done about all that is possible in our generation."

Lashley's contributions to psychology are accurately represented in a recently published volume of selected papers, *The Neuropsychology of Lashley.*[3] The reprinted articles reflect the four major divisions of Lashley's total scientific production: (1) laying the foundations, (2) the grand attack upon connectionism, (3) experimental studies of sensory representation (chiefly vision), and (4) general theory.

The earliest papers dealing with protozoans and coelenterates stem directly from Lashley's training as a biologist and geneticist, but among them are clear indications of his concern with problems of behavior. Such, for example, are his field studies with Watson of the reproductive and homing behavior of terns. After a brief period of work on Pavlovian conditioning Lashley began to concentrate more and more upon the study of neural mechanisms and learning. He quickly convinced himself that contemporary theories were erroneous, and that learning could never be explained in terms of the formation of simple connections within the brain. During the years at Minnesota and at the Behavior Research Fund, Lashley experienced his most productive period and his studies of learning and brain function culminated in the publication of the monograph, *Brain Mechanisms and Intelligence,* published by the University of Chicago Press in 1929. This was Lashley's longest single publication. He never wrote a book, and in fact sometimes, only half facetiously, pronounced his opinion that book writing should be left to those who could not or would not carry on research. In the 1929 monograph, in addition to the results of many careful experiments, Lashley enunciated his controversial concepts of "mass action" and "equi-

[3]McGraw-Hill Book Company, Inc., 1960.

potentiality." These were, in actuality, simply a summary of the experimental findings, and did not purport to serve as explanations. . . .

As is true of all first-rank scientists, Lashley's interests and insights ranged far beyond the boundaries encompassing his personal research. In 1920, as an assistant professor at Minnesota, he wrote to a prospective graduate student, outlining several potential thesis projects:

March 21, 1920

Dear Mr. Stone:

The discussion of plans and problems at long range will probably not be very satisfactory to either of us, but we shall have to make the best of a bad situation. I shall attempt now only a most general outline of possibilities. Then, when I know your interests somewhat better, we can take up specific problems.

Do you expect to come up for your doctorate next year? The selection of your problem will depend largely upon this. If you do, your choice is limited to problems in which the technique is pretty well worked out and a good many interesting possibilities are ruled out. If you have more time to spend you can produce a much more attractive and original thesis.

At present I am interested chiefly in the following fields:

1. Comparative anatomical and physiological studies of the sense-organs, especially in audition and color-vision. Work here will give immediate definite results but does not seem to attract much attention. An advantage for you would be the fact that you have the technique.
2. Effect of drugs, diet, starvation, hormones, etc. upon the learning process. Here the technique is simple and results are fairly certain.
3. The experimental control of instincts; the effects of internal secretions upon specific reactions—for example, attempts to induce maternal behavior in virgin females by injection or transplanting pregnant uterus. A great deal of preliminary work will be necessary here and I doubt that much could be done in a single year, but positive results would be pretty sure to make a man in psychology.
4. Physiology of the nervous system in relation to learning. You can get some idea of this field from my recent paper in Psychobiology. A few specific problems are—

   The formation of conditioned reflexes without the cerebrum. The best chance here is in work with decerebrate frogs or salamanders.

   The determination of the exact cortical path of visual or auditory habits; a more detailed application of the method which I used for the visual area in the rat.

The function of the motor cortex in habits; training an animal in a habit of manipulation, recovery from paralysis without practice in the habit, tests for retention of the habit—to determine whether the motor area functions in habit or only in tonic control.

Effects of maldevelopment of the brain upon intelligence and learning ability. Partial occlusion of carotids in infancy (rat). Production of abnormal development of brain in fish or amphibia.

5. General functional anatomy of the brain.

Correlation of excitable areas with cytoarchitecture. Combined stimulation and anatomical studies of the development of the motor cortex in young animals.

The determination of sensory projection areas in the rat by strychnine and extirpation methods.

Location of reflex paths of instincts by destruction of basilar regions. I think I have a technique for destroying minute areas of the thalamus, which may or may not give results.

Binocular and monocular vision of birds in relation to cerebral function.

These are the types of problems. Most of them demand some histological technique and if you have had experience in this it will help greatly. If by chance you have the string galvanometer technique there is a wealth of problems to be attacked at once. If you have a good foundation in chemistry, there are some important problems in the relation of efficiency to the chemistry of the blood which might be practicable. If we can get clinical material, which I doubt, you might work on a problem in re-education, or such a thing as the factors which modify tonic innervation in hemiplegia.

Let me know if any of the above problems seem attractive to you and I will give you a more detailed program with suggestions as to working up the technique. If you want to work in functional neurology you will have to have some surgical technique, and if you can pick it up this summer, so much the better. You can probably get a third year medic to help you out. Decide what animals you want to work with and get as familiar with their normal behavior as you can. If you have not done so, work out the gross anatomy of several brains, cat, sheep, and rabbit.

As for literature, there are very few suggestive books. Parker's Elementary Nervous System (forget exact title), Verworn-Irritability, Lucas-Conduction of Nerve Impulse, Gaskell-Auto-Funktionen der Nerven Centra Bd. 3. Von Monakow-Lokalisation im Gros hirn. Look up Von Monakow's articles and T. Graham Brown's in Ergebnisse der Physiologie. Run through recent volumes of Brain, Amer. J. of Physiol., Journal of Physiol. (British), and read whatever interests you. What can you find out about intra-uterine development of reflexes?

It is going to be rather difficult for you to work into a new field and to turn out a well rounded piece of work in one year, but we can try, at any rate. Let me have your reaction to these suggestions soon and do not hesitate to ask for more detailed programs or any help that I can give you.

Sincerely yours,

(signed) K. S. Lashley

The recipient of this letter was Calvin Stone who was, years later, elected to the National Academy of Sciences. Those who are familiar with developments in physiological psychology since the letter was written will find many of Lashley's suggestions impressively prophetic. He was then thinking more than a decade ahead of his time, and several of the lines of investigation which he mentioned have since been opened with fruitful and significant results.

Lashley's enduring interest in visual mechanisms resulted in a long series of publications representing basic contributions, not only to visual learning and its physiological basis, but also to the science of neuroanatomy. By studying degenerative changes in the lateral geniculate nucleus consequent to restricted destruction in the visual cortex, for example, he was able to demonstrate that different parts of the thalamic nucleus are connected to different areas in the striate region. There is, in fact, something approximating a point-for-point projection of the lateral geniculate upon the visual cortex. Lashley later went on to show that there is a similar projection of other thalamic nuclei to the cortex.

Another major contribution to neuroanatomy was made by Lashley and George Clark in 1946, when they reported their study of the cytoarchitecture of the primate cerebral cortex. Prior to this work various scholars had subdivided the cortex in different ways, basing their decisions upon apparent, local differences in the types, numbers, and sizes of cells present. Some specialists listed more than one hundred separate cortical areas. Brodmann, one of the most widely followed authorities, described forty-seven distinct areas in the human cortex.

Lashley and Clark's critical examination of the cortex of the spider monkey, *Ateles*, revealed that at most there are six, architectonically discriminable areas in the neopallium. As Hebb has said, the study was crucial and at one blow demolished the current reliance upon local differences in cellular composition as indices to major structural compartmentalism.[4] The results were so convincing that no refutation was even attempted, and Lashley received congratulations from several leading neuroanatomists including Lorente de Nó.

His fertile mind was ever on the alert for any facts that might throw light on how the nervous system works. A long-time sufferer from migraine, Lashley made careful records of the visual patterns and scotomata which accompanied his attacks, and from these data formulated a provocative hypothesis concerning concurrent activity within the striate cortex. He once calculated the speed of finger movements involved in playing a rapid cadenza on the piano, and compared this with the known speed of neural transmission. The comparison revealed that the intervals between successive finger movements were too short to support the theory that each movement is aroused by motor impulses which in turn are set off by sensory impulses derived from the preceding finger movement. There is not enough time for a sensory message from the finger to go to the brain and pass to the motor area and then for a motor impulse to return to the finger muscles. Lashley often cited this example in support of the notion of central patterning of complex motor sequences.

Lashley's attitude toward research was that it demands the complete, personal involvement of the investigator. In his beginning years as an experimenter he was interested in the acquisition of motor skills. One of the tasks investigated was that of throwing darts at a target. A single session lasted twenty-two hours and each subject, Lashley among them, was required to make a cast every few minutes. A table loaded with sandwiches stood in one corner of the laboratory, and the subjects marched from the throwing stand, around

[4] *American Journal of Psychology*, Vol. 72, No. 1 (1959), p. 148.

the table, grabbing a sandwich when necessary, thence back to the throwing line once more.

In later years Lashley continued to conduct his own experiments, and the system of employing assistants to make the actual tests found little favor in his scheme of things. It was his conviction that good research workers are rare and that money cannot buy inspiration and brains. In a letter written to John B. Watson in 1953, Lashley expressed himself as follows:

"The money available for research now is rather shocking. The man who doesn't have $20,000 per year for his research is probably intellectually honest. There are not enough competent men to spend the money. I recently attended a symposium on the training of graduate students at the Southern Society of Philosophy and Psychology. The discussion was entirely on training men for clinical practice. I finally blew up and delivered a speech to the effect that some research is needed as a basis for clinical practice and that I had heard rumors that graduate instruction might occasionally be concerned with training men for research, though one would never suspect it from the symposium. The head of the Civil Service was there and said that he cannot find competent research men, and thanked me for bringing up the subject. Membership in the A.P.A. is approaching 20,000, but I don't believe there are as many good research men in the field as there were in 1918."

Theory Building and Razing. A major source of motivation which influenced Lashley throughout most of his professional life was the desire to formulate a comprehensive theory of learning. He was, of course, certain that any tenable theory would have to be of a neurophysiological nature, and he made several attempts in this direction. Being convinced that simple connectionism would never explain learning, Lashley was inclined toward some form of field theory, but despite the brilliance of his speculations he was never satisfied with any of them for very long. As a matter of fact he was especially adept at marshalling convincing evidence which demolished every existing theory of learning, including his own.

In the 1920's he was persuaded by R. M. Elliott, who was editing the Century Psychology Series, to write a book on learning. The task was never completed. In 1928 Lashley wrote to Professor Elliott referring to the project and making the following comment:

"I am working on it intermittently. The difficulty is the final collapse of my whole neurological and psychological system. I am sure that none of the existing theories of learning is even relevant to the problem. I am coming to doubt that even the reflex is a valid statement of spinal mechanisms. I have no alternative hypothesis."

Ten years later, while at Harvard, Lashley wrote, "I am afraid the prospects for a book are not good. My bricks won't hang together without speculative straw that I know is hooey." . . .

In his Vanuxem Lectures, delivered at Princeton in 1952, Lashley enunciated a theory of shifting fields of excitation within the cerebral cortex as a basis for learning. In 1955 he wrote to John B. Watson as follows:

"I shall try to finish up a couple of books in the next year or two. The Vanuxem Lectures are giving me trouble; since I gave them my students and I have disproved most of what I said in the lectures—my theory of spreading neural patterns—and I have no alternative to offer."

Although he was unconvinced by his own theories, many of Lashley's formulations had significant impact upon contemporary thought and stimulated much original research. For example, demolition of connectionistic explanations opened the way for alternative hypotheses. Demonstration that certain visual habits lost after cortical injury could be relearned postoperatively pointed up the problem of vicarious function. An ingenious analysis of "pseudoaffective states" in brain-injured patients exploded current theories implicating the thalamus as the center for emotional experience.

Teacher, Friend, Associate. It was Lashley's professed philosophy that trying to teach people is useless, "Those who need to be taught can't learn, and those who can learn don't need to be taught." Nevertheless he could upon occasion be a stimulating lecturer, and he was particularly effective in informal seminars. A former student recalls Lashley's effect upon students at Minnesota very vividly:

"I saw Karl for the first time when I was taking a General Psychology course. An assembly lecture was given to all psychology classes once every two weeks, with different professors giving one lecture to about 200 students. Karl tall, lean, sardonic, held up a frog, made the muscles jump, grinned at us and talked informally in his rather precise voice. We learned more in 40 minutes from him than we had from the other eight professors and we all filed out of the hall wanting to know when we could take a course from this thin, splendid lecturer with the pince-nez on a black string. We quickly learned that we couldn't. He hated teaching formally and was available for only a few graduate students."

One of Lashley's colleagues during the Minnesota period remembers him as being always deep in research for what seemed to be eighteen hours of every day. Though thin as a rail and sometimes white as a sheet he was imbued with great zest and never seemed tired. At the bi-weekly departmental seminars Lashley's presentation of his own research always generated great excitement. When others made their own reports he spoke rarely, but when he did, "it would be hard to exaggerate the impact of his thinking and of his personality on his students and colleagues."

R. M. Elliott recalls that at Minnesota there was "always a small coterie of devoted students who practically lived with him in the laboratory." This was true also at the University of Chicago and later at Harvard. Lashley did a great deal of teaching, but this took place in small groups, the traditional coffee hour in his laboratory, or in individual conversations in his own office or the student's lab. He very rarely visited the research room of a subordinate, being a great believer in letting a student "go it alone"; but he was available for advice and consultation if the student sought him out. It is plausible that this attitude stemmed from Lashley's experiences at the University of West Virginia, when Reese simply told him to "work up" the anatomy of the sheep brain and then left him to his own devices.

The system worked with superior students, but others fell by the wayside, overwhelmed by a situation in which they were, for the first time in their college careers, offered unlimited freedom in research and expected to perform like mature scientists. The present writer used to argue with Lashley that a little more direction and guidance might help some students achieve independence and develop the ability to plan and execute their own research, but Lashley believed that anyone who needed this kind of support would never become a successful investigator and might as well be eliminated early in the game.

Within the limits just described Lashley gave willingly of himself in his relations with students and colleagues, but his intimates were few. He surrounded himself with a distinct reserve, which held no note of unfriendliness, but tended to discourage personal intimacy. He was, in a sense, aloof without being cold. . . . .

Of course, such a complex personality was, inevitably, perceived differently by different people, and one acquaintance who knew Lashley at Minnesota during the early twenties remembers him as being,

". . . very perceptive about people . . . sensitive to their states of mind and feeling . . . kind and generous to his friends, students and colleagues, but without harboring any sentimental illusions about them . . . his opinion of human nature was not at all flattering, yet he didn't want people to be hurt. He did not suffer fools gladly, but he did suffer them courteously and gently—except of course when they got in the way of something really important and then he disposed of them efficiently."

Remembering that as a child, Karl Lashley had very few playmates, associated predominantly with adults, and apparently spent more than the usual amount of time in solitude, wandering the woods and fields, working in his shop, reading—remembering these things one is inclined to wonder whether Lashley the man may not have found it difficult, embarrassing, or simply not worthwhile to make or accept those overtures which are essential to the eventual establishment of numerous friendships. A letter from one of the few men with whom he developed true intimacy describes Lashley as,

". . . a man who desired friendship and love, but was cautious when approached, similar to approaching a thing of wildness and timidity. As teacher and pupil, but more as friends and companions, we worked together for many years. At times I look back upon those years with longing."

The genuine friendships Lashley did form were deep and abiding. A former colleague, writing after Lashley's death, refers to the "sheer friendship and affection" he felt, and adds, "with him I felt at ease as with few other people." One psychologist, when asked to contribute information regarding Karl's life, declined because it would be too painful to delve into the past, and in any event, Lashley would not have wanted it done. This conclusion may be correct, for Lashley steadfastly refused to prepare an account of his life for publication in the semiofficial series entitled *A History of Psychology in Autobiography*. He also declined a request to contribute an autobiographical account to the volume *Perspectives in Biology and Medicine*.

His deep sense of personal privacy would have made it exceedingly difficult for Lashley to write about himself for public consumption. This sort of difficulty is revealed in the following note sent to the present writer after more than twenty years of association:

May 20, 1957

Dear Beach:

As usual we are having library trouble here. I would appreciate it, if you would get one of your students to look up the page citations in the enclosed list. I enclose a check to pay for his time. The references are from the translation of the papers of Lorenz and Tinbergen. The translation has served my purpose, at any rate, in that by it I have caught a wife.

Claire Schiller and I are to be married on June 9. We plan to drive to California this summer, then to live here for a couple of years, until Christina is ready for college. It was a surprise to me—that is, being accepted.

I hope you can find someone to do this job quickly, so the printers can get out the page proof before we leave.

Sincerely,

Lashley

It would be incorrect to portray Lashley as a withdrawn, unapproachable, overintellectualized sort of person. He was, on the contrary, possessed of a keen sense of humor, and was almost unable to refrain from embroidering a good story when confronted with an appreciative audience. One of his students recalls being, "duly warned not to depend too much on the absolute veracity of K. S.'s stories, since he loved to embellish any story that he might tell if he thought the listener was impressed."

Although he loved and appreciated good plays and music, with the exception of opera, Lashley was not averse to attending burlesque shows. He read widely and his taste was catholic including Icelandic sagas, Virgil, Bertrand Russell, Balzac, Ambrose Bierce, and nonsense poetry which he greatly enjoyed composing as well as reading. His wry humor is reflected in his account of having sent money to an ailing aunt whom he had never seen. He found later that instead of being indigent, the lady was well off, and when she died she left her estate to the Philadelphia Antivivisectionist Society; Lashley concluded his story by saying, "I had never expected to contribute to that organization."

In both his professional and his private life Lashley displayed a great zest and love of exploration and excitement. To ride with him in his car, which was usually a flashy convertible, was truly a hair-raising experience. He operated an automobile with supreme disdain, both for traffic regulations and for the mechanical limitations of the vehicle.

For years Lashley sailed in dangerous waters without bothering to learn to swim. He did finally master that skill at the age of sixty-seven. He disliked inactivity and particularly begrudged the time lost in sleep, saying that it was a waste of life.

Marriages. Lashley was married twice. In 1918 he married Edith Anne Baker, an accomplished musician who could have had a professional career had she not been chronically afflicted with a severe asthmatic condition. Her illness required expensive medication and frequent hospitalization during the early years of the marriage; and the medical bills for the first year exceeded Lashley's salary as an instructor.

A son born to the couple in 1919 died shortly after birth and the Lashleys remained childless thereafter.

They were very close, sharing, among other things, a deep love of music. In many ways Edith's personality complemented Karl's. He was completely impractical with respect to financial matters, and as likely as not to spend an entire quarterly stipend on the purchase of a new car without worrying about money for living expenses until the next payment arrived. Edith therefore handled all of the family finances, and Lashley used to say that he never knew whether they had ten dollars or ten thousand in the bank, and never cared.

One family friend has written that, "Edith not only did not understand science, but at times disliked it. She was, however, much interested in people of all types—including scientists." This interest plus great natural charm made her a gracious hostess, and an evening in the Lashley home was always a relaxed and pleasant occasion.

Edith died in 1948 and Lashley remained a widower for nine years. In 1957 he married Claire Imredy Schiller, widow of the brilliant Hungarian psychologist, Paul Schiller. This second marriage, while tragically short, was a very happy one, and had an obviously revitalizing effect upon Lashley. He and his bride traveled across the United States, and on their honeymoon revisited the scene of his boyhood year in Alaska. At the time of his death they were planning joint research in the area of linguistics, for Lashley had a theory that certain problems of brain function might be illuminated through the study of language.

Extraprofessional Interests. Lashley's chief recreational interests were sailing and music. In addition he enjoyed shopwork and chess, and could, when he wished, perform very creditably in the role of chef.

When he was eleven years old he had a few piano lessons, but found scale practice impossibly dull. According to his own account he "picked up the violin without instruction" when he was eighteen. Lashley first heard classical music at the age of twenty and was immediately fascinated by it. During his first year in Minneapolis he was introduced by his wife, Edith, to the literature of chamber music.

The Lashleys' circle of acquaintances included many professional musicians, and beginning in 1920, the couple and their friends devoted at least one evening each week to the playing of chamber music. Lashley had bought an inexpensive 'cello and learned to play it while he was at Hopkins. Later he acquired two excellent ones. He collected an extensive library of instrumental music and continued to play as long as he lived. After moving from Harvard he played with the Jacksonville Philharmonic Orchestra and organized a small group of musicians which met regularly at his home. He was a trustee and generous benefactor of the Jacksonville College of Music.

Lashley's interest in sailing stemmed from childhood when he often fashioned a simple raft by tying two logs together and paddled about on the river. He recalled this pastime as being one of his greatest joys. During his family's sojourn in Seattle they lived next door to a boat designer whose yard was littered with scale models. These fascinated young Karl and awakened an enduring passion for sailing.

During his years at Hopkins he acquired a canoe, equipped it with leeboards, and learned, by trial and error, to sail. When he and Edith moved to Chicago he bought the Banshee, a thirty-foot yawl. Though he owned six other boats at later times, including a thirty-six foot yawl, the Banshee held his greatest affection. A letter written in 1955 acknowledges that the motor sailer he then owned was much more comfortable, but did not "provide much excitement."

Lashley's skill and interest in woodworking and other types of shopwork traced back to his boyhood when his father gave him a jigsaw outfit to reduce the wear and tear on the family sewing machine. This talent was often put to practical use. His last boat, the Skidbladnir, carried many fittings and castings of Lashley's own design. At the time of his second marriage Lashley did a major job of remodeling his house, which stands on the bank of the St. John's River, with a boat dock in the back yard. In enlarging the house, he laid a parquet floor, put up the ceiling, paneled the walls with knotty pine, and installed closets and a window seat, and then built the furniture including a bed, dressing table, desk, and bookcases.

Extramural Service. Despite the fact that he hated to divert his energies from his research, Lashley did serve his profession in a number of extramural capacities. He was a member of the editorial boards of several scientific journals including the following: *Journal of Genetic Psychology, Journal of Comparative Psychology, Journal of Animal Behavior, Acta Biologica, Acta Psychologica, Quarterly Review of Biology,* and *Journal of the Philosophy of Science.*

At various times Lashley served on different private or governmental committees and boards. His longest term was spent as a member of the National Academy of Science—National Research Council's Committee for Research on Problems of Sex. The annual meetings of this body afforded opportunity for the renewal of old acquaintanceships, particularly with Adolf Meyer whose seminars at Johns Hopkins had stimulated Lashley during his graduate and postgraduate years. Eventually, however, Lashley resigned from this committee because, as he put it, "I found myself saying 'no' to everything."

He was Civilian Advisor to the Office of Scientific Research and Development, and earlier in his career was actively associated with the Research and Development Division of the Prosthetic and Sensory Aids Service.

Elections and Honors. Although he had little enthusiasm for attending large meetings or conventions, and rarely did so, Lashley was elected to many scientific and philosophical societies. The following is a list of his affiliations: American Psychological Association (Council member 1926–1928; President, 1929), Eastern Psychological Association (President, 1937), Society of Experimental Psychologists, British Psychological Association (Honorary Fellow), American Society of Zoologists, American Society of Naturalists (President, 1947), British Institute for the Study of Animal Behavior (Honorary Member), American Society of Human Genetics, American Physiological Society, Harvey Society (Honorary Member), National Academy of Sciences (elected in 1930), Royal Society, London (Foreign Member), American Philosophical Society, American Academy of Arts and Sciences, New York Academy of Sciences (Honorary Member), Florida Psychological Association.

Among many invited addresses, Lashley delivered the Hughlings Jackson Lectures at Montreal in 1937, and the Vanuxem Lectures at Princeton in 1952.

That his eminence as an investigator was officially recognized by psychologists, zoologists, and physiologists is attested by several major awards. In 1937 the Society of Experimental Psychologists honored Lashley with the Howard Crosby Warren Medal which signifies outstanding scientific contributions to psychology. The National Academy of Sciences, in 1943, awarded Lashley the Daniel Girard Elliot Medal in Zoology. From the Royal College of Physicians he received the William Baly Medal in Physiology. This occurred in 1953.

Lashley was awarded Doctor of Science degrees from the University of Pittsburgh (1936), the University of Chicago (1941), Western Reserve University (1951), the University of Pennsylvania (1955), and in 1953 the Johns Hopkins University honored Lashley with the degree LL.D. . . .

Lashley's last published article was entitled "Cerebral Organization and Behavior" (1958). In the words of its author, this article deals with, "the problem of how the brain knows that it knows; what characteristics of neural activity constitute mind." Steadfastly opposing any retreat into metaphysics, Lashley liberally documents his claim that study of "the organization of mental states does not reveal any operations which cannot be accounted for in principle by the mechanisms of the brain." His final conclusion deserves full quotation:

"Mind is a complex organization, held together by interaction of processes and by time scales of memory, centered about the body image. It has no distinguishing features other than its organization. The mental phenomena must be subjected to an analysis as complete and detailed as that which is being made of neural activities. Only as progress is made in such an analysis, and as the picture of the brain's activities is completed, will it be possible to make significant correlations between the two organized systems. Meanwhile, there is no logical or empirical reason for denying the possibility that the correlation may eventually show a complete identity of the two organizations (p. 542)." . . .

Illness and Death. In February of 1954, while doing his annual two-weekly stint of teaching at Harvard, Lashley collapsed, and, to his disgust, was hospitalized. The eventual diagnosis was acquired hemolytic anemia which might yield to splenectomy or to treatment with cortisone. Lashley's opinion of the medical profession was not high, and he resisted the notion of surgery. As soon as cortisone treatment made it possible he returned to Jacksonville where, as he put it, he could "control the doctors."

Months of cortisone administration resulted in softening of the vertebrae with attendant spinal dislocations and, in November of 1955, a splenectomy was performed. Lashley's subsequent recovery seemed complete, and he remained in comparatively good health until his trip to Europe with his wife, Claire, in 1958. His sudden passing was in accord with a wish he once expressed to a friend, namely the hope that at the end he would simply collapse at one of the street corners of the world. The rest of the wish was not fulfilled, and will not be. It was that he would then be forgotten. . . .

THE SIXTIETH BIRTHDAY CELEBRATION VOLUME[3]

Lashley's 60th birthday was celebrated on June 7, 1950. Nissen had earlier solicited letters of felicitation from colleagues and students in America and around the world, and a total of 100 letters were received. Most letters were written in English (American and British), but there were also wishes expressed in French, German, Spanish, and in Chinese. The list of contributors appears next. It reads like a *Who's Who* in the biological and behavioral sciences of the time.

Also solicited were photographs of Lashley shown at various milestones, at graduation and receiving his earned and honorary degrees; photographs of the various institutions in which he studied and worked; and copies of his university transcripts. All this material was bound in a single, quite fascinating volume titled *Lashley, 1950,* embossed in gold on the cover and presented to him on his birthday.

---

[3]I am indebted to Claire S. Lashley for permission to publish excerpts of letters from this volume.

Excerpts of selected letters are provided. Each contains a message about Lashley that is worth noting. Together they add to the portrait of Lashley that was attempted in this volume.

Contributors to Sixtieth Birthday Celebration Volume

Adrian, Edgar D.
Allport, Gordon W.
Arthur, Grace
Bailey, Percival
Ball, Josephine
Bartlett, Frederick
Beach, Frank A.
Beebe-Center, J. G.
Bender, Morris B.
Birch, Herbert G.
Bird, Charles
Blake, Francis G.
Blum, Josephine S.
Boring, Edwin G.
Brentlinger, Mrs. D. H.
Bromiley, Reg. B.
Bucy, Paul C.
Burrows, William
Carlson, Anton J.
Carmichael, Leonard
Chow, K. L.
Clark, George
Clark, Sam L.
Corner, George W.
Darrow, Chester W.
Denny-Brown, Derek
Dodson, John D.
Drew, G. C.
Elliott, Richard M.
Evarts, Edward V.
Fenn, Wallace O.
Frisch, Karl von
Fulton, John F.
Gavan, James A.
Ghiselli, Edwin E.
Gibson, Mrs. S. M.
Griffin, Donald R.
Halstead, Ward C.
Haskins, Caryl P.
Hayes, Keith
Hebb, Donald O.
Heidbreder, Edna
Herrick, C. J.
Hisaw, Frederick L.
Hoagland, Hudson
Hooten, Earnest A.
Hu, Chi-Nan
Hull, Clark L.
Hunter, Walter S.
Ingebritsen, Otis C.
Johnson, Harry M.
Kennard, Margaret A.
Kinder, Elaine F.
Klüver, Heinrich
Koehler, Wolfgang
Krech, David
Landis, Agnes T.
Landis, Carney
Langfeld, Herbert S.
Leeper, Robert W.
Levine, Jacob
Lewis, Nolan D. C.
Lorente de Nó, R.
Maier, Norman R. F.
Moore, Carl R.
Morgan, Clifford T.
Nissen, Henry W.
Paterson, Donald G.
Penfield, Wilder
Pieron, Henri
Pinto, Teresa
Polyak, Stephen
Pribram, Karl H.
Reese, Albert M.
Rey, André
Richter, Curt P.
Riesen, Austin H.
Russell, James T.
Schiller, Claire H.
Schneirla, T. C.
Shaklee, Alfred B.
Sherwood, Mrs. K. K.
Smith, Douglas E.
Sperry, Roger W.
Stevens, S. S.
Stone, C. P.
Taliaferro, Lucy G.
Taliaferro, W. H.
Thurstone, L. L.
Tsang, Yu-Chuan
Vaughn, Charles L.
Wade, Marjorie
Watson, J. B.
Weed, Lewis H.
Weiss, Paul
Wiley, Lester E.
Woodworth, Robert S.
Yerkes, Robert M.
Yoshioka, Joseph G.
Yum, K. S.

Excerpts of Selected Birthday Letters: June 7, 1950

Adrian: You have done more than anyone to direct research on the brain and to bring physiology and psychology together.

Allport: I want to thank you . . . for your stern practice of self-criticism, a trait that has influenced many more of us than you probably realize. You have taught us to scrutinize our results, replicate, admit error, and start afresh. Now this may be an habitual virtue in the older sciences, but it has not been a virtue in psychology—not until you introduced it by example.

Bailey: I am coming more and more to appreciate the value of your contributions to the understanding of the cerebral cortex. I believe today that much saner views are coming to be prevalent as the result of your unrelenting scientific endeavor.

Ball: You seemed to regard teaching as one of the unpleasant necessities of your life and [I] wondered why, because you were an outstandingly successful teacher. I do not know of anyone who has a more quietly devoted following. . . . Your belief that "it's no use to teach people because those that need teaching can't learn and those that can learn don't need to be taught" made you exactly the kind of teacher I wanted.

Beebe-Center: You have influenced me much. The key factor . . . has been your tremendous belief in *actual* experimental research as distinct from contemplation or rhetoric. . . . Somehow you have brought home to me the chasm that separates mere research-mindedness from productivity in research.

Birch: You were always available for counsel, but never attempted in any way to make those of us who were working under you accept . . . your ideas. . . . It was a great pleasure to play music with you and Mrs. Lashley and to indulge my enthusiasm for Lewis Carroll with a fellow enthusiast.

J. S. Blum: It was a lot of fun to fight with you about "neopavlovianism," architectonics, strychninization, etc., and I think it taught us more than any amount of study among people with prejudices similar to ours. We had to give up some of the dogmas, and the ones that are left are, I believe, held on more adequate grounds.

Boring: What a pity Franz is not here to write a letter. He held staunchly all along that you were the white hope of American psychology!

Darrow: I still occasionally turn something out on the old lathe to which you attached a foot switch. . . . My subject matter, the emotions, have moved from the periphery into the calvarium, even into the cortex, where they can better participate in the phenomena of Mass Activity. . . .

Denny-Brown: From the confusion of thought which characterizes most present-day writings by clinical neurologists, you will probably wonder if your work has made any impression on their thinking. Let me assure you that those of us who are groping for truth in this field lean heavily on the fruits of your labors, though we may appear to be inarticulate. May you long be spared to continue to inspire us.

Elliott: We kept your name on the door of your laboratory (in Minnesota) for 22 years. Then the door itself had to be moved to another part of the building, but we saw to it that the name went with it. Then, alas, a month ago, a janitor who knows no history took upon himself to remove it. Never mind, your publications are in our library and you are in our hearts!

Evarts: When I recall the eighteen thousand trials you gave to one spider monkey, I am unable to feel sorry for myself in contemplating the relatively few trials that at times have seemed arduous to me. . . . Your theory of teaching has not been to teach at all, but to allow the willing student to learn by observing and following.

Fulton: I don't know what the score will be as far as functional localization is concerned and I do not fully agree with you about area 8, but this is a minor matter, for your healthy skepticism is challenging and stimulating. I think one might say of you, as Asher said of Sherrington, that you are *the* philosopher of the nervous system.

Ghiselli: Some of us have long since left the field of physiological psychology. Nevertheless, within the limitations of our talents, our work inescapably bears the imprint of the solid foundation you provided us. . . .

Cathy, Keith, and Viki Hayes: May your seas be calm, may your cello be mellow, and may none of your monkeys ever talk back.

Hebb: Prediction: historians of psychology will speak somewhat as follows: "The main development between 1900 and 1950 were the (nontheoretical) development of test methods stemming from Binet; the (falsely theoretical) elaboration and dogmatization of Freud's important pioneer work; and, . . . the biologically oriented attack on psychological problems by . . . Watson, Pavlov and Kohler, which is . . . best exemplified in the work of Lashley because of his contribution to method, his broad attack on the problems of perception, memory, intelligence and instinct, and his full recognition of the extent of these problems to behavior." The prediction may be somewhat obvious, but I prefer betting on a sure thing when I can.

Hooten: To approach one's sixtieth anniversary while consorting mainly with apes rather than with professors is a privilege rarely given to a scientist.

Hull: I recall that one time you took Mrs. Hull and me . . . out on your sail-boat on Lake Michigan. It was most delightful. As a matter of fact, that was the only time in my life I was ever in a sail-boat. . . . One evening we sat in your apartment and talked about psychological theory. Even then we didn't agree very well, though I don't recall what we disagreed about.

Hunter: I think I have read everything that he has written since the early days. Only his position on equipotentiality has aroused my disagreement; and now after the work in my laboratory where we have tried to pin down the neural control of the rat's maze habit without much success, I think that he at least had grounds for the earlier conclusions!

Klüver: If you have read G. Orwell's "Nineteen Eighty-Four," you will recall his prediction that by 1984 there will be only two types of scientific research left: 1) how to determine, against his will, what another human being is thinking, and 2) how to kill, without forewarning, several hundred million people within a few seconds. This implies, according to Orwell, that there will be only two types of scientists: 1) a mixture of psychologist and inquisitor concerned with studying facial or other bodily expressions and analyzing the effects of drugs, electric shock, and various forms of torture, and 2) the biologist, physicist, or chemist concerned only with such branches of his specialty as are important for destroying life. In view of the fact that novelists have been more often correct in predicting the future than social scientists, not to mention social "psychologists," I do not know just what to wish today [that is, in 1950]—whether to wish that a novelist, one George Orwell, will be wrong or whether to hope that you will somehow manage to be quite happy in resigning yourself to seeing the promised land of 1984 from a comfortable distance.

Krech: To invert an aphorism, I have always found that the neurologists know you as an excellent neurologist and the psychologists know you as an excellent psychologist.

Landis: I count myself fortunate that I was infected early with the virus of your skeptical curiosity for which there is no antibiotic.

Maier: To learn about nature we must ask many questions and the answer we get helps us to ask more intelligent questions. You never settled for simple answers even when you liked them. Instead you kept on asking more questions. You never designed an experiment to prove a pet theory and so your mind has always been open and subject to change whenever nature gave you an answer that didn't seem quite to fit with others. You had to integrate all answers, not just those that made sense at the outset.

Nissen: I consider myself extremely fortunate to be among those for whom you have been an effective part of the E. The value of the product, $E \times H$ (or, if you prefer, $E \rightleftharpoons H$), has thereby been substantially enhanced.

Penfield: Though you have moved up the mammalian scale to the chimpanzee the gap to man is still wide and we clinicians still sometimes find it difficult to fit our fancies to your facts.

Russell: You will recall . . . the jumping apparatus that recorded the force of the jump, the rats reared in darkness. . . . What I liked was the freedom in try-out of ideas which you gave us. . . . We strolled on the boardwalk this morning and I saw a V of birds going north—a sight that reminded me of one of your lectures on the migration of birds.

Claire Schiller: When we came to this country three years ago, it was one of his [Paul's] dreams to do research work at the unique institution which you direct, and in particular, with your guidance. That this dream could come true seemed almost like a miracle, and it was one of my happiest thoughts that it was granted him to spend that time in collaboration with you, whom he admired so greatly. Perhaps I do not assume too much in believing that knowing him may have meant some stimulation to you, too.

Schneirla: You and your work have stimulated interest in experimentation in psychology, in and beyond the fields in which you have worked specifically. . . . Your example . . . has influenced large numbers of students and colleagues beyond those who have been fortunate enough to work directly with you.

Shaklee: In these days when so many elaborate but disappointing schemes are proposed for the enrichment of higher education, I find it amusing that some of the most challenging education took place in short conversations on afternoons when you drove me home from the Labs on the old sand road to Orange Park.

Thurstone: I recall the days when even I had some share in bringing you to Chicago. I suppose that you can still handle a sailboat, that you are still in a string quartet, and that you still drink those huge cups of coffee.

Tsang: We, your Chinese students . . . stand apart as a group who went across the Pacific to enjoy the privilege of working under your supervision. We have shouldered up a mission which we intended to fulfil in China, but we feel chagrined to say that we have failed so far, owing first of all to our incapability and to the circumstances in a war-torn country. We mean to carry on, and we need your further encouragement and criticisms. I sent you 6 papers some time ago and you will receive more soon.

Charles L. Vaughn: If it seems strange that one should wait for the beginning of a decade to extend best wishes, I hope you will excuse the delay. For, after all, isn't the tradition of thinking in terms of the ten fingers one has but another illustration of the principle you have done so much to clarify: that man's thinking is bounded by his anatomical make-up?

Watson: It has been fun working with you—in the old Hopkins lab where you baby-sat with our firstborn rhesus monkey—in the dry Tortugas where we made bird nests in the sand to study proximate orientation.

Wiley: While trying to write this I sit thinking of my life when it was a part of yours. The days I worked for and with you; the days we sailed and had fun together; the Banshee and the excitement of wind and water and the pranks we played on some of your guests.

Yerkes: As I review our relations since I first came to know about you as student of Jennings and Watson (the first letter in my file from you is dated November 15, 1915), it rather clearly appears that my role in our association has been consistently that of promoter and instrumenter almost regardless of personal consideration; yours with equal consistency that of independent, self-determining and fairly individualistic creative scholar, shunning administrative opportunities and demands and giving little heed to recognition and personal preferment. It is, as I now appraise it, an oddly impersonal picture of mutual supplementation and facilitation. Apart from what our cooperative relationship may have done for our institutions, for the advance of our fields of learning, and for the art of education, we have, I believe, been notably useful to one another over more than three decades and that despite, or perhaps partly because of, our obvious intellectual and temperamental differences. I am reminded by these reflections that in my eighth decade I value more highly than ever before breadth of sympathy and appreciation, and tolerance beyond one's acquired special interests.

REFERENCES

Bartlett, F. C. Karl Spencer Lashley, 1890–1958. *Biographical Memoirs of Fellows of the Royal Society*, 1960, *5*, 106–118.

Beach, F. A., Hebb, D. O., Morgan, C. T., & Nissen, H. W. *The Neuropsychology of Lashley*. New York: McGraw-Hill, 1960.

5 Students and Colleagues of Karl S. Lashley

Jack Orbach
Queens College
City University of New York

UNIVERSITY OF MINNESOTA, 1917–1918; 1920–1926

Ph.D. Candidates

*Stone, Calvin Perry The congenital sexual behavior of the young male albino rat, 1921.
*Landis, Carney Studies of emotional reactions. General behavior and facial expressions, 1924.
*Shirley, Mary Margaret Factors influencing the activity of the rat, 1927.
*Jacobsen, Carlyle Ferdinand A study of cerebral function in learning, 1928.
*Thorson (Landis), Agnes Perseverance in the preschool child, 1935.
†#Dodson, John Dillingham An experimental study of the relative values of reward and punishment in habit formation, 1918. Sponsor: Yerkes.
†Arthur, Mary Grace A group point scale for the measurement of intelligence, 1924. Sponsor: Undetermined.

Master's Candidates

*Hunter (Brentlinger), Dorothy A study in localization of a complex motor habit in the albino rat, 1926.

---

*Sponsored formally or informally by Lashley
†Advisee of Lashley
#Co-authored one or more papers with Lashley

*Thorson (Landis), Agnes Tongue movements in internal speech, 1934 (see above for Ph.D. thesis).

Undergraduate Assistants

#Ball, Josephine (Measurement of sex behavior in male rats, 1930, University of California, Berkeley. Sponsor: Undetermined.)
#McCarthy, Dorothea Agnes The language development of the preschool child, 1929, University of Minnesota. Sponsor: Goodenough.)

BEHAVIOR RESEARCH FUND, INSTITUTE FOR JUVENILE RESEARCH, 1926–1929; UNIVERSITY OF CHICAGO, 1929–1935

Ph.D. Candidates

*#Wiley, Lester E. The function of the brain in audition, 1931.
*Tsang, Yu-Chuan The function of the visual areas of the cerebral cortex of the rat in the learning and retention of the maze, 1934.
*Ni, Chung Fang An experimental study of the influence of punishment for errors during learning upon retention, 1933.
*Hu, Chi Nan The effects of brain injury upon retentiveness in the rat, 1934.
*Ingebritsen, Otis Clarence Coordinating mechanisms of the spinal cord, 1931.
*Beach, Frank Ambrose Jr. Effects of cortical lesions upon the maternal behavior pattern in the rat, 1940.
†#Russell, James Thomas Applicability of the probable error formulae to psychological data, 1931. Sponsor: Carr.
†#Frank, Margaret The effect of a rickets-producing diet on the learning ability of white rats, 1930. Sponsor: Undetermined.
†#Peters, Henry N. Mediate association, 1933. Sponsor: Carr.
†Yum, Kwang Sup An experimental test of the law of assimilation, 1930. Sponsor: Carr.
†#McDonald, W. T. Not determined.
†Vaughn, Charles Lee Factors in rat learning: An analysis of the intercorrelations between thirty-four variables, 1937. Sponsor: Thurstone.
†Hebb, D. O. Transferred to Harvard; see below.
†Smith, Douglas E. Transferred to Harvard; see below.

Postdoctoral Fellows

Yoshioka, Joseph G. (Weber's law in the discrimination of maze distance by the white rat, 1926, University of California, Berkeley.)

Maier, N. R. F. (Reasoning in white rats, 1928, University of Michigan.)
Schneirla, Theodore Christian (Learning and orientation in ants studied by means of the maze method, 1928, University of Michigan.)
Leeper, Robert Ward (The reliability and validity of maze experiments with white rats, 1930, Clark University.)
Krechevsky, Isadore (Studies of the pre-solution behavior of the rat in sensory discrimination learning, 1933, University of California, Berkeley.)
Pennington, Leon A. (The auditory localization behavior of the white rat in relation to the so-called auditory area of the cerebral cortex, 1934, Brown University.)

Professional Associates

Klüver, Heinrich
Koffka, Kurt
Herrick, C. J.
Polyak, Stephen

HARVARD UNIVERSITY, 1935-1942; IN ABSENTIA, 1942-1955

Ph.D. Candidates

*Hebb, Donald Olding The innate organization of visual perception in the rat, 1936.
*Smith, Douglas E. Cerebral localization in somaesthetic discrimination in the rat, 1937.
*Levine, Jacob Studies on the interrelations of central nervous structures in binocular vision, 1941.
*Griffin, Donald Redfield The homing ability of birds: A problem in sensory physiology, 1942.
*Chow, Kao-Liang Transferred to the Yerkes Laboratories; see below.

Postdoctoral Fellows

Drew, George C. (The function of punishment in learning, 1934, University College, London.)
Ghiselli, Edwin E. (Subcortical mechanisms in maze and visual discrimination habits, 1936, University of California, Berkeley.)
Beach, F. A. Transferred from University of Chicago; see above.
Rey, André Swiss student of Piaget.

Professional Associates

Morgan, Clifford T.
Anderson, Edward E.

YERKES LABORATORIES OF PRIMATE BIOLOGY ORANGE PARK, FLORIDA, 1942–1955

Ph.D. Candidates

*Blum, Robert A. The nature of delayed response deficit in relation to the locus and character of pre-frontal extirpations in primates, 1949, Yale University (Nissen).

**#Blum (Semmes), Josephine Cortical organization in somesthesis, 1949, Yale University (Nissen).

**#Chow, Kao-Liang Effects of partial extirpations of posterior association cortex on visually mediated behavior in monkeys, 1950, Harvard University.

*Orbach, J. Effects of removal of visual cortex on learning and retention in the monkey, 1955, Princeton University (Wever).

†Birch, Herbert George The relation of experience and motivation to problem solving in chimpanzees, 1944, New York University (Schneirla).

Predoctoral Fellows Influenced by Lashley

Shaklee, Alfred B. 1942-43 (Psychological effects of vitamin B1 supplements to a "normal" diet, 1943, University of Minnesota.)

#Wade, Marjorie 1944-48 (Not determined.)

Gavan, James 1950-53 with Nissen (Growth and development of the chimpanzee, a longitudinal and comparative study, 1953, University of Chicago.)

Thompson, Robert 1951-52 with Hayes (Transposition as a function of stimulus comparison in the white rat, 1955, University of Texas.)

Welker, Wallace I. 1952-54 with Hayes (Play and exploration in chimpanzees, 1954, University of Chicago.)

Fantz, Robert L. 1953-55 with Hayes and Nissen (Object preferences and pattern vision in newly hatched chicks, 1954, University of Chicago.)

Premack, David 1954-55 with Nissen (Influence of prior learning of one discrimination component on learning of the second component when the two components are presented in combination, 1955, University of Minnesota.)

Postdoctoral Fellows and Associates

Nissen, Henry W.	1929-58
Young, William C.	1939-43
Hebb, Donald O.	1942-47 (see above)
Riesen, Austin H.	1940-43; 1946-49
#Sperry, Roger W.	1942-46
Kinder, Elaine F.	1943-44
#Clark, George	1943-47
Gardner, L. Pearl	1945
Hayes, Keith	1947-55
Pribram, Karl H.	1947-48
Schiller, Paul H.	1947-49
Chow, Kao-Liang	1947-54 (see above)
Evarts, Edward V.	1949-50
Pinto-Hamuy, Maria	1950
Bromiley, Reg B.	1949-51
Jarvik, Murray E.	1951-52
Hutt, Paul J.	1952-54
Odoi, Hiroshi	1953-54
Robinson, John S.	1953-54
Orbach, J.	1955 (see above)

JOHNS HOPKINS UNIVERSITY, 1911-1917; SAINT ELIZABETH'S HOSPITAL, WASHINGTON, 1916-1917

Teachers and Associates

#Jennings, Herbert Spencer 1896, Harvard University
#Watson, John Broadus 1903, University of Chicago
Meyer, Adolf 1890, University of Zurich
#Mast, Samuel Ottmar 1906, Harvard University
#Hubbert (Caldwell), Helen Brewster 1915, Johns Hopkins University
#Franz, Shepherd Ivory 1899, Columbia University

6 The Functional Significance of Architectonic Subdivisions of the Cortex: Lashley's Criticism of the Traditional View

I. T. Diamond
Duke University

It is fitting that we meet now, 50 years after the publication of Lashley's first great work on the cortex. I am grateful to Jack Orbach for planning this volume and for inviting me to participate. This opportunity to honor Karl Lashley is very important to me, and I have given much thought to the selection of a topic. I have chosen as my subject the subdivisions of the cortex. The functional significance of architectonic subdivision was the central issue of the monograph, *Brain Mechanisms and Intelligence*, and the conclusions of that study influenced the direction of Lashley's research and thinking for the rest of his life.

It is crucial for my argument to distinguish two separate questions or issues that Lashley addressed under the general heading of cortical subdivisions.

1. Do architectonic subdivisions correspond with differences in connections; that is, do they have functional significance?
2. Can the traditional classification of architectonic areas into sensory, association, and motor areas be supported by the results of the behavioral ablation method?

Lashley's answer to the first question was no, and on this he was wrong. His answer to the second question serves as the subject matter of this chapter.

THE PREVAILING VIEW OF THE CORTEX AT THE TIME LASHLEY BEGAN HIS RESEARCH

I want to begin with the view of the cortex that prevailed in 1929, at the time *Brain Mechanisms and Intelligence* was published. The first principle was the concept of sensory areas of the cortex. Sensory pathways had been traced to the neocortex from the eye, the ear, and the spinal cord, using the Marchi method for tracing degenerated fibers or the Golgi method for staining normal cell bodies, dendrites, and axons. The general view was that a conscious sensation was the result of impulses reaching the sensory areas. It comes as no surprise that Cajal was one of the pioneers who discovered that sensory pathways ascend to the cortex after relaying in the dorsal thalamus. Figure 6.1 reflects our efforts to collate several of his drawings presented in 1906, at the time he received the Nobel prize. Of course the sensory path is defined by the direction of the arrows pointing *toward* the cortex; but also note Cajal's arrows pointing in the direction of impulses that travel in descending fibers from the deep layers of cortex to thalamus and brain stem. I argue later that the significance of *descending* projections from sensory cortex has been missed because of the dramatic discovery that electrical stimulation of a region of the frontal cortex elicits movements.

This brings me to the second principle of the traditional view, the concept of the motor cortex. Since stimulation of a given locus will always produce the same movements or movements of the same part of the body, the motor cortex can be mapped by designating the various parts of the body. Figure 6.2 shows the motor cortex of a chimpanzee according to Sherrington (1906).

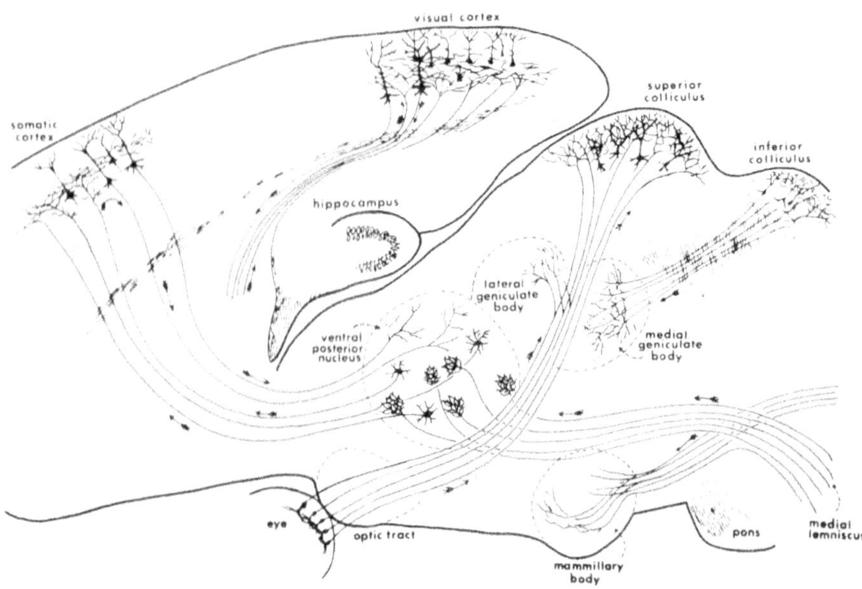

FIG. 6.1. Cajal's view of the sensory pathways to the cortex. The arrows indicate the direction of the nerve impulse. Note the medial lemniscus projecting to the ventral posterior nucleus, which in turn relays to the somatic cortex. Note also Cajal's view of the pyramidal cells in the deep layers of the cortex, with apical dendrites reaching close to the surface and the axons descending back to the ventral posterior nucleus.

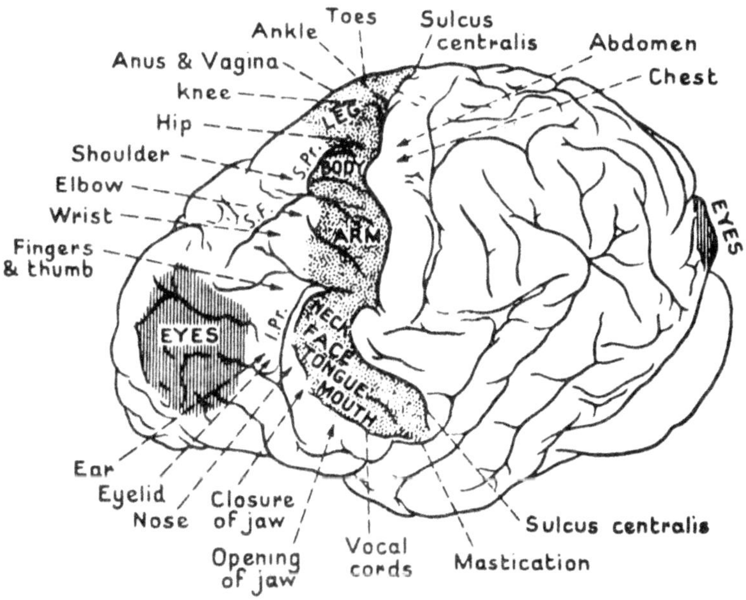

FIG. 6.2. Brain of a chimpanzee, taken from a figure in Sherrington's *Integrative Action of the Nervous System,* which in turn was taken from a paper by Grunbaum and Sherrington (see Sherrington, 1906). The following figure legend is taken from Sherrington: "Left hemisphere viewed from side and above so as to obtain as far as possible the configuration of the sulcus centralis area. The figure involves, nevertheless, considerable foreshortening about the top and bottom of sulcus centralis. The extent of the 'motor' area on the free surface of the hemisphere is indicated by the black stippling, which extends back to the sulcus centralis. Much of the 'motor' area is hidden in sulci; for instance, the area extends into the sulc. centralis and the sulc. precentralis, also into occasional sulci which cross the precentral gyrus. The names printed large on the stippled area indicate the main regions of the 'motor' area; the names printed small outside the brain, indicate broadly by their pointing lines the relative topography of some of the chief subdivisions of the main regions of the 'motor' cortex. But there exists much overlapping of the areas and of their subdivisions which the diagram does not attempt to indicate.

The shaded regions, marked 'EYES', indicate in the frontal and occipital regions respectively the portions of cortex which, under faradization, yield conjugate movements of the eyeballs. But it is questionable whether these reactions sufficiently resemble those of the 'motor' area to be included with them. They are therefore marked in vertical shading instead of stippling (as is the 'motor' area).

S.F. = superior frontal sulcus. S.Pr. = superior precentral sulcus. I.Pr. = inferior precentral sulcus."

The third principle followed from the belief that the regions intercalated between sensory and motor areas were devoid of incoming fibers from the thalamus. These areas were termed the *association areas*. The presumption was that they received fibers only from the sensory areas, and the fibers originating from the sensory areas of the cortex were called association fibers.

These three principles provided the starting point for studies of the evolution, embryology, and laminar organization of the cortex. The results of these sutdies in turn provided support for the principles.

Elliot-Smith (1910) and other pioneers of comparative neurology showed that there was little or no association cortex in primitive mammals, such as the opossum or hedgehog, and that the association areas expand with the evolution of primates. Figure 6.3 shows the location of the three sensory areas and the intercalated association areas in four mammals occupying different levels of the

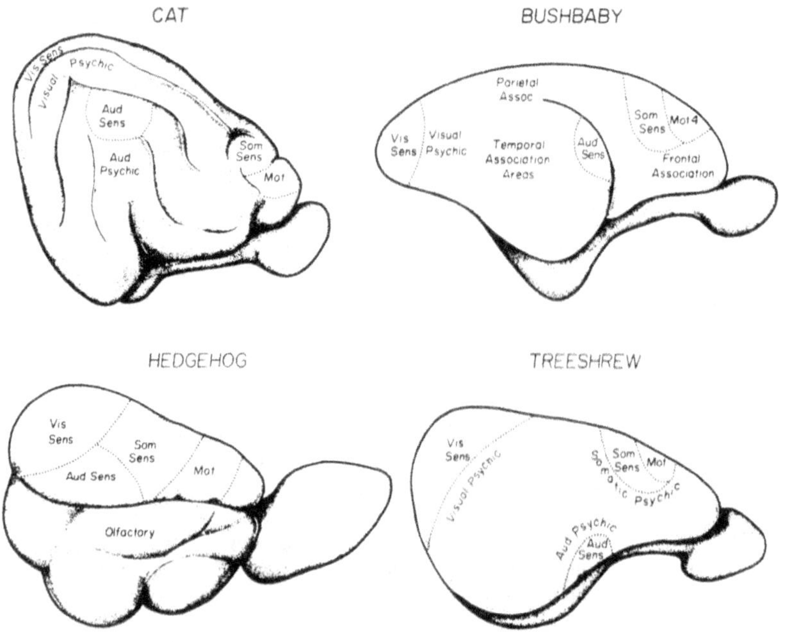

FIG. 6.3. The cortices of four mammalian species ranging in complexity from the most primitive, the hedgehog, to the more advanced cat and primate. The chief point is the location of the visual, auditory, and somatic sensory areas. In the bush baby, there is an extensive region intercalated between the sensory areas; on the other hand, in the hedgehog, the sensory areas are contiguous with each other. The location of the sensory areas in these four species is a very close approximation of the regions that would have been depicted by Campbell, Elliott-Smith, and Brodmann. I have taken certain slight liberties such as switching auditory sensory and auditory psychic in the cat—this for the sake of making the auditory sensory area closer to AI as this term is used today.

phylogenetic tree. Note that in the "lowly" hedgehog, no cortex is assigned to the association areas. This relation between phylogenetic level and the amount of association cortex supported the idea that the association areas serve an intellectual, as opposed to a sensory, function.

Neuroembryology also supported the classification into sensory, association, and motor areas. Flechsig (1901) had discovered that the sensory and motor areas develop myelin first, and this was taken as evidence of their more basic functions. In other words, the higher-level association areas cannot and do not need to function until the sensory and motor areas are already in operation.

That the cortex was layered was known in the middle of the 19th century, but it was not until the discovery of methods to stain cell bodies and fibers that the cortex was divided systematically on the basis of its laminar pattern. Brodmann and Campbell (1905) agreed that the sensory areas were similar to each other, sharing in common a highly developed fourth granular layer (for references to Brodmann's publications, see Sanides 1970, 1972). It was generally accepted that the several sensory areas had a common function, so it seemed natural that they shared in common the same architectonic features.

However, it is appropriate for us to ask: "What is this common function that was taken for granted 80 years ago?" At first glance, the sensations of "red," "burning pain," and "500 Hz" appear to have nothing in common. The answer is complicated and requires an understanding of the prevailing epistemology of the 19th century. According to our "senses," the external world consists of objects—a table, a chair, a pencil, etc. Surely we are not born with "table" and "chair" neurons; even less likely are the properties of objects recognized by the retina or cochlea. The bell is not in the ear. These perceptions of objects must be the result of experience. If we try to eliminate the effects of experience and learning, we might achieve a pure sensation devoid of meaning. Psychologists in the 19th century, and before them philosophers of the 18th century (Hume, for example), tried to identify these simple elements of the mind. The result of this concerted effort was a list of simple sensory qualities—for example, color, brightness, pitch, temperature. Thus a "pencil" is simply an oblong streak of yellow color. The significance of identifying *sensations* is that they should reflect the innate mechanisms inherent in sense organs and should therefore be the same for all persons with normal sense organs. Whenever the sensation does *not* conform to the physical energy impinging on the sense organ, the failure can be attributed to certain physiological mechanisms in the receptor. Thus, after looking at yellow light for a while, the retina does not immediately return to its original state; as a result, a physically gray card will appear blue. The most obvious examples of failures to sense a change in the stimulus can be attributed to limitations in the sense organ. The receptor has some threshold below which energy can produce no effect.

When pathways were discovered from the eye to the cortex, it seemed reasonable to *postulate* that the analysis achieved by the receptor was preserved and unaltered in the pathway to the cortex and that consciousness was the special contribution of the cortex. (I emphasize *postulate* to underscore the fact that it was hypothetical and that there was no physiological evidence that the relay centers did nothing to transform the message.) As a result, conscious sensation "corresponds" in some sense to the physiological processes of the receptor, which in turn correspond to the *physical* stimulus but not to the meaning or significance of the object. This correspondence must be taken with the qualification that there are certain obvious limitations, such as the threshold of the receptor, effects of fatigue, habituation, etc. In conclusion and for the reasons I have tried to review, color was assigned to the visual cortex; pitch to the auitory cortex; and touch, temperature, and pain to the somatic cortex. Further, it seemed that this assignment of roles amounted to giving the sensory areas the *same* function—*simple sensation*. It follows from this argument that the symptoms produced by ablating the sensory areas of the cortex should mimic lesions of the receptor itself, and indeed the term *cortical blindness* attempts to convey the idea that the only difference between this syndrome and blindness, in the strict sense, is that the receptor is preserved. It was conceded that some automatic reflexes, such as dilatation of the pupil, might be mediated by subcortical pathways.

By the time Lashley began his studies of the cortex, several pioneers—Schafer (1888), Ferrier (1886), and Munk (1890)—had identified by the ablation method the visual sensory area of the cortex. That is, they found an area whose removal seemed to produce cortical blindness. Not only did they identify visual cortex, they also fulfilled the expectations of the traditional interpretation of sensory cortex.

All that remained was to find some neural mechanisms whereby the conscious sensation is transformed to the ordinary perception of the objects of the world. What was sought was a mechanism for the *association* of temporally contiguous sensations. Beginning with Hume, object perception was attributed to the *association* of successive sensations: thus, "bright" followed by "hot" followed by "pain" becomes "fire." When it was claimed that the cortical areas adjacent to the sensory areas received fibers from the sensory areas of the cortex but *not* from the sensory pathways, it seemed likely that these cortico-cortical pathways were the basis of association and perception. The area adjacent to the visual cortex was called "visual psychic" to suggest that it had more to do with *visual* learning or *visual* perception. Still further association between different modalities was assigned to areas more remote from the primary sensory area. It follows that there should be a pure memory loss following ablation of the association areas. A human patient with such a lesion should see a yellow band but not recognize it as a pencil. Indeed, a loss of recognition of objects was a common finding in the neurological clinic. Although a pure memory loss was never produced by experimental ablation of cortex, Munk (1890) described a dog that could avoid obstacles and could follow moving stimuli but did not seem to recognize a familiar object. The animal also suffered a sensory defect in a part of the visual field; nevertheless, Munk's report satisfied the expectations of most researchers.

Campbell (1905) brought all these lines of evidence together in a monograph that is entitled "*Localization of Cerebral Function*," published in 1905. The chief purpose of his paper was to present his own data on architectonic subdivisions; but he also tried to relate his findings to the evidence from experimental ablation studies of cortex and to the prevailing view of anatomy. To give a flavor of Campbell's thinking and writing style, I quote a short passage that reflects beautifully his underlying assumptions about sensation and perception. After arguing that the calcarine area is devoted to visual sensation since it is the target of the visual pathway from the eye, Campbell (1905) writes: "Granted that the calcarine area is solely devoted to the reception of primary visual stimuli, the mere existence of a second area placed in such immediate contiguity suggests the likelihood that it is concerned with the sorting out and further elaboration of these stimuli [p. 146]." It is no surprise to Campbell that the visual psychic area develops later than the visuosensory area. Earlier in the text, he states: "In early infancy the tracts for the conveyance of visual impulses to the primary cortical centre are obviously active but the visuo-psychic processes, being in abeyance, there is no need for association fibres [p. 145]."

THE ROLE OF ARCHITECTONIC SUBDIVISIONS IN INTELLIGENCE: LASHLEY'S THEORY OF MASS ACTION

In the beginning, Lashley had no reason to doubt the validity of these ideas and fully expected to find sensory losses after lesions of sensory areas and memory losses after lesions of association areas. But he also wanted to resolve some unsettled issues about the localization of intelligence in humans. Some clinicians argued that intelligence was localized in the frontal association cortex, the part of the cortex that expanded so dramatically between the stages of evolution represented by apes and human beings. Others maintained that a general dementia resulted from any cortical lesion, wherever the locus.

The traditional distinction between sensory and association cortex was not designed with a view toward explaining individual differences or species differences. To be sure, one could point to the increasing size of association cortex in an ascending series of species and argue that intelligence is nothing more than the capability of forming cortico-cortical connections—that is, the capacity to form associations. But does this mean that mammals with little or no association cortex only have sensations and do not perceive the outside world as consisting of objects? Further, the increased behavioral complexity that is the hallmark of the higher mammals (for example, the complex social relations in the family or troop) seems to go beyond the formation of associations between sensory elements. Thorndike, an American psychologist, tackled these questions, and although his solutions did not resolve all the issues, the methods he used had a large influence on Lashley. Thorndike (1911) tried to overcome the obstacle to comparing species on the same scale by inventing tests of learning that did not depend on the unique repertoire of a given species. Both a cat and a monkey can be placed in a small chamber with no way to exit except by finding and pressing a small pedal. At first, the animal might take 10 minutes, until it pressed the bar by accident. But after a few sessions, the subject would go directly to the lever and escape in 2 seconds. There is nothing about the sensory or motor ability of a wide variety of species that would play any serious role in the speed of learning. In this way, learning ability of cats and monkeys could be compared on the same scale.

Thorndike's approach was innovative, but the results were disappointing inasmuch as different species could not be readily ranked on any simple test of learning. Lashley thought the next step would be to use this kind of an intelligence test in combination with cortical lesions.

Although ability to learn a puzzle box or a maze seems, as a first approximation, to measure intelligence, how can one be sure without a clear definition of intelligence? In addressing this question, Lashley relied on the landmark monograph of a British psychologist, Spearman. Spearman (1927) argued that measurements of intelligence in humans consisted of a "hodgepodge" of tests—including those of arithmetic, vocabulary, memory, and so on—without knowledge of whether more or less weight should be placed on one or another test. He then reached the surprising conclusion, however, that this chaotic approach really did not detract from the validity of the measure. Put very simply, the reason a hodgepodge could be used was that the various tests were found to be correlated with one another. Ultimately, this correlation permitted Spearman to identify a general intellectual ability, which he called "G."

Inspired by Spearman's mathematical arguments and Thorndike's ingenuity, Lashley sought a constellation of tests bearing some resemblance to tests of human intelligence that correlated with one another. The various mazes seemed to fit the bill, but the results were disappointing. In a normal population of rats, no correlation was found between scores on one maze and scores on another maze. Either the tests were not sufficiently sensitive, or there are no individual differences in intelligence in a *normal* population of rats. After cortical lesions, however, those animals that performed poorly on one test also fell below average on a second or third test.

Now comes the central question: Is the deficit related to the locus of the lesion? Lashley had hoped to show, indeed expected to show, the crucial role of association areas. Instead the deficit was related to the size of the lesion irrespective of locus. This conclusion proved to be a turning point in his career.

In the end, as the next section shows, he discredited the first principle of cortical subdivision—that architectonic subdivisions reflect differences in connections. As it turned out, history proved him wrong. What is more significant for my purpose is that he questioned the function of the association areas in memory.

Cortical Subdivision: 1929–1949. Lashley's conclusion that the most significant intellectual functions of cortex are not localized proved to be insufficient to overturn Campbell's view of localization of function. One of the reasons for the resilience of the prevailing view was the evidence for visual sensory loss after the ablation of the striate cortex, and I come back to that point. Later in his career, Lashley turned his attack to the reliability of the method of architectonic subdivisions. He and his collaborator, Clark (Lashley & Clark, 1946), each defined the borders of architectonic subdivisions in a primate, and the discrepancies between judgments about borders provided an opportunity to ridicule the idea that architectonic subdivisions had functional significance. Even the view that architectonic subdivisions reflect differences in connections was questioned. To complete his rejection of current doctrines, even the view that architectonic subdivisions increase with the evolution of primates was challenged. It must be admitted that the architectonic method had become stagnant since the time of Campbell, and the main issues for further research seemed trivial and nitpicking; for example: "Is each architectonic subdivison entirely uniform?" or "How many features must change in order to establish a border?"

No sooner did Lashley's criticism gain the notice of researchers than did new discoveries reestablish architectonics, and cytoarchitectonics in particular, to its earlier high position. In the 1930s the method of evoked potentials had furnished another way of defining sensory areas of the cortex (see Adrian, 1947). The borders of these new maps corresponded well with the borders established by connectional and architectonic criteria. Then came the dicovery that each receptor surface—the body, the retina, the basilar membrane—was topographically represented not once but at least twice on the cortical surface, and these second maps also corresponded to architectonic borders (see Woolsey & Walzl, 1942). A picture of these first and second sensory areas is shown in Fig. 6.4. From that point in history (1949) to the present, the evidence has mounted that each architectonic subdivision corresponds with differences in connections.

It is one thing, however, to say that every architectonic division reflects some difference in connections and quite another to maintain the traditional view that every architectonic area receives fibers from just one thalamic nucleus, that there are no *overlapping* projections in the cortex, and that each sensory system consists of a *single* pathway with a single target in the cortex.

In my view, Lashley had identified a basic flaw in the traditional view. It is my thesis that the classification of architectonic areas into sensory areas, motor areas, and association areas reflects the philosophic distinction between sensation and perception much more than the brilliant anatomical discoveries of the 19th and early 20th centuries. In the remainder of this chaper, I trace the historical steps that take away whatever anatomical support there was for the distinction

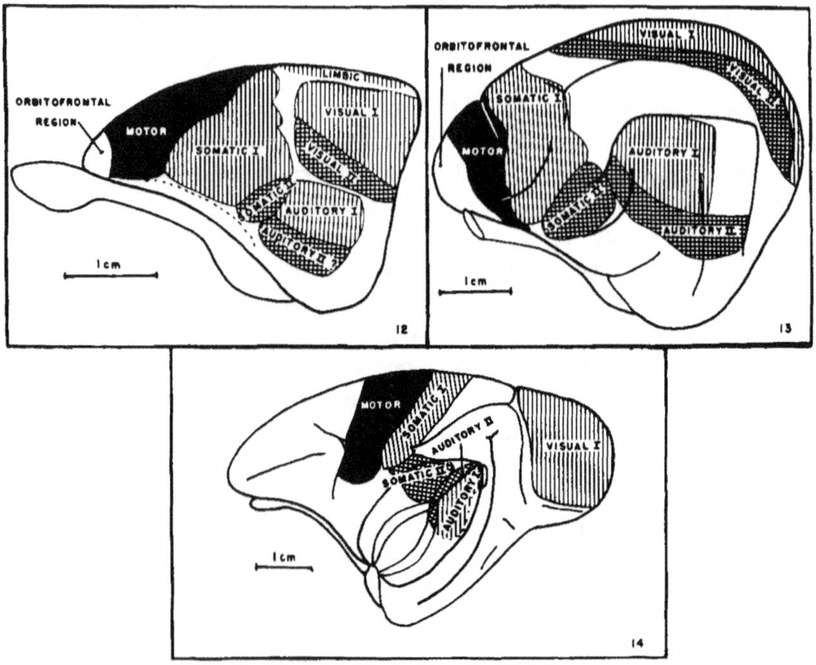

FIG. 6.4. The first (I) and second (II) sensory areas in a rabbit (upper left), cat (upper right), and monkey (bottom) (after Rose Woolsey, 1949). There are two principal points to be made by these drawings: that each sensory surface has two topographic representations in the cortex as revealed by the method of evoked potentials; and that, the amount of cortex intercalated between the sensory representations is minimal in the rabbit, maximum in the monkey, and intermediate in the cat.

between sensory and association areas. I argue that a revision in the traditional view of cortex is required, and because of the nature and purpose of this volume, I rely, to some extent, on my own research in pointing to the possibility of an alternative classification of architectonic subdivisions.

The Association Areas May Not Be Association Areas After All

Flechsig's view that the association cortex can be defined as the areas devoid of thalamic input was refuted in the 1930s by the retrograde degeneration studies of Walker (1938) and LeGros Clark (see for example LeGros Clark & Northfield, 1939). In fact, long before these experimental studies and as early as 1900, suggestions of a pulvinar projection to parietal and temporal lobes were made by Probst and Dejerine. In any case, by the mid 1930s, both Walker and LeGros

Clark had demonstrated in primates that the pulvinar complex undergoes retrograde degeneration after experimental lesions of the association cortex of the temporal, parietal, and occipital lobes.

The significance of these projections remained obscure until very recently. But even without an understanding of the function of these projections, it is reasonable to wonder how the distinction between sensory and association areas could survive for almost 50 years. The answer is that if the thalamus itself is divided into sensory and association nuclei, then there is a way of preserving a

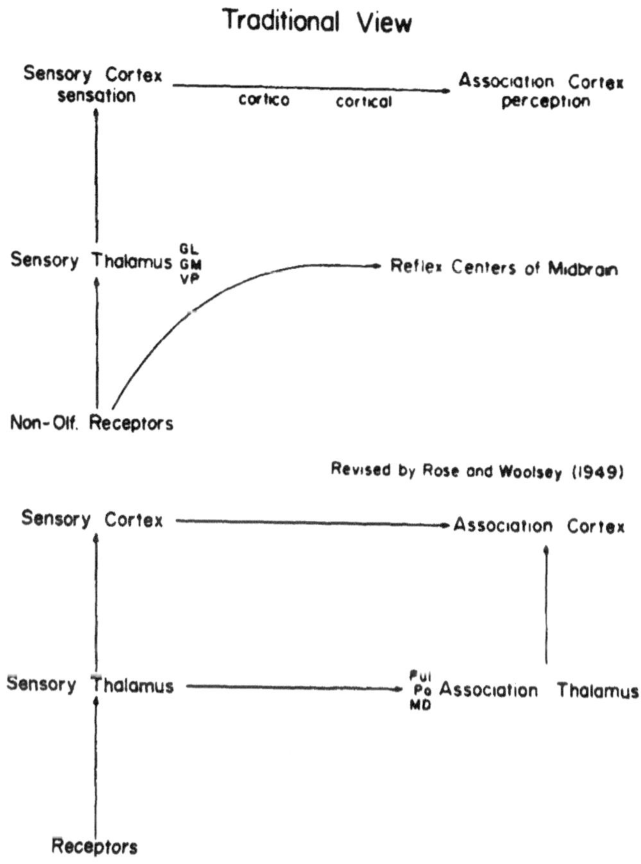

FIG. 6.5. Diagram showing the connections of the sensory and association cortex according to the traditional view and, below, the revision made by Rose and Woolsey (1949). All three neocortical sensory pathways relay in the thalamus. Rose and Woolsey's modification is that the sensory thalamus or relay nuclei project to the association thalamus, which in turn projects to the association cortex. Abbreviations in the diagram are as follows: GL, lateral geniculate body; GM, medial geniculate body; MD, medial dorsal nucleus; Po, posterior nucleus; Pul, pulvinar nucleus; VP, ventral posterior nucleus.

distinction between *primary* sensory areas of cortex—areas that receive fibers from sensory relay nuclei—and *secondary* areas that correspond to the association areas and that receive fibers from the association thalamic nuclei, the pulvinar and mediodorsal nuclei. This was the solution offered by Rose and Woolsey in 1949, and Fig. 6.5 contrasts their proposal with the original concept of sensory pathways. These authors called the relay nuclei "extrinsic" and the association nuclei "intrinsic."

THE DISCOVERY OF SENSORY PATHWAYS RELAYING IN THE INTRALAMINAR NUCLEI

In the late 1940s the study of the cortex was revolutionized by the discovery that electrical stimulation of the reticular formation could change the EEG from a high-voltage, slow alpha rhythm to low-voltage, fast activity, thus mimicking the effect of a real stimulus in the outside world that alerts or activates an individual from a drowsy, relaxed, and inattentive state (see Moruzzi & Magoun, 1949). But the pathways from the reticular formation to cortex remained unspecified. The route taken by the reticular activating system did not seem to depend on the known sensory pathways through the relay nuclei of the thalamus. There was evidence that the intralaminar nuclei of the thalamus had access to wide areas of neocortex (see Dempsey & Morison, 1942), and an argument was made that the reticular formation utilizes the intralaminar nuclei for the final relay in its pathway to neocortex. The trouble was that the intralaminar nuclei did not undergo retrograde degeneration after cortical lesions (Rose & Woolsey, 1949). Therefore, when Moruzzi and Magoun published their landmark paper in 1949, the intralaminar nuclei were not thought to project to the cortex at all, let alone to the whole of the cortex. I am sure you have heard more about this phase of history from Donald Lindsley, whose contribution to this inquiry is well known.

The next step in the study of cortical subdivisions required a new method for tracing connections, and this was achieved by Nauta's discovery of a way to trace terminal degeneration of small, unmyelinated fibers; see, for example, Nauta and Whitlock (1954); Nauta and Kuypers (1958); Mehler, Feferman, and Nauta (1960); and Killackey and Ebner (1972). The principal achievement of the Nauta method was the revelation of sensory pathways that could not have been imagined by the anatomists of the 19th century. The lateral column system was found to project to the reticular formation, which in turn was found to project to the intralaminar nuclei, which were found to project to the neocortex after all.

For the purpose of discussing the issue of cortical subdivisions, the crucial point is that the projections of any one of the intralaminar nuclei extended across borders between architectonic subdivisions. Long before the demonstration of the projections of the intralaminar nuclei, Cajal, and later his student Lorente de No (1938), had described thalamic axons that ascend to layer I of the cortex, travel parallel to the cortical surface, and emit collaterals to several architectonic subdivisions. To contrast these projections from those projections that terminate in layer IV of just one architectonic subdivision, they were called "diffuse." When the projections of the intralaminar nuclei were traced to the cortex by anterograde degeneration, they were found to terminate principally in layer I (Killackey & Ebner, 1972). So it is reasonable to conclude that the fibers seen by Cajal and Lorente de No originated from intralaminar nuclei or nuclei functionally similar to the intralaminar nuclei. (Whether a diffuse projection should be taken to mean a projection to all of the neocortex is a question that is discussed later.)

The evidence that some thalamic nuclei project to several architectonic subdivisions suggests, first, that there must be an overlap in projections, and presumably in function, in at least some cortical subdivisions; and, second, that there are likely to be some functions that are not restricted to single subdivisions. I am sure it has not escaped your notice that both ideas are congenial to Lashley's criticism of the traditional view.

Can we form any idea of the functions of the "diffuse" thalamic projections? Of course, insofar as the intralaminar thalamic nuclei are at the disposal of the reticular activating system, this function may have to do with attention. In the next section I describe a "diffuse" projection from a nucleus not usually regarded as a member of the intralaminar class. My purpose is to set the stage for a review of behavioral studies.

The Organization of the Auditory Cortical Field

As the cortex continued to be explored by the method of evoking potentials to auditory stimuli, new auditory areas were discovered. Thus, the borders of auditory cortex kept expanding at the expense of the traditional association cortex. Eventually the auditory cortex in the cat, the favorite subject of physiologists, extended from the middle suprasylvian sulcus to the rhinal fissure and contained many subdivisions that became widely known by these common abbreviations: AI, AII, Ep, Ins, Temp, AIII, etc. Figure 6.6 shows Rose and Woolsey's earlier version of auditory cortex in the cat and next to this a later version, with additional areas defined by evoked responses to auditory stimuli (see Woolsey, 1961). The thalamic projections to these areas were, of course, studied by the method of thalamic retrograde degeneration. Only in one cortical subdivision, AI, did small lesions result in severe retrograde degeneration in the medial geniculate body (GM), and then it was restricted to one part of GM, the ventral division (GMv); other parts of GM—for example, the magnocellular division (GMmc)—were spared. However, when huge lesions were made, comprising all or most of the subdivisions, then retrograde degeneration in the thalamus was more extensive and included the magnocellular division; see Rose and Woolsey (1958); Daimond, Chow, and Neff (1958); and Neff and Diamond

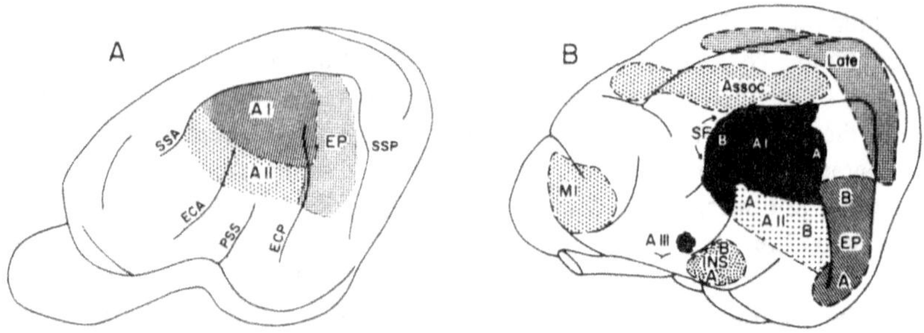

FIG. 6.6. Two diagrams of the auditory cortex in the cat. (A) is an earlier version that shos AI and AII in addition to a third area called EP. Abbreviations in (A) are as follows: EP, posterior ectosylvian area; SSA, anterior suprasylvian sulcus; ECA, anterior ectosylvian sulcus; PSS, pseudosylvian sulcus; ECP, posterior ectosylvian sulcus; SSP, posterior suprasylvian sulcus. (B) shows a later version of the auditory cortex. Each area represents a projection of the basilar membrane, with A standing for the apex and B standing for the base. Thus in AI the projection from rostral to caudal is from base to apex. In AII the projection from rostral to caudal is from apex to base. In addition to AI and AII, note the presence of a projection to EP, a fourth projection to the suprasylvian fringe (SF), a fifth projection to the insular area (INS), and a sixth projection called AIII.

(1958). Rose interpreted this result as reflecting the widespread projection of collaterals from the magnocellular division. Assuming that cells are sustained by any one of the collaterals, all cortical subdivisions that are targets of collaterals must be removed to see degeneration.

Recently, my colleagues and I have repeated the earlier retrograde degeneration studies using the new method of retrograde transport of horseradish peroxidase (HRP) (Winer, Diamond, & Raczkowski, 1977). Presumably, HRP can be transported by any one of the collaterals of a cell body, so the method is potentially capable of identifying projections of neurons that could be missed by retrograde degeneration. As is shown in the summary chart of Fig. 6.7, the results supported the earlier conclusion that GMv projects just to AI and that GMmc projects to every one of the subdivisions of the auditory field. The evidence showed that some few, scattered labeled cells were found in GMmc, whatever area was injected with HRP. In contrast, only with AI injections were cells of GMv labeled, and these took the form of narrow curved ribbons or columns. These ribbons of labeled cells were predictable from the way the neurons of GMv and their dendrites are aligned as revealed by the Golgi studies.

The chart also shows that other subdivisions of the auditory thalamus project to two or more subdivisions. They are not as "diffuse" as GMmc and not as "specific" as GMv. Thus there are three kinds of auditory relay nuclei: The first projects to only one area, the area that would have been called sensory by Campbell and that was later called AI; the second, GMmc, seems to resemble the nuclei of the intralaminar class and projects widely to the belt around the core

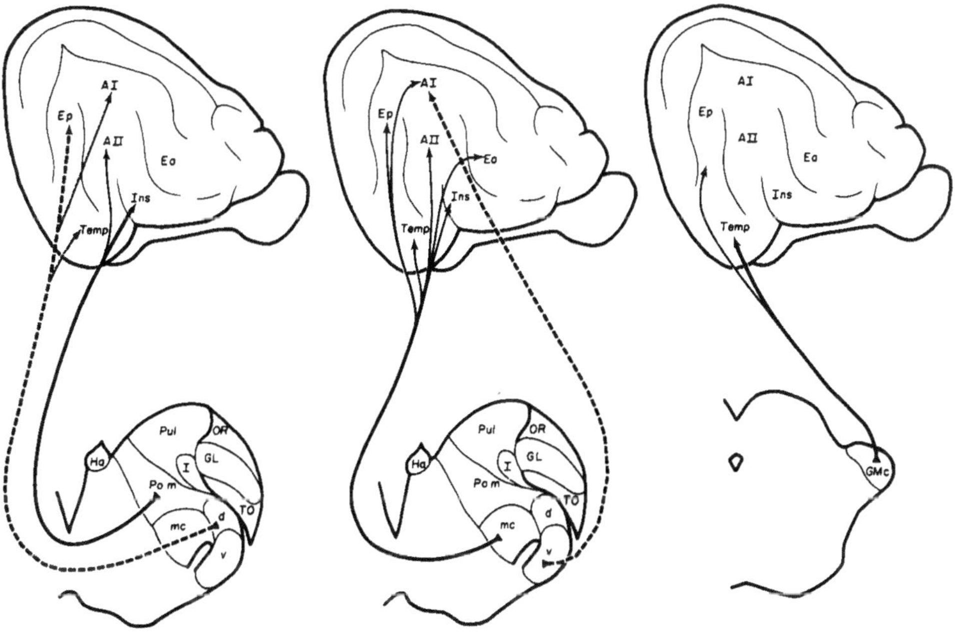

FIG. 6.7. A schematic picture of the connections of the thalamus to the auditory cortex in the cat. The chief point is made in the middle diagram: The ventral division of the medial geniculate body (v) projects just to AI (broken line). The magnocellular division of the medial geniculate body (mc) projects to all of the various auditory subdivisions, including AI, AII, the insular area (Ins), the temporal area (Temp), and the anterior and posterior ectosylvian areas (Ep and Ea). Further abbreviations in the thalamus are as follows: d, dorsal division of the medial geniculate body; Pom, medial division of the posterior nucleus; Pul, pulvinar nucleus; I, inferior division of pulvinar nucleus; Ha, habenula nucleus; GL, lateral geniculate body; TO, optic tract; OR, optic radiations; GMc, caudal division of medial geniculate body.

area as well as to AI; third, there are nuclei that fall between these two extremes and project to two or three cortical subdivisions.

A very similar organization can be found in the somatic field. Recall that in Lashley's time, just the ventral posterior nucleus (designated Vb in Fig. 6.8) was assigned the function of relaying somatosensory impulses to cortex. Then came the evidence that centre median (CM) must be relaying somatosensory impulses, since centre median receives fibers directly and indirectly from the lateral columns. There was also evidence that parts of the posterior group (Po) projected to the somatic cortex. In 1962, Chow and I tried to summarize the available evidence for parallel somatosensory pathways (Diamond & Chow, 1962). Chow is a "Lashley Ph.D." and a contributor to this volume. The figure that we published in 1962 is reproduced here (Fig. 6.8) for two reasons. First, it shows three

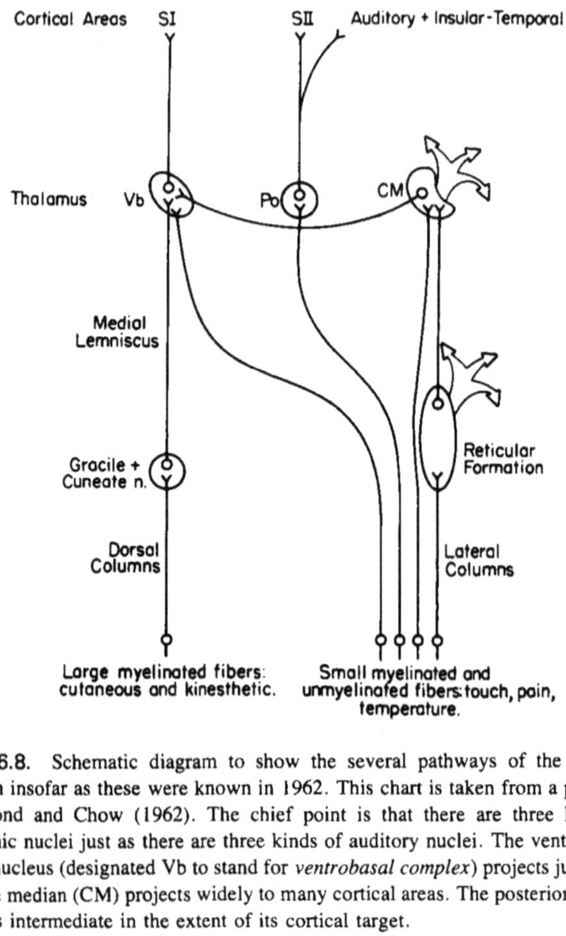

FIG. 6.8. Schematic diagram to show the several pathways of the somatic system insofar as these were known in 1962. This chart is taken from a paper by Diamond and Chow (1962). The chief point is that there are three kinds of thalamic nuclei just as there are three kinds of auditory nuclei. The ventral posterior nucleus (designated Vb to stand for *ventrobasal complex*) projects just to SI. Centre median (CM) projects widely to many cortical areas. The posterior nucleus (Po) is intermediate in the extent of its cortical target.

different types of thalamic relay nuclei: most specific, most diffuse, and intermediate; this, of course, exactly parallels the organization found in the auditory system. Second, in the somatic system it is possible to trace parallel pathways back to their origin in receptors. Whether or not parallel visual and auditory pathways can be traced back to different retinal ganglion cells or different cells of the cochlear nuclei is beyond my present purpose.

In more recent studies of *Galago*, employing the newer method of retrograde transport of HRP, we confirm, as expected, the idea that the ventral posterior nucleus projects solely or principally to koniocortex—that is, to area 3b (see Nowakowski & Penny, 1979; Penny & Nowakowski, 1979). But there are nuclei of intralaminar class—in particular, CIN and CM—that project not only to 3b but to all areas in an extensive belt around 3b. Note that we included area 4, or the

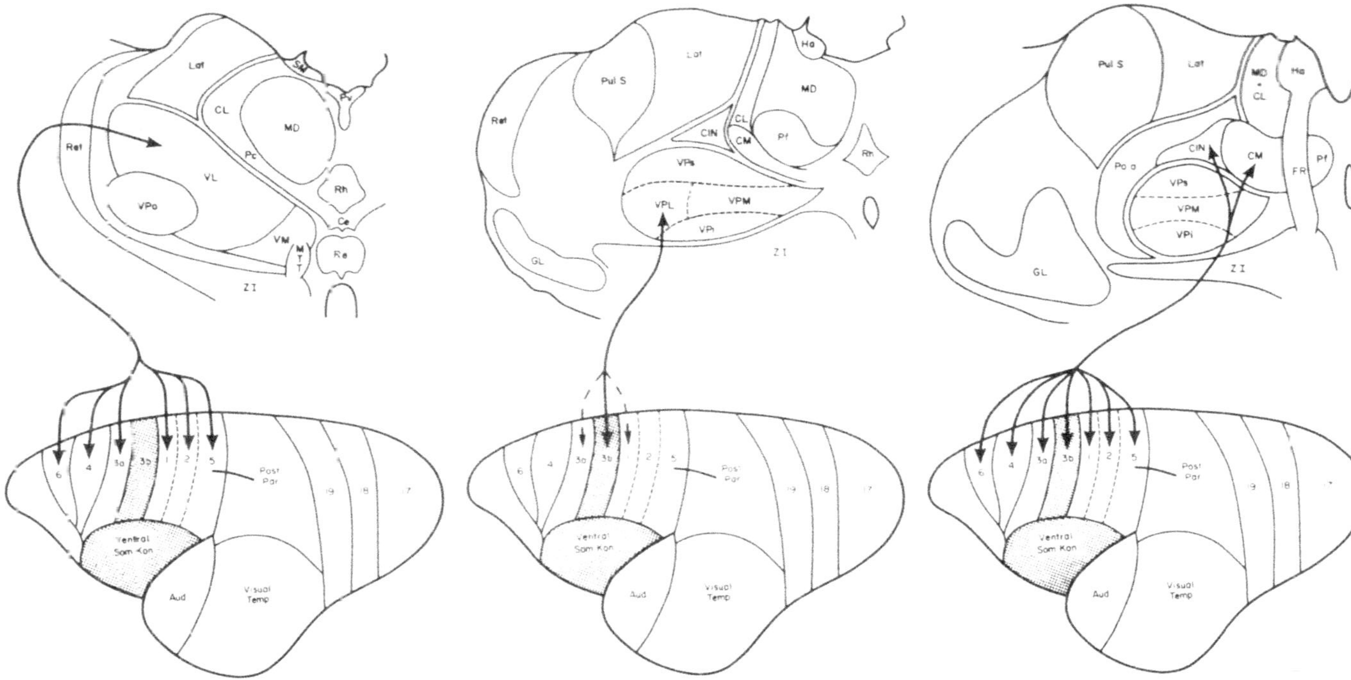

FIG. 6.9. The projections from the thalamus to the somatic field in the prosimian primate, *Galago senegalensis*. The connections between the thalamus and cortex are depicted by arrows aiming in both directions to suggest that these connections are reciprocal. Note that VPL projects to a restricted part of the cortex, whereas VL, CIN, and CM project to many areas of the somatic field. The abbreviations in this figure are as follows: Aud, auditory field; Ce, central nucleus; CIN, central intralaminar nucleus; CL, central lateral nucleus; CM, center median; FR, fascicular retroflexus; GL, lateral geniculate body; Ha, habenula; Lat, lateral nucleus; MD, medial dorsal nucleus; MTT, mammilo thalamic tract; Pc, pericentral nucleus; Pf, parafascicular nucleus; Po a, anterior portion of the posterior nucleus; Pul S, superior division of pulvinar nucleus; Pv, paraventricular nucleus; Re, reuniens nucleus; Ret, reticular nucleus; Rh, rhomboidal nucleus; SM, stria medullaris; Ventral Som Kon, ventral somatic koniocortex; Visual Temp, visual temporal field; VL, ventral lateral nucleus; VM, ventral medial nucleus; VPi, inferior division of the ventral posterior nucleus; VPL, ventral posterior nucleus, lateral sector; VPM, ventral posterior nucleus, medial sector; VPo, ventral posterior nucleus, oral division; VPs, ventral posterior nucleus, superior division; ZI, zona incerta.

motor area, as a part of the belt of the somatic field, and I return to this point later. (See legend of Fig. 6.9 for abbreviations.) In view of Lashley's criticism of the reliability of the architectonic method, I think it is appropriate to show a photomicrograph of a sagittal section through the somatic cortex of the *Galago*. Figure 6.10 shows that the absence of sulci in this species makes the borders of the subdivisions easier to locate.

Just as in the case of the auditory field, there are several additional nuclei—for example, VA and VL—whose projections are more extensive than those of the most restricted nucleus but less extensive than those of the most diffuse nucleus.

In conclusion, I have tried to show that both the auditory cortex and the somatosensory cortex consist of a group of subdivisions lying contiguous to one another. Since all of the subdivisions in the group can be identified principally with a single modality, they probably constitute a functional unit in some sense. We can call this unit a *field,* with the qualification that the word does not carry any of the meaning it has either in physics or embryology. The various subdivisions of a field share some connections in common; notably, they receive projections from one particular thalamic nucleus and reciprocate with descending projections to that nucleus. Later I show that almost half of the neocortex in the prosimian primates consists of the visual field.

The Function of the Auditory Field. Just after the war, W. D. Neff came to the University of Chicago to begin a study of the auditory cortex by the method of ablation, and I had the opportunity to work in the laboratory he established for a number of years—from 1947 to 1957. The main conclusion, for the present purpose, of that early work was to show that cats are by no means deaf after bilateral removal of the entire auditory field, including not just the sensory core area, AI, but the extensive belt surrounding AI. Deprived of this entire field, cats can still respond to changes in pitch or intensity or to a change from a left-ear to a right-ear simulus. Even when deficits were uncovered, the nature of the defect

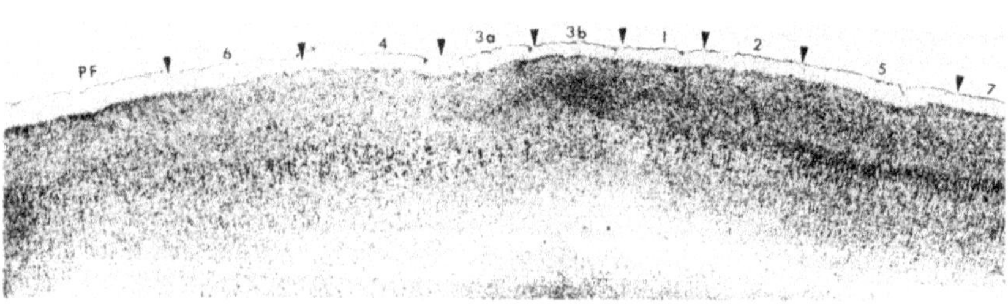

FIG. 6.10. Photomicrograph of a sagittal section of the cortex of *Galago senegalensis* to show the different architectonic subdivision. The lack of sulci makes it easier to determine borders between subdivision. PF stands for prefrontal cortex.

could not be attributed to a sensory loss (see Butler, Diamond, & Neff, 1957; Masterton & Diamond, 1964; Neff & Diamond, 1958).

This leaves only the effects of visual cortex ablation to support the traditional view of functions of sensory areas. I should say that Heinrich Kluver (1942), a longtime friend and colleague of Lashley, repeated the pioneer studies of Schafer (1888), Ferrier (1886), and Munk (1890) except that Kluver used a much more elaborate and exhaustive battery of tests for visual discrimination. His main conclusions supported the studies of the 19th century. The monkeys behaved as if they were blind; they bumped into obstacles in unfamiliar environments; they failed to discriminate between patterns or between colors; and they failed to track or localize visual objects. The monkeys were not entirely blind and still had the residual vision to detect changes in luminous flux. Of course, Lashley himself had studied the visual cortex of the rat and had concluded that only brightness discrimination remains preserved after visual ablation.

I was struck by the difference between the effects of auditory cortex ablations and visual cortex ablations and decided to reinvestigate vision after striate cortex removal. I chose a series of species, including hedgehog, tree shrew, and prosimian primate. I do not now explain my choice of species or describe differences between species (see Diamond, 1973); instead, I concentrate on the principal conclusions as these bear on the concept of the cortical field.

STUDIES OF THE VISUAL CORTEX IN TREE SHREW, *TUPAIA GLIS:* THE DISCOVERY OF THE TECTOPULVINAR PATHWAY

The striate cortex of the tree shrew is very distinctive, and there could hardly be any disagreement between observers as to the border between areas 17 and 18. Incidentally, Lashley conceded that the borders of the striate cortex in primates were an exception to the rule that different observers will fail to agree on borders between divisions. When the striate cortex was removed in a number of experiments, the tree shrew—which normally is very active—continued to circle its home cage at a lively pace and showed no obvious deficits in localizing stimuli, tracking moving stimuli, or avoiding obstacles. The animals could run and jump with accuracy in an unfamiliar environment. Neither did they show any lasting deficits in learned discriminations of pattern or color (see Diamond & Hall, 1969; Snyder & Diamond, 1968). When deficits were finally revealed, they could hardly be described as a simple *sensory loss,* as that term was used in the traditional view of sensory cortex. However, when the lesion was enlarged to include the posterior two-thirds of the neocortex, the animals suffered severe deficits in pattern discrimination (see Figs. 6.11 and 6.12). Even this symptom may not reflect a simple sensory loss, but that is a question I do not wish to debate for the present. The chief implication of these findings is that there must

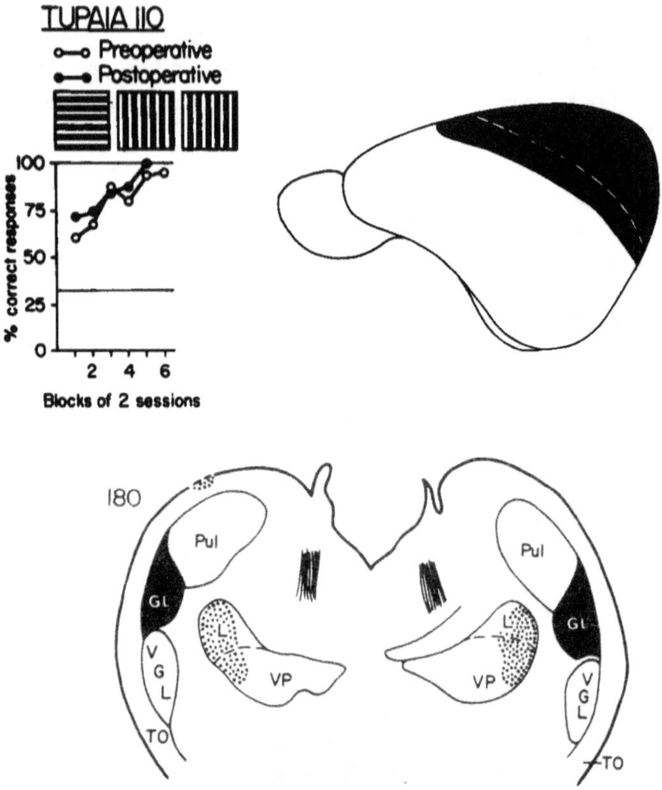

FIG. 6.11. The effects of ablation of striate cortex in the tree shrew. The lesion is depicted in black on a lateral view of the cerebral hemisphere. The border of the striate cortex is indicated by a dashed line. The effects of this ablation on the thalamus are depicted in a diagram that shows complete retrograde degeneration of the lateral geniculate body. Severe retrograde degeneration is shown in black, and slight degeneration is shown by stippling. The learning curves before and after surgery are shown in the upper left diagram. The animal's task is to choose horizontal stripes and to reject two alternative cards bearing vertical stripes. It only required 10 sessions for the animal to recover a 100% level of performance.

be a belt of cortex adjacent to the striate area that is the recipient of one or more parallel visual pathways that are *not* relayed in the lateral geniculate body. Of course, if the extrastriate areas depended entirely on the striate cortex for their input, they would be rendered useless after striate cortex ablation, in which case the deficits after the large lesions should not be greater than those produced by the lesions of the striate cortex alone.

Since the intralaminar nuclei had been shown earlier to receive sensory fibers, it seemed natural to suppose that other thalamic nuclei hitherto regarded as intrinsic were in fact extrinsic, or relay centers. The most probable source of visual input to the thalamus seemed to be the superior colliculus, and the most probable target of the superior colliculus seemed to be the pulvinar nucleus. Before our studies of tree shrew, Chow and I made this argument simply on the strength of the principle of parallel pathways. Using the Nauta method of anterograde degeneration, we looked for and found projections from the superficial layers of the superior colliculus to the pulvinar nucleus in the tree shrew (see Fig.

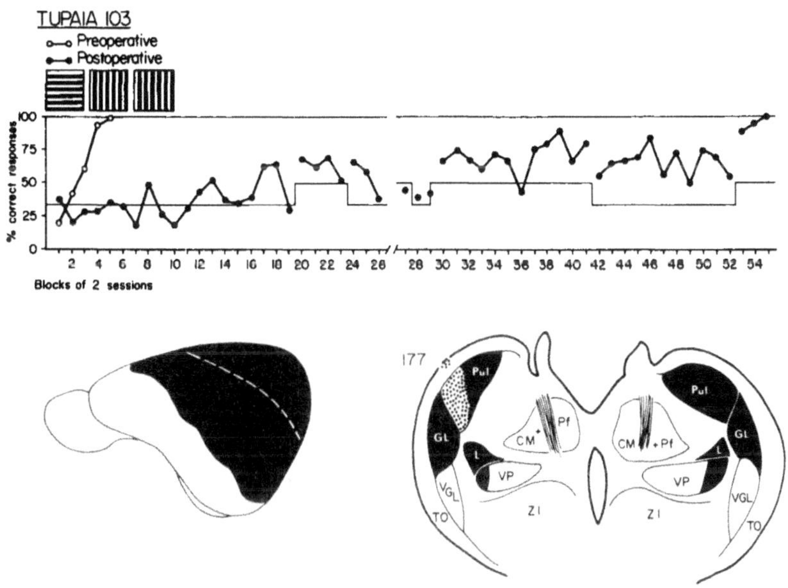

FIG. 6.12. The record of *Tupaia* 103, an animal that suffered a much more extensive lesion, extending as far rostral as the auditory and somatic fields and, in fact, invading the somatic field, as is reflected by retrograde degeneration in the ventral posterior nucleus. In addition to the complete degeneration of the lateral geniculate body, severe retrograde degeneration was found in the pulvinar nucleus, which—later studies have shown—projects to an extensive region adjacent to the striate cortex. The postoperative learning curve can be compared with that shown in Fig. 6.10. After 108 sessions and various special procedures, the animal eventually was able to attain a 100% level of performance. The chance level is shown by a horizontal line that is either at the 33% mark (when there were three stimulus cards) or the 50% mark (when there were two cards). The animal never did learn the problem with three cards. Abbreviations in this and the previous figures are as follows: CM, centre median; GL, lateral geniculate body; L, lateral nucleus; Pf, parafascicular nucleus; Pul, pulvinar nucleus; TO, optic tract; VGL, ventral lateral geniculate body; VP, ventral posterior nucleus; and ZI, zona incerta.

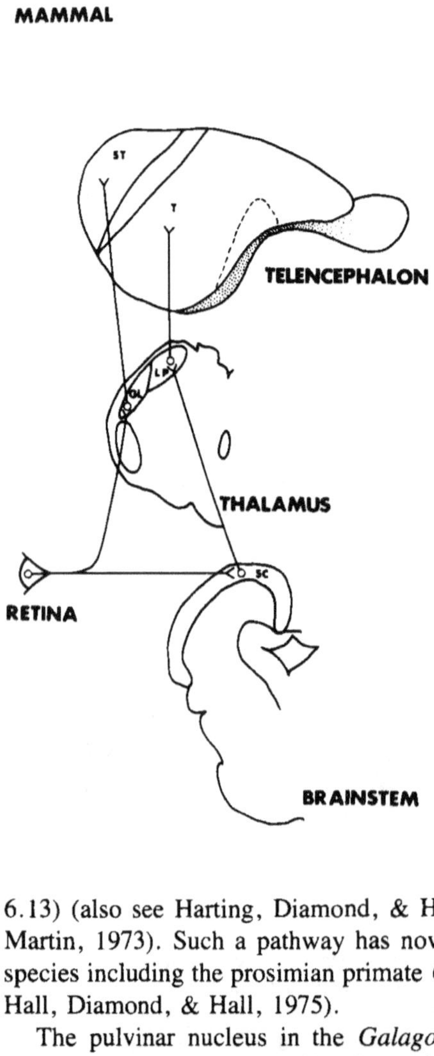

FIG. 6.13. Schematic diagram of the visual connections in the generalized or prototypical mammal. The chief point is that the retina projects to both the lateral geniculate body in the thalamus and to the superior colliculus (SC). The lateral geniculate body relays impulses to the striate cortex (ST). The superior colliculus initiates a parallel pathway through the thalamus. LP stands for lateral posterior nucleus or the pulvinar nucleus, which in turn projects to the temporal cortex (T).

6.13) (also see Harting, Diamond, & Hall, 1973; Harting, Hall, Diamond, & Martin, 1973). Such a pathway has now been identified in a number of other species including the prosimian primate *Galago senegalensis* (see Glendenning, Hall, Diamond, & Hall, 1975).

The pulvinar nucleus in the *Galago* projects to a vast area of neocortex including the striate cortex (Raczkowski & Diamond, 1980). In the striate area, the pulvinar projections, of course, overlap with the projections of the lateral geniculate body. Earlier I pointed out that when projections from a diffuse thalamic nucleus overlap with the projections of a specific thalamic nucleus, the diffuse projections terminate in Layer I whereas the specific projections terminate in layer IV. The striate cortex is no exception. The lateral geniculate body projects to layer IV of the striate cortex, whereas the pulvinar nucleus projects to layer I of the striate cortex. In the next section, I describe experiments that demonstrate pulvinar projections to layer I of striate cortex by means of restricting HRP to layer I (see Carey, Fitzpatrick, & Diamond, 1979).

You have, no doubt, anticipated the conclusion of this argument. The pulvinar nucleus in the visual system bears some resemblance to the magnocellular division of the medial geniculate body in the auditory system and to the intralaminar nuclei in the somatic system. The target of the pulvinar nucleus can be defined as the visual field. So defined, the visual field lies adjacent to the auditory field, and the auditory field lies adjacent to the somatic field. These three fields are shown in the cortex of the prosimian primate in Figs. 6.14 and 6.15.

Electrophysiological and anatomical studies in the cat also show three huge fields in the neocortex; the visual field extends from area 17 on the medial wall to the middle suprasylvian sulcus (see Palmer, Rosenquist, & Tusa, 1978). That marks the beginning of the auditory field, which extends ventrally to the old olfactory cortex and rostrally to the somatic field. These three sensory fields of the cat are also drawn in Fig. 6.15.

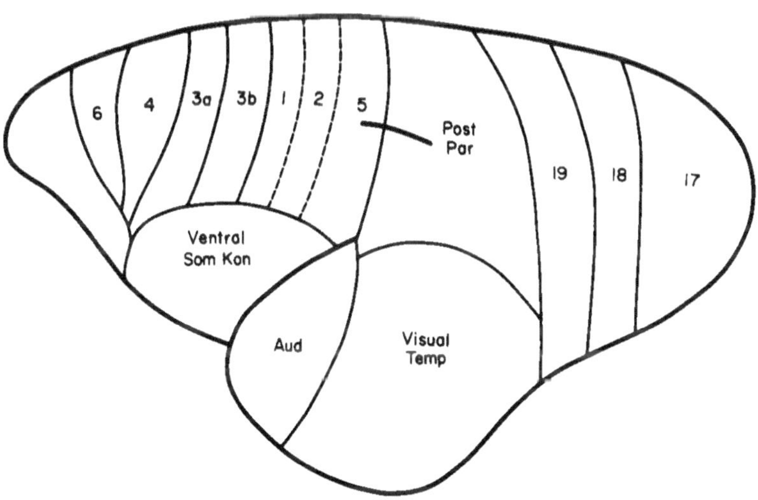

FIG. 6.14. The various subdivisions of the cortex in the prosimian primate, *Galago senegalensis*. The auditory field (Aud) is shown at the rostral pole of the temporal lobe. The visual field includes, in addition to area 17, areas 18 and 19 and the visual temporal field (Visual Temp). The caudal half of the posterior parietal region (Post Par) also belongs to the visual field. Most of the rest of the neocortex consists of the somatic field, which is divided into the following subdivisions: areas 6, 4, 3a, 3b, 1, 2, and 5 and the ventral somatic koniocortex (Ventral Som Kon), which constitutes a representation of the face.

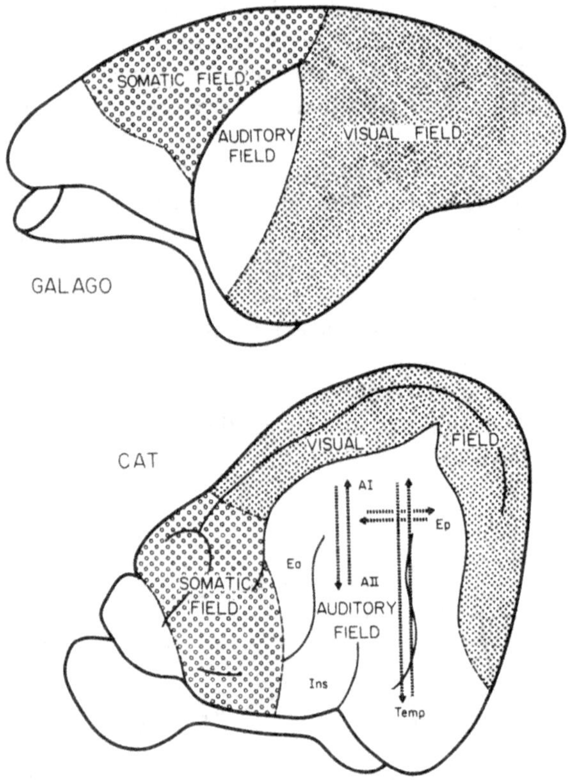

FIG. 6.15. The three principal fields in the cortex of the *Galago* (above) and the cat (below). The chief point is that the three sensory fields meet one another, leaving no intercalated areas to be assigned for association. In both species the cortex of the frontal lobe, which is the target of the medial dorsal nucleus, is not classified. Any further discussion of this frontal granular cortex is beyond our present purpose.

In the picture of the cat cortex, an attempt was made to convey extensive interconnections between the various subdivisions of the auditory field. For example, arrows show that AI projects to AII and that AII sends a reciprocal projection back to AI. Abbreviations for this figure are as follows: AI, auditory area I; AII, auditory area II; Ea, anterior ectosylvian area; Ep, posterior ectosylvian area; Ins, insular area; and Temp, temporal area.

HOW SHOULD WE CLASSIFY MOTOR CORTEX?

In the traditional view, the pathways for conditioned reflexes or for responding to complex learned perceptions (all "perceptions," of course, are learned, in contrast to "sensations") involve, first, a projection from sensory areas to association areas and, second, cortico-cortical projections from association areas to the motor cortex. Lashely, of course, was suspicious of this scheme, as you might guess. In 1950 he wrote:

> I first became sceptical of the supposed path of the conditioned reflex when I found that rats trained in a differential reaction to light showed no reduction in accuracy of performance when almost the entire motor cortex along with the frontal poles of the brain was removed. The observation led to a series of experiments designed to test the part played by the motor cortex in the retention of various habits. The matter can be tested either by removing motor cortex or by severing its connections with the sensory areas of the brain [p. 456].

Lashley went on the discuss the main conclusions of this inquiry. When the visual areas of the rat were separated from the motor areas by a deep incision, the animals were able to learn complex visuomotor habits as readily as do normal animals. Further, when monkeys were trained to open various latch boxes, the removal of motor cortex produced a temporary paralysis; but after this paralysis recovered sufficiently, the animals immediately opened the boxes without any random exploratory movements. Thus the removal of the motor area did not produce any loss of memory for the movement. These experiments seem to rule out the motor cortex as containing any part of the conditioned reflex arc. Later, Lashley and one of his most illustrious students, Roger Sperry, made multiple incisions through the cortex of both rats and monkeys, with the result that the cortex was essentially crosshatched (see Sperry, 1947). Such lesions had no effect on memory unless the primary afferent pathways to the sensory areas were transected, and the animals did not even show any postoperative incoordination of the movements necessary for their habitual performances. These results led Lashley to conclude that associative connections or memory traces of the conditioned reflex did not extend across the cortex as well-defined pathways.

In the light of our concept of a sensory field, how do we classify the *motor cortex* as this term was used by the neurophysiologists who discovered it? And if there is no evidence for pathways from sensory cortical areas to motor cortical areas, what is the pathway for sensory motor habits?

First I should say that studies of cortico-cortical connections provide little support for the traditional view. According to the traditional view, the auditory koniocortex (AI) should project to the surrounding association cortex, but few if any association fibers should reciprocate. In fact, our studies of cortico-cortical pathways in the auditory field demonstrate the existance of reciprocal connections and refute the idea of a one-way flow of impulses from AI to its surround (Diamond, Jones, & Powell, 1968). I have tried to convey the reciprocal character of cortico-cortical connections in the diagram shown in Fig. 6.15. A similar argument can be made for the visual field. The striate cortex projects to the extrastriate belt, but there is ample evidence of reciprocal projections returning to the striate area (Tigges, Spatz, & Tigges, 1973). Indeed all of the subdivisions within a field are interconnected with one another, insuring an interaction between the various parallel pathways (Spatz & Tigges, 1972).

At the same time there is relatively little crossing of the borders between one field and the next. It is surprising how few fibers in the cat pass from AI and the auditory suprasylvian fringe under the depths of the suprasylvian sulcus into the visual cortex. The functional unity of a sensory field could be defended on the basis of cortico-cortical fibers alone. So few are the fibers passing between fields that the question arises: How is multimodal integration achieved? Surely there must be convergence, and if the site is not in the temporal association cortex or motor cortex, where is it?

I come back to this point, but first let me try to dispose of the question of motor area 4. No doubt motor area 4 is unique in its number of direct connections to the spinal cord. But it is one thing to say that motor area 4 is the area most directly connected with the motor cells of the spinal cord and quite another to say that area 4 is the motor area of the cortex. Motor area 4 is sensory cortex inasmuch as it receives sensory fibers from the thalamus. That these thalamic fibers are conveying cutaneous sensory impulses has been demonstrated by recording unit potentials in the primary motor cortex of the rhesus monkey (Wise, 1980). These impulses are probably relayed by VL and CM, and Fig. 6.9 diagrams the projections from VL and CM to area 4 based on our evidence obtained in *Galago*. At the same time, the areas caudal to motor area 4, sensory areas 3a, 3b, 1 and 2 are motor inasmuch as they also project to the spinal cord. This projection was shown years ago by the Nauta method (see Liu & Chambers, 1964), but the separation between the classes "sensory" and "motor" was so firmly and rigidly held that the significance of these projections was missed. Descending cortical projections were believed to play a role chiefly in gating ascending sensory pathways.

Whatever the functional significance is of corticospinal fibers, every area of the somatic field is only one or two synapses removed from the ventral horn cells. The recent transport methods permit experiments that identify the very cells of origin for corticospinal fibers. The results show that when the spinal cord is injected with HRP, cortical cells are labeled throughout the entire somatic field, and they are not restricted to the so-called motor area (Murray & Coulter, 1981). All of these cells prove to be in layer V, and this provides the starting point for my final section. In conclusion, motor area 4 is one of the subdivisions of the somatic field, no more deserving of the term *motor* than is area 3 and no less deserving of the term *sensory* than is area 3.

LAMINAR ORGANIZATION OF THE CORTEX

The retrograde transport of HRP and the anterograde transport of tritiated amino acids have provided new opportunities to study the laminar organization of the cortex, and in this closing section I try to show how these new findings bear on our central question of the subdivisions of the cortex.

I pointed out before that experiments using the method of anterograde degeneration have shown that the intralaminar nuclei project to the cortex and that these projections terminate in layer I. The anterograde transport of tritiated amino acids has revealed additional projections to layer I. For example, Ogren and Hendrickson in 1977 injected the pulvinar nucleus of the monkey and found a dense population of silver grains in layer I of the striate cortex. Later we restricted HRP to layer I of the striate cortex in the *Galago* and found that the HRP had been transported in a retrograde direction to both divisions of the pulvinar complex. Figure 6.16 shows that the labeled cells are distributed in two curved ribbons, one in each subdivision of the pulvinar complex. This fine detail in the organization of the projections could never have been seen by retrograde degeneration. The implication is that the layer I projection is not diffuse in the sense of being "scattered about." This kind of evidence supports the conclusion that where projections overlap, the "diffuse" nuclei terminate in layer I whereas the "specific" nuclei terminate in layer IV.

There is a corresponding difference in the reciprocal projections from the cortex to the thalamus. If HRP is injected into the ventral division of the medial

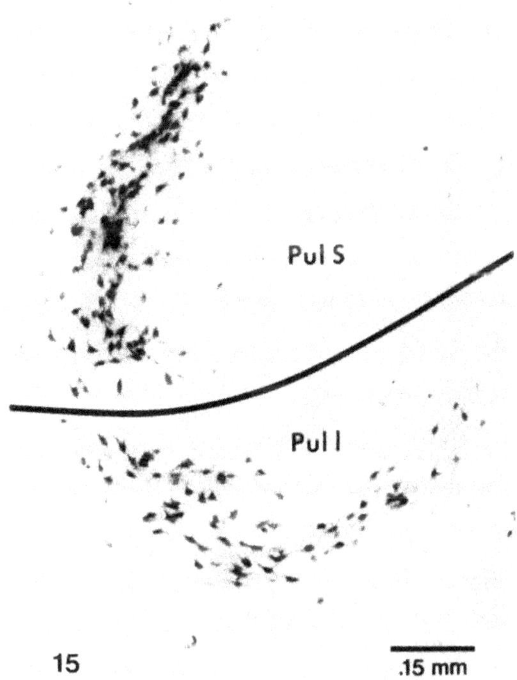

FIG. 6.16. Photomicrograph to show HRP-filled neurons in the pulvinar complex of the *Galago* after HRP was injected into the superficial layers of the striate cortex. The labeled cells constitute two ribbons or bands that meet at the border between the two subdivisions. Note that the cells are oriented parallel to the tangent at every point in the two arcs. Abbreviations in this figure: Pul I, inferior division of the pulvinar nucleus; Pul S, superior division of the pulvinar nucleus.

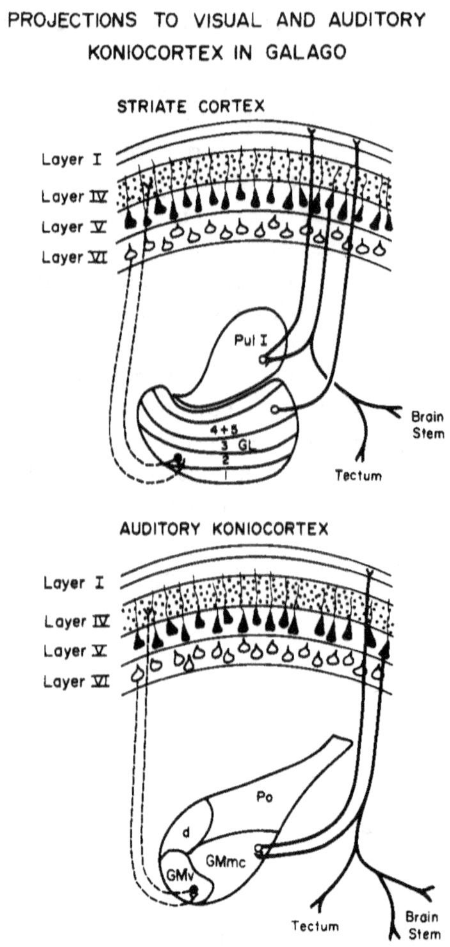

FIG. 6.17. This diagram is an attempt to show the symmetry in the organization of the connections of the auditory and visual koniocortex. Each cortical area receives projections that terminate in layer IV and projections that terminate in layer I—these two originating from different thalamic nuclei. Each cortical area reciprocates the ascending projections to layer IV by descending fibers from layer VI and reciprocates ascending projections to layer I by descending projections from layer V. The descending projections from layer V also continue to the tectum and brain stem. Abbreviations for this figure are: d, dorsal division of the medial geniculate body; GL, lateral geniculate body; GMmc, magnocellular division of the medial geniculate body; GMv, ventral division of the medial geniculate body; Po, posterior nucleus; and Pul I, inferior division of the pulvinar nucleus.

geniculate, then the cortical cells from which originate descending projections to GMv are labeled. All of these labeled cells are restricted to layer VI of area AI. On the other hand, if the magnocellular division in the *Galago* is injected with HRP, labeled cells are found in AI as well as all of the other subdivisions of the auditory field. Further, all of these cells are found in layer V. Figure 6.17 shows a diagram of the connections of the auditory koniocortex that tries to illustrate the rule that a layer IV projection is reciprocated by a layer VI neuron and a layer I projection is reciprocated by a layer V neuron. There is a symmetry between the organization of the visual and auditory systems, with the pulvinar nucleus playing the role of the magnocellular division, as I discuss in the next paragraph.

It seems to be the rule in biology that as soon as classes are distinguished, individual cases will appear to fall between classes. The pulvinar nucleus projects to layer I of the striate cortex, a point I have belabored; but the pulvinar projections to the temporal lobe and to the extrastriate belt terminate in layer IV—not layer I. Further, these two projections turn out to be collaterals of the same axon. Therefore, one collateral of a pulvinar neuron is of one class, and the other collateral is of a second class. The question posed by this organization is: "What is the origin of cells that reciprocate the two kinds of collaterals?" The answer is shown in an experiment that is illustrated in Fig. 6.18. If HRP is injected into the pulvinar nucleus in *Galago*, the labeled cells in the cortex form two populations—one of them in the temporal lobe and one in the striate cortex. All of the cells in the striate cortex are in layer V. All of the cells in the temporal lobe are in layer VI.

The difference between layer V neurons and layer VI neurons goes beyond different targets in the talamus. All of the projections from layer V to the thalamus are probably collaterals of axons that continue to descend to the tectum, the pons, the reticular formation, and, in the case of the somatic field, to the spinal cord (c.f. Kawamura & Diamond, 1978). To illustrate this point and to provide further support of my concept of a sensory field, I have selected an experiment of Denis Raczkowski's thesis (1978), in which HRP was injected into the superior colliculus of the *Galago*. In *Galago* 1321L (see Fig. 6.19) the HRP covered the superficial layers above stratum opticum and just reached the deeper layers below stratum opticum. Cells were labeled in cortical areas 17, 18, 19, all divisions of the temporal lobe, and the caudal half of the posterior parietal area. In other words, cells were labeled in evey subdivision of the visual field, and no cells were labeled outside the visual field—with the notable exception of a small population at the rostral extremity of the somatic field, an area that likely corresponds to the frontal eye fields.

In other experiments with injections of the deep layers of the superior colliculus, cells were labeled throughout the somatosensory field but were restricted to this field; or cells only in the auditory field were labeled. In some cases with injections not necessarily larger than the ones that labeled a single field, two fields—or even all three fields—contained labeled cells. When two fields contained labeled cells, the cells were not distributed in a patch on the border but were distributed throughout both fields. These experiments involving tectal injections were done in both tree shrew and *Galago*, with the same results (see Casseday, Jones, & Diamond, 1979). Thus the deeper layers of the superior colliculus are the targets of converging fibers from all three sensory fields. The significance of this conclusion is that the deep layers of the superior colliculus have access directly or indirectly to motor cells.

It is very likely that the same neurons that project to the deep tectum send collaterals to the pons and reticular formation. Even the striate area itself sends descending projections to the pons (Glickstein, King, & Stein, 1972). All of these targets have access to motor cells and can be regarded as a part of the motor system. If one insists on defining "the motor cortex," layer V throughout most of the neocortex seems to be a good candidate.

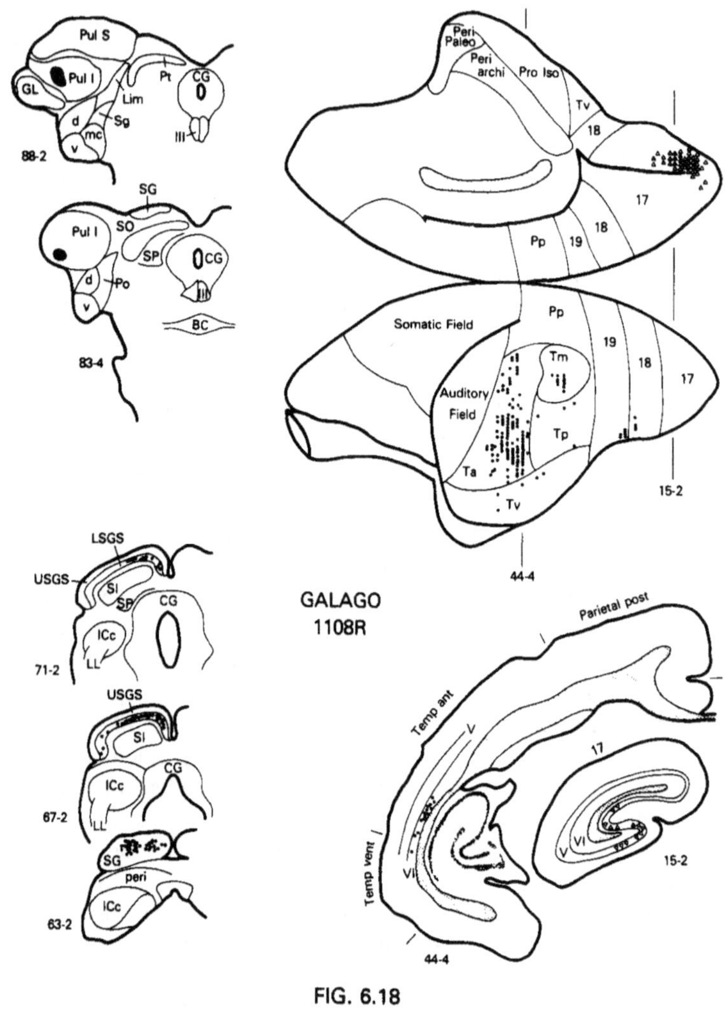

Pul S
GL
Pul I
Pt
CG
Lim
d
Sg
mc
v
III
88-2
SG
Pul I
SO
SP
CG
d
Po
v
III
BC
83-4
LSGS
USGS
SI
SP
CG
ICc
LL
71-2
USGS
SI
ICc
CG
LL
67-2
SG
peri
ICc
63-2
Peri Paleo
Peri archi
Pro Iso
Tv
18
17
Pp
19
18
Somatic Field
Pp
Tm
19
18
17
Auditory Field
Tp
Ta
Tv
15-2
44-4
GALAGO
1108R
Parietal post
Temp ant
V
17
Temp vent
VI
V
VI
15-2
44-4

FIG. 6.18

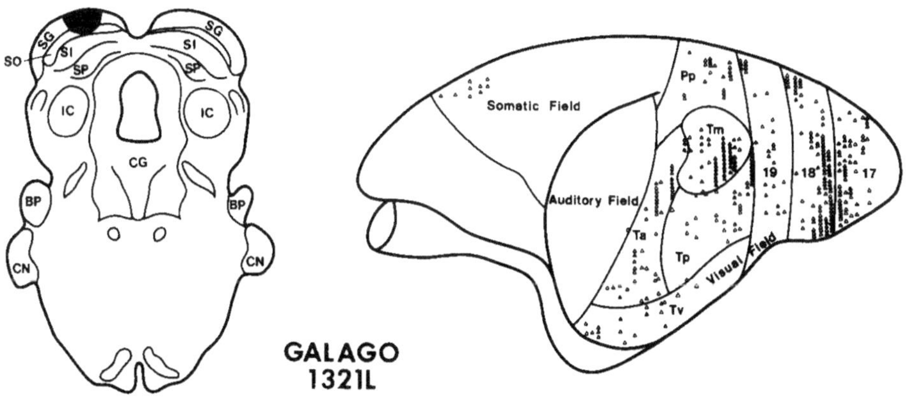

FIG. 6.19. The distribution of cortical cells in the *Galago* after an HRP injection into the superior colliculus. The extent of the diffusion of HRP is shown by the black region on the left drawing. The chief point concerns the distribution of labeled cells in the cortex, which are shown by triangles on a lateral view of the cortex. Except for nine cells at the frontal extremity of the somatic field, all the labeled cells are in the visual field. The nine exceptional cells probably correspond to the frontal eye fields.

FIG. 6.18. (*Opposite page*) Diagram of experimental results in *Galago* 1108R, in which HRP was injected into the inferior division of the pulvinar complex. The injection site is depicted in the upper left corner by black spots indicating the extent of the diffusion of HRP. Labeled cells are depicted by dots, and in the lower left frontal sections through the superior colliculus show many cells in the lower tier of the two superficial layers of the superior colliculus. Labeled cells in the cortex are divided into two populations; the first population is distributed mainly in area Ta, and all of these cells are found in layer V, which is depicted by dots. The second population is on the medial wall of the striate area, and all of these cells are in layer V, which is depicted by triangles. Abbreviations for this and Fig. 6.19 are as follows: BC, brachium conjuctivum; BP, brachium pontis; CG, central grey; CN, cochlear nucleus; d, dorsal division of the medial geniculate body; GL, lateral geniculate body; IC, inferior colliculus; ICc, inferior colliculus, central nucleus; Lim, nucleus limitans; LL, lateral lemniscus; LSGS, lower stratum griseum superficiale; mc, magnocellular division of the medial geniculate body; Parietal post and Pp, posterior parietal cortex; peri, pericentral nucleus of the inferior colliculus; Peri archi, periarchi cortex; Peri Paleo, peripaleo cortex; Po, posterior nucleus; Pro Iso, proiso cortex; Pt, pretectum; Pul I, inferior division of the pulvinar nucleus; Pul S, superior division of the pulvinar nucleus; SG, superficial layers of superior colliculus; Sg, suprageniculate nucleus; SI, intermediate layers of superior colliculus; SO, stratum opticum; SP, deep layers of superior colliculus; Ta and Temp ant, anterior temporal area; Tm, middle temporal area; Tp, posterior temporal area; Tv and Temp vent, ventral temporal area; USGS, upper tier of stratum griseum superficiale; v, ventral division of the medial geniculate body; III, nucleus of the third cranial nerve.

SUMMARY

I have tried to show that the traditional classification of cortical areas into three groups—sensory, motor, and association areas—was a synthesis of some landmark anatomical discoveries on one hand and some brilliant philosophic speculation initiated by David Hume on the other. Lashley devoted much of his scientific life to testing some of the chief implications of this classification. He could not find evidence from ablation studies in support of the prevailing view of the function of association and motor areas. Lashley thus rejected the traditional view and, in its place, conceived of the cortex acting as a single functional unit, at least for learning and higher intellectual functions. He even rejected the idea that architectonic subdivisions had any functional significance. Subsequent research has shown that he was wrong in arguing that architectonic subdivisions are not related to differences in connections. On the other hand, the traditional view that cortical pathways from sensory areas to association areas serve as the basis for the transformation from sensation to perception and cortical pathways from association areas to motor areas serve to transform perception to action had very little anatomical basis even in Lashley's time, and it still remains unsupported by anatomy. New evidence leads to an entirely different classification of architectonic subdivisions into three sensory fields (see Diamond, 1979).

Each field is the target of not one but several parallel pathways. I have presented both behavioral and anatomical evidence that demonstrate the existence of the tectopulvinar path in parallel to the geniculostriate path. No doubt the various pathways are functionally distinct, and the differences in function may even be traced to different receptors, as in the case of the somatosensory system. However, it is not possible, because of the organization of these parallel pathways, to identify one cortical architectonic area with one pathway.

First, there is at least one pathway in every sensory system that terminates in a number of contiguous cortical areas, and there is at least one area in each sensory field that is the target of several pathways. Thus the striate cortex is the target of both the geniculostriate and the tectopulvinar pathways. Perhaps this complexity contributes to the difficulty in defining the functional significance of cortical subdivisions by the ablation method.

In general I have distinguished three kinds of pathways in terms of a classification of thalamic nuclei.

1. One class, consisting of VP, GL, and GMv, projects only to one cortical subdivision; these cortical subdivisions correspond to the sensory areas of the traditional view and have been called koniocortex (see Sanides 1970, 1972). The projections from this class terminate in layer IV.

2. One class, including some intralaminar nuclei, GMmc, and the pulvinar complex, projects to *every* subdivision in a sensory field. The projections of this class terminate in layer I, at least in the koniocortex, where they overlap with nuclei of the first class.

3. Some nuclei or thalamic subdivisions project to two or three cortical subdivisions. That is, these projections are intermediate in extent between projections in class 1 and class 2.

4. There may be other thalamic nuclei that project to more than one field, and if such projections exist in all mammals, they probably originate from nuclei of the intralaminar and midline class. To argue this point, however, and to discuss fine details such as projections to layer VI of cortex would take me beyond the limits of my purpose and the time and space allotted.

According to the traditional view, the *sensory* path terminated when impulses first reached the sensory cortex. I have tried to show that the sensory cortex is only the first step in a series of loops or circuits involving descending projections to the thalamus and tectum. For example, the striate cortex projects to the lateral geniculate body, forming a cortico-thalamo-cortical loop. The striate cortex also projects to the superficial layers of the superior colliculus, which project to the pulvinar complex, and the circuit is completed by projections from pulvinar back to the striate area. The pulvinar nucleus also projects to the cortex of the temporal lobe, which in turn projects to the deep superior colliculus. These neurons of the deep layers of the superior colliculus send descending fibers to the motor centers but also send ascending fibers that return to the thalamus. On top of this complex interaction between parallel pathways, between the thalamus and cortex, and between tectum and cortex, countless fibers pass from one cortical subdivision to other subdivisions of the sensory field. The challenge remains as it was in Lashley's time: How can the function of the parts of this complex system of interrelated centers and pathways be understood by the behavioral ablation method?

ACKNOWLEDGMENTS

I thank Pamela Madren and Susan Havrilesky for their help in preparing this manuscript, which was supported by NIMH research grant 04849 and NSF research grant BNS 79-15780.

REFERENCES

Adrian, E. D. *The physical background of perception*. London: Oxford University Press, 1947.

Butler, R. A., Diamond, I. T., & Neff, W. D. Role of auditory cortex in discrimination of changes in frequency. *Journal of Neurophysiology*, 1957, *20*, 108–120.

Cajal, S. R. The structure and connexions of neurons. In *Prix Nobel*, 1906.

Campbell, A. W. *Histological studies on the localization of cerebral function*. Cambridge: Cambridge University Press, 1905.

Carey, R. G., Fitzpatrick, D., & Diamond, I. T. Layer I of striate cortex of *Tupaia glis* and *Galago senegalensis:* Projections from thalamus and claustrum revealed by retrograde transport of horseradish peroxidase. *Journal of Comparative Neurology*, 1979, *186*, 393–438.

Casseday, J. H., Jones, D. R., & Diamond, I. T. Projections from cortex to tectum in the tree shrew, *Tupaia glis*. *Journal of Comparative Neurology*, 1979, *185*, 253–292.

Dempsey, E. D., & Morison, R. S. The production of rhythmically recurrent cortical potentials after localized thalamic stimulation. *American Journal of Physiology*, 1942, *135*, 293–300.

Diamond, I. T. The evolution of the tectal-pulvinar system in mammals: Structural and behavioral studies of the visual system. *Symposium of the Zoological Society of London*, 1973, *33*, 205–233.

Diamond, I. T. The subdivisions of neocortex: A proposal to revise the traditional view of sensory, motor and association areas. In J. M. Sprague & A. N. Epstein (Eds.), *Progress in psychobiology and physiological psychology* (Vol. 8). New York: Academic Press, 1979.

Diamond, I. T., & Chow, K. L. Biological psychology. In S. Koch (Ed.), *Psychology: A study of a science* (Vol. 4). New York: McGraw-Hill, 1962.

Diamond, I. T., Chow, K. L., & Neff, W. D. Degeneration of caudal medial geniculate body following lesions ventral to auditory area II in cat. *Journal of Comparative Neurology*, 1958, *109*, 349–362.

Diamond, I. T., & Hall, W. C. Evolution of neocortex. *Science*, 1969, *164*, 251–262.

Diamond, I. T., Jones, E. G., & Powell, T. P. S. The association connections of the auditory cortex of the cat. *Brain Research*, 1968, *11*, 560–579.

Elliott-Smith, G. Some problems relating to the evolution of the brain. *Lancet*, 1910, *1*, 1–6.

Ferrier, D. *The functions of the brain*. New York: Putnam, 1886.

Flechsig, P. Developmental (myelogenetic) localization of the cerebral cortex in the human subject. *Lancet*, 1901, *2*, 1027–1029.

Glendenning, K. K., Hall, J. A., Diamond, I. T., & Hall, W. C. The pulvinar nucleus of *Galago senegalensis*. *Journal of Comparative Neurology*, 1975, *161*, 419–458.

Glickstein, M., King, R., & Stein, J. Visual input to the pontine nuclei. *Science*, 1972, *178*, 1110–1111.

Harting, J. K., Diamond, I. T., & Hall, W. C. Anterograde degeneration study of the cortical projections of the lateral geniculate and pulvinar nuclei in the tree shrew (*Tupaia glis*). *Journal of Comparative Neurology*, 1973, *150*, 393–440.

Harting, J. K., Hall, W. C., Diamond, I. T., & Martin, G. F. Anterograde degeneration study of the superior colliculus in *Tupaia glis:* Evidence for a subdivision between superficial and deep layers. *Journal of Comparative Neurology*, 1973, *148*, 361–386.

Kawamura, S., & Diamond, I. T. The laminar origin of descending projections from the cortex to the thalamus in *Tupaia glis*. *Brain Research*, 1978, *153*, 333–339.

Killackey, H. P., & Ebner, F. F. Two different types of thalamo-cortical projections to a single cortical area in mammals. *Brain, Behavior, and Evolution*, 1972, *6*, 141–169.

Kluver, H. Functional significance of the geniculo-striate system. *Biological Symposio*, 1942, *7*, 253–299.

Lashley, K. S. In search of the engram. In *Physiological Mechanisms in Animal Behaviour. Symposium of the Society for Experimental Biology*. New York: Academic Press, 1950.

Lashley, K. S., & Clark, G. The cytoarchitecture of the cerebral cortex of Ateles: A critical examination of architectonic studies. *Journal of Comparative Neurology*, 1946, *85*, 223–305.

LeGros Clark, W. E., & Northfield, D. W. G. The cortical projection of the pulvinar in the macaque monkey. *Brain*, 1939, *60*, 126–142.

Liu, C. N., & Chambers, W. W. An experimental study of the corticospinal system in the monkey (*Macaca mulatta*). *Journal of Comparative Neurology*, 1964, *123*, 257–284.

Lorente de No, R. Cerebral cortex: Architecture, intracortical connections, motor projections. In J. F. Fulton (Ed.), *Physiology of the nervous system*. New York: Oxford University Press, 1938.

Masterton, R. B., & Diamond, I. T. Effects of auditory cortex ablation on discrimination of small binaural time differences. *Journal of Neurophysiology*, 1964, *27*, 15–36.

Mehler, W. R., Feferman, M. E., & Nauta, W. J. H. Ascending axon degeneration following anterolateral cordotomy. *Brain*, 1960, *83*, 718–750.

Moruzzi, G., & Magoun, H. W. Brain stem reticular formation and activation of the EEG. *Electroencephalography and Clinical Neurophysiology*, 1949, *1*, 445-473.

Munk H. Of the visual area of the cerebral cortex, and its relation to eye movements. *Brain*, 1890, *13*, 45-70.

Murray, E. A., & Coulter, J. D. Organization of corticospinal neurons in the monkey. *Journal of Comparative Neurology*, 1981, *195*, 339-365.

Nauta, W. J. H., & Kuypers, H. G. J. M. Some ascending pathways in the brain stem reticular formation. In H. H. Jasper, L. D. Proctor, R. S. Knighton, W. C. Noshay, & R. T. Costello (Eds.), *Reticular formation of the brain*. Boston: Little, Brown, 1958.

Nauta, W. J. H., & Whitlock, D. G. An anatomical analysis of the nonspecific thalamic projection system. In E. D. Adrian (Ed.), *Brain mechanisms and consciousness*. Springfield, Ill.: C. C. Thomas, 1954.

Neff, W. D., & Diamond, I. T. The neural basis of auditory discrimination. In H. F. Harlow & C. N. Woolsey (Eds.), *Biological and biochemical bases of behavior*. Madison, Wisconsin: University of Wisconsin Press, 1958.

Nowakowski, R. S., & Penny, G. R. Thalamocortical connections of the somatic field of the prosimian, *Galago senegalensis*. *Anatomical Records*, 1979, *193*, 638.

Ogren, M. P., & Hendrickson, A. E. The distribution of pulvinar terminals in visual areas 17 and 18 of the monkey. *Brain Research* 1977, *137*, 343-350.

Palmer, L. A., Rosenquist, A. C., & Tusa, R. J. The retinotopic organization of lateral suprasylvian visual areas in the cat. *Journal of Comparative Neurology*, 1978, *177*, 237-256.

Penny, G. R., & Nowakowski, R. S. Thalamo-cortical interconnections of the somatic field of the prosimian, *Galago senegalensis*. *Neuroscience Abstracts*, 1979, *5*, 711.

Raczkowski, D. *An anatomical study of the tecto-pulvinar path in the prosimian* Galago senegalensis. Ph.D. dissertation, Duke University, 1978.

Raczkowski, D., & Diamond, I. T. Cortical connections of the pulvinar nucleus in Galago. *Journal of Comparative Neurology*, 1980, *193*, 1-40.

Rose, J. E., & Woolsey, C. N. Organization of the mammalian thalamus and its relation to the cerebral cortex. *Electroencephalography and Clinical Neurophysiology*, 1949, *1*, 391-404.

Rose, J. E., & Woolsey, C. N. Cortical connections and functional organization of the thalamic auditory system of the cat. In H. F. Harlow & C. N. Woolsey (Eds.), *Biological and biochemical bases of behavior*. Madison, Wisconsin: University of Wisconsin Press, 1958.

Sanides, F. Functional architecture of motor and sensory cortices in primates in the light of a new concept of neocortex evolution. In C. R. Noback & W. Montagne (Eds.), *The primate brain*. New York: Appleton-Century-Crofts, 1970.

Sanides, F. Representation in the cerebral cortex and its areal lamination patterns. In G. H. Bourne (Ed.), *Structure and function of nervous tissue* (Vol. 5). New York: Academic Press, 1972.

Schafer, E. A. Experiments on special localization in the cortex cerebri of the monkey. *Brain*, 1888, *10*, 362-380.

Sherrington, C. S. *The integrative action of the nervous system*. New Haven, Conn.: Yale University Press, 1906.

Snyder, M., & Diamond, I. T. The organization and function of the visual cortex in the three shrew. *Brain, Behavior and Evolution*., 1968, *1*, 244-288.

Spatz, W. B., & Tigges, J. Experimental-anatomical studies on the "middle temporal visual area (MT)" in primates. *Journal of Comparative Neurology*, 1972, *146*, 451-464.

Spearman, C. *The abilities of man*. New York: Macmillan, 1927.

Sperry, R. W. Cerebral regulation of motor coordination in monkeys following multiple transection of sensorimotor cortex. *Journal of Neurophysiology*, 1947, *10*, 275-294.

Thorndike, E. L. *Animal intelligence*. New York: Macmillan, 1911.

Tigges, J., Spatz, W. B., & Tigges, M. Reciprocal point-to-point connections between parastriate and striate cortex in the squirrel monkey (Saimiri). *Journal of Comparative Neurology*, 1973, *148*, 481-490.

Walker, A. E. *The primate thalamus*. Chicago: University of Chicago Press, 1938.

Winer, J. A., Diamond, I. T. & Raczkowski, D. Subdivisions of the auditory cortex of the cat: The retrograde transport of horseradish peroxidase to the medial geniculate body and posterior thalamic nuclei. *Journal of Comparative Neurology*, 1977, *176*, 387-418.

Wise, S. P. Personal communication and papers in press, 1980.

Woolsey, C. N. Organization of cortical auditory system. In W. A. Rosenblith (Ed.), *Principles of sensory communication*. Cambridge, Mass.: MIT Press, 1961.

Woolsey, C. N., & Walzl, E. M. Topical projections of nerve fibers from local regions of the cochlea to the cerebral cortex of the cat. *Johns Hopkins Hospital Bulletin*, 1942, *71*, 315-344.

7 Current Concepts on the Mechanism of Vision: A Lashley Heritage

Pedro Pasik and Tauba Pasik
Department of Neurology,
Mount Sinai School of Medicine
of The City University of New York

INTRODUCTION

It was during our earliest contact with psychology that we first heard of Karl Spencer Lashley, almost 40 years ago, in Argentina. There was nothing particularly positive about what we were taught. Public education, although secular, was strongly influenced by the ultra-conservative church of Pious XII, and as a result, the required psychology course contained an entire section entitled "Critique to Psychometrics." Through a series of purely metaphysical arguments, it attempted to prove the actual foolishness of the subject on the grounds that psychological phenomena by their very nature were immeasurable. The major attack against Wundt expanded to include, among others, a fellow by the name of Lashley, who not only claimed to do these measurements but dared to talk about intelligence in rats! Fifteen years later we had already embarked in neuropsychological research and were privileged to meet Lashley and hear his last public address at the convention of the Association for Research in Nervous and Mental Disease in December of 1956. It was indeed reassuring that during his lecture, Lashley reaffirmed in characteristically biting terms his unreadiness to accept what he called the "doctrines of scientific despair and Christian hope" (Lashley, 1958, p. 2).

Just after the appearance of the monograph celebrated in the present lectures, Lashley published a series of 18 articles under the common title *The Mechanism of Vision*, encompassing the period between 1930 and 1948. In them, he set the ground rules for the analysis of visually guided behavior using the ablation technique. First and most important was the strict reconstruction of the lesion from serial histologic sections, which he had described in detail earlier in his monograph (Lashley, 1929). Second was the critical evaluation of the behavioral tests. In the words of the outstanding electrophysiologist Ragnar Granit, when these basic rules are followed, the "ablation experiment becomes a salubrious antidote against overinterpretation of single-cell data" (Granit, 1975, p. 329). For the past 20 years we have applied these rules to explore the properties of so-called extrageniculostriate vision in rhesus monkeys—that is, the visual capacities that remain after total bilateral excision of the striate cortex. In the last 10 years we became concerned also with the synaptic architecture of the lateral geniculate nucleus. In fact, the roots of most of our research can be found in Lashley's *The Mechanism of Vision,* where he explored the behavior of rats with similar lesions as well as some anatomical aspects of the visual system of this animal; and in Heinrich Klüver's pioneering investigations on the behavior of the normal and occipital lobectomized monkey (Klüver, 1933, 1936, 1937, 1941, 1942). The mutual influence of these two giants transpires in their publications and becomes apparent in the discussion that follows.

The purpose of this presentation is to review some of our research in the light of Lashley's *The Mechanism of Vision*. The studies were made on over 100 monkeys, and it is with gratitude that we acknowledge the stimulating collaboration of our students, Drs. T. Feinberg, M. Miller, P. Schilder, S. Solomon, and J. Wininger, in some of the behavioral aspects. In addition, the anatomical work was carried out in collaboration with Dr. J. Hámori and Professor J. Szentágothai of Semmelweis University in Budapest.

METHODOLOGY AND NORMAL DATA

The Mechanism of Vision contains two papers dealing with methodology and the behavior of the normal rat (Lashley, 1930a, 1938b). The development of the jumping stand technique led to the discovery that the rat could discriminate visual patterns almost as well as the primate. The success of this method can be compared with Klüver's pulling-in technique, which this author invented for the monkey (Klüver, 1933). A remarkable parallelism can be drawn between the results in the monkey (Klüver, 1933) and in the rat (Lashley, 1938b), particularly because of the use by the latter investigator of Klüver's method of equivalent stimuli and "critical trials" (trials with no differential reward). Following this tradition, we adopted similar strategies with the pulling-in apparatus to study visually guided behavior in the monkey. One of the variants of the testing situation is depicted in Fig. 7.1, where only the food wells approach the animal while stimuli remain *stationary*. Under this condition, we could demonstrate that normal monkeys may utilize total luminous flux cues to solve a classically defined brightness discrimination problem (Schilder, Pasik, & Pasik, 1967). These monkeys were trained first to select the brighter of two equal-area squares, which, therefore, emitted the greater flux. When the positive stimulus was paired

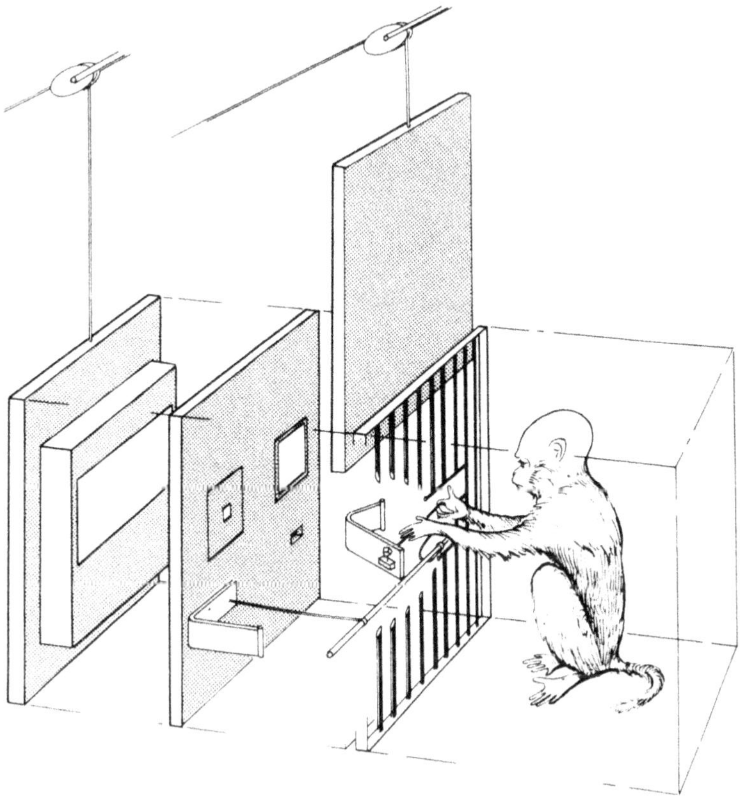

FIG. 7.1. Pulling-in apparatus with stationary stimuli. Opaque enclosure indicated by broken lines. From left to right: light source, panel containing the stimulus apertures and movable food wells, opaque guillotine door, and animal cage. A portion of the front of the cage has been omitted for clarity (from Schilder, Pasik, & Pasik, 1967).

with a larger square of the same brightness in "critical trials," the animal switched to the new target, which this time was the one emitting the greater flux. Subsequently, full retraining was required when the original positive stimulus was opposed to a larger and dimmer target in a flux-equated situation. This testing method, however, was found rather ineffective for pattern discrimination problems and was soon replaced in our studies by the pulling in of *movable* stimuli, illustrated in earlier publications (Pasik & Pasik, 1980; Schilder, Pasik, & Pasik, 1971).

Two more articles in *The Mechanism of Vision* pertain to visual acuity and refractive power of the rat's eye (Lashley, 1930c, 1932). The discrimination of vertical versus horizontal square-wave gratings of various spatial frequencies was used for the first measurement, which was found to be between 26 and 52 minutes of arc for the pigmented rat and two to five times higher for the albino. With respect to the focal range, Lashley discovered a "marked myopia" in all eyes examined, which contradicted the view, current at the time, that rats were hypermetropic. Klüver determined visual acuity in a cebus monkey with the pulling-in technique in terms of *minimum visibile* and obtained figures as low as 0.3 minutes of arc (Klüver, 1933). Subsequent investigations in rhesus monkeys using square-wave gratings gave values between 0.6 and 1.1 min of arc (Cowey & Ellis, 1967; Weinstein & Grether, 1940; Weiskrantz & Cowey, 1963). Our data (Miller, Pasik, & Pasik, 1980), derived from the contrast sensitivity functions of sinusoidal gratings of four monkeys, indicate a mean acuity value equivalent to 0.7 min of arc ($SD = 0.02$). The same monkeys were examined with an automated, computerized retinoscope that measures 2000 samples of the far point in various meridians in 3 seconds (Safir, 1972). The animals were found to have one emmetropic eye (± 0.50 diopter—D) and the other, slightly myopic (−0.7/1.3 D) or hyperopic (+0.9 D). In addition they all had some degree of astigmatism in a particular meridian varying from 1.6 to 2.4 D.

EXTRAGENICULOSTRIATE VISION

A major group of papers in *The Mechanism of Vision* series have as a central theme the testing of rats with destruction of the visual cortical areas. Lashley (1931) found that rats with practically complete striatectomy jumped readily and oriented to visual targets. They adjusted the force of the jump to various distances but were less accurate than normals and rats reared in darkness (Lashley & Russell, 1934). Operated animals relearned to jump to a white target and solved a size discrimination problem but failed it when targets were equated for total luminous flux, a measurement referred to by Lashley as total luminosity. Pattern tests were also failed except for one animal that could discriminate horizontal from vertical stripes as narrow as 2.9°. It is interesting that this was the only subject with verified 100% bilateral destruction of striate cortex. The ablation did not influence the rate of formation of a light versus no-light discrimination habit, but the differential "intensity" threshold was increased (Lashley, 1930b). In view of these findings, he used aphakic rats to find out whether learning with or without visual cortex utilized different aspects of the stimuli. These animals lacked pattern vision even before the destruction of the striate cortex, and therefore the postoperative loss of the "brightness" habit could not be attributed to interference with detail vision and the forced use of some different visual modality (Lashley, 1937a). Partial striatectomies gave little evidence of differential effects in relation to the region ablated except for a small anterolateral portion that appeared crucial for pattern vision. It was later proven, however, that the deleterious effects of its resection were due to damage to the optic radiations

(Lashley & Frank, 1932). The retention of a preoperatively learned pattern discrimination required at least 8% of striate cortex (Lashley & Frank, 1934) and the consequent preservation of 400 to 700 geniculate neurons (Lashley, 1939). Most of the qualitative observations of these studies applied also to the destriated monkey, according to the extensive analysis of Klüver (1936, 1937, 1941, 1942), who concluded that total luminous flux was the only effective visual cue for this animal. This interpretation was based on the results of "critical trials" showing no differential response to figures differing in brightness and area but equated for flux.

Our initial observations on monkeys deprived of striate cortex (Pasik, Pasik, & Schilder, 1969) confirmed Klüver's findings, but in addition, with continued training on flux-equated figures using differential reward, all the animals eventually solved the problem, requiring about 2000 trials to reach the established criterion for successful performance. (Our procedures call for up to 6000 or 7000 trials before a failure is recognized.) These results did not necessarily negate Klüver's conclusion, since destriated monkeys might still detect differences in the rate of change of luminous flux during eye, head, and/or body movements, particularly when either target was being partially excluded from the sampled space. Thus, the rate of change during a horizontal scanning was higher when a small bright target, as opposed to a large dim target, was being eliminated from the visual field. In addition to this possibility, it was necessary to rule out the suggested role of the amount of contour (Weiskrantz, 1963) before ascertaining the occurrence of a straightforward brightness and/or area discrimination. For this purpose, monkeys were trained on four successive tasks containing the same brightness difference (Schilder, Pasik, & Pasik, 1971): (1) a small dim circle versus a small bright circle of equal area, differing in both brightness and total luminous flux; (2) a large dim circle versus the same small bright circle, differing in brightness, area, and contour and equated for flux; (3) the same large dim circle versus a bright annulus with the outside diameter equal to that of the opposing target and the same area and brightness as the small bright circle of Tests 1 and 2 (these targets had the same differences in brightness and area as in Test 2; the relative amount of contour was the reverse of test 2; and the overall surface and flux were equated); and (4) the same large dim circle versus another annulus of the same area but with the sum of outer and inner circumferences equal to the circumference of the opposing target. (These figures differed in brightness, area, and overall surface and were equated for contour and flux.) The first test was solved on the basis of flux differences since the second test had to be relearned with no transfer effects. The other three tests, however, with no flux differences present, were mastered with decreasing numbers of errors and almost perfect transfer across them. The targets of the third test, by covering the same overall surface, minimized the possibility of solving the problem utilizing different rates of change in flux during eye, head, and/or body movements. The fourth test eliminated the amount of contour as the differential cue. The conclusion was inescapable that brightness and/or area discrimination had been established with some degree of perceptual "constancy" present in the situation.

By this time, it became clear that we had a powerful behavioral paradigm to demonstrate visual capacities in the absence of striate cortex, and we decided to attempt the training of destriated monkeys on color and pattern discrimination (Pasik & Pasik, 1971; Schilder, Pasik, & Pasik, 1972). In this study, operated monkeys succeeded in mastering three tests with equated-flux figures without previous training with flux-differing targets. These tasks were a small bright versus a large dim circle, a circle versus triangle, and a red versus green discrimination. In addition, one other animal solved a red versus achromatic discrimination problem, the two targets being behaviorally equated for brightness. These least expected results were backed by extensive controls given as "critical trials." They stand in direct contradiction to the findings of both Lashley in the rat and Klüver in the monkey and have recently been confirmed in another laboratory (Keating, 1979; Dineen & Keating, 1981).

A further step in understanding extrageniculostriate vision was geared to find out the nature of the remaining pattern vision. Psychophysical and electrophysiological experiments have suggested that certain elementary stimulus attributes are important for normal pattern recognition. These characteristics are the spatial frequencies extractable by Fourier analysis from the edges present in the target, together with their contrasts and orientations (Campbell, 1974). In fact, the striate cortex is especially suited for these functions since its neurons apparently receive both orientation and spatial frequency information in an overlapping, three-dimensional lattice arrangement (Maffei & Fiorentini, 1977). In view of the demonstration of residual pattern vision in destriated monkeys after prolonged training, it became important to determine their discriminative capacities for orientation and spatial frequency as well as their limits at various contrasts. The experiments were conducted in the same pulling-in apparatus with movable, transilluminated stimuli using a three-stage forced-choice psychophysical procedure. The animals were trained to criterion on a maximal difference (vertical vs. horizontal luminous line; homogeneous target vs. sinusoidal gratings of high contrast equated for mean luminance), followed by estimation of the threshold according to an adaptive staircase procedure, and ending with the determination of the limen by the method of constant stimuli with seven values pivoting around the previous estimate. One hundred responses were accumulated for each step, and the resultant psychometric functions straighten on a transformed probability scale. The threshold was derived from a linear least-squares solution as the value eliciting 75% correct responses. Figure 7.2 depicts the psychometric function for bar orientation in one illustrative monkey before and after the ablations. The stimuli were narrow bars of about $16° \times 0.3°$. It was indeed remarkable that a monkey without striate cortex could still disciminate a

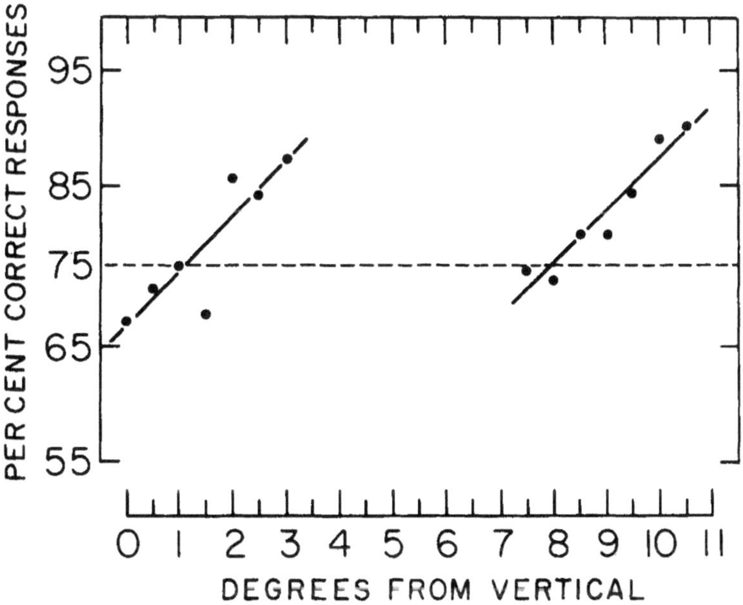

FIG. 7.2. Psychometric functions for orientation of luminous bar. The ordinate represents the number of correct responses in 100 trials given with each orientation on a probability scale transformed so that $z = 0$ at the 75% level instead of the standard 50% level. Left and right functions were obtained before and after complete striatectomies, respectively. Note that threshold values increase from approximately 1° to 8°

bar deviating from the vertical by as little as 8° (Pasik, Pasik, Nolan & Solomon, 1976).

In a more recent study, contrast sensitivity functions were determined again before and after total striatectomy (Miller et al., 1980). This experiment was required to define the contrast thresholds for detection of sinusoidal gratings with spatial frequencies of 0.5, 1.0, 2.0, 4.0, 8.0, 16 and 32 cycles per degree (cy/deg) of visual angle, using contrast values between 79% and 0.6%. Figure 7.3 illustrates the findings in one of the animals. It is apparent that the normal monkey could master the discrimination of all gratings at maximum contrast, whereas the operated animal could only solve the problem with gratings between 0.5 and 4.0 cy/deg or, at most, 8.0 cy/deg when the criterion for successful performance was set at a lower value (84% instead of 90% correct responses). The highest frequency cutoff level—that is, the highest spatial frequency detected at maximum contrast, determined by extrapolation—gave an estimate of classical visual acuity. It is seen that in this monkey, the ablations reduced the value from 41 to 13 cy/deg. Using a half cycle as the minimal discriminable

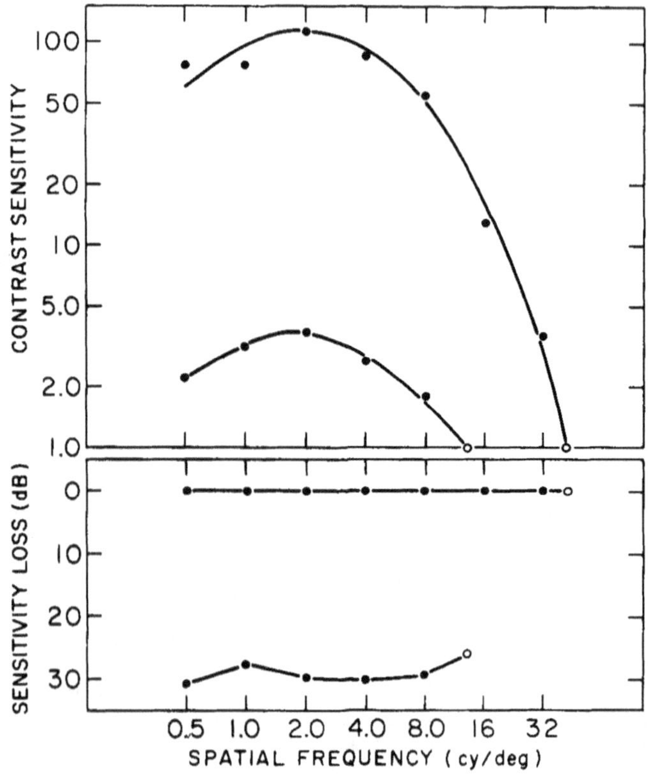

FIG. 7.3. Contrast sensitivity function (above) before (top curve) and after (bottom curve) complete striatectomies. Note the decrease of the highest frequency cutoff point and the marked depression of the remaining function. Sensitivity loss (below) expressed as 20 times the logarithm of the preoperative/postoperative sensitivity ratio. The bottom values reflect an almost flat loss of approximately 30 db (from Miller, Pasik, & Pasik, 1980).

difference, this destriated animal had an acuity of about 2.3 minutes of arc, representing about 20/80 vision on the Snellen chart. The most important finding, however, was the loss of sensitivity for the perceivable gratings, so that considerably more contrast was necessary for detection as compared to the normal. The loss was approximately 30 db at all frequencies (Fig. 7.3). These results cannot be attributed to changes in refractive power, since postoperative values were similar to those obtained preoperatively (see preceding). It is tempting to conclude that persistent, albeit reduced, sensitivity to bar orientation and to spatial frequency and contrasts of gratings are important factors supporting the residual capacity for pattern discrimination in the destriated monkey.

The jumping accuracy of Lashley's destriated rats can be interpreted as a relatively preserved visual space localization. Although this ability was not discovered in similarly operated monkeys (Klüver, 1942), there were indications from work on one such animal with incomplete ablations that it could localize visual events in space (Humphrey, 1974). We pursued this matter in monkeys with histologically verified total excision of the striate cortex and found that, indeed, they could be trained to reach accurately for a rather small (2°) and low-contrast (11%) target consisting of an apple cube on a white background (Feinberg, Pasik, & Pasik, 1977, 1978; Solomon, Pasik, & Pasik, 1979). A concurrent investigation showed further that at least one totally destriated monkey succeeded in reaching accurately to the source of a 110-msec flash (Weiskrantz, Cowey, & Passingham, 1977). This latter finding ruled out the role of eye movements in locating the target by proprioceptive feedback, since the duration of the stimulus was below the latency for visually elicited saccades.

CRITICAL STRUCTURES FOR EXTRAGENICULOSTRIATE VISION

The Mechanism of Vision also comprises several articles concerned with the subject of critical structures for extrageniculostriate vision. From the several possible candidates responsible for the reacquisition of so-called brightness discrimination habits (in fact, the discriminanda differed also in total luminous flux), Lashley quickly disposed of the lateral geniculate nuclei because they degenerated completely after striatectomy (Lashley, 1935). In the same publication, he also ruled out other structures on the basis of the preservation of the habit after additional ablations of peristriate cortex and of other cortical areas. It should be noted that he failed to recognize the crucial role of total luminous flux, as opposed to brightness (luminance), in guiding the visual behavior of the operated rats, although he was aware of this factor in the earlier size discrimination experiments (Lashley, 1931). The only additional lesion that eliminated the habit was the destruction of the so-called optic thalamus. This designation meant something different than the classic definition of the term, which was equivalent, in the anatomy texts of that time, to the entire dorsal thalamus or the thalamus proper of today (Gray, 1930). In any event, Lashley included in his "optic thalamus" a group of nuclei identified currently within the pretectum: "pretectile nucleus," lateral region of the nucleus of the posterior commissure, "large-celled nucleus of Clark" (probably the olivary nucleus of the pretectum), and the pars posterior of the lateral nucleus, which he believed was the homologue of the pulvinar. A confounding factor, however, was that damage to these nuclear masses also destroyed the optic tracts and, with them, the visual input to the superior colliculus. Lashley (1935) concluded that "in the absence of the striate cortex the reaction to light is dependent upon some part of the complex of structures included in the optic thalamus and colliculi [p. 68]." In the same publication, he dismissed the accessory optic system because the effective additional lesions destroying the optic tracts were located such that the accessory tracts had already separated from the main pathway and, therefore, were presumably spared. The earlier suggestion that the critical structures were the superior colliculi (Lashley, 1931) was subsequently disproven by Lashley's students (Ghiselli, 1938; Layman, 1936). In further studies on the role of the "optic thalamus" and superior colliculi, Lashley found that estimation of distance was maintained after destruction of these regions if the geniculostriate system was preserved. He recognized, however, that total ablation of those structures had not been achieved (Lashley, 1937b).

Finally, Lashley (1942) offered some evidence against simple serial processing of visual information at successively linked cortical fields. Deficits even in rather complex tests, such as the so-called conditional reaction, could be accounted for only by large central scotomata due to lesions of the striate cortex and/or by a motor disturbance interfering with the response requirements of the tests—namely, jumping. This functional autonomy of the visual cortex with respect to other cortical areas received further support in the last and only article in the series utilizing primates (spider monkeys, *Ateles geoffroyi*) (Lashley, 1948). In this study, ablation of at least 60% of prestriate cortex failed to produce visual discrimination deficits except in both conditional and delayed reactions in some of the animals. The conclusions were that the possible influence of the striate cortex on other cortical areas involved in visual processes was mediated through indirect pathways via subcortical structures. However, Lashley cautiously pointed out that a crucial region could not be ruled out, because the cortex along the occipitotemporal and collateral sulci had been spared in his animals. Apparently, the controversy has lasted until present times, as can be found in recent excellent reviews (Dean, 1976; Gross, 1973).

Our own work on critical structures for extrageniculostriate vision in the monkey attempted first to explain the discrepancy between our results (see preceding) and the conclusions of Klüver (1942). From sources discussed elsewhere (Pasik & Pasik, 1971), it became apparent that Klüver's monkeys had more ample lobectomies, probably at the level of the ascending limb of the superior temporal sulcus as opposed to the lunate sulcus. Indeed, we were able to show that monkeys with such extensive removals could discriminate equal-area figures differing in brightness but failed to distinguish the same brightness differences when the figures were equated for flux by appropriately enlarging the dimmer one. It was suggested, therefore, that the circumstriate cortex, which was totally destroyed in these animals, was critical for solving problems with flux-equated targets. The next subject of inquiry was the source of visual information to the circumstriate cortex in the absence of the geniculostriate system. It is known that the superior colliculus projects to the inferior pulvinar, which in turn is the origin of afferent fibers to the circumstriate cortex (Benevento & Rezak, 1976). In a series of experiments we trained monkeys on the same two tests of the previous study before and after the standard occipital lobectomy, which removes the striate totally but the circumstriate cortex, only partially. In a second stage, either the superior colliculi (Pasik, Pasik, Schilder, & Wininger, 1973) or the inferior pulvinars were destroyed (unpublished results). The effects in all were comparable to those of the extended lobectomies; that is, the monkeys could discriminate flux-differing figures and failed when the targets were equated for flux. In a more recent study we also demonstrated that the superior colliculi were essential for space localization in the absence, but not in the presence, of striate cortex (Solomon et al., 1979). Apparently, the colliculus may be sufficient for this capacity since it survives ample removals of striate and circumstriate cortices (Keating, 1980).

Although the previous experiments emphasized the importance of the superior colliculi for many manifestations of extrageniculostriate vision, the fact remained that monkeys without striate cortex *and* superior colliculi could still perform a visual discrimination if the targets differed in total luminous flux. It is obvious that there must be other structures mediating this residual elementary capacity. The search succeeded in earlier investigations (Pasik & Pasik, 1973a, 1973b) using a much simpler behavioral paradigm, as illustrated in Fig. 7.4. Monkeys were trained to press the lighted one of a pair of neon bulbs arranged horizontally. When the habit was reestablished after striatectomies, bilateral lesions were made in one of several structures considered to participate in the visual process; inferotemporal cortex, posterior parahippocampal cortex, pulvinars, pretectum, superior colliculi. None of these additional destructions abolished the habit permanently. Only when a large lesion was made in the mesodiencephalic junction involving the superior colliculi and the medial and lateral pretectal regions did the performance of the test remain close to chance for 6000 trials. It was also noted that as a result of the damage, there was severe degeneration of a nucleus located ventral to the brachium of the inferior colliculus, presumably representing the caudal portion of the lateral terminal nucleus of the accessory optic tract (Pasik & Pasik, 1980). We further showed that this region receives optic fibers from both the contralateral eye and the ipsilateral eye (Pasik, Pasik, & Hámori, 1973). When this nucleus was destroyed bilaterally, with minimal damage to the superior colliculi, in addition to total striatectomies, the animals also failed the test in 6000 trials. This finding strongly suggested that visual input through the accessory optic system is essential for the ability of destriated monkeys to discriminate differences in total luminous flux (Pasik & Pasik, 1973a). The discrepancy with the conclusions of Lashley (1935) that the integrity of the accessory optic tract was not sufficient to maintain extrageniculostriate vision is difficult to resolve since no detailed description of his lesions is available. It is very possible, for example, that the accessory optic tracts were spared but that their terminal nuclei were destroyed by the massive lesions of the "optic thalamus" and superior colliculi (Lashley, 1935).

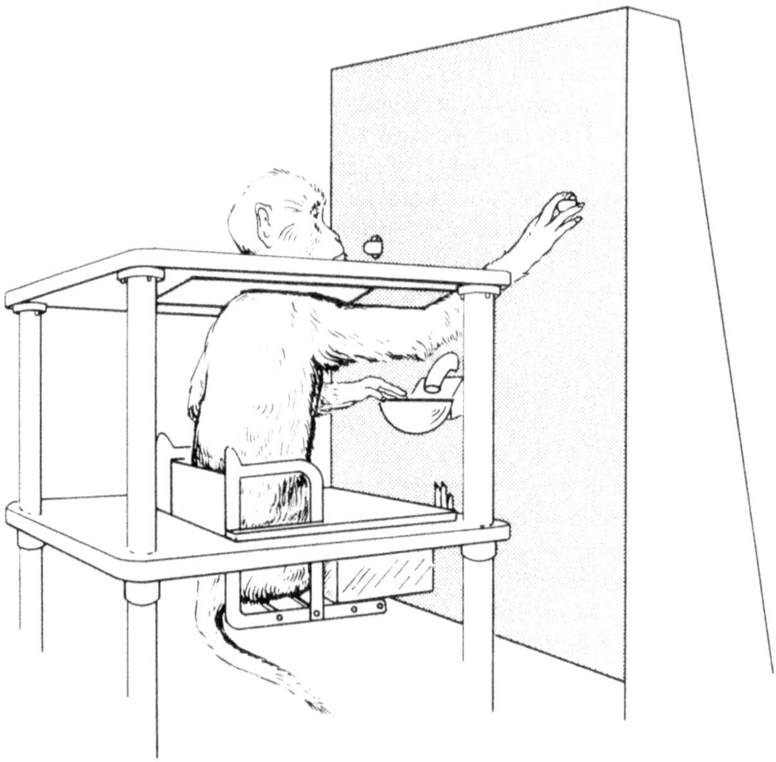

FIG. 7.4. Testing situation for light versus no-light discrimination. Either the right or the left pilot light is lit in each trial according to Gellerman schedules. Pressing the "on" stimulus results in delivery of a glucose pellet into the reward cup. The monkey and the stimulus panel are enclosed in an isolation booth (not shown) (from Pasik & Pasik, 1973b).

ANATOMICAL CONSIDERATIONS

The last subject covered in *The Mechanism of Vision* is strictly anatomical and involves studies on the structure and image-forming power of the eye (Lashley, 1932), already commented upon earlier, as well as on the sites of termination of retinal fibers (Lashley, 1934a) and the cortical projections of the lateral geniculate nucleus (Lashley, 1934b). In addition, there is a quantitative analysis of numerical relationships along the visual pathway (Lashley, 1938a), fortunately reviewed in a later publication (Lashley, 1939). The original article was unavailable to the present authors from libraries in New York and New Jersey as well as from the National Library of Medicine. Of direct relevance to our own research are the studies on the pars dorsalis of the lateral geniculate nucleus (LGNd), which were made essentially by causing retrograde degeneration through circumscribed resections of the striate cortex (Lashley, 1934b). Based on thionin-stained material, only one type of neuron was recognized in the normal nucleus. In two rats, 3 months after total destruction of the striate cortex, Lashley found about 40% remaining neurons, but "not a single normal ganglion cell could be identified" (Lashley, 1934b, p. 60). Abnormalities were described as shriveled nuclei and failure of both nuclei and cell bodies to stain sharply. It is possible that the proportion of residual neurons was overestimated because the overall shrinkage of the degenerated nucleus apparently was not taken into consideration. Statements as to the condition of the LGNd after striate ablation varied in subsequent papers. Without specifying survival time, it is said, for example, that after partial cortical lesions, the geniculate ganglion cells disappeared completely from a limited region (Lashley, 1939) or that normal cells could occasionally be seen either scattered in the degenerated areas (Lashley & Frank, 1934) or along the margin of the pars ventralis (Lashley, 1935).

In the monkey, we have always seen few remaining neurons in the LGNd after resection of the entire striate cortex. These observations led to a change in the classic criterion for complete ablation. Instead of the "total" degeneration of the LGNd (Lashley & Frank, 1934; Polyak, 1957), we adopted the actual examination of the remaining cortical tissue for verifying the absence of striate cortex. It is of interest that Lashley ignored evidence available at the time that pointed to the existence of short-axoned cells in the LGNd, in addition to the principal or projecting neurons (for review, see Polyak, 1957). This was probably because the 1930s were a dormant period in the use of the Golgi method, and not enough significance was being given to the observations made with it. There is no question today that essential components of the LGNd organization are Golgi Type II cells or interneurons, some of which are still present after chronic resection of striate and circumstriate cortices (Pasik, Pasik, Hámori, & Szentágothai, 1973). Figure 7.5 depicts these findings in Nissl preparations, similar to those illustrated by Lashley (1934b) but showing a surviving cell in the midst of the gliotic stroma of a "totally" degenerated LGNd. The information on these neurons in the monkey LGNd at the light-microscopy level remains scanty and limited to few incidental observations (Ball', Portugalov, & Shkol'nik-Yarros, 1964; Campos-Ortega, Glees, & Neuhoff, 1968; Pasik, Pasik, Hámori, & Szentágothai, 1973; Szentágothai, 1973). Moreover, their characterization at the electron microscopy level is only inferential, since no direct correlation has ever been made between light and electron microscopic pictures of the same interneurons. The ultrastructure and synaptic articulations of these cells, however, have been studied intensely on the basis of indirect evidence. They appear to have scanty cytoplasm which is poor in all common organelles but displays synaptic vesicles and presynaptic sites in all regions—namely, the soma, proximal and distal dendrites, as well as the axon hillock, axon initial segment, and terminal boutons (Hámori, Pasik, & Pasik, 1978; Pasik, Pasik, & Hámori, 1976) (Figs. 7.6 and 7.7). The existence of so-called presynaptic dendrites and somata—that is, post-

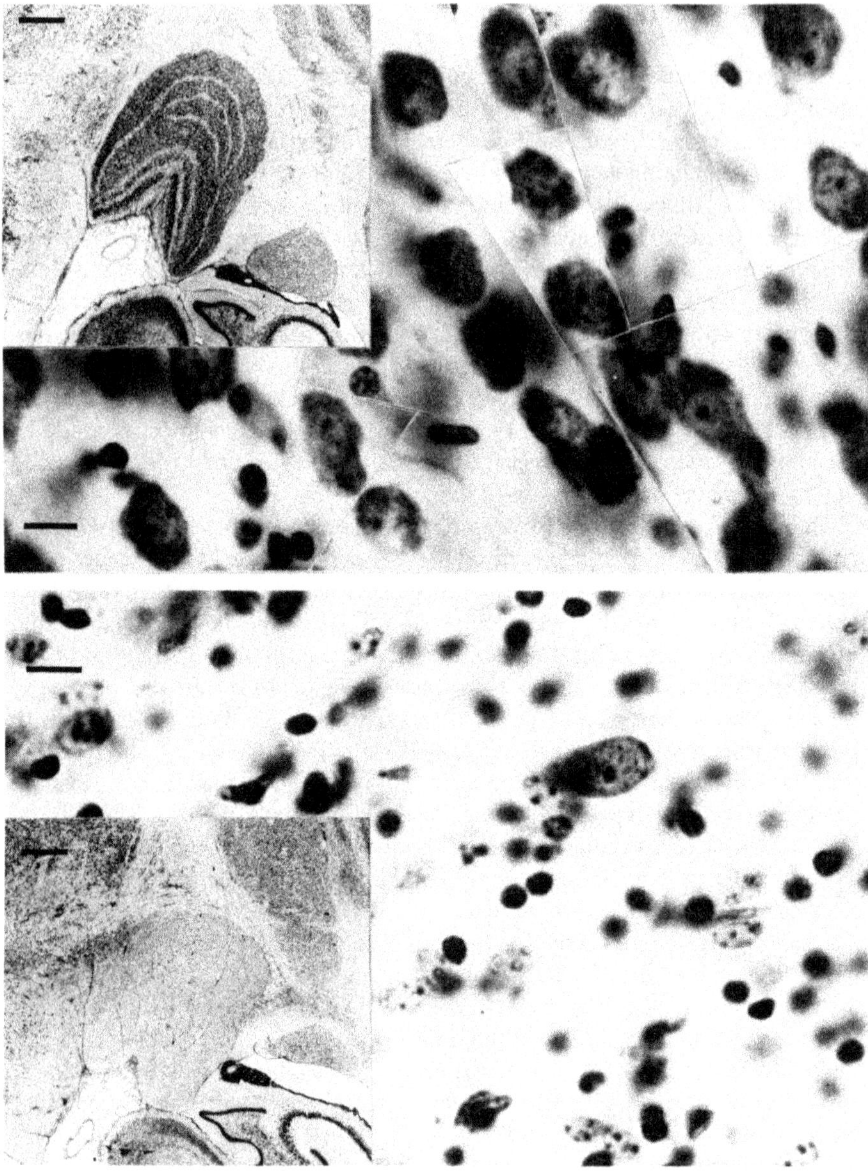

FIG. 7.5. Lateral geniculate nucleus in the normal (top) and 16 months after total removal of striate cortex (bottom)—cresyl violet stain. Low-magnification photographs show the general appearance of the nuclei (scale: 1 mm). High magnification reveals the normal neuronal population at the top and the presence of an apparently normal neuron amidst glial proliferation in the "totally" degenerated nucleus at the bottom (scale: 10 μm.).

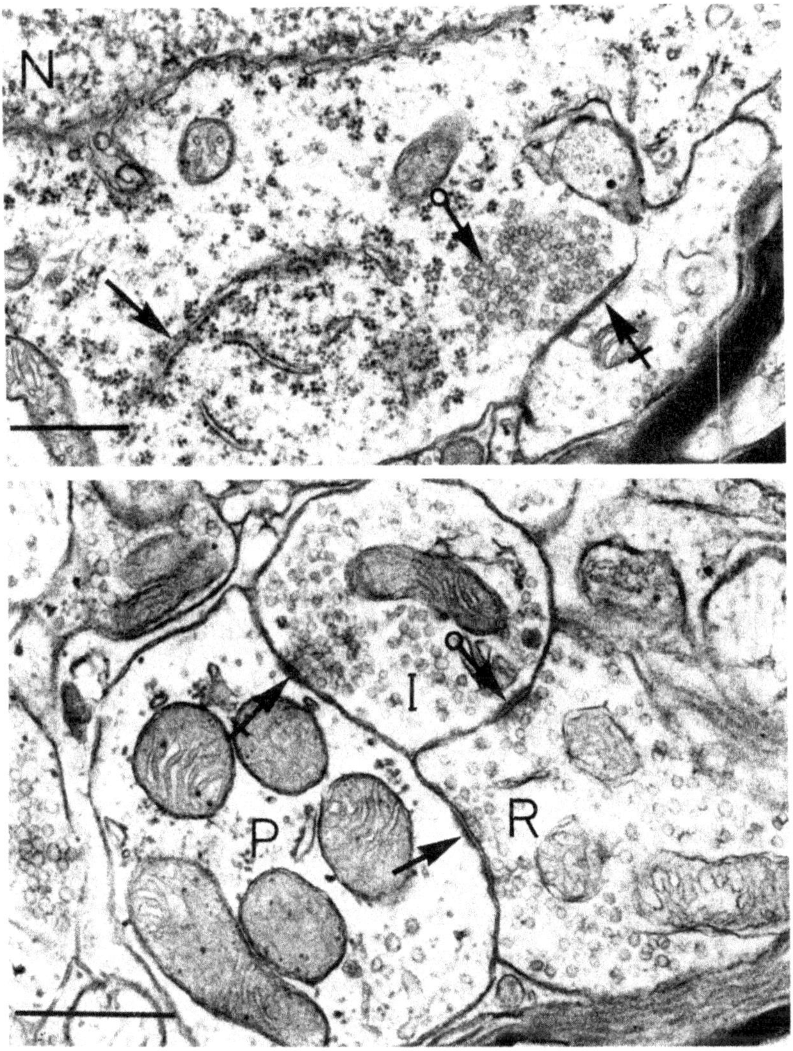

FIG. 7.6. Electron micrograph of LGNd. Top: Part of the soma of an interneuron with nucleus (N), rough endoplasmic reticulum (arrow), and an accumulation of synaptic vesicles (ringed arrow). There is a somatodendritic synapse (crossed arrow) with a profile probably belonging to a dendrite of another interneuron, also containing a few vesicles (scale: 0.5 μm.). Bottom: Synaptic triad made by a retinal terminal (R), recognized for its mitochondria with wide intercrestal spaces and spheroid vesicles. This profile is presynaptic to a principal cell dendrite (P) at arrow and to an interneuron dendrite (I) at ringed arrow, in turn presynaptic to the same principal cell profile at crossed arrow (scale: 0.5 μm) (from Hámori, Pasik, & Pasik, 1975).

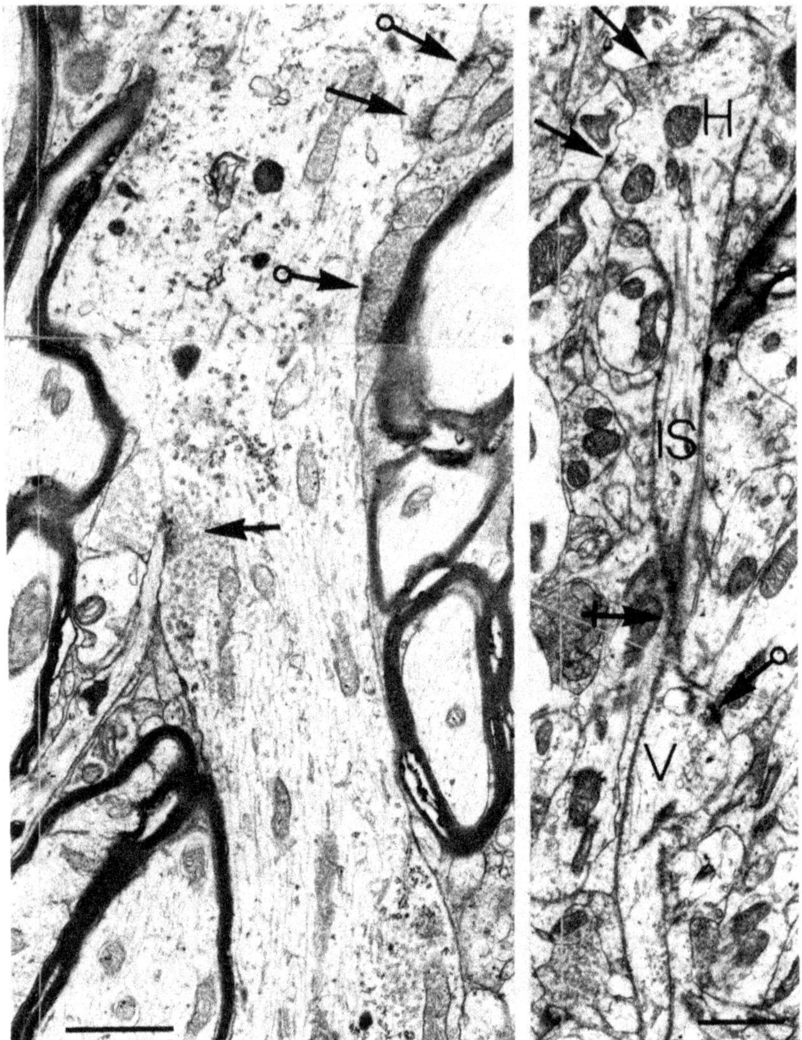

FIG. 7.7. Electron micrographs of LGNd. Left: Proximal dendrite of an interneuron containing synaptic vesicles and showing presynaptic (arrows) and postsynaptic sites (ringed arrows) (scale: 1 μm) (from Hámori, Pasik, & Pasik, 1975). Right: Axon hillock (H) and axon initial segment (IS) of an interneuron. The hillock contains vesicles and is presynaptic at arrows. The IS shows fasciculation of microtubules and subaxolemmal density that is interrupted at a varicosity (V) filled with vesicles and is presynaptic to another profile (ringed arrow). Continuity of the two elements at crossed arrow was verified in serial sections (scale: 1 μm) (from Hámori, Pasik, & Pasik, 1978).

synaptic elements that, in the immediate vicinity, are also presynaptic—gives rise to a multiplicity of complex synaptic arrangements. The most common is the *triadic* synapse where a retinal terminal is presynaptic to a principal cell dendrite and to an interneuron dendrite, the latter being, in turn, presynaptic to the same principal cell element (Fig. 7.6). The input to the triad, instead of a retinal terminal, may be of cortical origin or a part of another interneuron (Pasik & Pasik, 1979; Pasik, Pasik, & Hámori, 1977). Similarly, the output element, instead of belonging to a principal cell, may be an interneuron dendrite. Simpler but less frequent arrangements are *serial* synapses where an input element is presynaptic to an interneuron presynaptic dendrite, which in turn is presynaptic to an output element. Finally, although rare, there are also *reciprocal* synapses where both polarities are present within the same synaptic plaque between two interneuron profiles. This complex synaptology of triadic, serial, and reciprocal articulations offers multiple possibilities for processing the visual information given by the spatial and temporal characteristics of the stimuli. The capabilities of the neuronal networks are even more enhanced when one considers, for example, that several triads can be coupled either through a single presynaptic dendrite common to all of them or through synaptically connected elements of different interneurons (Lábos, 1977).

CONCLUDING REMARKS

The preceding review summarized Lashley's viewpoints on the mechanism of vision. It was not intended to be unbiased. On the contrary, Lashley's concepts were critically evaluated in the light of our own research. Some of his basic ideas still stand, others have been superseded. In addition to strictly morphologic matters, we have given some answers to "what" and "with what" the destriated monkey sees. The lasting question is "how?" It is appropriate to close with Lashley's own words: "Always the question How? punctures the bubble of theory, and the answer is to be sought in analysis and ever more analysis" (Lashley, 1933, p. x).

DEDICATION

We wish to dedicate this presentation to Professor Morris B. Bender, our inspiring teacher, on the occasion of his 75th birthday.

ACKNOWLEDGMENTS

All of our work reviewed here has been made possible by the generous and uninterrupted support of the National Institute of Mental Health through Research Grant #MH-02261. Our thanks are also due to Minerva Feliciano for her invaluable secretarial help and to Victor Rodriguez for technical assistance.

REFERENCES

Ball', T. V., Portugalov, V. V., & Shkol'nik-Yarros, E. G. On the structural and histochemical characteristics of the lateral geniculate body in monkeys. *Zhurnal vysshei nervoi Deyatel'nosti imeni I. P. Pavlova,* 1964, *4,* 707–713 (in Russian).

Benevento, L. A., & Rezak, M. The cortical projections of the inferior pulvinar and adjacent lateral pulvinar in the rhesus monkey (Macaca mulatta): An autoradiographic study. *Brain Research,* 1976, *108,* 1-24.

Campbell, F. W. The transmission of spatial information through the visual system. In F. O. Schmitt & F. G. Worden (Eds.), *The neurosciences third study program.* Cambridge, Mass.: M.I.T. Press, 1974.

Campos-Ortega, J. A., Glees, P., & Neuhoff, V. Ultrastructural analysis of individual layers in the lateral geniculate body of the monkey. *Zeitschrift fur Zellforschung und mikroscopische anatomie,* 1968, *87,* 82–100.

Cowey, A., & Ellis, C. M. Visual acuity of rhesus and squirrel monkeys. *Journal of Comparative and Physiological Psychology,* 1967, *64,* 80–84.

Dean, P. Effects of inferotemporal lesions on the behavior of monkeys. *Psychological Bulletin,* 1976, *83,* 41–71.

Dineen, J., & Keating, E. G. The primate visual system after bilateral removal of striate cortex. Survival of complex pattern vision. *Experimental Brain Research,* 1981, *41,* 338-345.

Feinberg, T., Pasik, P., & Pasik, T. Visually mediated space localization in monkeys without striate cortex. *Federation Proceedings,* 1977, *36,* 507.

Feinberg, T. E., Pasik, T., & Pasik, P. Extrageniculostriate vision in the monkey. VI. Visually guided accurate reaching behavior. *Brain Research,* 1978, *152,* 422–428.

Ghiselli, E. E. The relationship between the superior colliculus and the striate area in brightness discrimination. *Journal of Genetic Psychology,* 1938, *52,* 151-157.

Granit, R. A. Half a century in the neurosciences: Personal comments on choices and decisions. In F. C. Worden, J. P. Swazey, & G. Adelman (Eds.), *The neurosciences: Paths of discovery.* Cambridge, Mass.: M.I.T. Press, 1975.

Gray, H. *Anatomy of the human body* (W. H. Lewis, Ed., 22nd Ed.). Philadelphia: Lea & Febiger, 1930.

Gross, C. G. Visual functions of inferotemporal cortex. In R. Jung (Ed.), *Central processing of Visual Information: Handbook of Sensory Physiology* (Vol. VII/3 B). Berlin, Heidelberg, and New York: Springer, 1973.

Hámori, J., Pasik, P., & Pasik, T. Postnatal differentiation of "presynaptic dendrites" in the lateral geniculates nucleus of the rhesus monkey. In G. W. Kreutzberg (Ed.) *Physiology and pathology of dendrites. Advances in Neurology,* Vol. 12, 1975.

Hámori, J., Pasik, T., & Pasik, P. Electron microscopic identification of axonal initial segments belonging to interneurons in the dorsal lateral geniculate nucleus of monkey. *Neuroscience,* 1978, *3,* 403–412.

Humphrey, N. K. Vision in a monkey without striate cortex: A case study. *Perception,* 1974, *3,* 241-255.

Keating, E. G. Rudimentary color vision in the monkey after removal of striate and preoccipital cortex. *Brain Research,* 1979, *179,* 379–384.

Keating, E. G. Residual spatial vision in the monkey after removal of striate and preoccipital cortex. *Brain Research,* 1980, *187,* 271-290.

Klüver, H. *Behavior mechanisms in monkeys.* Chicago: University of Chicago Press, 1933.

Klüver, H. An analysis of the effects of the removal of the occipital lobes in monkeys. *Journal of Psychology,* 1936, *2,* 49–61.

Klüver, H. Certain effects of lesions of the occipital lobes in monkeys. *Journal of Psychology,* 1937, *4,* 383-401.

Klüver, H. Visual functions after removal of the occipital lobes. *Journal of Psychology,* 1941, *11,* 23–45.

Klüver, H. Functional significance of the geniculostriate system. *Biological Symposia*, 1942, *7*, 253-299.
Lábos, E. Theoretical considerations of local neuron circuits and their triadic synaptic arrangements (TSA) in subcortical sensory nuclei. *Journal of Neuroscience Research*, 1977, *3*, 1-10.
Lashley, K. S. *Brain mechanisms and intelligence. A quantitative study of inquiries to the brain*. Chicago: University of Chicago Press, 1929.
Lashley, K. S. The mechanism of vision: I. A method for rapid analysis of pattern-vision in the rat. *Journal of Genetic Psychology*, 1930, *37*, 453-460. (a)
Lashley, K. S. The mechanism of vision: II. The influence of cerebral lesions upon the threshold of discrimination for brightness in the rat. *Journal of Genetics Psychology*, 1930, *37*, 461-480. (b)
Lashley, K. S. The mechanism of vision: III. The comparative visual acuity of pigmented and albino rats. *Journal of Genetic Psychology*, 1930, *37*, 481-484. (c)
Lashley, K. S. The mechanism of vision: IV. The cerebral areas necessary for pattern vision in the rat. *Journal of Comparative Neurology*, 1931, *53*, 419-478.
Lashley, K. S. The mechanism of vision: V. The structure and image-forming power of the rat's eye. *Journal of Comparative Psychology*, 1932, *13*, 173-200.
Lashley, K. S. Introduction to Klüver, H. *Behavior mechanisms in monkeys*. Chicago: University of Chicago Press, 1933.
Lashley, K. S. The mechanism of vision: VII. The projection of the retina upon the primary optic centers in the rat. *Journal of Comparative Neurology*, 1934, *59*, 341-373. (a)
Lashley, K. S. The mechanism of vision: VIII. The projection of the retina upon the cerebral cortex of the rat. *Journal of Comparative Neurology*, 1934, *60*, 57-79. (b)
Lashley, K. S. The mechanism of vision: XII. Nervous structures concerned in the acquisition and retention of habits based on reactions to light. *Comparative Psychology Monographs*, 1935, *2*, 43-79.
Lashley, K. S. The mechanism of vision: XIII. Cerebral function in discrimination of brightness when detail vision is controlled. *Journal of Comparative Neurology*, 1937, *66*, 471-480. (a)
Lashley, K. S. The mechanism of vision: XIV. Visual perception of distance after injuries to the cerebral cortex, colliculi, or optic thalamus. *Journal of Genetic Psychology*, 1937, *50-51*, 189-207. (b)
Lashley, K. S. The mechanism of vision: IX. The numerical relations of cells in the visual system of the rat. *Ukrainskii Psikhonevrologicheskii Akademia*, 1938. (a)
Lashley, K. S. The mechanism of vision: XV. Preliminary studies of the rat's capacity for detail vision. *Journal of Genetic Psychology*, 1938, *18*, 123-193. (b)
Lashley, K. S. The mechanism of vision: XVI. The functioning of small remnants of the visual cortex. *Journal of Comparative Neurology*, 1939, *70*, 45-67
Lashley, K. S. The mechanism of vision: XVII. Autonomy of the visual cortex. *Journal of Genetic Psychology*, 1942, *60*, 197-221.
Lashley, K. S. The mechanism of vision: XVIII. Effects of destroying the visual "associative areas" of the monkey. *Genetic Psychology Monographs*, 1948, *37*, 107-166.
Lashley, K. S. Cerebral organization and behavior. In H. C. Solomon, S. Cobb, & W. Penfield (Eds.), *The brain and human behavior (Research Publications of the Association for Research in Nervous and Mental Diseases*, Vol. 36). Baltimore, Md.: Williams & Wilkins, 1958.
Lashley, K. S., & Frank, M. The mechanism of vision: VI. The lateral portion of the area striata in the rat: A correction. *Journal of Comparative Neurology*, 1932, *55*, 525-529.
Lashley, K. S., & Frank, M. The mechanism of vision: X. Postoperative disturbances of habits based on detail vision in the rat after lesions in the cerebral visual areas. *Journal of Comparative Psychology*, 1934, *17*, 355-392.
Lashley, K. S., & Russell, J. T. The mechanism of vision: XI. A preliminary test of innate organization. *Journal of Genetic Psychology*, 1934, *45*, 136-144.
Layman, J. D. Functions of the superior colliculi in vision. *Journal of Genetic Psychology*, 1936, *49*, 33-47.

Maffei, L., & Fiorentini, A. Spatial frequency rows in the striate visual cortex. Vision Research, 1977, *17*, 257-264.

Miller, M., Pasik, P., & Pasik, T. Extrageniculostriate vision in the monkey. VII. Contrast sensitivity functions. *Journal of Neurophysiology*, 1980, *43*, 1510-1526.

Pasik, P., & Pasik, T. Extrageniculostriate vision in the monkey. V. Role of the accessory optic system. *Journal of Neurophysiology*, 1973, *36*, 450-457. (b)

Pasik, P., & Pasik, T. Circuitos neuronales con participación de dendritas presinápticas en el núcleo geniculado lateral dorsal del mono. *Revista de Microscopía Electrónica*, 1979, *6*, 255-263.

Pasik, P., Pasik, T., & Hámori, J. Synapses between interneurons in the lateral geniculate nucleus of monkeys. *Experimental Brain Research*, 1976, *25*, 1-13.

Pasik, P., Pasik, T., & Hámori, J. Neuronal circuits with "presynaptic dendrites" in dorsal lateral geniculate nucleus (LGNd) of monkeys. *Neurosciences Abstract*, 1977, *3*, 572.

Pasik, P., Pasik, T., Hámori, J., & Szentágothai, J. Golgi type II interneurons in the neuronal circuit of the monkey lateral geniculate nucleus. *Experimental Brain Research*, 1973, *17*, 18-34.

Pasik, P., Pasik, T., Nolan, J. T., & Solomon, S. J. Bar orientation discrimination in normal and destriated monkeys. *Neuroscience Abstracts*, 1976, *2*, 1130.

Pasik, P., Pasik, T., & Schilder, P. Extrageniculostriate vision in the monkey: Discrimination of luminous flux-equated figures. *Experimental Neurology*, 1969, *24*, 421-438.

Pasik, T., & Pasik, P. The visual world of monkeys deprived of striate cortex: Effective stimulus parameters and the importance of the accessory optic system. In T. Shipley & J. E. Dowling (Eds.), *Visual processes in vertebrates* (Vision Research, Supplement No. 3). Oxford: Pergamon Press, 1971.

Pasik, T., & Pasik, P. Extrageniculostriate vision in the monkey. IV. Critical structures for light vs. no-light discrimination. *Brain Research*, 1973, *56*, 165-182. (a)

Pasik, T., & Pasik, P. Extrageniculostriate vision in primates. In S. Lessell & J. T. W. van Dalen (Eds.), *Neuro-ophthalmology*. Amsterdam: Excerpta Medica, 1980.

Pasik, T., Pasik, P., & Hámori, J. Nucleus of the accessory optic tract: Light and electron microscopic study in normal and eye-enucleated monkeys. *Experimental Neurology*, 1973, *41*, 612-627.

Pasik, T., Pasik, P., Schilder, P., & Wininger, J. Extrageniculostriate vision in the monkey: Effect of circumstriate cortex or superior colliculi ablations. *Excerpta Medica*, 1973, Int. Congr. Series No. 296, 201-202.

Polyak, S. *The vertebrate visual system* (H. Klüver, Ed.). Chicago: University of Chicago Press, 1957.

Safir, A. Automatic measurement of the refractive properties of the eye. *Medical Research Engineering*, 1972, *11*, 12-20.

Schilder, P., Pasik, P., & Pasik, T. Total luminous flux: A possible response determinant for the normal monkey. *Science*, 1967, *158*, 806-809.

Schilder, P., Pasik, P., & Pasik, T. Extrageniculostriate vision in the monkey. III. Circle vs. triangle and "red vs. green" discrimination. *Experimental Brain Research*, 1972, *14*, 436-448.

Schilder, P., Pasik, T., & Pasik, P. Extrageniculostriate vision in the monkey. II. Demonstration of brightness discrimination. *Brain Research*, 1971, *32*, 383-398.

Solomon, S. J., Pasik, T., & Pasik, P. Effects of striate cortex and/or superior colliculi ablations on accurate reaching by monkeys. *Neuroscience Abstracts*, 1979, *5*, 808.

Szentágothai, J. Neuronal and synaptic architecture of the lateral geniculate body. In R. Jung (Ed.), *Handbook of sensory physiology* (Vol. 7/B). Berlin: Springer, 1973.

Weinstein, B., & Grether, W. F. A comparison of visual acuity in the rhesus monkey and man. *Journal of Comparative Psychology*, 1940, *30*, 187-195.

Weiskrantz, L. Contour discrimination in a young monkey with striate cortex ablation. *Neuropsychologia*, 1963, *1*, 145-164.

Weiskrantz, L., & Cowey, A. Striate cortex lesions and visual acuity of the rhesus monkey. *Journal of Comparative and Physiological Psychology*, 1963, *56*, 225-231.

Weiskrantz, L., Cowey, A., & Passingham, C. Spatial responses to brief stimuli by monkeys with striate cortex ablations. *Brain*, 1977, *100*, 655-670.

8 Development and Plasticity in the Visual System

Kao Liang Chow, Ph.D.
Department of Neurology,
Stanford University School of Medicine

> If an animal is trained to choose the larger of two circles he will spontaneously choose the larger of any pair of figures. The reaction is not differentiated for form. If he is trained with two different forms, he is undisturbed by wide variations in the size of the figures. So, in every discrimination habit the response is not to a specific pattern but to some property which distinguishes the two figures and which must be differentiated before the motor responses can be associated with it. Furthermore, when the nature of these differentiating properties is tested, they turn out to be relational: relative size, relative direction, proportions, and the like. Such evidence, I believe, disposes of the theory that reactions to relational properties are due to irradiation of conditioned reactions to absolute properties.
>
> These lines of evidence from the animal work support the conclusion already reached by the members of the Gestalt school, that the fundamental organization in perception is innate. And this organization has very definite characteristics, a preference, as it were, for certain specific arrangements of the physical elements of stimulus [Lashley, 1938, p. 450].

In the preceding paragraphs, Lashley set forth his position regarding visual discrimination learning and the innateness of perceptual organization, a position I believe he held unwaveringly throughout his later years. At the time he wrote the passage I quoted, Lashley had already demonstrated—by means of quantitative behavioral experiments similar to those detailed in the 1929 monograph—normal depth perception in dark-reared rats. Hebb's (1937) report on the learning abilities of dark-reared rats also suggested that some elements of perceptual organization are innate. While I was at the Yerkes Laboratories of Primate Biology, working as a student assistant for the Riesen–Nissen chimpanzee dark-rearing project, Lashley followed with interest the development of specific visual pattern preferences in our animals; but he nevertheless remained ambivalent about the significance of our visual deprivation results.

During the last two decades, of course, the study of the visual system has undergone an explosive development, brought about by the advent of single-unit microelectrode recording and, more recently, by new anatomical methods such as autoradiography and horseradish peroxidase histochemistry. Data regarding many aspects of the normal development of the mammalian visual system, as well as visual deprivation's effects on this development, are rapidly accumulating. No doubt these data, obtained from sophisticated experimental techniques unavailable to him, would have fascinated Lashley. In his inimitable fashion, he would also have been vastly amused by the difficulties confronting any simplistic hypotheses or generalizations about the visual developmental process and its underlying mechanisms.

At the risk of provoking Lashley's posthumous amusement, I shall begin by proposing five generalizations that I think represent a useful assessment of the significance of recent experiments concerning the normal and abnormal development of the visual system in the monkey, cat, hamster, rat, mouse, opossum, and rabbit (Barlow, 1975; Blakemore, 1977; Chalupa & Rhoades 1978; Daniels & Pettigrew, 1976; Dräger, 1978; Grobstein & Chow, 1976; Hirsch & Leventhal, 1978; Hubel, 1979; Hubel, Wiesel, & LeVay, 1977; Rhoades & Chalupa, 1978; Rocha-Miranda & Lent, 1978; Shaw, Yinon, & Auerbach, 1975; Wiesel & Hubel, 1963). They are offered here to take stock of what has been accomplished, what is generally agreed upon, and what remains controversial. After that, I present data from my colleagues' and my work on the rabbit and utilize these data to evaluate some of the generalizations. The extensively reviewed literature on visual development of the cat and monkey, as well as the relatively few studies of the rat and hamster, are alluded to only occasionally in what follows.

GENERALIZATIONS

Any generalization about a still evolving field of inquiry is inevitably confronted by exceptions of fact and conflicting interpretations of results. The following are offered to extract from the large number of publications some schema that can be used to organize one's thoughts and to direct the future search for explanatory mechanisms:

1. The visual system continues to grow both physiologically and morphologically after the animal is born. This statement is probably true of all mammalian species.
2. There is a brief period after the animal is born, or after the animal's eyes open, during which the distribution of normal visual stimulation alters visual

development. The timing and duration of this "critical period" when the visual system is susceptible to visual deprivation varies from species to species but probably exists in all mammals.

3. There are conflicting results and opinions about the possibility of recovery from the abnormal visual development following visual deprivation. Many factors appear to be relevant to the recovery process; each must therefore be examined on a case-by-case basis. Some of the relevant factors are the type of deprivation effects, the particular species used, the timing of visual deprivation, the length of visual deprivation, and the kind of postdeprivation visual environment.

4. The normal visual environment may play a positive role in the development of the visual system. Experiments that test this proposition are difficult to design, and the results obtained so far are controversial.

5. The developing visual system appears to exhibit a limited degree of compensatory growth following neonatal injury. Experimental demonstrations of morphological and physiological plasticity are beginning to reveal the complexity of the issues involved.

NORMAL DEVELOPMENT OF RECEPTIVE FIELD CHARACTERISTICS

Neurons in the visual system are specified with respect to their retinotopic locations, their responses to specific stimulus features, and—where binocularity is present—their responses to stimulation of each eye. Cells exhibiting these properties exist in animals before their eyes open. For example, cells responsive only to an oriented line stimulation or cells that can be binocularly activated are found in the visually naive kitten's striate cortex (Hubel & Wiesel, 1963; Wiesel & Hubel, 1974), and cells that respond differentially to specific features of visual stimuli appear in the central visual system of newborn rabbits (Fox, Chow, & Kelly, 1978; Mathers, Chow, Spear, & Grobstein, 1974; Rapisardi, Chow, & Mathers, 1975). Like most neonatal neurons, these cells have a low background discharge rate, and their response to stimulation habituates rapidly. Also, they have a less refined receptive field organization than adult neurons. Otherwise, they are essentially like adult brain cells, and their presence indicates that functional connections have been formed before visual experience begins. At the same time, however, cells also exist that do not respond to any stimulus or respond to light stimulation in a haphazard, inconsistent way. Therefore, the question is not simply whether single cells display highly organized behavior without prior visual stimulation—they certainly do—but also whether different types of cells are present in a given structure in adultlike proportions. Thus, a population approach provides an additional criterion for interpreting the unit data: A structure may not be considered matured until all neurons or neuronal groups reach not only their final stages of morphological and physiological development but also the same proportions found in the adult. When viewed this way, the visual pathways of rabbit and cat appear to develop continuously long after the animals' eyes first open.

Before the cat's eyes open, its superior colliculus contains a large number of cells responsive only to stationary light stimulation. These cells progressively decrease in number; their decrease coincides with an increase, lasting up to 50 days, of neurons responsive to movement as well as to stationary light. The proportion of binocular cells also progressively increases, reaching the adult level at about 50 days after birth (Norton, 1974; Stein, Labos, & Kruger, 1973). The increase of binocular cells and sharpening of binocular disparity in cat striate cortex takes place weeks after eye opening (Daniels & Pettigrew, 1976). As for the rabbit, a recent report of the gradual increase in size from an initially small central region to the entire retinotopically arranged visual field in its striate cortex may be interpreted as reflecting the addition of new cells responsive to light stimulation in the maturing animal (Choudbury, 1978). Our studies of the rabbit visual system, explicitly based on the population approach, clearly demonstrate the development after eye opening of neurons with different receptive field characteristics (Fox et al., 1978; Grobstein & Chow, 1976; Mathers et al., 1974; Rapisardi et al., 1975).

One essential requirement for using the population approach to study receptive field development is that every cell recorded electrophysiologically in each electrode penetration be classified. It is assumed that the cells thus sampled adequately represent the entire population. Samples of cells from animals differing in age or in the experimental conditions under which they were reared may then be compared, and any differences obtained are presumed to reflect developmental differences. I have previously discussed in detail the justifications for these assumptions together with other methodological considerations (Grobstein & Chow, 1976). Suffice it to say here that even though the possibility of electrode bias in such sampling cannot conclusively be ruled out, the regularity of the neuronal growth curves derived from our data (see following) make it clear that complicated and ad hoc explanations are necessary to account for our results in terms of electrode-sampling biases.

Neurons in the rabbit visual system, like those in other animals, respond differentially to specific stimulus features and can thus be classified into several receptive field types. Investigators, using different criteria and testing methods, have studied the receptive fields of visual neurons in many different animals and have described several receptive field types common to all, including the monkey, cat, hamster, rat, mouse, and opossum. Except for some variations in detail, our classification of rabbit neurons conforms to these general classes (Chow, Masland & Stewart, 1971; Masland, Chow, & Stewart, 1971; Stewart, Chow, & Masland, 1971). We have consistently employed the following classificatory scheme for receptive field types. The receptive field types in the dorsal nucleus of the lateral geniculate body (LGN) are the familiar concentric type, which has an excitatory or inhibitory center with an antagonistic surround; the uniform type, which has only a well-defined on or off region but no surround; the motion-sensitive type, which responds best to a moving light in any direction; and the directionally selective type, which responds best to a light or dark stimulus moving across the field in one direction but shows either no response or a suppression of background activity to movement in the other direction. The first three types are grouped as cells with nonoriented field. There are no, or very few, cells that are unresponsive to light stimulation in the LGN. Besides the four types of cells already listed, three additional types can be distinguished in the striate cortex: simple cells, which have an elongated excitatory region bordered on one or both sides by an inhibitory region and which are best excited by a stationary bar oriented within the excitatory zone; complex cells, which also have elongated fields but require movement of a properly aligned edge through the long axis of the field to excite them; and oriented-directional cells, which have elongated fields and respond only to a light or dark bar that is oriented parallel to the long axis of the field and moved through this axis. These three types are collectively termed oriented receptive field cells. In addition, some cortical cells either respond to strong whole eye illumination or respond erratically to stimuli in a local area; these are classified as cells with indefinite field. The cells in superior colliculus (SC) consist of the three nonoriented cell types and the directionally selective, oriented-directional, and indefinite cells.

The rabbit's eyes normally open at about 10 days of age. Our results showed that as early as 5 to 6 days after birth, about 30% of geniculate cells and about 10% of striate cortical cells could be excited by light stimulation. The proportions of cells responsive to any sort of light stimulation grew to about 80% at the time of eye opening and continued to increase for another 10 to 20 days before reaching adult levels. Figure 8.1 shows the development of the proportions of all light-excitable cells in the LGN, SC, and striate cortex. The displacement of the LGN curve to the left indicated that geniculate cells developed earlier than collicular and cortical cells by about 2 days (Fox et al., 1978; Mathers et al., 1974; Rapisardi et al., 1975; Spear, Chow, Masland, & Murphy, 1972).

The development of the individual receptive field types in these structures is plotted separately in Fig. 8.2. The developmental curves of the three types of nonoriented cells were comparable. For the sake of clarity, the three were combined in the collicular and cortical graphs. Similarly, the three oriented cell types in the cortex were combined. (The directionally selective cells were not included in this and following figures.) These graphs clearly showed that the development of specific feature extraction was a continuous process, starting well before the animal's eyes open for cells displaying nonoriented fields and after eye opening for cells with oriented fields. Both these types increased in relative numbers over the subsequent weeks. The indefinite cells were an exception. These cells have a complex growth pattern: Their relative numbers first increased to a peak at, or slightly after, eye opening and progressively decreased to the adult proportion.

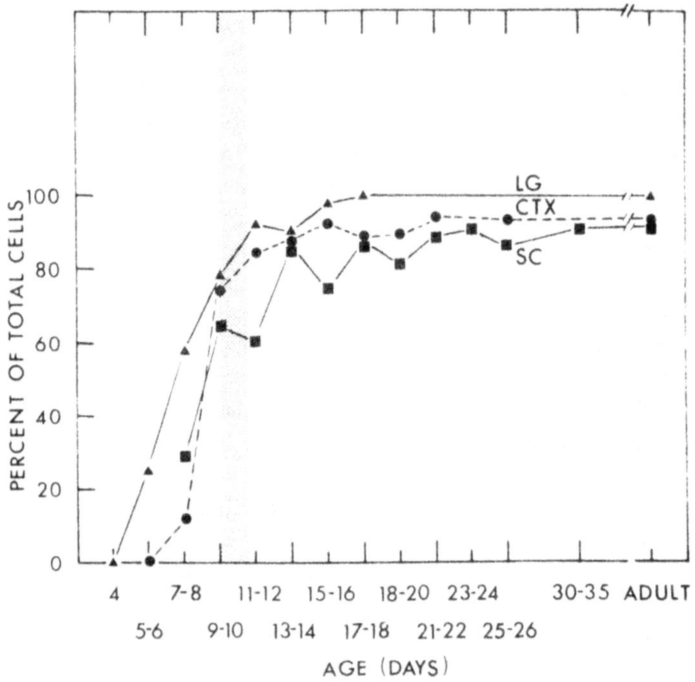

FIG. 8.1. Postnatal development of responsive cells in the rabbit's lateral geniculate nucleus (LG), superior colliculus (SC), and striate cortex (CTX). Percentages of cells responsive to any light stimulation are plotted as a function of age. In this and the following two figures, the shaded column indicates the time when the eyes normally open.

The declining phase of their growth curve appeared to be the reciprocal of the inclining phase of the oriented cells' curve in the striate cortex.

To summarize this series of studies: Neurons responsive to light stimulation exist in the rabbit's central visual system before the animal's eyes open. The earliest such cells appear at 5 to 6 days of age—that is, at about the time of the first appearance of receptor outer segments and synaptic contacts among bipolar, amacrine, and ganglion cells (McArdle, Dowling, & Masland, 1977). It is therefore possible that the limiting factor in the appearance of the light-responsive cells may be the maturation of the retina. The number of light-responsive cells is small in the beginning, but it progressively increases to reach that of the adult at 10 to 20 days after eye opening. The biphasic growth pattern of the indefinite cells raises the question of what underlies the decline of these cells during the immediate post-eye-opening period. Do they disappear, thereby constituting simply another instance of cell death during development? Are they actively inhibited? Or are they transformed into neurons with specific receptive field properties, particularly the oriented cells?

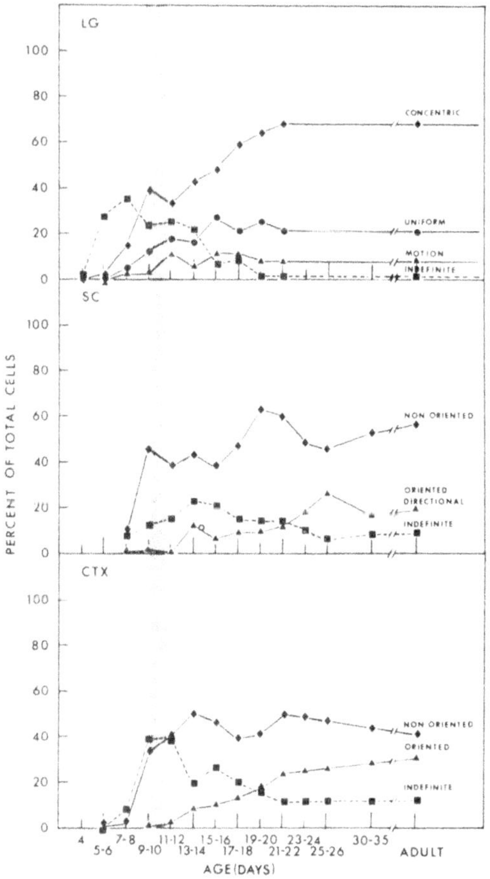

FIG. 8.2. Time course of receptive field development in the rabbit's LG, SC, and CTX. The percentages of cells exhibiting various receptive field characteristics are plotted as a function of age. The concentric, uniform, and motion-sensitive receptive fields are grouped under nonoriented cells. The simple, complex, and oriented-directional receptive fields are grouped under oriented cells.

EFFECTS OF VISUAL DEPRIVATION

Many methods have been used to alter normal visual stimulation in newborn animals. That most frequently used is to suture the eyelids together, thereby cutting off patterned stimulation and drastically reducing the amount of light transmitted to the eye. We have used monocular lid suturing extensively in our rabbit studies. Here the eyelids of one eye are sutured shut before eye opening; the eyelids of the other are allowed to open at the usual time. Because of the almost complete crossing of retinal projections, and hence the large monocular fields, unit recordings may be confined to monocular regions of the brain. The development of the largely deprived side of the brain can thus be compared with that of the other, ''control'' side in the same animal.

The adverse effects of visual deprivation have been demonstrated in many species. However, most of our studies have been concerned with an aspect of visual development seldom addressed by other investigators: how monocular deprivation's length affects the development of the different types of receptive fields. The following summarizes the results of our systematic studies on collicular and cortical cells, together with some preliminary data on geniculate neurons.

The development of receptive field characteristics of the rabbit's geniculate cells appeared to be complete by about 20 to 25 days of age (Baumbach & Chow, 1978; Rapisardi et al., 1975). At that time, the relative proportions of different cell classes reached the adult status (Fig. 8.2). When the animal was monocularly deprived during this period, the distribution of the receptive field types changed; that is, the distribution of receptive fields in the deprived LGN was significantly different from that obtained in the control LGN ($P < 0.001$, χ^2 test). Table 8.1A shows that there were significantly more unresponsive and indefinite cells in the deprived LGN—that is, 24% in the deprived structure versus 2% in the control LGNd ($P < 0.001$, test for differences between proportions corrected for discreteness, two-tailed test)—and that there was a corresponding lack of uniform cells in the deprived LGNd. When deprivation was continued to the young adult age (82-116 days), such abnormal distributions persisted but were less severe than those obtained by shorter deprivation periods. Table 8.1B shows that there was still a higher proportion of unresponsive and indefinite cells than were seen in the undeprived structure, and this difference was significant ($P < 0.001$). But the proportion (16%) of such cells was considerably lower than the proportion (24%) obtained from the 20-25-day deprivation group. There was also a slight

TABLE 8.1
Percentages of Cells in Each Receptive Field Category Recorded in the LGN of Monocularly Deprived Rabbits

	A (21-25 Days)		*B (82-116 Days)*[a]	
No. of Cells	*Deprived* 100	*Control* 103	*Deprived* 102	*Control* 191
Unresponsive	15	1	9	0
Indefinite	9	1	7	0
Concentric	53	52	55	68
Uniform	9	27	17	21
Motion	11	15	10	8
Directional	3	4	2	3

[a]The control data in B were those from Stewart et al. (1971).

increase of the uniform cells, from 9% in the group deprived until 20 to 25 days of age to 17% in the group deprived until 82 to 116 days of age.

Three general conclusions can be drawn from these data, which appear to apply also to the results from our collicular and cortical studies. First, visual deprivation significantly alters the relative proportions of receptive fields; second, this alteration takes the form of a sharp increase of unresponsive and indefinite cells at the expense of some other specific field types (in the case of the LGNd, it is at the expense of the uniform cells); third, the longer the visual deprivation, the less anomalous the distribution becomes.

A timed series study was made to examine the effects of visual deprivation on collicular cells (Fox et al., 1978). Monocularly deprived rabbits in successive age groups, from 9 to 10 days until 35 days after birth, were used to reveal the complexity of the abnormal receptive fields' development. These results are illustrated by the series of graphs in Fig. 8.3. It should be noted that by definition, experimental deprivation was not possible before the animals' eyes opened. Therefore, the curves for the deprived superior colliculus began at Days 11-12.

The top graph shows that the increase in percentages of all light-responsive neurons in the deprived colliculus did not differ from that in the control colliculus. Similarly, there was no difference in development between the non-oriented cells. However, quite a different picture emerged in the development of the oriented-directional cells. These cells showed an initial growth rate that was identical in the deprived and normal colliculus for about 3 weeks; but starting at Day 21-22, a precipitous decrease in the percentage of oriented-directional cells occurred in the deprived colliculus. These cells reached a high of 12% at Days 19-20, but fell to a low of 4% at Days 25-35 and maintained that level to the end of the 5th week. The difference between the percentages of the oriented-directional cells in the deprived and cortical data was statistically significant for the final three age groups (χ^2 test, $P < 0.05$). No experiments with longer deprivation periods were performed. Therefore, it remains possible that the percentages of these cells would show further changes.

The curves for the indefinite cells also show that there were complex changes in the development of these cells—changes that were highly correlated with those that were seen in the development of the oriented-directional cells. The percentages of the indefinite cells grew normally for 3 weeks. But beginning at Days 21-22, an abnormal increase occurred in the deprived colliculus in contrast to the continued decrease seen in the control colliculus. At the end of 5 weeks, a significant difference existed between the percentages (16% vs. 6%) of indefinite cells in the deprived and control colliculi. Both these groups of deprived cells, the oriented-directional and the indefinite cells, appeared to grow normally after eye opening but then abruptly departed from the normal course. This suggests that the oriented-directional cells were somehow transformed into indefinite cells.

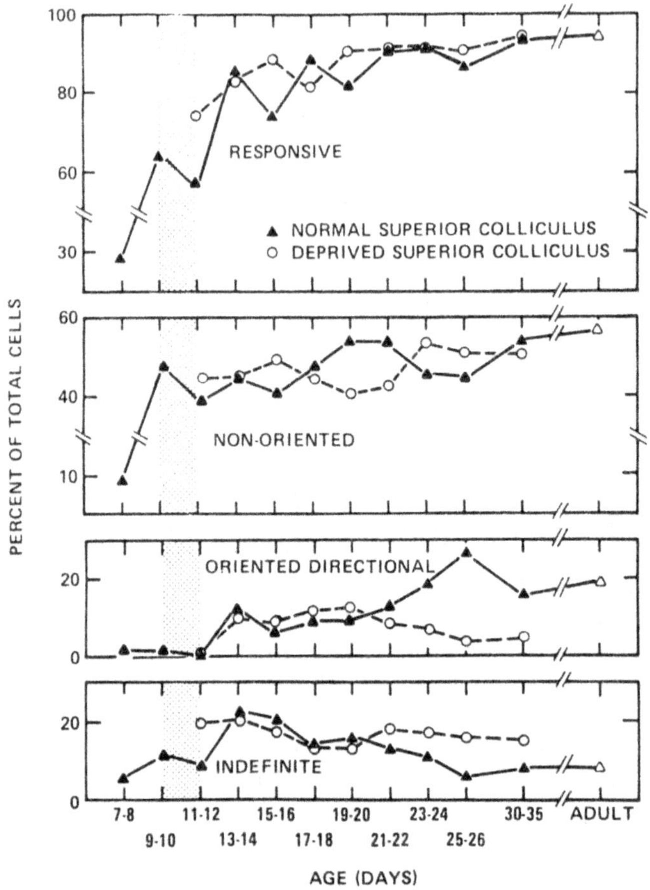

FIG. 8.3. Comparison of the postnatal development of responsive cells in the rabbit's SC receiving either normal light stimulation or inputs from a sutured eye. The solid lines are the normal data and the interrupted lines, the data from the deprived colliculus. The top panel depicts the percentages of cells responsive to any light stimulation. Note the differences between the two sets of curves evident in the lowest two panels, which represent the oriented-directional cells and the indefinite cells.

The effect of visual deprivation on striate cortical cells was less extensively studied (Grobstein & Chow, 1976, and unpublished data). Only four groups of neonatal rabbits were used. The lengths of deprivation ranged from 20 to 25 days to 3 to 14 months. In this series, we have not sampled the cells on the nondeprived side of the cortex; instead we have used data from normal animals for comparison. Figure 8.4 illustrates the results. The open bars are the percentages of cortical cell types in normal 9-to-10-day-old rabbits and adults. The filled bars represent the percentages found in the deprived animals. In normal rabbits, the

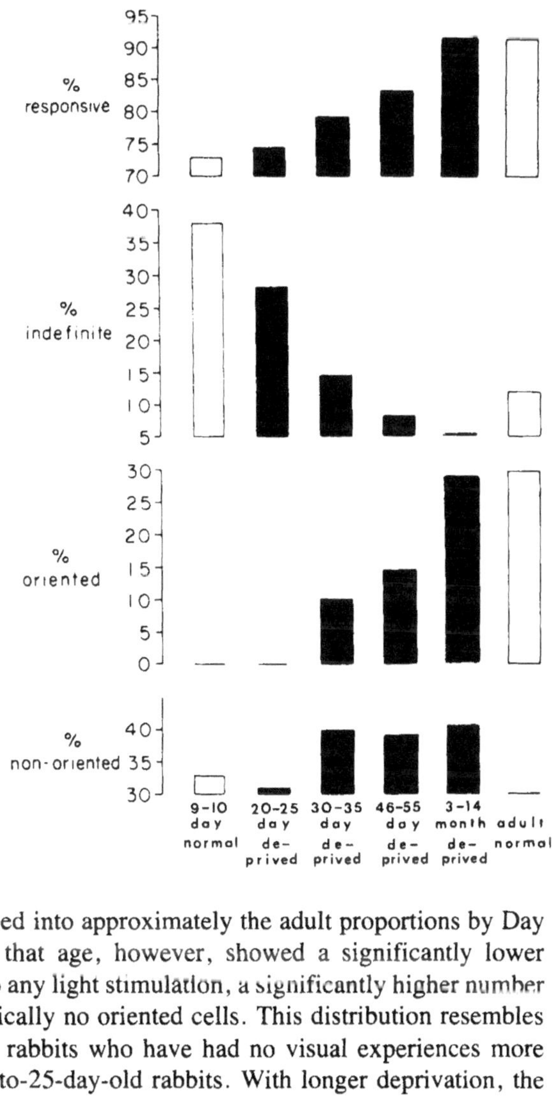

FIG. 8.4. Postnatal development of cortical cells responsive to any light stimulation and of those exhibiting specific receptive field characteristics in rabbits monocularly deprived for various lengths of time. The four sets of solid bars are the cortical data from four groups of rabbits deprived for 20 to 25 days, 30 to 35 days, 46 to 55 days, and 3 to 14 months. The open bars are the data collected from normal 9-to-10-day-olds and normal adult rabbits.

receptive field types developed into approximately the adult proportions by Day 25. The deprived group at that age, however, showed a significantly lower number of cells responsive to any light stimulation, a significantly higher number of indefinite cells, and practically no oriented cells. This distribution resembles that seen in 9-to-10-day-old rabbits who have had no visual experiences more than that seen in normal 20-to-25-day-old rabbits. With longer deprivation, the relative frequency of the receptive fields progressively changed toward the normal adult level. This trend is clearly shown in Fig. 8.4. By 3 to 14 months, the distribution of cell types in the deprived cortex looks very much like that in the normal adult except that there were still more nonoriented cells and fewer indefinite cells. It seems that striate cortical cells possess the capability of maturing normally without visual stimulation. However, visual experience may have a supportive function that hastens the rate of development. Whether still longer deprivation would damage the cells permanently, as has been demonstrated in the case of binocular cells in the cat's cortex, remains to be studied.

That the duration of visual deprivation is an important variable in the development of the rabbit's visual cells is well documented by these studies. They show that visual deprivation affects only certain types of receptive fields. The affected cells' rate of development is altered in a complex way that cannot be easily explained by any single mechanism.

Several related aspects of the receptive field development in rabbits should be noted in passing. Lid suturing in the adult does not affect geniculate or cortical cells, which suggests that a critical period for the deprivation effect exists. No attempt to delineate such a period, however, has been made. The problem of recovery from deprivation's effects is complicated by the fact that at least in the LGNd and cortex, these effects abate as deprivation is prolonged. Finally, only one study has attempted to examine whether normal visual environment plays a positive role in receptive field development in the rabbit. In contrast to the results reported for the cat's visual cortex (Hirsch & Leventhal, 1978), Mize and Murphy (1973) failed to obtain changes in the orientation specificity of oriented cortical cells in rabbits reared so as to restrict their visual experiences to either horizontal or vertical stripes. In view of the paucity of such studies of the rabbit, and the recent conflicting results reported for similar studies of the cat (Blakemore, 1977; Stryker & Sherk, 1975; Stryker, Sherk, Leventhal, & Hirsch, 1978), any speculation regarding the possible role of normal visual experiences should probably be reserved for the future.

MORPHOLOGICAL DEVELOPMENT OF SUPERIOR COLLICULUS AND STRIATE CORTEX

The morphological development of the rabbit's collicular and cortical cells has been studied by Vrensen and by Mathers and his colleagues (Mathers, 1977, 1979; Mathers, Mercer, & Marhsall, 1978; Vrensen, 1978; Vrensen, De Groot, & Nunes-Cardoza, 1977). They have collected a wealth of quantitative data using Golgi-stained and electron microscopic materials. One is impressed by the vigor of growth and the complexity of the processes involved and particularly by the variety of neuronal types and neuronal components. How this aggregate of anatomical changes, occurring after birth and after eye opening, relates to the functional development of this system remains uncertain.

The following data are selected to illustrate the growth rates of some anatomical features. The dendritic spines of Cortical Layer 5 pyramidal cells and Layer 4 stellate cells showed rapid growth right after eye opening and reached maximum growth at 25 days. A similarly rapid growth of spines appeared in the periform and stellate cells in the upper layers of colliculus, but they had an earlier growth peak at 15 to 20 days. The rapid development of synapses in the cortical neurons also started at about 10 days and reached its maximum at 25 days. However, both the number of dense projections and the number of synaptic vesicles per synaptic contact zone increased gradually from birth to about 27 days. In the colliculus, the synapses started to increase at 5 days and followed a slower rate of growth, reaching their peak at 20 days. In both cases, the number of synapses containing spherical vesicles increased at a faster rate than the number of synapses containing flattened vesicles.

These data show that most of the development of dendritic spines and synaptic terminals started at about the time of eye opening and reached the adult level at about 20 to 25 days. This time course more or less paralleled the development of certain receptive field types. One specific case was the development of spines on the intrinsic cells, the periform and stellate cells; this development coincided with that of oriented-directional cells in the colliculus (Mathers, 1977). One probably should not read too much into these results. Nevertheless, these anatomical data provide useful foundations for the further identification of structural-functional correlates at the cellular level.

Our own preliminary studies on the development of the uncrossed retinotectal projections also demonstrate that this system underwent considerable postnatal development. In adult rabbits the uncrossed fibers projected to a small lateral border region in the second quartile of the rostral colliculus. Figure 8.5A shows dark-field autoradiographs of coronal sections of the colliculus of an adult rabbit who had tritiated proline projection into one eye 7 days before it was killed. The uncrossed retinotectal fiber terminals appear as the light patches, which is shown in detail in Fig. 8.5B. Reconstruction of the surface view of these projections is shown in Fig. 8.5C. These results show a wider distribution of the uncrossed fibers than that revealed by the Fink-Heimer fiber degeneration method following monocular enucleation. The contralateral colliculus was completely covered by the labeled terminals (not shown).

In newborn rabbits the uncrossed retinotectal projections occupied a much wider area. The results from autoradiographs obtained from a 1-day-old rabbit are shown in Fig. 8.6. The labeled terminals appeared in both the rostral and medial regiors of the colliculus. These areas were clear of any label in the adult rabbit, as is shown in Fig. 8.5. The colliculus of the newborn rabbit is naturally much smaller than that of the adult, and thus the same amount of fiber distribution may appear to be larger. That this is not the case can easily be seen by comparing the surface reconstructions of the adult and the newborn colliculi shown in Figs. 8.5A and 8.6A. There was an absolute increase of the size of the labeled region in the colliculus of the newborn rabbit. The data of another 6-day old rabbit showed an intermediate amount of terminal distribution.

These results corroborate the recent report by Land and Lund (1979), which showed that in newborn rats, the retinotectal pathway from each eye was distributed to the entire contra- and ipsilateral colliculus. The uncrossed projections later retracted to the small, adult pattern within 10 days. Other instances of anomalous fibers in newborn animals that later retract, leaving the adult pattern, are the callosal projections of the rabbit's striate cortex (Chow, Baumbach, &

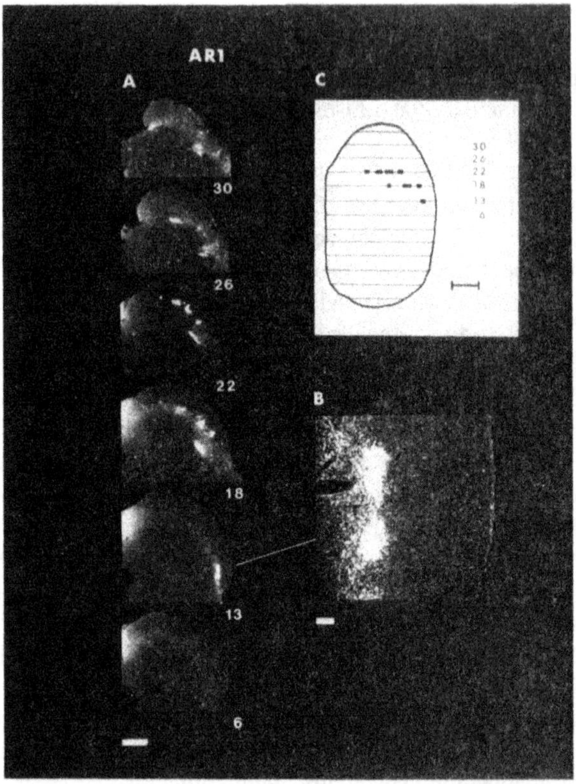

FIG. 8.5. A. Dark-field autoradiographs of coronal sections of the anterior half of the superior colliculus of an adult rabbit. Only the colliculus ipsilateral to the injected eye is shown. The bright patches shown in Sections 22, 18, and 13 are the radioactively labeled retinotectal terminals. B. A detailed view of the labeling is shown. Other bright patches of labeling in Sections 30 to 18 are terminals in the pretectal nucleus and nucleus of the optic tract. C. Reconstruction of the dorsal surface of the colliculus showing the location and extent of the uncrossed retinotectal projections in black. In this and the following two figures, the coronal sections were cut at 52μ, and every other section was saved and processed for ARG. The numbers referred to the ARG sections. Calibration bars in A and C—1.0 mm; in B—0.1 mm.

Lawson, 1981) and the ipsilateral retinogeniculate projections of the hamster (So, Schneider, & Frost, 1978). A redistribution of afferent fibers during development also occurs in the monkey striate cortex: In newborn animals the input from two eyes is intermingled but later becomes segregated into ocular dominance columns (Hubel, 1979; Hubel et al., 1977).

These anatomical studies clearly indicate that just as the receptive fields of neurons continue to develop postnatally, many morphological aspects of the visual system also show marked structural changes many days after birth.

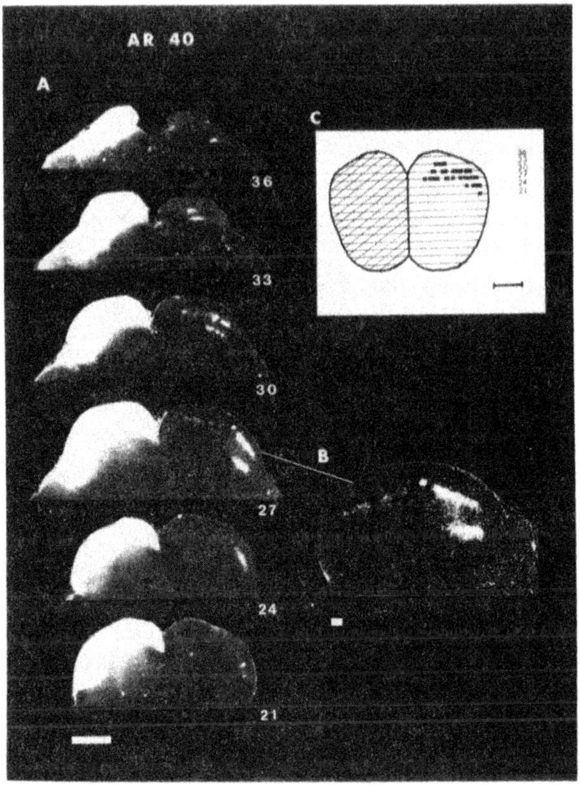

FIG. 8.6. A. Dark-field autoradiographs of coronal sections of the superior colliculus of a 1-day-old rabbit. The bright patches of the labeled terminals cover most of the anterior third of the colliculus. B. A detailed view of the terminal labeling is shown. C. Reconstruction of the dorsal surface of the colliculus to show the location and extent of the uncrossed retinotectal projections in black. The contralateral colliculus is completely covered by labeled terminals, as depicted by hatching. Calibration bars in A and C—1.0 mm; in B—0.1 mm.

THE ANOMALOUS, UNCROSSED RETINOTECTAL PROJECTIONS

Another aspect of the postnatal maturational process is the anomalous growth of fiber projections into a novel region in animals who have sustained local brain lesions at birth. This abnormal growth suggests the presence of some plastic mechanisms in the developing nervous system capable of compensating for the early injury. Several instances of such compensatory growth have been reported (Lund, 1978). One example pertaining to the developing visual system is the dramatic increase of the small, uncrossed retinotectal terminals that cover almost entirely the colliculi of rats and hamsters monocularly enucleated at birth (Cunningham & Speas, 1975; Finlay, Wilson, & Schneider, 1979; Frost & Schneider, 1976; Lund, Cunningham, & Lund, 1973). These anomalous retinal fibers are functional; that is, they form normal retinotopic maps, albeit sometimes with disoriented axes, and the activated collicular cells show more or less normal receptive field characteristics.

In view of the recent report, cited previously, that the widespread distribution of the uncrossed retinotectal terminals occurs normally in the newborn rat and rabbit, the interpretation of these results at present is uncertain. The absence of large numbers of crossed retinal fibers following neonatal enucleation may induce a compensatory growth or rerouting of the few uncrossed fibers to occupy the now vacant territory; or their absence may instead result in a lack of competition that allows the original fibers to remain. Possibly both these mechanisms are involved.

Our study of the neonatally enucleated rabbit confirms the spreading of the uncrossed retinotectal fibers. However, in contrast to the rat and hamster, the expansion of the fiber terminals in our Fink–Heimer-stained material was rather limited: They spread only a little distance from the normal anterolateral border to the rostral and middle part of the colliculus. Furthermore, cells within this expanded zone were not activated by either light stimulation of the eye or electric shock of the optic nerve head (Chow, Mathers, & Spear, 1973). One factor that might account for the conflicting results is that these animals may be at different maturational stages at the time of enucleation. That is, the rabbit's visual system may be more mature at birth than that of the rat and hamster and therefore has less potential for compensatory reorganization.

In order to test this possibility, we performed monocular enucleation of the rabbit fetus. The rabbit gestation period is 31 days. The surgery was done at 20 or 25 days of gestation—that is, at a fairly immature stage. The status of the uncrossed retinotectal projections was examined when these animals were about 2 to 3 months old. Tritiated proline was injected into the remaining eye, and autoradiography was performed to delineate the distribution of the uncrossed retinotectal fibers' terminals. Microelectrode recordings were carried out to test whether the collicular cells would be excited by these anomalous retinal fibers. In some cases, both the autoradiographic and electrophysiological studies were performed on the same animal; in others, only electrophysiological recordings were performed. Results obtained from the two groups of animals were essentially similar and are considered together.

The autoradiographic data showed that after monocular enucleation, the uncrossed retinotectal terminals occupied a much wider area. They were distributed over the entire anterior one-third of the colliculus, including the rostral tip and the medial margin. Figure 8.7A is a series of coronal sections of the colliculus ipsilateral to the proline-injected eye of a rabbit enucleated at Gestational Day 25. These autoradiographs show heavy labeling at the lateral half of the colliculus and clumps or patches of labeling toward the medial border. The con-

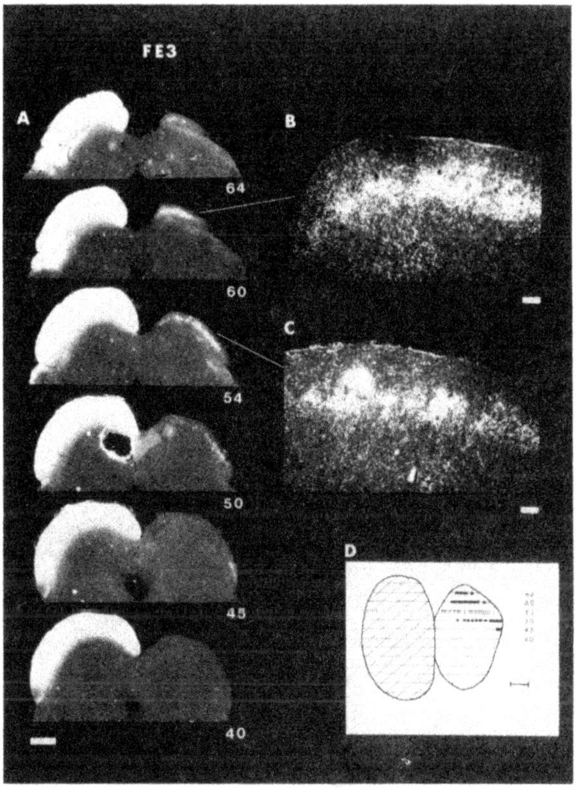

FIG. 8.7. A. Dark-field autoradiographs of coronal sections of the superior colliculus of rabbit Fe3, monocularly enucleated at Gestational Day 25. The hole in Section 50 is an artifact. B,C. Detailed view of the labeled retinotectal terminals in Sections 60 and 54. D. Reconstruction of the dorsal view of the colliculus with the labeled region marked by black. Calibration bars in A and D—1.0 mm; in B and C—0.1 mm.

tralateral colliculus was completely covered by the labeling. Figure 8.7D is a reconstruction of the dorsal surface of the colliculus showing the locations of the labeled terminals. These morphological results demonstrate that an immature brain has more potential than a mature brain to restructure itself following local lesions. It should be noted that even the fetally enucleated rabbit's enlarged retinotectal distribution does not approach the almost complete innervation of the colliculus by anomalous retinotectal fibers seen in rats and hamsters enucleated at birth.

Results from recordings of collicular cells judged to be well within the terminal distribution of the uncrossed fibers were disappointing. Only 7 out of 87 cells had normal receptive field characteristics. They were recorded from two electrode penetrations (in two different animals), each of which was situated at the lateral edge of the colliculus. Moreover, the receptive fields of these normal cells were located at the extreme nasal field, practically in front of the animal's nose. From these considerations, we conclude that they represent cells innervated by the small, ipsilateral retinotectal projection present in normal animals. A reconstruction of one of these two penetrations is shown in Fig. 8.8, Penetration 4. The cells in Penetration 3 that were clearly within the uncrossed fiber projection did not respond to any light stimulation. (Serial coronal sections and the surface-view reconstruction of the colliculus of this animal is shown in Fig. 8.7.) Another 5 cells showed indefinite responses. Of these, 2 were located at the lateral border zone, as shown in Fig. 8.8. The other 3 were more medially located. It is not clear whether they were cells innervated by the medial extension of the normal uncrossed retinal fibers or cells that had acquired new functional connections with the aberrant fibers.

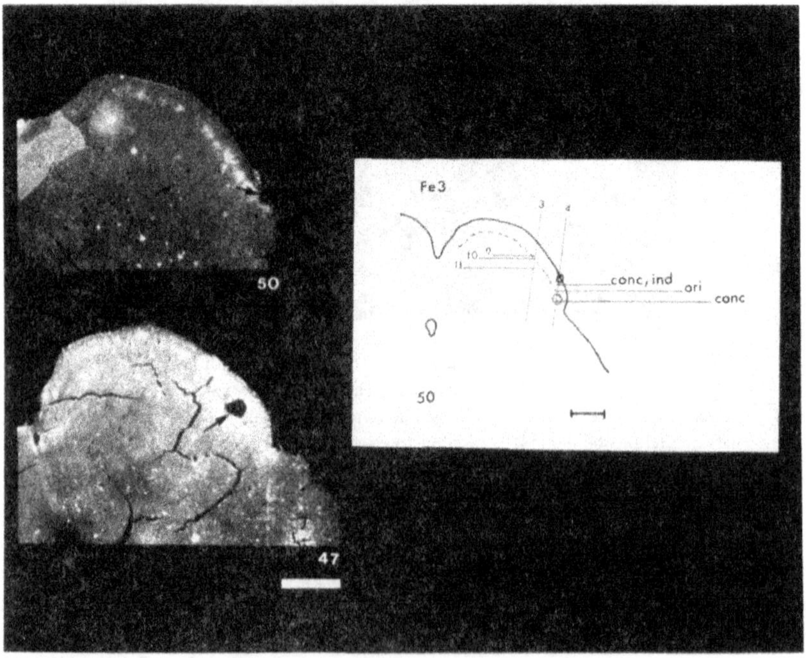

FIG. 8.8 Reconstruction of units recorded in the colliculus of rabbit Fe3. The arrows in the dark-field audioradiographs indicate the electrode burn marks. They are superimposed in the outline drawing (open circles). The neurons in Penetration 4 showing normal responses to light stimulation were judged to be within the normal uncrossed retinotectal projection zone. Units 9 to 11 did not respond to any light stimulation. Calibration bars—1 mm. (Conc = concentric; ind = indefinite; ori = oriented receptive field.)

Equally disappointing were the results obtained from electric shock stimulation of the optic nerve head. Only 4 out of 31 cells could be driven. They were recorded from one animal that had been monocularly enucleated at Gestational Day 20. The locations of these cells are marked by black dots on the reconstructed electrode track of Fig. 8.9. In this figure, Units 6 to 26 were tested with light stimulation but failed to respond. Electric shocks were used to test Units 32 to 52. Figure 8.9A shows two consecutive shock-evoked responses of Unit 34.

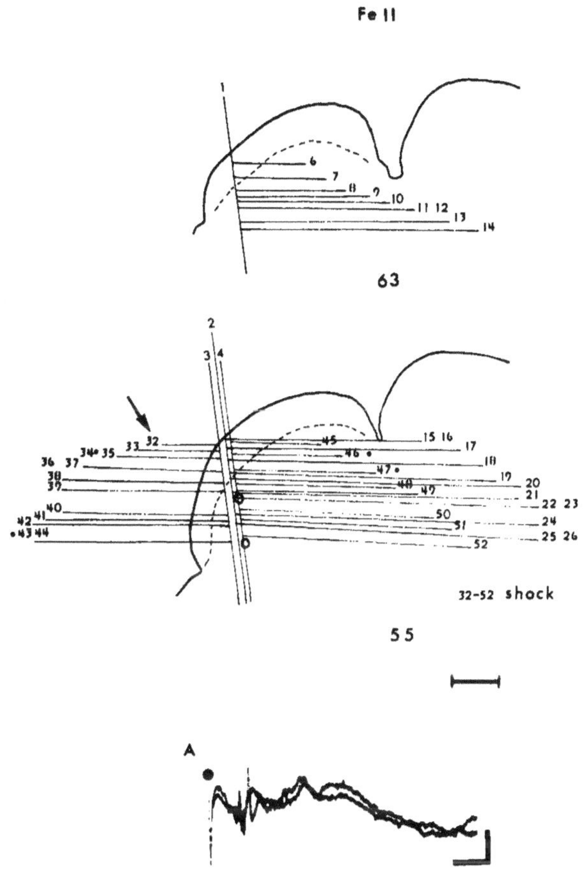

FIG. 8.9. Reconstructive of units recorded in rabbit Fe 11, monocularly enucleated at Gestational Day 20. Open circles are electrode burn marks. Units 6 to 26 failed to respond to light stimulation. Units 32 to 52 were tested for their responses to electric shock of the optic nerve. Four units indicated by dots were driven by shock. Calibration bar—1 mm. A. Two consecutive traces of the responses of Unit 34 to shock (0.1 ms, square wave, and 2 mA). Single spikes are superimposed on the field potentials. Calibration—100 μV and 10 ms.

The spike discharges are superimposed on the field potentials. All the recorded units in this animal were well within the rostrolateral region of the colliculus.

The main findings of these studies is that in contrast to those of the rat and hamster, the anomalous uncrossed retinal fibers of the rabbit fail to form significant functional connections with collicular cells. Autoradiographic-electron-microscopic data are needed to be certain of the existence of synaptic terminals on collicular cells within the enlarged, uncrossed retinal fiber distributions. The few cells with indefinite receptive fields, and the cells located at the middle of the colliculus that responded to electric shock, may represent the beginnings of such connections. Whether still earlier enucleation—say, at Gestational Day 15—would alter these results is problematic. (There is also some question whether such early enucleates could survive.) Another issue that has not been addressed in this type of research is the significance of species differences; for example, the brain of a rodent may have more potential for reorganization than that of a lagomorph.

The comparison of the fetally enucleated and the newborn animals described in the previous section indicates that there is a wider distribution of the uncrossed retinotectal fibers in the former than in the latter (compare Fig. 8.6 and Fig. 8.8). No data on the uncrossed retinal fibers of rabbit fetus at Day 20 of gestation are available. Therefore, there remains the possibility that elimination of the massive crossed fiber projection following monocular enucleation does not promote the regrowth or rerouting of the uncrossed fibers but, rather, allows these fibers to persist in their prenatal state.

CONCLUDING REMARKS

This series of studies on the development of the rabbit's visual system provide support to the five general conclusions I listed at the beginning of this chapter. The data from these studies point to the complex and interdependent nature of the maturational processes involved. Differences exist in the time course of the postnatal development of the different receptive field types. In some cases the data suggest a reciprocal development relationship between receptive field types. The length of monocular deprivation appears to influence deprivation's effects on development. Especially noteworthy is the recovery toward normalcy of striate cortical cells after long-term visual deprivation. Some aspects of these results corroborate data obtained from other animals, but similar systematic studies are few. The postnatal increase of dendritic spines and synaptic terminals on collicular cells and the reduction of uncrossed retinotectal projections are examples of the dynamics of morphological growth. The lack of significant functional connections between the anomalous uncrossed retinal fibers and collicular cells in the fetally enucleated rabbit, in contrast to the situation in the rat and hamster, points to the need for more comparative studies.

In summarizing these results I am reminded of one of Lashley's legacies in neuropsychological research—his penchant for using pragmatic and eclectic approaches to dispose of simplistic theories of brain functions. I hope that these discussions will help to subject current hypotheses and generalizations regarding the development of the visual system to similar examination.

ACKNOWLEDGMENTS

The preparation of this paper and the research reported here has been supported by NIH Grants NS 18512, NS 12151, and EY 00691. I would like to acknowledge the extensive contributions of the postdoctoral fellows with whom it has been my good fortune to be associated: Richard Masland, David Stewart, Peter Spear, E. Hazel Murphy, Lawrence Mathers, Gian Mascetti, Arthur Douville, Salvatore Rapisardi, Paul Grobstein, Patricia Fox, Amy Kelly, Dale Baumbach, John Crabtree, and Louis Ostrach. I thank James Aase, Robin Lawson, and Otto Bernegger for the histological material and Cheryl Joo for secretarial assistance.

REFERENCES

Barlow, H. B. Visual experience and cortical development. *Nature (Lond)*, 1975, *258*, 199-205.

Baumbach, H. D., & Chow, K. L. Receptive field development in the dorsal lateral geniculate nucleus in rabbits subjected to monocular eyelid suture. *Brain Research* 1978, *159*, 69-83.

Blakemore, C. Genetic instructions and developmental plasticity in the kitten's visual cortex. *Philosophical Transactions of the Royal Society, Series B* 1977, *278*, 425-434.

Chalupa, L. M., & Rhoades, R. W. Modification of visual response properties in the superior colliculus of the golden hamster following stroboscopic rearing. *Journal of Physiology (London)*, 1978, *274*, 571-592.

Choudbury, B. P. Visual field representation in the newborn rabbit's cortex. *Brain Research*, 1978, *153*, 27-38.

Chow, K. L., Baumbach, H. D., & Lawson, R. *Callosal projections of the striate cortex in the neonatal rabbit*. Experimental Brain Research, 1981, *42*, 122-126.

Chow, K. L., Masland, R. H., & Stewart, D. L. Receptive field characteristics of the striate cortical neurons in the rabbit. *Brain Research*, 1971, *33*, 337-352.

Chow, K. L., Mathers, L. H., & Spear, P. D. Spreading of uncrossed retinal projection in superior colliculus of neonatally enucleated rabbits. *Journal of Comparative Neurology*, 1973, *151*, 307-322.

Cunningham, T. J., & Speas, G. Inversion of anomalous uncrossed projections along the mediolateral axis of the superior colliculus: Implications for retinocollicular specificity. *Brain Research*, 1975, *88*, 73-79.

Daniels, J. D., & Pettigrew, J. D. Development of neuronal responses in the visual system of cats. In G. Gotlieb (Ed.), *Studies of the development of behavior and the nervous system* (Vol. 3). New York: Academic Press, 1976.

Dräger, U. C. Observations on monocular deprivation in mice. *Journal of Neurophysiology*, 1978, *41*, 28-42.

Finlay, B. L., Wilson, K. G., & Schneider, G. E. Anomalous ipsilateral retinotectal projections in Syrian hamsters with early lesions: Topography and functional capacity. *Journal of Comparative Neurology*, 1979, *183*, 721-740.

Fox, P. C., Chow, K. L., & Kelly, A. S. Effects of monocular lid closure on development of receptive field characteristics of neurons in rabbit superior colliculus. *Journal of Neurophysiology*, 1978, *41*, 1359-1372.

Frost, D. O., & Schneider, G. E. Normal and abnormal uncrossed retinal projections in Syrian hamsters demonstrated by Fink-Heimer and autoradiographic techniques. *Neuroscience Abstracts*, 1976, *2*, 812.

Grobstein, P., & Chow, K. L. Receptive field organization in the mammalian visual cortex: The role of individual experience in development. In G. Gotlieb (Ed.), *Neural and behavioral specificity* (Vol. 3). New York: Academic Press, 1976.

Hebb, D. O. The innate organization of visual activity. I. Perception of figures by rats reared in total darkness. *Journal of Genetic Psychology*, 1937, *51*, 101-126.

Hirsch, H. V. B., & Leventhal, A. G. Functional modification of the developing visual system. In M. Jacobsen (Ed.), *Handbook of sensory physiology* (Vol. 10). New York: Springer Verlag, 1978.

Hubel, D. H. The visual cortex of normal and deprived monkeys. *American Scientists*, 1979, *67*, 532-543.

Hubel, D. H., & Wiesel, T. N. Receptive fields of cells in striate cortex of very young, visually inexperienced kittens. *Journal of Neurophysiology*, 1963, *26*, 994-1002.

Hubel, D. H., Wiesel, T. N., & LeVay, S. Plasticity of ocular dominance columns in monkey striate cortex. *Philosophical Transactions of the Royal Society of London, series B*, 1977, *278*, 377-409.

Land, P. W., & Lund, R. D. Development of the rat's uncrossed retinotectal pathway and its relation to plasticity studies. *Science*, 1979, *205*, 698-700.

Lashley, K. S. Experimental analysis of instinctive behavior. *Psychological Bulletin*, 1938, *45*, 445-471.

Lund, R. D. Development and plasticity of the brain. Oxford: Oxford University Press, 1978.

Lund, R. D., Cunningham, T. J., & Lund, J. S. Modified optic projections after unilateral eye removal in young rats. *Brain, Behavior, and Evolution*, 1973, *8*, 51-72.

Masland, R. H., Chow, K. L., & Stewart, D. L. Receptive-field characteristics of superior colliculus neurons in the rabbit. *Journal of Neurophysiology*, 1971, *34*, 148-156.

Mathers, L. H. Postnatal maturation of neurons in the rabbit superior colliculus. *Journal of Comparative Neurology*, 1977, *173*, 439-456.

Mathers, L. H. Postnatal dendritic development in the rabbit visual cortex. *Brain Research*, 1979, *168*, 21-30.

Mathers, L. H., Chow, K. L., Spear, P. D., & Grobstein, P. Ontogenesis of receptive fields in the rabbit striate cortex. *Experimental Brain Research*, 1974, *19*, 20-35.

Mathers, L. H., Mercer, K. L., & Marshall, P. E. Synaptic development in the rabbit superior colliculus and visual cortex. *Experimental Brain Research*, 1978, *33*, 353-369.

McArdle, C. B., Dowling, J. E., & Masland, R. H. Development of outer-segment and synapses in the rabbit retina. *Journal of Comparative Neurology*, 1977, *175*, 253-273.

Mize, R. R., & Murphy, E. H. Selective visual experience fails to modify receptive field properties of rabbit striate cortex neurons. *Science*, 1973, *180*, 320-323.

Norton, T. T. Receptive field properties of superior colliculus cells and development of visual behavior in kittens. *Journal of Neurophysiology*, 1974, *37*, 674-690.

Rapisardi, S. C., Chow, K. L., & Mathers, L. H. Ontogenesis of receptive field characteristics in the dorsal lateral geniculate nucleus of the rabbit. *Experimental Brain Research*, 1975, *22*, 295-305.

Rhoades, R. W., & Chalupa, L. M. Receptive field characteristics of superior colliculus neurons and visually guided behavior in dark-reared hamsters. *Journal of Comparative Neurology*, 1978, *177*, 17-32.

Rocha-Miranda, C. E., & Lent, R. (Eds.). *Opossum neurobiology* [*Neurobiologia do Gamba*]. Rio de Janeiro: Academia Brasileria de Ciencis, 1978.

Shaw, C., Yinon, U., & Auerbach, E. Receptive fields and response properties of neurons in the rat visual cortex. *Vision Reseach,* 1975, *15,* 203-208.

So, K. F., Schneider, G. E., & Frost, D. O. Postnatal development of retinal projection to the lateral geniculate body in Syrian hamsters. *Brain Research,* 1978, *142,* 343-352.

Spear, P. D., Chow, K. L., Masland, R. H., & Murphy, E. H. Ontogenesis of receptive field characteristics of superior colliculus neurons in the rabbit. *Brain Research,* 1972, *45,* 67-86.

Stein, B. E., Labos, E., & Kruger, L. Sequence of changes in properties of neurons of superior colliculus of the kitten during maturation. *Journal of Neurophysiology,* 1973, *36,* 667-679.

Stewart, D. L., Chow, K. L., & Masland, R. H. Receptive field characteristics of lateral geniculate neurons in the rabbit. *Journal of Neurophysiology,* 1971, *34,* 139-147.

Stryker, M. P., & Sherk, H. Modification of cortical orientation selectivity in the cat by restricted visual experience: A reexamination. *Science,* 1975, *190,* 904-906.

Stryker, M. P., Sherk, H., Leventhal, A. G., & Hirsch, H. V. B. Physiological consequences for the cat's visual cortex of effectively restricting early visual experience with oriented contours. *Journal of Neurophysiology,* 1978, *41,* 896-909.

Vrensen, G. Ontogenesis of the visual cortex of rabbits and the effect of visual deprivation. In M. A. Corner, R. E. Baker, N. E. Van de Pol, D. F. Swaab, & H. B. M. Uylings (Eds.), *Maturation of the nervous system.* Amsterdam: Elsevier, 1978.

Vrensen, G., De Groot, D., & Nunes-Cardoza, J. The postnatal development of neurons and synapses in the visual and motor cortex of rabbits: A quantitative light and electron microscopic study. *Brain Research Bulletin,* 1977, *2,* 405-416.

Wiesel, T. N., & Hubel, D. H. Single-cell responses in striate cortex of kittens deprived of vision in one eye. *Journal of Neurophysiology,* 1963, *26,* 1003-1017.

Wiesel, T. N., & Hubel, D. H. Ordered arrangement of orientation columns in monkeys lacking visual experience. *Journal of Comparative Neurology,* 1974, *158,* 307-318.

9 Two-Way Streets of the Mammalian Cerebral Cortex

Austin H. Riesen
Department of Psychology
University of California

Karl Lashley was a man of strong opinions. He took sides on issues. Once he stated on which side he stood, he was quite capable of softening or qualifying an extreme position. In *Brain Mechanisms and Intelligence*, his full appreciation of qualifying or limiting conditions appears in the body of the chapters. His conclusions at the ends of the chapters or in summary statements elsewhere are generally overstatements, and therefore in some disagreement with the expanded text. He preferred oversimplifications. Among these was one I heard him repeat verbally, but not in writing: "All scientific journals published before 1920 should be thrown out of the libraries. What's in them is generally wrong, anyway, or no longer important."

Lashley was an avowed "innater" even as he engaged in research on learning. He also claimed atheism, dislike of ministers and medical doctors, and a disaffection for Pavlovian conditioning especially in applications to Watsonian behaviorism. He is best known for his support of the doctrine of "mass action" in cortical functioning and the corollary principle of "vicarious functioning."

Lashley advised students against tackling complex research issues. Emotion was an area that he felt was not ready for research answers. Effects of dark-rearing, as shown by behavioral and neurophysiological arrested development, were frowned upon as topics for research, especially by graduate students, because clear-cut hypotheses were difficult to support and outcomes were not supportive of either an all-out innate or all-out environmental set of determining conditions.

In 1942, when Robert M. Yerkes retired, Lashley inherited me as a Research Associate attached to the Infant Studies Program (Nissen, 1942) at the Laboratories of Primate Biology in Orange Park, Florida. Nissen and I had been using a manual of behavior items that was based on studies of human infants. Arnold Gesell, M.D., and Helen Thompson, Ph.D., had collaborated in the production of this manual, which clearly carried the implied interpretations of nativism (Gesell & Thompson, 1934). Postural items proved to be quite applicable to chimpanzee babies, as did those relevant to visual perception. Our results, as published in Riesen and Kinder (1952) and Riesen (1970), showed that human infants developed postural abilities later postnatally than the chimpanzees, but were quite close in ages of appearance to the young apes when perceptual items were compared. The latter findings formed the background for the decision by Nissen and me to blindfold a newborn chimpanzee. We wanted to find out, and we were quite open-minded about possible outcomes, just what a major change in environment would do to visual development.

Quite frankly, as a Yale graduate student, I was more impressed with Professor Hull's environmentalism than I was with Dr. Gesell's nativism. I was prepared to find some effects, however temporary, of the dark-rearing. Neither Nissen nor I was quite prepared to handle the degree of difficulty we had in keeping our infant, Jent, from loosening his blindfold. We hoped to exclude vision until Jent was 16 weeks old, but by 12 weeks we felt defeated by his manual dexterity. Early on many mornings he was peeking alongside a nostril with a favored left eye. This may explain a strong convergent squint (strabismus) that appeared after 1 year of age and became permanent. At 12 weeks there was no recognition of feeding bottle, spoon, or food. With blindfolds removed, Jent's selective visual fixations improved, and he began gradually to anticipate contact from visual objects and to respond discriminatively to them. Unfortunately, World War II changed priorities for us, and further studies were delayed. Lashley and his good friend, Paul Weiss of the University of Chicago, supported my appointment as an officer in the Altitude Training program of the United States Army Air Corps.

The late Dr. Herbert Birch was a key person in instituting new and more successful procedures when the work was resumed. Dark-rearing was substituted for the blindfold procedure. Hoods that could quickly be slipped on and off gave secure control of visual input when animals were brought into daylight. Lashley was astonished, if not disappointed, to witness the lack of visual orienting, the absence of reaching for, or avoidance of, objects that had become tactually discriminated by subjects Snark and Alfalfa. He suggested a procedure, long a favorite of his, for combining reward and punishment in order to motivate visual discriminating behaviors. By this time Dr. Birch had returned to New York City, and it was Hebb, Nissen, and I who followed Lashley's suggestion.

We decided on a schedule of daily trials in which the feeding bottle was shown, then the subject rewarded if it approached the bottle by allowing several sucks and swallowing of baby formula. In contrast, a black-and-white-striped circular plaque was presented, to be followed when the subject approached it by mild shock on the mouth region (Fig. 9.1). Compared with other nursery-reared

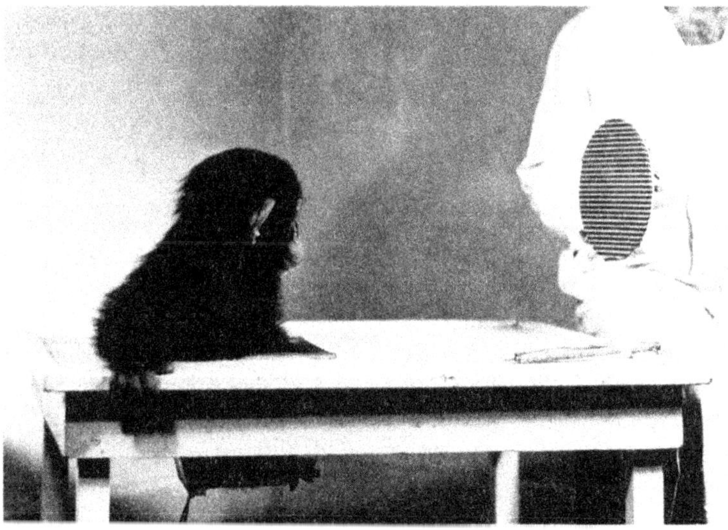

FIG. 9.1. Target at standard distance for visual approach-avoidance learning with young chimpanzee subject.

infants of similar age, who learned quickly, the dark-reared required many trials (Riesen, 1958, pp. 435 ff.).

Once the plaque versus feeding bottle discrimination had been established, we proceeded to train a differentiation of horizontal from vertical stripes. The wide stripes were then gradually narrowed, and we tested for the acuity thresholds. Prolonged, early dark-rearing had resulted in a long-term deleterious effect on visual acuity (Riesen, 1958, 1965).

Such findings raised questions about possible changes in the anatomy and physiology of the eye as well as the visual nervous system. A most cooperative, interested, and helpful ophthalmologist, Dr. W. J. Knauer, examined our young chimpanzees on repeated visits to the laboratories and in his Jacksonville office. Retinoscopy showed some refractive errors, but the most dramatic finding was a considerable disc pallor. In these early infants reared in the dark, the persistence of this index of nerve atrophy pointed to irreversible effects in the retina. Other infants, reared with daily exposures to diffused light, recovered from milder degrees of disc pallor and showed much recovery of visually guided behavior (Riesen, 1950, 1958).

At this point in the research two very different interpretations of the results appeared. Hebb (1949) saw them as corroborating the von Senden (1960) review of human congenital cataract literature. He supported a theory of the development of form perception that emphasized early learning. Lashley, in opposition, saw disc pallor as indicating severe retinal atrophy. Thus, the data in his view did not violate nativism. He could hold out for genetic neural organization as fundamental to perception. Perceptual processes were the consequence of how neuronal pathways and brain ''fields'' developed—a one-way street from genes to behavior.

VICARIOUS FUNCTIONING—EVIDENCE FOR PLASTICITY

The principle of *equipotentiality*, or, in a less extreme form, *vicarious functioning*, was attributed by Lashley (1929) to clinical neurologists—that is, to Bianchi, Goldstein, Monokow, and others. Lashley's work served to channel the concept into neuropsychology, where it continues to gain experimental support, as in a recent study by Howarth, Meyer, and Meyer (1979). The current volume has notable and detailed evidence in Chapter 7, by Pasik and Pasik, for vicarious functioning in visual projection systems. This form of visual plasticity was well supported in terms of behavior and electrophysiology by Stewart and Riesen (1972). Visual placing, visual cliff avoidance, and visual exploratory behaviors were retained in rabbits following ablation of striate cortex done at 5 days of age, but not in adult operates. Mean latencies of evoked responses in lateral (V-II) cortex dropped from 29.8 to 23.7 as a consequence of this ''reorganization.''

Kennard's monkeys (1938) in a much earlier study showed vicarious assumption of function following lesions of motor cortex. Again this happened in very young monkeys but failed in older animals. In general, early age at cortical loss followed by environmental demands for exercising the function are key factors that work toward behavioral recovery.

Inasmuch as retina evolves from cortex as well as projecting to cortex, the research proposal of Ms. Dale Zilbert a few years ago seemed eminently worth pursuing. She suggested that central visual projections might take over innervation from adjacent intact retina after laser lesions of the visual streak in *young* rabbits but would fail to do so in *older* animals. With assistance and equipment made available by Dr. Robert V. Shearer of Loma Linda University School of Medicine, Loma Linda, California, the experiments were carried out (Zilbert & Riesen, 1971). Postoperative recovery was tested 2 to 4 months after the retinal lesions had been placed. Adult rabbits proved to have reduced acuity as a result of the lesions, whereas rabbits in which lesions were placed at 2 to 3 weeks of age showed normal levels of acuity.

FIELD THEORY VERSUS PATHWAYS AND CONNECTIONS

Development or recovery in cortical function may best be explained in terms of synaptic reorganization (i.e., connections newly established) rather than in terms of vague references to cortical fields, as Lashley preferred. Single-unit recording has reestablished the multiple pathway and ''cell assembly'' concepts (Hebb,

1949) as fundamental to the neuropsychology of perception and motor functions. Also generally accepted are findings that pathways, and the synapses underlying them, are highly determined by innate organizing factors. How such factors operate and how environments confirm or modify them remain major, unsolved problems in developmental neurobiology. Lashley would find both comfort (in evidence for innate organization) and distress in modern single-cell work. He had thoroughly rejected (1929) "the old notion of elementary ideas located in single cells of the brain. . . . this is clearly not the principle of neural organization [p. 162]."

Genetic determination is not sufficient to organize and maintain visual perception to its fullest. Anatomic, physiological, and behavioral studies are in agreement that perceptual processing requires two-way streets. Lashley preferred to conceptualize such brain mechanisms as one-way and as field determined, not as pathways nor as multidirectional.

When Lashley (1929) found correlations between amount of cortical tissue removed and degree of maze-performance deficits, he was unable to relate this set of results to stimulus–response concepts. Much earlier, in 1917, he had made a most convincing argument for organization within a brain region that could only reflect (1) sensory learning within and between sense modes such as hearing and vision, and (2) motor learning of action patterns that did not require immediate sensory feedback. Corollary to these positive requirements was the demonstration that S–R learning theories were by themselves inadequate. I acknowledge a great indebtedness to Lashley and to Hebb for straightening out my own thinking on this subject. Sight-reading a musical arpeggio, Lashley pointed out, and executing same on a musical instrument require such speed of neuronal processing that local brain circuitry must, after patient and oft-repeated rehearsal, program the percept of the arpeggio as a unit and its execution in motor terms before there is time for sensory feedback from muscles. Lashley made frequent reference to this example of his in conversation and in classroom or seminar discussions. The following quotation from a University of Wisconsin symposium contribution of mine (Riesen, 1958) illustrates my indebtedness:

> I conceive of the development of form vision as requiring a sensory-sensory integration that involves learning according to a contiguity principle. My basic premise is in this respect the same as that of Hebb (1949). Such development, the evidence reviewed above indicates, must await differential excitation from contours, corners, and edges. These insure that certain loci in the retina, and hence certain cells in the projection areas, are maximally active while others remain relatively inactive. When there is consistency and repetition in the patterns of these loci, sensory-sensory conditioning takes place. The probability of the participation of certain cells in an activation sequence increases, and that of other cells remains the same or decreases. Some relatively permanent structural modifications must result which register the effects of, and *constitute*, the intrasensory associative patterning. Hebb has gone to some pains to develop neuropsychological constructs which are applicable to simultaneous and sequential patterns of this kind.

Since S-S learning is more difficult to measure than S-R learning, psychology with a behavioristic orientation tends to minimize consideration of it or to deny it. Hull's concept of afferent neural interaction would be broad enough to include it, but Hull would prefer to handle any modification of sensory-sensory relationships by inserting a hypothetical response between Ss to provide S-R-S sequences. Lashley (1929) has argued that there is not time for all the responses that would be necessary to account for fast-moving behavior in accordance with an S-R-S schema. One reason that sensory-sensory integrations are so slighted in psychology lies in the loose definition of "stimulus" employed. The S-R theorists accept any complex combination of sensory energies, such as is inherent in a visual form or a tactual proprioceptive pattern, as *a* stimulus. Tacit acceptance of the organism's capacity to make unity out of diversity is general, especially since Gestalt psychology asserted that such a capacity is innate. This has not led to an understanding of how the unique inter-relations within each unity are integrated into a unique unit.

In responding to the uniqueness of patterns which can only be discriminated (or identified) on the basis of subtle differences in contour, hue, and brightness relationships within the pattern, the sophisticated perceiving organism also *isolates* the pattern within a massive afferent flux. "Meaningful" segments of spatial mosaics in the visual environment are abstracted by selective "attention." Our visually naive subjects are apparently meeting neither the integrative nor the selective requirements of form perception effectively. They do show certain limited, innate predispositions to isolate and unify. They can cope with a "real" environment only after frequent contiguities of specific combinations of sensory energies greatly expand the selective and integrative processes.

With cumulative visual exposure to spatial patterns our chimpanzee subjects show gradually increasing facility for discriminating complex forms. It is highly significant that horizontal vs. vertical striation should have proved relatively easy for Chow to discriminate. These stimuli carry the same differentiating cues repetitively over the visual field. At the other extreme is the very late appearance of discriminations for faces. Here, the discrimination must be based on subtle differences in the relative angular, curvilinear, and areal dimensions. Memories of familiar faces must serve as reference standards. These involve sensory-sensory integrations (associations) developed over many hours of experience [pp. 445–446].

PLASTICITY IN EARLY VISUAL DEVELOPMENT

Following the dark-rearing of Snark and Alfalfa, Nissen, K. L. Chow, J. Semmes, R. Fantz, and I further pursued the questions of early optic atrophy as opposed to central (CNS) organizing mechanisms. To learn whether the dark-rearing produced atrophy only during a critical age, we raised Debi (No. 136) from birth to 7 months and Faik (No. 101) from 8 to 24 months in the darkroom. To our surprise, both animals developed disc pallor. Debi recovered normal retinal and disc appearance by 18 months, but Faik was like Snark in that his retina never recovered normal appearance under the ophthalmoscope. Years later, when Snark and Faik were enucleated (Chow, Riesen, & Newell, 1957), we were able to determine that a major portion of the retinal ganglion cells had disappeared. We continue to regard this as evidence for a disturbance of protein synthesis in underused neurons and in supporting metabolic systems. We were able, to show (Rasch, Swift, Riesen, & Chow, 1961), that retinal neurons and receptor cells are markedly depleted in RNA concentrations when stimulation is withheld. Cats did not lose ganglion cells, however, with prolonged dark-rearing. Kandy (No. 140) did not develop pallor of the optic nerve heads (discs) by 3 months. Her visual behaviors were slow in developing, but by 7 months of age she behaved normally and was discriminating strangers from familiar persons (Riesen, 1958, p. 431).

Chimpanzees 125 and 142 were the first two of three infants that we reared under a daily program of diffused light. Chow was born on 2/5/50. Five days after birth he was moved into the darkroom. Beginning at 2 weeks of age Chow received 1½ to 2 hours daily of diffused light through a white Plexiglas dome. Kora (No. 142) was similarly exposed to unpatterned light but without the delay, so that she was never without a daily exposure of 90 min. When each of these chimpanzees was 7 months of age, it was brought into a normally patterned visual environment. They showed no photophobia (lid closure in bright light) such as the dark-reared infants showed. They had lively pupillary reflexes, both simple and consensual. The fundus and disc were normal for Kora, but in Chow the fundus was, according to Dr. Knauer, "a little bit pale, but does not have the white appearance of optic nerve atrophy." Also, "the nerve head appears somewhat flattened." Retinoscopy at 1 m gave rather similar results: +2:00 in each eye for Kora, and +2:50 in each eye for Chow. (These determinations were not made until about 6½ weeks after termination of visual deprivation.)

Both Chow and Kora showed spontaneous nystagmus in episodes of 1 to 5 jerks, predominantly in a horizontal direction. They also exhibited cover nystagmus toward the side of the uncovered eye. There was no eyeblink to an approaching object and no steady fixation, and heterotropia was obvious. This was strongly exo- in Chow and moderately so in Kora.

The first eyeblinks to object-approaching-face occurred 9 days after Chow came into lighted environments. For Kora this appeared a day earlier, and for both infants movement across the visual field was also likely to produce startle with eye closure. Contact of face produced a startle response, clearly indicating that there was no visual awareness or anticipation of the contact. First visual pursuit of a moving object occurred on Day 11 with Chow and Day 13 with Kora. These pursuit movements were jerky, not smooth-flowing as in normal infants of like age. First visual fixations of persons appeared at approximately 2 weeks post-dark-rearing (with diffused light).

Both infants required many days to orient toward, and pursue with proper head orientation, their white feeding bottle with brown nipple attached. At 3 weeks (nearly 8 months of age) Kora was recorded to have responded as follows: "Protrudes lip as follows bottle, but shows very little response to distance. Gives only slight forward extension of neck while protruding lips, and makes no effort to reach forward farther, regardless of nearness of bottle, until contact is made. Then she will follow nipple forward for considerable distance if it is pulled slowly away." The clear discrimination of the bottle from a variety of other objects required still another 3 to 4 weeks. For Chow this required nearly 10 weeks of full daytime visual experience.

Our nursery-reared chimpanzee babies that were reared in a visual environment normally gave initial avoidance responses to strange objects and strange persons beginning in the 4th month after birth. Chow and Kora began to show object avoidance during their 9th month, or after 35 and 38 days in lighted surroundings. Fear of strange persons did not appear in Chow until 5 months in light. Kora consistently "trusted" all persons. Hers appeared to be a case of unusual social motivation, not a matter of acuity.

When acuity tests were done with Chow, he showed at 11½ months of age that he could resolve vertical versus horizontal striations with widths of ⅓ mm, or the equivalent of a visual angle of 3 min, a highly satisfactory performance (Riesen, 1958, p. 437). By this stage Chow showed only infrequent episodes of spontaneous nystagmus, and his fixation and binocular convergence were greatly improved. When an object was brought to within about 4 in. of his face, the convergence was lost and exotropia reappeared.

Difficulties of visual fixation as exhibited by Chow and Kora were reduced but not eliminated with another infant. Wenka (No. 168) was raised with simple visual spot targets available during her 90 min under the illuminated dome, and two intermittently lighted "stars" were put into the darkroom.

BINOCULARITY IN VISUAL DEVELOPMENT

When infant chimpanzees emerged at 7 months into normal daylight and day-night conditions (from dark-rearing or diffused light), they invariably had fixation problems. Exotropia, spontaneous nystagmus, and eye alternation were only very gradually reduced and not always completely eliminated. The most sensitive period for developing binocularity appeared to be over by 7 months of age. With infant Wenka, whose environment contained simple fixation targets, the development of binocular convergence came about more rapidly than for three other infants, but the availability of such simple light-on-dark and dark-on-light spots was not nearly equivalent to a normally patterned visual world. Table 9.1 shows comparisons in terms of the number of days beyond 7 months that were required for developing increasing proficiencies in convergence eye movements.

After many months into the 2nd year, these early deprived animals showed nystagmus and exotropia in episodic form when they became either fatigued or

TABLE 9.1
Numbers of Days in Normal Visual Environment and Counting from 7 Months of Age Until Convergence Eye Movements Could Be Elicited by Approaching Visual Target. (Based on Riesen, 1958, p. 441.)

	Condition of Rearing and Animal					
	Total Darkness	*Diffused Light*		*Diffused Light with Fixation Spots*	*Holder Only*	*Free-moving*
Eye Movements	*No. 136 Debi*	*No. 125 Chow*	*No. 142 Kora*	*No. 168 Wenka*	*No. 148 Mita*	*No. 119 Lad*
First convergence	58	40	59	5	8	0
to 5 in.	76	74	59	17	40	0
to 3 in.	93	124	107	63	82+	0
to lip contact	117	131	385+	86	301	9

overly excited. For example, on January 1, 1956, when Wenka was 19 months of age, the following entry was made in her diary:

> Lateral, vertical, and oblique fixation nystagmus appeared during initial period of some tension in unfamiliar surroundings. This was particularly evident when she looked up toward the ceiling light fixture. After 5 minutes she became well relaxed. She looked up toward the light periodically and showed no nystagmus.

And further, during Gesell-Thompson testing:

> Showed fixation of pellet but interest remained centered on bottle. . . . Other test situations given and performance was well within range of nursery-reared infants of her age. Manipulation was on a par with the infants showing best emotional adjustment to the testing procedure. . . . She became playful and good ocular coordination returned. But within 2 or 3 minutes she quieted down, exotropia occurred twice as she was watching my face. Left eye maintained fixation.

Dark-reared infant Debi appeared to develop good binocular vision during her 2nd year. She easily maintained fixation and convergence when an object was brought closer until it touched her lips. However, by February 1956, when she was 9 years old, Debi had become strongly esotropic. Diary entries by Riesen indicate that she fixated monocularly with either eye, the other deviating sharply inward. Nystagmus had also returned: "Left eye fixates, right eye shows inward squint. She cocks head to her right and peers from left canthi. Eyes show isolated, or groups of, fast jerks to the right [2/25/56]."

Chow also went through stages of improving binocular fixation and a return to more frequently manifested exotropia; then, during his 5th year, he became a convergent squinter:

> Strong "squint" persisted during 5 minutes while Chow was excitedly playful and sociable at 9:00 A.M. today. He frequently cocked his head around toward the right shoulder, looked at me with the right eye, which was in nasal corner of orbit. Other eye meanwhile was in center of orbit. At other times he fixated briefly and alternatingly, the esotropic strabismus being quite strong all the while [11/24/54].

Kora was still showing episodes of exotropia when she died at the age of 2 years and 9 months. Her extremely brief terminal illness was diagnosed as meningitis. The sequence of shifting from exotropia to esotropia is in agreement with results in cats following many months of recovering from binocular lid suturing (Cynader, Berman, & Hein, 1976).

Whether dark-reared or regularly exposed to diffused light, none of the chimpanzees deprived of pattern vision from birth to 7 months gained uncomplicated binocularity. We conclude, therefore, that the critical period for the development of normal binocular vision is less than the age period of birth to 7 months. Extrapolation of this finding to human infants would indicate that by 1 year of age, normal binocularity must be established if it is not to suffer inadequacies.

REQUIREMENTS FOR EARLY VISUAL FIXATION AND PURSUIT

Sensory-motor-sensory feedback loops must depend upon environmental supports for the development of binocular vision. The findings already reviewed strongly suggest such a conclusion. Dr. Jack Orbach proposed in 1953 that a way to test this conclusively would be to raise an infant in an environment rich in room patterns, with illumination provided only in brief flashes. This would give the visual system patterned stimulation without the opportunity for visual refixations or eye movement "confirmation." This clearly requires a two-way street of information exchange and a memory system that improves the two-way coordination as usage is repeated. Even "two-way" is an oversimplification.

Mack (No. 145) was a male infant born October 5, 1954. From October 11 until May 6, 1955, this infant chimpanzee lived in a room that was fully illuminated every 8 sec with a flash of 1/15 sec duration. Beginning at 6 weeks of age Mack was also exposed to homogeneous light for 90 min per day through the translucent dome, as earlier with Kora and Chow. In Orbach's words: "The darkroom was enriched with multi-shaped objects in the crib and suspended from the ceiling [visible during each flash]. During the last month of dark-rearing, the square test plaque was suspended from the ceiling about four feet from the crib. He was taken out (of darkroom) at seven months" (Diary notes, 1954).

In the absence of fixation or pursuit opportunities, Mack developed visual abilities no better than those of Debi, Chow, or Kora. He had exotropic strabismus, episodes of nystagmus, and by 15 months an unreliable ability for convergence responses to approaching objects. He learned a set of pattern discrimination habits only after 163 sessions, given two per day. (This training was carried out by Orbach and by Robert Fantz.) In this respect Mack did no better or worse than Chow (Riesen, 1958, p. 436). Wenka had learned to the same criterion level in 109 sessions, apparently having benefited from simple fixation targets during the first 7 months. In experiments using monkeys, Orbach and Miller (1969) fully confirmed the need for an early environment containing visual patterns if adequate binocular skills and eye–hand coordinations are to be seen later.

PATTERN RECOGNITION AFTER EARLY PATTERN DEPRIVATION

Multiple and redundant line orientation stimuli such as we used to measure visual acuity have proved quite easy for visually deprived chimpanzees and cats to learn (Riesen, 1965). This result agrees well with data from single-cell recording, since cortical units selective for orientation are found to be plentiful at an early age and survive *bi*nocular deprivation quite well (Ganz, Hirsch, & Tieman, 1972). Form discriminations are more difficult for pattern-deprived animals to learn (Wilson & Riesen, 1966). Animals exposed to patterns while restrained also have greater difficulty than unrestrained, pattern-experienced animals (Riesen, 1965). Further analyses of the nature of these difficulties in visually deprived animals were recently provided in a study by Tees (1979). Visually experienced animals (rats) were found to discriminate pattern irregularities and contour separations more readily than dark-reared animals.

EARLY VISUAL DEPRIVATION AND INTEROCULAR TRANSFER

In 1950 two of my graduate students at Chicago and I began to experiment with cats to determine whether visual experience is necessary for developing interocular equivalence of learned discrimination habits. K. L. Chow, D. O. Hebb, Henry W. Nissen, and I had discussed this question over lunch in Orange Park. In his 1949 book, Hebb challenged the notion that interocular equivalence was innately guaranteed, citing evidence for failure of such in birds that J. Levine, a Lashley student, had published 4 years earlier (1945). Experiments with infant chimpanzees utilized monocular deprivation of patterns with diffused light exposure. The other eye experienced room patterns for 90 min per day. Results of these and other procedures are fully reported in a paper by Chow and Nissen (1955). Three different habits were learned by Sally (No. 164)—two with the diffused-light eye and the other with the pattern-experienced eye. No immediate interocular transfer occurred, although fewer trials were needed for the second eye in each case. These results and results with our cats (Riesen, Kurke, & Mellinger, 1953) fully confirmed Hebb's expectations. In both sets of studies normally reared control animals showed immediate transfer of habits learned by the same techniques.

Implications of these transfer studies include the clear confirmation that two-way streets are involved in organizing the visual nervous system. The chimpanzees and cats receiving stable visual patterns in their early postnatal weeks gain central neural organization from this experience. Sensorimotor feedback or reafference or (more likely) both are operating to assure a high degree of equivalence between the two eyes. Years later, another of my graduate students, Dale Schissler, clearly determined that some degree of independence remains even in normally reared cats (Schissler & Riesen, 1969). Rabbits are essentially monocular even after much visual experience and even with visual intensity discriminations that in cats readily transfer without early patterned light (Aarons, Halasz, & Riesen, 1963; Dickerson & Riesen, 1977; Riesen & Aarons, 1959). Species differ in the constraints placed on early visual plasticity.

RESTRAINT DURING EARLY VISION DISRUPTS MOVEMENT PERCEPTION

Are stable visual patterns enough? Elimination of nystagmus and poor fixation skills might be sufficient to assure good pattern vision. A comparison between two rearing conditions that we used for chimpanzee infants in 1949 to 1951 indicated that stable visual patterns are not sufficient for normal visual development. Both infants, Lad (No. 119) and Mita (No. 148), were reared to 7 months while receiving 90 min of the lighted environment daily. Lad was permitted free movement about the crib, whereas Mita was supine in the holder (without the dome in position) during the 90 min of exposure to the indoor environment. As can be seen from data tabulated for the Wisconsin symposium (Riesen, 1958), Mita developed visual responses more poorly than did Lad, who was in most respects similar to a normally seeing animal.

For his doctoral dissertation at the University of Chicago, Aarons (1957) proposed that visual movement, like intensity of light, might be expected, as a primitive and basic visual process, to provide quicker learning and immediate interocular transfer in kittens reared with exposure only to diffused light. Results with kittens reared with free movement and those reared while restrained were dramatically different, as we reported in 1959 (Riesen & Aarons, 1959). Both groups learned intensity discriminations and showed transfer, but the restrained kittens failed to learn to discriminate movement from nonmovement. Interocular transfer tests were thus not possible. The conclusion is clear: Perception of visual movement requires experience with active as well as passive movement. The reafference principle is once again validated.

ONCE ESTABLISHED, IS PRIMATE VISION DURABLE?

We ask next whether movement perception, object recognition, and accurate eye–hand coordinations can survive even after these are well developed if a period of visual deprivation intervenes. Ethics would dictate against asking such a question experimentally of a human being, although prison conditions and records have sometimes been cited (e.g., by Gordon Walls in *The Vertebrate Eye,* 1942). The implications are frightening.

In a symposium paper presented at the annual convention of the American Psychological Association in September 1959, I reported two experiments—one with a monkey and one with a chimpanzee (Riesen, 1961). The monkey was in darkroom quarters from 5 to 10 months of age. The chimpanzee was in diffused light from the age of 10 to 18 months. I quote from my symposium paper (Riesen, 1961):

> Both animals showed loss of recognition for food or food containers. In each case approximately eight days were required before these animals regained the clear discriminations between pieces of food and inedible objects which they had shown with complete accuracy before the deprivation period.
>
> Both animals showed inaccuracies of distance and direction when making protective eyelid responses and when approaching and reaching for objects. These improved rapidly during the first three days post-deprivation.
>
> During initial hours of return to the visually structured environment these animals showed, in addition to the eye–hand inaccuracies, some peculiarities of eye movement and binocular coordinations. A pendular nystagmus of rapid (8 per second) rate appeared in the chimpanzee youngster and moments of exotropia. . . . The monkey showed occasional eye and head oscillations [p. 24].

Recovery of binocular coordination and steady fixation required less time, a matter of hours, than did some of the object discriminations. Basically, we may conclude that well-established early oculomotor and perceptual habits are durable. Visual problems after cataract removal in mature individuals are relatively transient when adequately treated.

ELECTROPHYSIOLOGICAL INDICATORS AFTER DEPRIVATION

Karl Lashley's Board of Scientific Advisors to the Yerkes Laboratories of Primate Biology suggested in 1948 that we do some comparisons of deprived and nondeprived visual systems by using ERG (electroretinography), alpha rhythm, and evoked cortical potentials. In accord with this recommendation, two dark-reared chimpanzees were taken to Jacksonville in June 1948 to the neurology clinic of Dr. William H. McCullagh. Debi was 7 months of age and received her first exposure to light since the day of birth as a part of the electroencephalography procedures. Frontal and parietal leads gave slow, large-amplitude waves with small-amplitude irregularities superimposed. ''All of four differently placed occipital electrodes showed very rapid low amplitude waves (30–50 per second), and sharp spikes at the rate of 2–3 per second. Six per second alpha rhythm was also recorded.'' (Diary notes, 1948). Exposure to light produced no clear change. Snark at 40 months of age and after 7 months in lighted surroundings showed a 7- to 8-per-sec alpha. His acuity at this time was testing very low: striations of 8 mm in width were required for horizontal versus vertical grid discriminations. This width was 20 times greater than normal. (Snark had earlier discriminated 5-mm stripes; his visual acuities continued to deteriorate over a period of years.)

Working with dark-reared kittens, one of my students, Bruce Baxter (Baxter & Riesen, 1961), found that the b-wave of the ERG was slow to recover when flashes of high intensity were used. Ramsey and I (Riesen, 1965) found similar effects in rhesus monkeys. In both species recovery occurred with a week or more in normal diurnal lighting conditions.

To evaluate physiological properties of visual cortex, Siegel, Coleman, and I (1973) recorded evoked responses from young cats. Following rearing to 6 months in diffused light, the cortical flash-evoked responses were the same as in control animals. Pattern-evoked responses showed different response conformations in normally reared cats, but not in those reared in diffused light. Longer latency components of the normal kittens' responses differentiated the two groups. Where no pattern is involved, as also in flicker-induced evoked potentials, even dark-rearing did not impair cortical following of the stimulus frequency in Baxter's earlier study (1966).

CHANGES IN CELLS OF THE VISUAL CORTEX FOLLOWING DEPRIVATION

Visual deprivation by dark-rearing is a technique with a long history. Berger used it in 1900 to study changes in cells of the occipital cortex in dogs and cats. More recently Gyllensten, Malmfors, and Norrlin (1965) found retarded growth of cell diameters and of internuclear material in mice with 4 to 8 weeks of dark-rearing, and Valverde (1967) reported reduced numbers of spines on apical dendrites of pyramidal cells.

Thinking in terms of reduced connections in the visual cortex as a consequence of visual deprivation, Paul Coleman and I (1968) elected to measure the development of dendritic branching in layer IV stellate cells. Since more branching would be expected to correlate with more synaptic microstructures, we anticipated finding fewer branchings in dark-reared cats at 6 months. Our results for pyramidal cells of the cingulate cortex where visual input is received, as well as striate cortex, supported our expectation. The data were more consistent for cingulate gyrus neurons than for the sample from striate cortex. In both areas the second- and third-order dendrites were larger in numbers for the cats reared in lighted rooms. Dark- versus light-rearing conditions did not have significant effects on layer V pyramids as measured on basilar dendrites.

Using environmental complexity as the experimental manipulation, Greenough and Volkmar (1973) and Greenough, Volkmar, and Juraska (1973) have reported selective effects on dendrites in the occipital cortex related to enriched versus impoverished conditions of rearing. These studies provide extensions of the earlier studies by Holloway (1966), by Schapiro and Vukovich (1970), and by our study with cats. Sensory stimulation versus deprivation is the common experimental variable (Riesen, 1966, pp. 125–126).

Growth-promoting effects of stimulation have been measured in various other ways to show anatomically (Fifková, 1974; Globus, 1975) and physiologically (Blakemore & Van Sluyters, 1975; Peck & Blakemore, 1975) that developmental neurobiology has much to gain by careful study of these function-related changes. It is beyond the purpose of this chapter to review the field in a comprehensive manner.

STIMULUS GENERALIZATION IN NAIVE MONKEYS

In a paper they published in 1946, Lashley and Wade challenged the position of Pavlov and of Hull (1939) with regard to stimulus generalization gradients. Paradoxically, Hull's nativistic position was challenged by that of Lashley and Wade in which one of two alternatives emphasized prior experience with the relevant stimulus dimension. In brief, Lashley and Wade predicted that naive organisms would show broad and flat generalization. After differential reinforcement of S^d and S^Δ, a steeper gradient should develop.

In a study using hue as the stimulus dimension, Ganz and Riesen (1962) found the flat gradient in dark-reared macaque monkeys on the 1st day of testing, with steeper slopes thereafter until they averaged during 7 days of testing significantly steeper gradients than hue-experienced animals. This steepness developed in the absence of differential reinforcement, since all testing was done under an extinction procedure. A subsequent and related study showed innate stimulus generalization of a form discrimination in form-naive monkeys, with transfer to new retinal locations also strongly present. These results were obtained with conditions of stabilized images by the Riggs–Ditchburn technique. Hence, form-naive animals showed generalization of form without contouring eye movements (Ganz & Wilson, 1967). Lashley would have been pleased with such fine support for his nativism.

EFFECTS OF SOMATOSENSORIMOTOR DEPRIVATION

Thalamic and midbrain sensory nuclei respond at least as much as does the cerebral cortex to enriched or impoverished environmental rearing conditions. Modalities other than vision have been studied less, but documentation is now ample to show the generality of the phenomenon. Very recently the cerebellum became implicated in studies on the rat (Pysh & Weiss, 1979) and on Old World monkeys (Floeter & Greenough, 1979). Effects of isolation-rearing in monkeys and chimpanzees are by now well documented (Mason, 1968; Riesen, 1971). Impaired social skills are profound as are abilities in tool using and problem solving (Davenport, Rogers, & Rumbaugh, 1973; Menzel, Davenport, & Rogers, 1970). Early somatosensory deprivation must be considered as a most important factor in such long-term behavioral deficits (Prescott, 1971). Body contact, warmth, passive movement, opportunities for grasping and clinging, and other forms of vestibular and muscle, tendon, and joint stimulation are implicated. Perhaps these are significant factors in early human development even in variations that do not severely violate life-support requirements.

My students and I resolved several years ago to test this supposition by studying stumptail monkeys during and following rearing under four conditions of environmental support, three of which involved social isolation. We have reported preliminary findings in terms of behavioral and brain changes (Riesen, Dickerson, & Struble, 1977; Struble & Riesen, 1978). Our behavioral data are largely in agreement with studies that have been concerned with effects of social isolation on stereotyped motor patterns, self-directed stimulation, excessive fear and avoidance, and aggressive behaviors, which become not only asocial but severely antisocial (Mitchell, 1970).

Our infant monkeys (*Macaca arctoides*) were born in the colony established by Rhine in 1968 (Rhine & Hendy-Neely, 1978). After birth, each was left for 1 week with its mother in a stabilized and supportive social group. Infants reared in Conditions 1, 2, and 3 were separated from their mothers at 1 week. They were moved singly to Plexiglas cages situated along one side of a colony cage in which a social group lived. Each of the clear Plexiglas cages had a stainless steel grid floor. For the 2nd week after birth a heating pad was placed on the grid. Meanwhile assistance was given to help the infant monkey feed from a bottle of Similac with nipple protruding into the cage. Within 2 or 3 days the monkey was able to secure the nipple without assistance.

Condition 1 was conducted in a cube cage 30 cm on each edge. In addition to the feeding bottle, a food hopper containing soaked monkey Chow was mounted on the front surface.

Condition 2 was also conducted in a cube cage with sides nearly four times longer. Equipment on the front surface was identical with that for Condition 1.

Condition 3 was identical in overall space to Condition 2. It was enriched with play objects and two ladders (one inclined and the other horizontal) and a swing.

From each of these three living spaces, infants could see each other and the colony animals. The colony animals climbed to the level of the Plexiglas cages frequently and touched the outside surfaces. Sounds and air circulation moved readily through slots in the top and side surfaces of the Plexiglas. Surfaces accessible to the colony animals were not slotted.

Condition 4 was the "social control" situation. Here the infants remained with their mothers in the colony. They were breast-fed until, gradually, they began to eat the solid foods provided in large amounts to the members of the colony. The colony varied in number of infants present from zero to three; adult females numbered four or five; there were two adolescent animals and one adult male who had "alpha" status throughout.

Once or twice a week as required, each infant in the isolation conditions was transferred to a Plexiglas carrying cage. This permitted home-cage cleaning and weighing of the infant.

Behavioral Observations

For 1 hour daily, 5 days per week, each infant was scored for presence within a 30-sec interval of any of 25 behavior items. Differences due to rearing conditions began to appear reliably during the 3rd month of life. Stereotyped behaviors developed under Conditions 1, 2, and 3, including self-clutch, self-bite, hop in place, digit suck, body jerk, and bizarre body orientations. These behaviors all appeared with low frequencies in the Condition 4 (mother-reared) infants. By contrast, no significant effects of rearing condition appeared for active, passive, grimace, rock, and other items. *Depart other,* occurred with high frequency only under Condition 4. *Auto,* defined as normal self-manipulation, scratching, and rubbing, was highly significantly related to rearing condition. It was relatively infrequent under Condition 4 by comparison with the three isolation conditions.

In order of decreasing mean values for body weight at 6 months of age, the infants ranked as follows in terms of rearing condition: 1>2>3>4. Heart weight and gonad weight followed the same sequence. Brain weights and adrenal weights were, on the average, highest for Condition 3 animals. These differences did not reach significance.

Measures of Dendritic Branching in Cortical Layer IV Stellate Cells

Six cortical areas were sampled for the study of cells in layer IV of the cerebral cortex. For Condition 4 five mother-reared animals were sampled at 6 months of age. Four animals were used for each of the other conditions. However, in frontal and in motor II cortex, only three animals from Condition 1 could be adequately studied, and there were three available from Condition 3 for somatosensory II.

From each animal for each cortical area 20 stellate cells were drawn. Drawings were done blind by the use of code designations so that drawers did not know from which animals or conditions their slides were derived. Spiney stellates and cutoff pyramids were eliminated from consideration. The samples used were independent of those drawn for the study reported earlier (Struble & Riesen, 1978), in which we compared effects of Conditions 1 and 4.

The Golgi–Cox method with tungstate modification was used. The tissue was in staining solution for 4 weeks, embedded and mounted, and cut normal to the pia at a thickness of 120 μ. Drawings of individual cells were made at a magnification of 500 $\times$.

Scoring of dendrites and their branching used the method of Coleman and Riesen (1968) as adapted from Clendinnen and Eayrs (1961). First-order dendrites arising from the cell body were followed to the first branch. The two second-order branches were each followed, and so on through the fifth order. Branches beyond this were ignored. In the accompanying figures, average values and their standard errors are presented. Analyses of variance and covariance were determined using computer program BMDP2V of the Health Sciences Computing Facility, University of California, Los Angeles, revision of December 1977. Individual branching points were then subjected to Scheffé tests (Kirk, 1968).

In the visual cortex (area 17) no significant differences due to rearing condition were found. Neither were there significant effects in our samples from the prefrontal cortex (frontolateral surface).

For somatosensory I cortex the effects of rearing conditions were highly significant. Analysis of variance for condition ($F = 12.53$; $df = 3, 13$; $p = .0001$) and for order $\times$ condition interaction ($F = 5.64$; $df = 12, 53$; $p = .0001$) justified using Scheffé tests. This showed that the grand mean of branch counts for Condition 3 exceeds those for Conditions 1 or 2 at the .01 level. Condition 4 branching exceeds that for Condition 1 at the .05 level. At branch order 4 (Fig. 9.2) Condition 3 exceeds Condition 1 at the .01 level. Other individual branch order comparisons did not reach significance (.05 or better).

Rearing Condition 3 also resulted in significantly greater branching ratios overall than each of the other conditions ($p = .01$). Taken individually at order 4 Condition 3 was higher than Condition 1 at the .01 level.

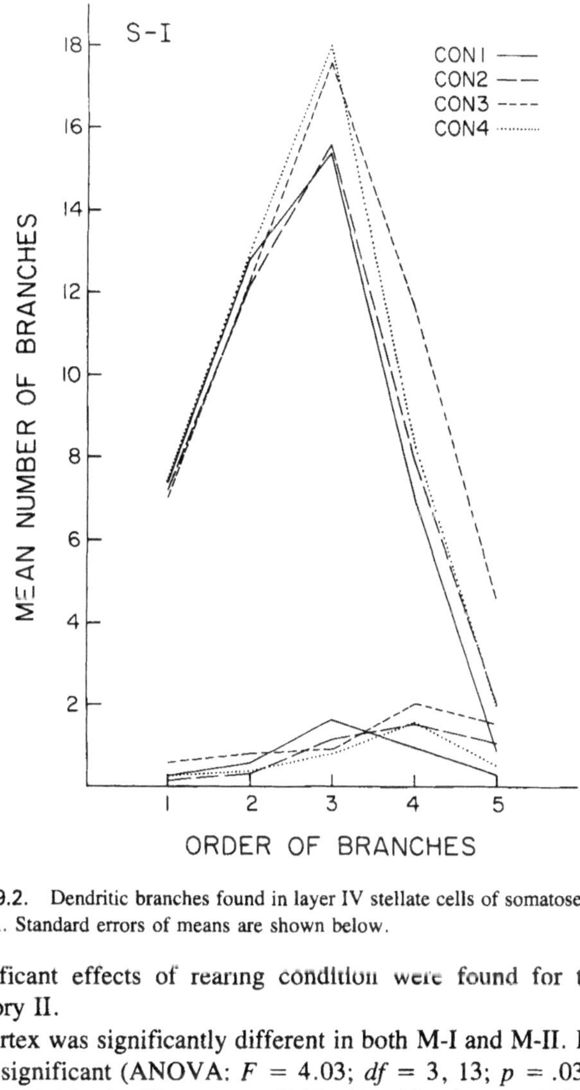

FIG. 9.2. Dendritic branches found in layer IV stellate cells of somatosensory I cortex. Standard errors of means are shown below.

No significant effects of rearing condition were found for the cortex in somatosensory II.

Motor cortex was significantly different in both M-I and M-II. In M-I condition proved significant (ANOVA: $F = 4.03$; $df = 3, 13$; $p = .031$). Order by condition was highly significant ($F = 7.40$; $df = 12, 52$; $p = .0001$). Figure 9.3 shows that the differences lay primarily in third- and fourth-order dendrites. The only comparison at a single branch point that reached significance was at order 3 in which Condition 3 exceeded Condition 1 ($p < .05$).

Branching ratios overall showed that M-I cortex for Condition 3 animals was higher than Condition 1 ($p < .05$) and Condition 4 higher than 1 ($p < .01$). Ratio 2 (order 3 over 2) showed Conditions 3 or 4 each to be significantly greater than Condition 1 at better than the .01 level.

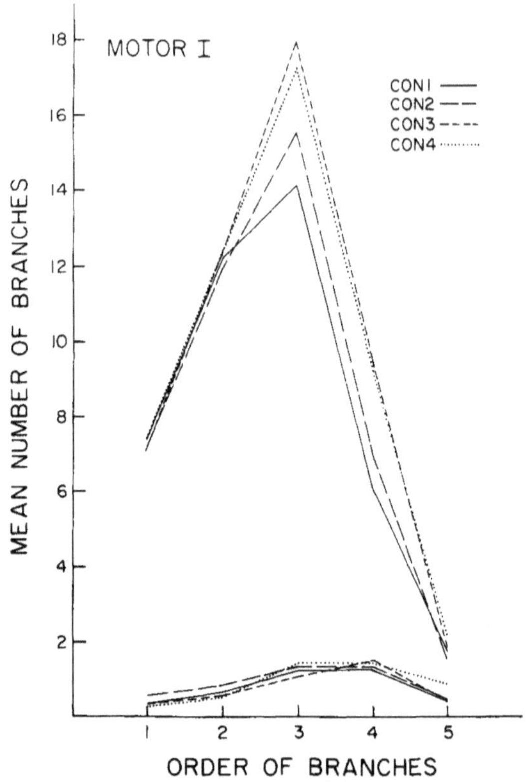

FIG. 9.3. Mean values in motor I cortex for number of branches of each order at 6 months in monkeys reared under four environmental conditions.

Again in M-II cortex (Fig. 9.4) the differential effects of condition on number of dendritic branches appeared in the third- and fourth-order branches. The ANOVA showed an overall effect of condition ($F = 3.82$; $df = 3, 11$; $p = .04$) and an order × condition interaction ($F = 2.61$; $df = 12, 44$; $p = .01$). Condition 1, overall, was less than Condition 4 ($p < .05$). Differences in variance are also of interest. Data for Condition 3 were most variable, and those for Condition 4 (mother-reared) were notably low in variance.

Layer IV stellate cells represent initial stages of processing by the cerebral cortex in primary sensory areas. Motor cortex may or may not be developing efferent motor coordinations at this midlayer level. Since these stellates are thought to be inhibitory in mode of action, they may be best regarded as "sharpening" the information that arrives from thalamic nuclei or through U fibers from neighboring cortical regions.

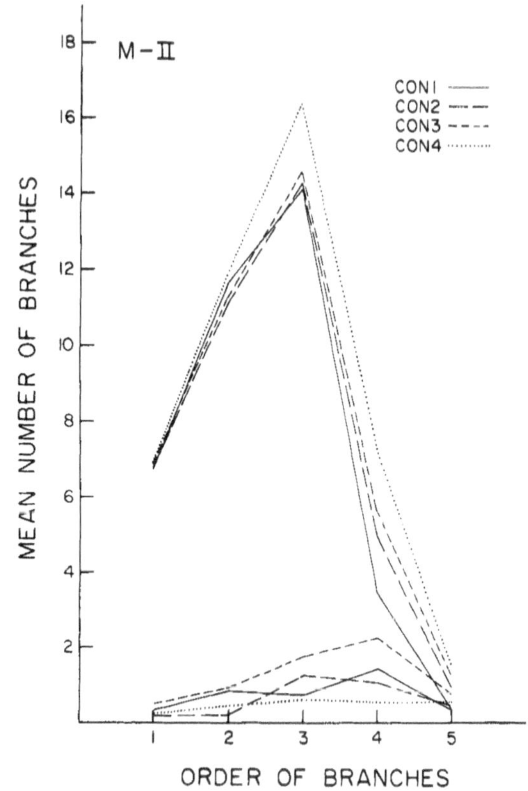

FIG. 9.4. Mean numbers of dendritic branches of each order in motor II cortex under four rearing conditions.

We (B. J. Sonnier, M. Stell, and others) are currently working on dendritic branching studies of additional layers of cortex and on pyramidal cells to see whether all cortical layers participate in the changes thus far seen in layer IV. As we expected from the recent work in the literature, our preliminary findings are telling us that some of them do. Now the questions to be answered include: Which layers, what cells, and at what age periods? And is there a more sensitive time period within the 6 months for which our data with the infant monkeys now speak? (Riesen, Sonnier, Struble, & Lehr, 1981)

Progress in the developmental neuropsychology of the two decades since 1960 has been phenomenal. Lashley would no longer have to say that from what we know about the nervous system, learning should be impossible. Anatomy and physiology, coupled with studies of environmental effects (learning), point toward an array of intercorrelated changes. Neurochemistry has much to tell us about mechanisms. The challenge now is to refine the vast array of correlations into event sequences. What behavior causes which changes in the nervous system? Once a change has been structured, how does it function in behavior? Understanding this two-way process is really what Lashley was seeking all along. Those he inspired to continue the search are not seeking in vain.

REFERENCES

Aarons, L. *Visual movement and intensity discrimination in cats after early restriction and deprivation of pattern vision*. Doctoral dissertation, University of Chicago, 1957.

Aarons, L., Halasz, H. K., & Riesen, A. H. Interocular transfer of visual intensity discrimination after ablation of striate cortex in dark-reared kittens. *Journal of Comparative and Physiological Psychology*, 1963, *56*, 196–199.

Baxter, B. L. The effect of visual deprivation during postnatal maturation on the electrocorticogram of the cat. *Experimental Neurology* 1966, *14*, 224-237.

Baxter, B. L., & Riesen, A. H. Electroretinogram of the visually deprived cat. *Science*, 1961, *134*, 1626-1627.

Berger, H. Experimentall-anatomische Studien über die durch den Mangel optischer Reize veranlassten Entwicklungshemmungen in Occipitallappen des Hundes und der Katze. *Archiv fur Psychiatrie und Nervenkrankheiten*, 1900, *33*, 521-567.

Blakemore, C. The conditions required for the maintenance of binocularity in the kitten's visual cortex. *Journal of Physiology (London)*, 1976, *261*, 423–444.

Blakemore, C., & Van Sluyters, R. C. Innate and environmental factors in the development of the kitten's visual cortex. *Journal of Physiology (London)*, 1975, *248*, 663–716.

Chow, K. L., & Nissen, H. W. Interocular transfer of learning in visually naive and experienced infant chimpanzees. *Journal of Comparative and Physiological Psychology*, 1955, *48*, 229–237.

Chow, K. L., Riesen, A. H., & Newell, F. W. Degeneration of retinal ganglion cells in infant chimpanzees reared in darkness. *Journal of Comparative Neurology*, 1957, *107*, 27–42.

Clendinnen, B. G., & Eayrs, J. T. The anatomical and physiological effects of prenatally administered somatotropin on cerebral development in rats. *Journal of Endocrinology*, 1961, *2*, 183–193.

Coleman, P. D., & Riesen, A. H. Environmental effects on cortical dendritic fields. I. Rearing in the dark. *Journal of Anatomy*, 1968, *102*, 363–374.

Cynader, M., Berman, N., & Hein, A. Recovery of function in cat visual cortex following prolonged deprivation. *Experimental Brain Research*, 1976, *25*, 139–156.

Davenport, R. K., Rogers, C. M., & Rumbaugh, D. M. Long-term cognitive deficits in chimpanzees associated with early impoverished rearing. *Developmental Psychology*, 1973, *9*, 343–347.

Dickerson, G. P., & Riesen, A. H. Interocular transfer of a luminous flux discrimination in the rabbit. *Vision Research*, 1977, *17*, 25–27.

Fifková, E. Plastic and degenerative changes in visual centers. In G. Newton & A. H. Riesen (Eds.), *Advances in psychobiology* (Vol. 2). New York: Wiley Interscience, 1974.

Floeter, M. K., & Greenough, W. T. Cerebellar plasticity: Modification of Purkinje cell structure by differential rearing in monkeys. *Science*, 1979, *206*, 227–229.

Ganz, L., Hirsch, H. V. B., & Tieman, S. B. The nature of perceptual deficits in visually deprived cats. *Brain Research*, 1972, *44*, 547–568.

Ganz, L., & Riesen, A. H. Stimulus generalization to hue in the dark-reared macaque. *Journal of Comparative and Physiological Psychology*, 1962, *55*, 92–99.

Ganz, L., & Wilson, P. D. Innate generalization of a form discrimination without contouring eye movements. *Journal of Comparative and Physiological Psychology*, 1967, *63*, 258–269.

Gesell, A., & Thompson, H. *Infant behavior: Its genesis and growth*. New York: McGraw-Hill, 1934.

Globus, A. Brain morphology as a function of presynaptic morphology and activity. In A. H. Riesen (Ed.), *The developmental neuropsychology of sensory deprivation*. New York: Academic Press, 1975.

Greenough, W. T., & Volkmar, F. Pattern of dendritic branching in occipital cortex of rats reared in complex environments. *Experimental Neurology*, 1973, *40*, 491–504.

Greenough, W. T., Volkmar, F. R., & Juraska, J. M. Effects of rearing complexity on dendritic branching in frontolateral and temporal cortex of the rat. *Experimental Neurology*, 1973, *41*, 371–378.

Gyllensten, L., Malmfors, T., & Norrlin, M.-L. Effect of visual deprivation on the optic centers of growing and adult mice. *Journal of Comparative Neurology*, 1965, *124*, 149–160.

Hebb, D. O. *The organization of behavior*. New York: Wiley, 1949.

Holloway, R. L., Jr. Dendritic branching: Some preliminary results of training and complexity in rat visual cortex. *Brain Research*, 1966, *2*, 393–396.

Howarth, H., Meyer, D. R., & Meyer, P. M. Perinatal injuries to the visual cortex enhance the significance of extravisual cortex for performance of a visual habit. *Physiological Psychology*, 1979, *7*, 163–166.

Hull, C. L. The problem of stimulus equivalence in behavior theory. *Psychological Review*, 1939, *46*, 9–30.

Kennard, M. A. Reorganization of motor function in the cerebral cortex of monkeys deprived of motor and premotor areas in infancy. *Journal of Neurophysiology*, 1938, *1*, 477–496.

Kirk, R. E. *Experimental design: Procedures for the behavioral sciences*. Belmont, Calif.: Brooks/Cole, 1968.

Lashley, K. S. The accuracy of movement in the absence of excitation from the moving organ. *American Journal of Physiology*, 1917, *43*, 169–194.

Lashley, K. S. *Brain mechanisms and intelligence*. Chicago: University of Chicago Press, 1929.

Lashley, K. S., & Wade, M. The Pavlovian theory of generalization. *Psychological Review*, 1946, *53*, 72–87.

Levine, J. Studies in the interrelations of central nervous structures in binobinocular vision. II. The conditions under which interocular transfer of discriminative habits takes place in the pigeon. *Journal of Genetic Psychology*, 1945, *67*, 131–142.

Mason, W. A. Early social deprivation in the nonhuman primates: Implication for behavior. In D. C. Glass (Ed.), *Biology and behavior: Environmental influences*. New York: Rockefeller University and Russell Sage Foundation, 1968.

Menzel, E. W., Davenport, R. K., Jr., & Rogers, C. M. The development of tool using in wild-born and restriction-reared chimpanzees. *Folia Primatologica*, 1970, *12*, 273–283.

Mitchell, G. Abnormal behavior in primates. In L. A. Rosenblum (Ed.), *Primate behavior: Developments in field and laboratory Research* (Vol. 1). New York: Academic Press, 1970.

Nissen, H. W. Studies of infant chimpanzees. *Science*, 1942, *95*, 159–161.

Orbach, J., & Miller, M. H. Visual performance of infrahuman primates reared in an intermittently illuminated room. *Vision Research*, 1969, *9*, 713–716.

Peck, C. K., & Blakemore, C. Modification of single neurons in the kitten's visual cortex after brief periods of monocular visual experience. *Experimental Brain Research*, 1975, *22*, 57–68.

Prescott, J. W. Early somatosensory deprivation as an ontogenetic process in the abnormal development of the brain and behavior. In I. E. Goldsmith & J. Moor-Jankowski (Eds.), *Medical primatology*. New York: Karger, 1971.

Pysh, J. J., & Weiss, G. M. Exercise during development induces an increase in Purkinje cell dendritic tree size. *Science*, 1979, *206*, 230–232.

Rasch, E., Swift, H., Riesen, A. H., & Chow, K. L. Altered structure and composition of retinal cells in dark-reared mammals. *Experimental Cell Research*, 1961, *25*, 348–363.

Rhine, R. J., & Hendy-Neely, H. Social development of stumptail macaques (*Macaca arctoides*): Momentary touching, play, and other interactions with aunts and immatures during the infants' first 60 days of life. *Primates*, 1978, *19*, 115–123.

Riesen, A. H. Arrested vision. *Scientific American*, 1950, *183*, 16–19.

Riesen, A. H. Plasticity of behavior: Psychological aspects. In H. F. Harlow & C. N. Woolsey (Eds.), *Biological and biochemical bases of behavior*. Madison: University of Wisconsin Press, 1958.

Riesen, A. H. Studying perceptual development using the technique of sensory deprivation. *Journal of Nervous and Mental Disease*, 1961, *132*, 21–25.

Riesen, A. H. Effects of visual deprivation on perceptual function and the neural substrate. In J. de Ajuriaguerra (Ed.), *Désafférentation expérimentale et clinique* (Symposium Bel Air II). Geneva: Georg & Cie, 1965.

Riesen, A. H. Sensory deprivation. In E. Stellar & J. M. Sprague (Eds.), *Progress in physiological psychology* (Vol. 1). New York: Academic Press, 1966.

Riesen, A. H. Chimpanzee visual perception. In G. Bourne (Ed.), *The chimpanzee* (Vol. 2). Basel and New York: Karger, 1970.

Riesen, A. H. Nissen's observations on the development of sexual behavior in captive-born, nursery-reared chimpanzees. In G. Bourne (Ed.), *The chimpanzee* (Vol. 4). Basel and New York: Karger, 1971.

Riesen, A. H., & Aarons, L. Visual movement and intensity discrimination in cats after early deprivation of pattern vision. *Journal of Comparative and Physiological Psychology*, 1959, *52*, 142–149.

Riesen, A. H., Dickerson, G. P., & Struble, R. G. Somatosensory restriction and behabehavioral development in stumptail monkeys. *Annals of the New York Academy of Sciences*, 1977, *290*, 285–294.

Riesen, A. H., & Kinder E. F. *Postural development of infant chimpanzees*. New Haven: Yale University Press, 1952.

Riesen, A. H., Kurke, M. I., & Mellinger, J. C. Interocular transfer of habits learned monocularly in visually naive and visually experienced cats. *Journal of Comparative and Physiological Psychology*, 1953, *46*, 166–172.

Riesen, A. H., Sonnier, B. J., Struble, R. G., & Lehr, P. Branching differences in stellate cells related to cortical area and rearing environment of monkeys. In J. W. Prescott (Ed.), *Consequences of social isolation upon primate brain development and behavior*. New York: Academic Press, 1981.

Schapiro, S., & Vukovich, K. R. Early experience effects upon cortical dendrites: A proposed model for development. *Science*, 1970, *167*, 292–294.

Schissler, D. R., & Riesen, A. H. Partial interocular transfer of visual discriminations in cats. *Developmental Psychobiology*, 1969, *2*, 81–86.

Senden, M. von [*Space and sight*] (P. Heath, trans.). London: Methuen, 1960.

Siegel, J. M., Coleman, P. D., & Riesen, A. H. Pattern evoked response deficiency in pattern-deprived cats. *Electroencephalography and Clinical Neurophysiology*, 1973, *35*, 569–573.

Stewart, D. L., & Riesen, A. H. Adult versus infant brain damage: Behavioral and electrophysiological effects of striatectomy in adult and neonatal rabbits. In G. Newton & A. H. Riesen (Eds.), *Advances in psychobiology* (Vol. 1). New York: Wiley-Interscience, 1972.

Struble, R. G., & Riesen, A. H. Changes in cortical dendritic branching subsequent to partial social isolation in stumptailed monkeys. *Developmental Psychobiology*, 1978, *11*, 479–486.

Tees, R. C. The effect of visual deprivation on pattern recognition in the rat. *Developmental Psychobiology*, 1979, *12*, 485–497.

Valverde, F. Apical dendritic spines of the visual cortex and light deprivation in the mouse. *Experimental Brain Research*, 1967, *3*, 337–352.

Walls, G. L. *The vertebrate eye and its adaptive radiation.* Bloomfield Hills, Mich.: Cranbrook Institute of Science, 1942.

Wilson, P. D., & Riesen, A. H. Visual development in rhesus monkeys neonatally deprived of patterned light. *Journal of Comparative and Physiological Psychology,* 1966, *61,* 87–95.

Zilbert, D. E., & Riesen, A. H. A comparison of the effects of infant and adult retinal lesions upon visual acuity in the rabbit. *Experimental Neurology,* 1971, *33,* 445–458.

10 Functional Organization of the Rat Brain

Robert Thompson
Fairview State Hospital
Costa Mesa, California and
University of California
Irvine Medical Center
Orange, California

INTRODUCTION

One of the most puzzling problems in neuropsychology concerns the whereabouts of the brain memory trace. Does it inhabit a given sector of the cerebrum or brain stem, or is it diffusely represented throughout the cerebrum and/or brain stem? Lashley, who has been associated with the quest for the engram more than any other individual in the history of neuropsychology, was torn between these two views. In his 1929 monograph, for example, he reported: "The maze habits show no definite localization when formed; the brightness habit is clearly associated with the area striata . . . and the problem box with the frontal region [p. 132]." And again, in his famous 1950 article on the search for the engram, he stated that "it is impossible to demonstrate the isolated localization of a memory trace anywhere within the nervous system. Limited regions may be essential for learning or retention of a particular activity, but within such regions the parts are functionally equivalent. The engram is represented throughout the region [p. 478]." Thus on one hand, Lashley was faced with data (on maze habits that show the mass action effect) indicating that the trace is not to be found within a discrete region of the brain. At the same time, however, he faced another set of data (on visual discrimination and problem-box habits that do not show the mass action effect) suggesting that a localized region of the brain may house the memory trace.

Lashley attempted to resolve this dilemma by assuming that the neural mechanisms (and the locus of the engrams) underlying the performance of simple habits of the conditioned-reflex type—associating a single sensory stimulus with a simple motor response—are different from those underlying the performance of complex habits, such as a eight-cul maze. In the former case, only the relevant sensory cortical receiving area would be involved. In the latter case, where the mass action effect is observed, virtually the entire cerebral surface would be involved. It is interesting to note that this notion that different neural mechanisms support different classes of learned responses has recently been offered by some investigators (Norman, 1973; Thompson, 1979a) to account, at least in part, for the confusion and contradictions surrounding the experimental animal literature on the neural substrates of memory.

Another issue related to the anatomical localization of the memory trace is whether the trace resides within the cerebral cortex or within the internal regions of the brain. On this issue, Lashley faced no dilemma, for the data available to him indicated that the cerebral cortex was the dominant level of the nervous system when it came to the performance of previously learned responses. When the rat is trained on a maze, visual discrimination, or problem-box task, extensive damage to neocortical tissue would abolish the habit. Lashley's dismissal of the importance of extracortical formations in the expression of learned responses was also reinforced by the findings that cerebellar damage failed to interfere with a maze habit (Lashley & McCarthy, 1926) and that basal ganglia lesions failed to alter visual discrimination performance (Lashley, 1921).

Lashley did not altogether deprive subcortical regions of memorial functions. Rats sustaining extensive neocortical damage, for example, could learn a simply light-dark discrimination or a simple maze habit (Lashley, 1929). In the intact animal, however, Lashley argued that those mechanisms concerned with the execution of learned responses must reside within the depth of the cerebrum, as evidenced by the fact that a normal animal loses these habits in the presence of extensive neocortical destruction.

Research within the past three decades suggests that the interior parts of the brain may have more important functions in learning and memory than Lashley supposed. It remains to be seen, however, whether the functions of these subcortical formations are subservient to, or separable from, neocortical processes.

Another point that is of some relevance to the anatomical localization of the memory trace concerns the lesion method that Lashley developed to study the locus of memories. Although Lashley used the lesion method throughout his investigative career for the purpose of tracing pathways underlying learning and memory, he cautioned against attributing retention losses induced by brain damage to the simple destruction of engrams. Amnestic effects resulting from surgical intervention could arise from a disturbance in set or attention, a weakening of motivation, a derangement of a space-coordinate system, or a disorder in some other known or unknown cognitive function.

This word of caution raised by Lashley stresses the fact that the performance of a learned activity is not simply a matter of the reception of a signal followed reflexively by the elicitation of a response. Rather, the execution of a goal-directed response would appear to be the product of a series of complex operations, ranging from the expectancy of a reward or punishment that can facilitate the activation of a memory trace system to the presetting of a response program that can regulate the motor act independent of sensory control.

And finally, it is important to emphasize that Lashley's theoretical approach to the understanding of brain function as a whole was a holistic one. He was not inclined to view the brain as a composite of tightly knit units having diverse functions. At the same time, however, he did admit to a limited degree of cerebral localization. In his monograph (1929), for example, he stated: "The direct evidence on cerebral organization in the rat and also many results from brain lesions in higher forms indicate that there is a correspondence of structural and functional differentiation only between the grosser units of anatomy and behavior" and ended the paragraph by concluding that "there is a definite limit to the possible dissociation of functions [p. 157]."

The results of my own investigations on the search for the anatomical pathways and nuclear masses concerned with the expression of learned responses in the rat have been viewed by some as an extension of Lashley's research program. A further similarity of greater importance is that the data that have come from my laboratory are, I believe, most satisfactorily interpreted in terms of the holistic approach that Lashley favored. That is, emphasis has been placed on the functions of groups (blocks) of neural structures rather than on the subfunctions of the component parts. The inclusion of subcortical formations within these functional blocks would represent a departure from Lashley's theoretical formulations.

MAPPING BRAIN SYSTEMS UNDERLYING LEARNED RESPONSES

My objective is to discuss the functional significance of a number of brain systems recently identified by the lesion method that are presumed to play a role in the maintenance of certain previously learned, goal-directed responses in the rat. The reader is referred back to the cited research papers for the original data supporting the interpretations offered.

Whereas Lashley focused on the problem of mapping cortical systems supporting learned responses, I have endeavored to map complete brain (cortico-subcortical) systems supporting learned responses. This has been accomplished by sampling many different cortical and subcortical sites with lesions (using different groups of rats for different lesion placements) and then testing the rats' retention of a preoperatively acquired response (see Fig. 10.1). The distribution of individual lesions found to induce serious amnestic effects (zero or negative error savings scores) would constitute a lesion-defined functional system governing the performance of that acquired response.

The visual discrimination habit was the initial target of this research effort (Thompson, 1969, 1976b; Thompson & Massopust, 1960), but other learned responses have since been charted, including an incline plane (vestibulo-

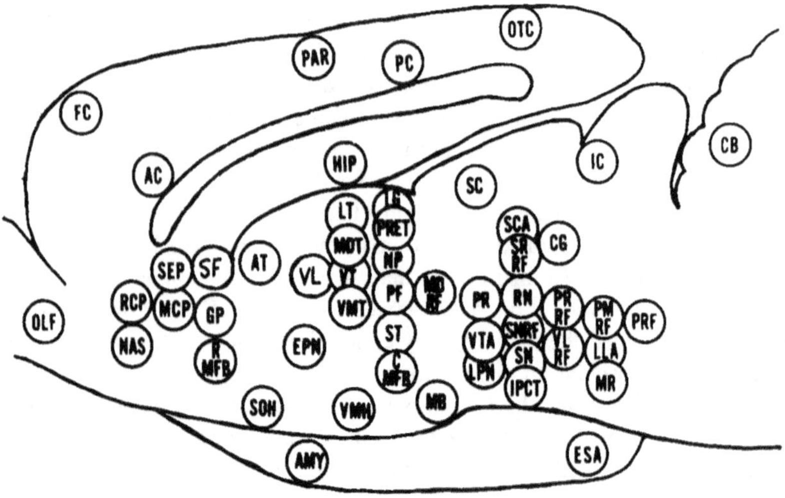

FIG. 10.1. Schematic drawing of a parasagittal section of the rat brain showing the relative positions of 52 sites where lesions were separately placed for the purpose of charting functional systems governing learned responses. Modified from Thompson (1978a).

kinesthetic) discrimination (Thompson, Arabie, & Sisk, 1976), a maze problem (Thompson, 1974), active and passive avoidance responses (Thompson, 1978b), and latch-box habits (Spiliotis & Thompson, 1973; Thompson, Gates, & Gross, 1979).

By comparing the maps of critical structures associated with each of the foregoing learned tasks, it has been possible to isolate six groups of brain sites (functional blocks) that appear to be selectively involved in the expression of

TABLE 10.1
Functional Blocks Critical for Retention of Various Learned Tasks in the Rat

	Learned Task					
Functional Block	*Sim. Visual Discrimination*	*Inclined-Plane Discrimination*	*Succ. Visual Discrimination*	*Maze*	*Active Avoidance*	*Latch Box*
Integrating	X	X	X	X	X	X
Visual	X		X			
Proprioceptive-kinesthetic		X	X	X	X	X
Cognitive map				X	X	
Fear-initiating response					X	
Skilled response						X

particular kinds of goal-directed learned activities. Some learned responses, such as simultaneous visual discrimination habits, require the engagement of only two of these functional blocks, whereas others (active avoidance tasks) seem to involve the recruitment of at least four of these functional blocks (see Table 10.1).

The balance of this chapter is devoted to a discussion of these functional blocks underlying learned responses followed by a discussion of the implications of these functional blocks on the locus of the engram. These discussions may, as Lashley (1950) once remarked of his own results, "obscure rather than illuminate the nature of the engram, but they serve at least to illustrate the complexity of the problem and to reveal the superficial nature of many of the physiological theories of memory that have been proposed [p. 455]."

FUNCTIONAL BLOCKS OF THE RAT BRAIN

Integrating Block

This block is conceived to consist of most components of the basal ganglia (red nucleus, substantia nigra, subthalamic nucleus, entopeduncular nucleus, globus pallidus, and caudal portion of the caudoputamen), ventral portions of the brain stem reticular formation (including its extension into the posterolateral hypothalamus, parafascicular nucleus, nucleus posterior thalami, and pretectum) and a major part of what Nauta (1958) has termed the "limbic midbrain area" (ventral tegmental area of Tsai and interpedunculo-central tegmento-median raphe complex). The most distinguishing feature of this block from a functional standpoint is that lesions that destroy any one of its constituent nuclei tend to produce serious amnestic effects (zero or negative savings scores) on a wide variety of learned tasks including visual and nonvisual discriminations, mazes, active avoidance responses, and latch-box problems (Spiliotis & Thompson, 1973, Thompson, 1978a, 1978b). By virtue of these generalized amnestic effects, the term *integrating* has been used to describe this functional block.[1]

[1]Two problems arise in relation to the composition of the integrating block. First, lesions of the median raphe are not apt to interfere with the performance of previously learned active avoidance responses (Thompson, 1978b). This finding, however, is to be interpreted with caution since raphe-lesioned rats usually "learn" active avoidance responses faster than controls. The second problem has to do with the omission of the entorhino-subicular area from the integrating block. There is evidence that bilateral damage to this area disrupts retention of a broad range of learned responses, with the possible exception of difficult latch-box tasks (Thompson, 1976a). Since generalized retention deficits are not associated with hippocampal lesions (Thompson, 1978a), the significance of the entorhino-subicular area for the performance of certain tasks (visual and inclined-plane discriminations) must be sought in pathways that do not terminate within hippocampal tissue. Since these extrahippocampal targets of entorhino-subicular efferents are not yet worked out, I chose not to discuss the entorhino-subicular area in this chapter.

It should be noted that all the foregoing tasks susceptible to interference of discrete lesions to this integrating block require the subject to move from one locus within the environment to another to obtain a reward. The only task investigated to date that does not require the integrity of many constituents of this block for its preservation is the passive avoidance response (Thompson, 1978b). Passive avoidance conditioning is, of course, unique among learned activities in that the subject is rewarded (avoids a noxious event) contingent on *not* moving from one designated position within the environment to another. Based upon these observations, I am led to speculate that this block serves a bewilderingly complex role in motor control.

In an intriguing article, David G. Russell (1976) has proposed that the performance of skilled movements in the human may be mediated by a "central response organization system" that generates motor impulses that reduce the discrepancy between currently perceived position of a limb and desired position of a limb, the latter being stored or predicted within a space-coordinate system. I propose to extend Russell's central response organization system in the service of all goal-directed learned activities and to view the integrating block as its neural substrate.

Consider the theoretical position of Bindra (1976) that all goal-directed learned activities are roughly a matter of approaching a succession of increasingly "attractive" (hedonically more positive or less negative) positions in space, the most attractive being that occupied by the goal object. According to this conceptualization, learning does not involve any strengthening of a bond between the stimulus features of the environment and a response. It does, however, involve the formation of conditioned incentive stimuli (through the strengthening of the bond between the stimulus features of the environment and the goal object) in such a way that the stimulus features of spatial positions close to the goal object will be endowed with greater incentive value than those distant from the goal object. A central response organization system (integrating block) would then serve the function of generating motor impulses that would reduce the discrepancy between currently perceived position in space and the most desired position in space.

It should be emphasized that the basal ganglia, brain stem reticular formation, ard limbic midbrain area contain anatomical and functional characteristics that would be essential for supporting the activities of Russell's central response organization system. First, its extension into the lower parts of the neuraxis would provide escape routes necessary to control and sequence motor acts organized at caudal brain stem levels (Berntson & Micco, 1976). Second, many components of the integrating block are recipients of corticifugal projection systems (Valverde, 1962; Webster, 1961); thus this block is provided with cortically processed sensory information necessary for peripheral guidance of motor acts. And finally, this block contains functional elements involved in arousal (Moruzzi & Magoun, 1949), motivational (Ungerstedt, 1971), inhibitory

(Thompson, 1978b), motor (Kornhuber, 1974), and reward (Routtenberg, 1973) processes that would be fundamental to the initiation, maintenance, and plasticity of goal-directed motor acts.

Although customarily conceptualized as being anatomically and functionally distinct, the extent of interconnectivity existing among the basal ganglia, brain stem reticular formation, and limbic midbrain area (see Fig. 10.2) clearly allows for the possibility that these three morphological systems combine to serve a common function. The anatomical studies of Shute and Lewis (1967); Lynch, Smith, and Robertson (1973); Miller, Richardson, Fibiger, and McLennan (1975); and Reubi and Emson (1978) particularly underscore the potential for interactions among the basal ganglia, brain stem reticular formation, and limbic midbrain area.

To those who do not find the notion of a subcortical integrating mechanism very appealing, it must be pointed out that there is increasing evidence that surgical decortication does not preclude acquisition (or even retention) of certain simple, goal-directed response sequences in laboratory animals. According to Lashley (1929), removal of about 80% of the neocortex in rats only slightly impairs mastery of a position habit acquired in a single-unit *T* maze. This finding

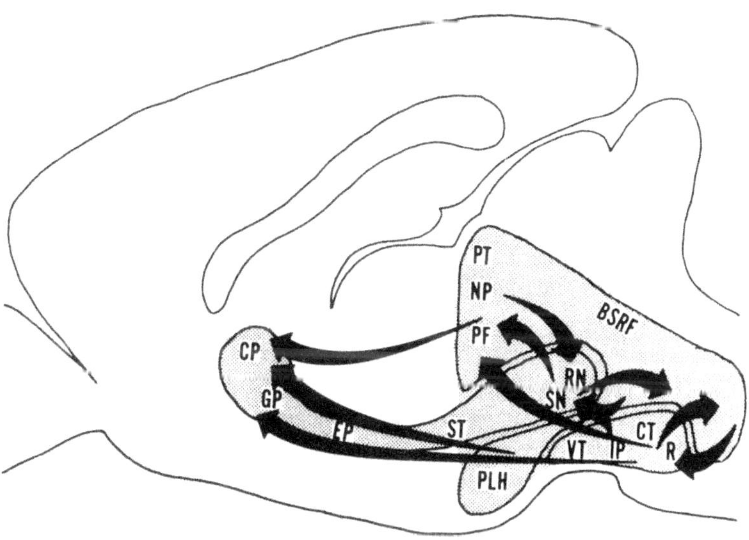

FIG. 10.2. Schematic drawing of a parasagittal section of the rat brain showing some of the interconnecting pathways of the integrating block (stippled areas). Abbreviations: BSRF = brain stem reticular formation, CP = caudal caudoputamen, CT = central tegmentum, GP = globus pallidus, EP = entopeduncular nucleus, IP = interpeduncular nucleus, NP = nucleus posterior thalami, PF = parafascicular nucleus, PLH = posterolateral hypothalamus, PT = pretectum, R = median raphe, RN = red nucleus, SN = substantia nigra, ST = subthalamus, VT = ventral tegmental area.

has since been confirmed (Thompson, 1959). Swann (1935), in an article that is rarely referred to, reported that lesions of up to 85% of the neocortical surface do not seriously interfere with retention of an odor discrimination in rats. (I have recently gathered data in support of Swann's work to the extent that large frontal, parietal, or occipitotemporal ablations have no deleterious effects on the performance of a tap water–acetone discrimination in rats.) Oakley and Russell (1977) have presented convincing evidence that certain classes of Pavlovian conditioning are preserved following decortication in rabbits. Furthermore, rabbits lacking most of their cerebral cortex can be trained to lever press for food (Oakley, 1971), and decorticate cats can acquire a simple maze habit (Bjursten, Norrsell, & Norrsell, 1976) or a simple avoidance response (Meyer, 1963). Dr. A. Grant Young, at Louisiana State University, and I have shown that decorticate rats can be trained (or retrained) to lever press for a sucrose solution, to displace a stimulus card, or to rotate a button latch to obtain water and to avoid entering a small, dark compartment under threat of foot shock. All of these studies clearly establish the existence of a self-sufficient mechanism within the interior regions of the brain that can mediate simple, goal-directed learned responses. It is by no means unreasonable to propose that this mechanism mainly comprises the basal ganglia, brain stem reticular formation, and limbic midbrain area. Parenthetically, the fact that complex laboratory tasks cannot readily be established in decorticate preparations could be explained, at least in part, in terms of deficits in the processing of fine-grained sensory information upon which the performance of complex tasks usually depends.

Visual Block

This block consists, in part, of the retina, lateral geniculate nucleus, and occipital cortex. As expected, this block comes into play in the performance of visually guided behaviors.

After reviewing his research on visual discrimination performance in brain-damaged rats, Lashley (1950) concluded: "The conduction of impulses is from the retina to the lateral geniculate nuclei, thence to the striate areas, and from them down to some subcortical nervous mechanism. The pathway beyond the striate cortex is unknown. It may be direct to the spinal cord [p. 467]." The subcortical nervous mechanism to which Lashley referred is proposed to consist of the integrating block discussed in the preceding section. Retention of both brightness and pattern discrimination habits has been found to be severely compromised by lesions to any one component part of this integrating block (Thompson, 1976b). The key problem, however, concerns the identification of those conduction pathways beyond the striate (occipital) cortex that functionally relates the visual block with the integrating block. On the strength of the most recent experimental findings, it now appears that these two blocks are functionally connected by at least three separate descending conduction pathways. They include the occipito-incertal pathway, the occipito-reticular pathway, and the occipito-caudoputamenal pathway (see Fig. 10.3).

According to Nauta and Bucher (1954), the occipital cortex of the rat sends a modest projection to the zona incerta of the subthalamus. Since the zona incerta is intimately connected with other elements of the basal ganglia, it is a likely candidate to serve as a link between the visual block and the integrating block. Support for this possibility has come from the findings that bilateral lesions to the zona incerta produce retention deficits on a visual discrimination habit but fail to produce retention deficits on an equally difficult nonvisual discrimination habit (Thompson & Bachman, 1979b).

Valverde (1962) has reported that one contigent of occipitofugal fibers takes a descending course through the lateral half of the cerebral peduncle and, at approximately the level of the substantia nigra, leaves the peduncle at right angles to terminate in the ventrolateral quadrant (nucleus cuneiformis) of the mesencephalic reticular formation and nucleus reticularis pontis oralis. These two brain stem areas to which occipital efferents terminate are constituents of the integrating block. That this pathway relates the visual block with the integrating block is suggested by the findings that lateral pedunculo-nigral lesions (which would disjoin the occipito-reticular pathway) profoundly impair visual discrimination

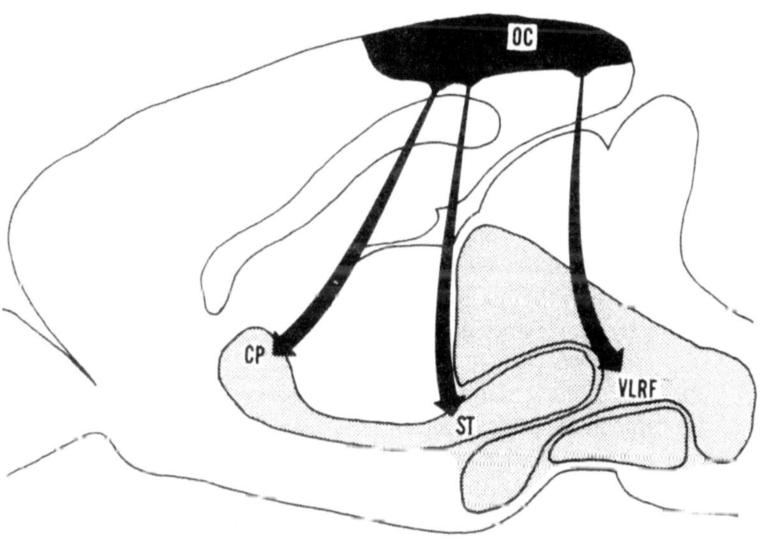

FIG. 10.3. Schematic drawing of a parasagittal section of the rat brain showing the connections of the occipital cortex (blackened areas) with the integrating block (stippled areas). Abbreviations: CP = posterior caudoputamen, OC = occipital cortex, ST = subthalamus, VLRF = ventrolateral midbrain reticular formation.

performance while having only slight effects on nonvisual discrimination performance (Thompson & Craddock, 1972; Thompson & Peddy, 1979).

Webster (1961) has shown that the anterior cortical areas of the rat brain tend to project to the anterior portions of the caudoputamen, whereas the posterior (occipitotemporal) cortical areas give rise to projections to the posterior portions of the caudoputamen. That an occipito-striate (and/or temporo-striate) connection may play a significant role in visually guided behavior was first suggested by the findings that lesions to the tail of the caudate nucleus interfere with visual discrimination performance in monkeys (Divac, Rosvold, & Schwarcbart, 1967). More recently, Livesey and Muter (1976) have reported retardation in visual discrimination reversal in rats receiving stimulation of the posterior caudoputamen. Further evidence implicating the occipito-caudoputamenal connection in visual discrimination performance has been reported by Thompson and Bachman (1979a). They found that electrolytic lesions destroying the posterior division of the caudoputamen induced significantly greater retention losses on a horizontal-vertical discrimination than on an equally difficult inclined-plane (nonvisual) discrimination.

The foregoing pathways may not be the only functional links uniting the visual block with the integrating block. For example, occipital efferents are known to terminate within the pretectum (Goodman & Horel, 1966; Nauta & Bucher, 1954), a region of the brain stem that is part of the integrating block. And not to be ignored is the observation that the brain stem reticular formation sends collaterals to the lateral geniculate nuclei (Scheibel & Scheibel, 1958).

Proprioceptive-Kinesthetic Block

This block largely consists of the parietal cortex; the cingulate cortex; the anterior, lateral (ventrolateral), ventromedial, and ventrobasal thalamic nuclei; and the cerebellum (Fig. 10.4). There is no need to elaborate on the interconnectivity of this block except to say that the component parts are either directly or indirectly associated with the receipt of proprioceptive-kinesthetic impulses arriving from spinothalamic, lemniscal, and spinocerebellar tracts (Zeman & Innes, 1963).

This functional block was first identified when those brain sites critical for visual discrimination performance were compared with those critical for inclined-plane-discrimination performance (Thompson et al., 1976). (The inclined-plane problem usually consists of training blinded subjects to choose a pathway that slopes upward and to avoid an adjacent pathway that slopes downward.) The similarities between the two maps of critical brain sites were observed in connection with the basal ganglia, brain stem reticular formation, and limbic midbrain area (integrating block). With respect to the differences, the visual habit included the retino-geniculo-occipital complex (visual block), whereas the inclined-plane habit included the parietal and cingulate cortices; the

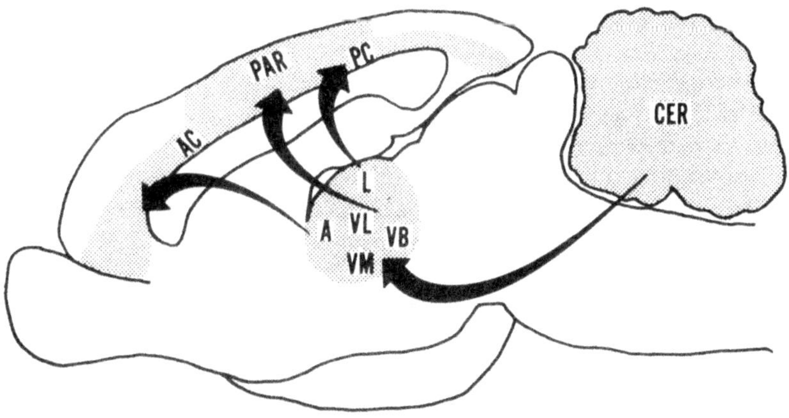

FIG. 10.4. Schematic drawing of a parasagittal section of the rat brain showing the components (and some of the interconnecting pathways) of the proprioceptive-kinesthetic block (stippled areas). Abbreviations: A = anterior thalamus, AC = anterior cingulate cortex, CER = cerebellum, L = lateral thalamus, PAR = parietal cortex, PC = posterior cingulate cortex, VB = ventrobasal thalamus, VL = ventrolateral thalamus, VM = ventromedial thalamus.

anterior, lateral, ventromedial, and ventrobasal thalamic nuclei; and the cerebellum (proprioceptive-kinesthetic block).[2]

What is remarkable about this comparison is that the expression of the inclined-plane discrimination requires the integrity of many more brain structures than is required for the expression of the visual discrimination. My initial reaction to such a complex block mediating the inclined-plane problem (as opposed to that mediating a visual problem) was to suggest that *all* nonvisual habits depend on a mechanism that processes proprioceptive-kinesthetic cues for the purpose of directing and monitoring movements in nonvisual space (Thompson et al., 1976). Such a mechanism would certainly embrace many more neural elements than those associated with afferent pathways to the thalamus and thence to the appropriate cortical receiving areas. This notion now appears to be incorrect in light of the recent finding that a nonvisual odor discrimination habit (approach a stimulus object containing water-soaked sponges and avoid an adjacent stimulus object containing acetone-soaked sponges) survives following destruction of any one component of the proprioceptive-kinesthetic block (Thompson, 1980).

---

[2]The inclined plane problem is also disrupted by lesions to the medial longitudinal fasciculus, a principal ascending pathway of the vestibular system (Brodal, 1974). Thus the inclined-plane habit is supported by three functional blocks rather than only two. No other task investigated in my laboratory has been found to be susceptible to interference by lesions to the medial longitudinal fasciculus.

Perhaps the complexity of this block can be understood in terms of the number of functions that it potentially serves. Not only do proprioceptive-kinesthetic signals convey information about body position, as in the case of the inclined-plane problem, but they may also be essential for the central control of movement, for perception of the body schema, and for spatial discriminations as well. Because of these diverse functions, the processing of proprioceptive-kinesthetic impulses would conceivably involve an ensemble of structures not limited to the classical ascending pathways of the somatosensory system.

Support for this possibility comes from the finding that the proprioceptive-kinesthetic block seems to be necessary for the normal expression of a wide range of learned tasks that are not obviously related except for the possibility that they may have a proprioceptive-kinesthetic basis (see Table 10.1). These tasks include a maze (Thompson, 1974), active and passive avoidance responses (Thompson, 1978b), latch-box problems (Thompson et al., 1979), and a successive visual discrimination (Thompson, Bernard, & Hale, 1980): Go left in the presence of two black cards, and go right in the presence of two white cards.

If subsequent studies confirm the central role of this block in mazes, avoidance conditioning, and left–right discriminations, then it may be necessary to re-examine the notion that maze learning (Watson, 1907) and avoidance conditioning (Konorski, 1967; Mowrer, 1960) have a proprioceptive-kinesthetic basis. The involvement of the proprioceptive-kinesthetic sensory systems in the execution of skilled movements seems to be well established (Konorski, 1967; Luria, 1966).

Cognitive Map Block

This functional block is envisioned to consist of the occipital cortex, hippocampal formation, septofornix area, and mammillary bodies (Fig. 10.5). It is well established that both the hippocampal formation and the septal area send projections to the mammillary bodies and that the septal area and hippocampal formation are richly interconnected (Swanson, 1978). The anatomical link between the occipital cortex and the hippocampo-septo-mammilary complex very likely is consummated either directly by occipital efferents to the presubiculum (Nauta & Bucher, 1954) or indirectly by cortical association fibers to the entorhinal cortex (Van Hoesen, Pandya, & Butters, 1972).

This functional block was first recognized in a lesion study dealing with the performance of a three-cul maze habit (Thompson, 1974). At that time, it was speculated that this block constituted a central mechanism concerned with left–right discriminations rather than being concerned with some spatial mapping system, as proposed by Nadel and O'Keefe (1974; O'Keefe & Nadel, 1978) and later by Olton (1977). However, a recent study has demonstrated that rats prepared with hippocampal or occipital lesions are severely impaired in relearning a ladder maze (devoid of left and right turns) and show about the same degree of retention loss as other hippocampal or occipital rats tested on a conventional left–right maze (Thompson, 1979b). It appears, therefore, that this block is in

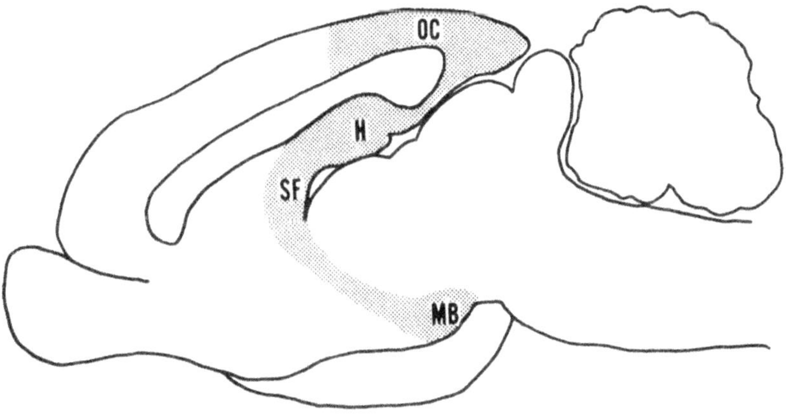

FIG. 10.5. Schematic drawing of a parasagittal section of the rat brain showing the components of the cognitive map block (stippled areas). Abbreviations: H = hippocampus, MB = mammillary bodies, OC = occipital cortex, SF = septofornix area.

some way implicated in spatial mapping of environmental objects in both the horizontal and vertical planes.

At first glance, it may come as a surprise to associate the occipital cortex functionally with the hippocampo-septo-mamillary body complex. It should be remembered, however, that Lashley (1943) demonstrated a nonvisual function of the occipital areas in maze performance by showing that rats with occipital ablations are inferior to blinded rats in retention of a maze habit. This observation has since been confirmed in rats (Thompson, 1977, 1979b), cats (Winer & Lubar, 1976), and monkeys (Orbach, 1959). The nonvisual function of the occipital areas has also been disclosed in an avoidance conditioning situation (Lubar & Middaugh, 1971; Lubar, Schostal, & Perachio, 1967; Thompson, 1977)

The nature of the nonvisual function of the occipital cortex has not been investigated to the degree it deserves. According to Lashley (1950), the role of the occipital cortex in maze performance is derivable from his theory of mass action—each part of the cerebral cortex contributes a facilitative effect to the functioning of other parts of the cerebral cortex. I would suggest as an alternative view that the nonvisual function of the occipital cortex is intimately associated with the spatial functions of the hippocampo-septo mammillary body complex.[3]

[3]Based upon the findings that a stylus maze habit (as opposed to a locomotor maze habit) is spared in monkeys prepared with visual cortical ablations, Orbach (1959) has likewise been disenchanted with Lashley's notion that the striate cortex exerts a general facilitative effect on other cortical regions. Orbach has suggested that the nonvisual function of the striate cortex may be related to "nonvisual orientation involving a locomotor sequence." This view is not remarkably different from the ones recently expressed by O'Keefe and Nadel (1978) and by Olton (1977) with reference to the functions of the hippocampus.

This view is based on the finding that lesions of the occipital cortex induce the same pattern of retention deficits on nonvisual tasks (losses on maze and active avoidance, but no losses on inclined-plane or latch-box problems) as do lesions of the hippocampus, septofornix area, or mammillary bodies (Spiliotis & Thompson, 1973; Thompson, 1978a, 1978b).

Fear-Initiating Response Block

This functional block is composed of a "posterior" division involving the dorsal midbrain (colliculi, tegmentum immediately medial to the medial geniculate nucleus, and portions of the central gray substance) and an "anterior" division involving the amygdala, mediodorsal thalamic nucleus, rostral parts of the medial forebrain bundle and caudoputamen, nucleus accumbens, and lateral convexity of the frontal (motor) cortex (Fig. 10.6). The spinomesencephalic and spinothalamic "pain" pathways, which terminate in or pass through the dorsal midbrain (Mehler, 1969), are perhaps the most relevant connections of the posterior division of this functional block. Pathways interconnecting some of the components of the anterior division have been described in the literature (Knook, 1965; Krettek & Price, 1977; Swanson & Cowan, 1975). Presumably, thalamic and hypothalamic routes unite these two divisions.

This block was uncovered after a lesion study was completed focusing on passive and active avoidance responses formed in the rat (Thompson, 1978b). Since avoidance behavior is customarily conceptualized as being motivated by

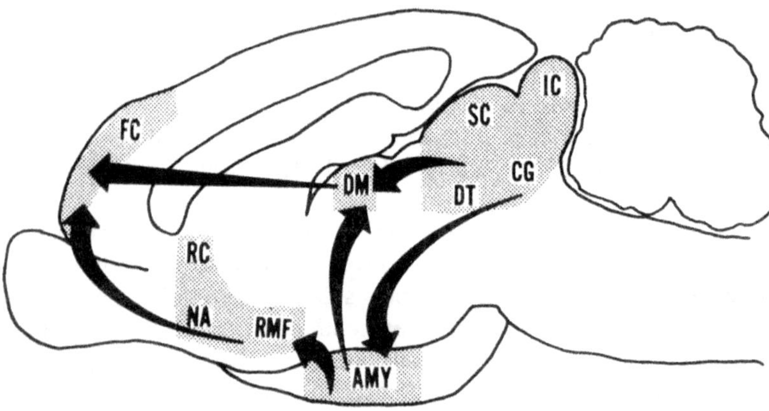

FIG. 10.6. Schematic drawing of a parasagittal section of the rat brain showing the components (and some of the interconnection pathways) of the fear-initiating response block (stippled areas). Abbreviations: AMY = amygdaloid complex, CG = central gray, DM = mediodorsal thalamic nucleus, DT = dorsal tegmentum, FC = frontal cortex, IC = inferior colliculus, NA = nucleus accumbens, RC = rostral caudoputamen, RMF = rostral medial forebrain bundle, SC = superior colliculus.

fear and reinforced by fear reduction, it is likely that this functional block plays a complex role in the elaboration of the fear motive.

Curiously, damage to any one of the constituents of this functional block fails to impair performance of two-choice (visual or vestibulo-kinesthetic) discriminations or a three-cul maze habit learned under the motive of escape-avoidance of foot shock (Thompson, 1974, 1976b; Thompson et al., 1976). In these situations, only response accuracy is monitored—choice of the positive stimulus object or correct alley. In active and passive avoidance situations, on the other hand, response latency (time between the onset of a signal and the occurrence or nonoccurrence of the correct response) is monitored rather than response accuracy. This suggests the possibility that the function of this block in avoidance learning is related to the initiation or mobilization of fear-motivated responses and has nothing to do with the direction or composition of the fear-motivated response (Thompson, 1979a).

Skilled-Response Block

The final functional block to be considered in this chapter is the smallest one, consisting of the lateral convexity of the frontal (motor) cortex and possibly some region of the dorsomedial thalamus that has not been fully identified.

This block was encountered in lesion studies aimed at elucidating the neural mechanisms underlying latch-box performance in the rat (Spiliotis & Thompson, 1973; Thompson et al., 1979). Most areas of the brain were canvassed with lesions after thirsty rats were trained on at least two latch-box tasks to obtain water. The first task required the rat to rotate a button latch in a clockwise direction to open a door leading to the goal box. The second task, which was more difficult than the first, consisted of sliding a bolt latch to the right to open the door. The retention test disclosed that those rats suffering lesions to components of either the integrating or proprioceptive-kinesthetic block generally showed relearning disturbances on the more difficult second problem. In addition, rats with lesions to the motor cortex or mediodorsal thalamic nucleus exhibited serious retention deficits, particularly on the second task (Thompson et al., 1979).

Because the mediodorsal thalamic nucleus has not been traditionally viewed as having a significant role in the production of skilled movements, it seemed prudent to reexamine the effects of lesions to this nucleus on retention of the two latch-box tasks. Of the 10 new brain-damaged rats tested, 7 were found to have lesions largely confined to the mediodorsal thalamic nucleus—these animals showed a significant loss on the button latch but not on the bolt latch. (The remaining 3 rats had more ventrally placed lesions damaging both the mediodorsal and ventromedial thalamic nuclei—they showed significant deficits on both latch-box tasks.) Until these conflicting findings can be resolved, it is reasonable to conclude that the skilled-response block comprises the motor cortex alone.

For over a century, neurological thinking has been dominated by the notion that voluntary movements are initiated and controlled by the motor cortex and that the corticospinal tract is the sole link between the volitional activities of the cerebrum and the spinal motor mechanisms. Lashley (1924, 1935, 1950) was one of the first investigators to amass experimental evidence inimical to this traditional view. For Lashley (1950), the motor cortex functions as "part of the vast reflex postural system which includes the basal nuclei, cerebellum and vestibular system [p. 458]." As it turns out, this view is not remarkably different from the one recently presented by Thompson, Gates, and Gross (1979)—that the motor cortex is a special extension of the proprioceptive-kinesthetic block.

Evidence that the motor cortex, rather than participating in the execution of voluntary action, may function primarily in the sensorimotor regulation of discrete movements of the distal musculature has been reviewed by Kornhuber (1974). This theory seems to be quite compatible with the neurobehavioral data gathered on the rat. Thus lesions to the rat's motor cortex, though disturbing digit (Castro, 1972), tongue (Castro, 1975), and rhinarium (Thompson, 1978a) usage in various problem-solving contexts, have little effect on the expression of locomotor tasks, such as maze and discrimination problems.

Granting that movements are not organized within the motor cortex raises the question of the whereabouts of the neural substrate that is responsible for this function. Based on a review of the literature, Berntson and Micco (1976) have advanced the view that the lower brain stem contains those assemblies of neurons that are fundamental to the expression of complex and coordinated behavioral patterns characteristic of the species under investigation. According to this view, neocortical and other forebrain systems are conceived to exert modulatory influences on the lower brain stem, to subordinate the lower brain stem to finer sensory control, and to contribute refinement to the final integration of the behavioral act.

In light of the recent findings on latch-box performance in the rat, the conceptualization of Berntson and Micco can be refined by interposing the integrating block between the forebrain sensory system (proprioceptive-kinesthetic block and skilled-response block) and the lower brain stem motor mechanism for the production of acquired skilled movements.

THE LOCUS OF THE ENGRAM RECONSIDERED

Choosing the cerebral cortex as the site of the memory trace was, for Lashley, more or less the outcome of a process of elimination. Little information was available to him concerning the contributions of subcortical formations to the learning process. Furthermore, Lashley's analysis of the records of rats with combined cortical and subcortical lesions failed to disclose any additional performance deficit that might be attributable to subcortical invasion.[4]

The situation is quite different today. It is reasonably well established, for example, that hippocampo-septal damage impairs maze performance (Carey, 1968; Kaada, Rasmussen, & Kveim, 1961; Niki, 1962; Thomas, 1971; Thompson, 1979b), that amygdaloid lesions disrupt avoidance habits (Horvath, 1963; Nagel & Kemble, 1976; Thompson, 1978b; Ursin, 1965), that red nucleus lesions interfere with visual discrimination performance (McNew, 1968; Smith, 1970; Thompson, 1969), and that brain stem reticular formation lesions disturb a wide variety of learned activities (Hernández-Peón & Brust-Carmona, 1961; Myers, 1964; Sprague, Levitt, Robson, Liu, Stellar, & Chambers, 1963; Thompson & Thorne, 1973). The results presented in the preceding sections of this chapter also implicate a broad range of subcortical formations in the performance of learned responses.

Perhaps the most convincing evidence that the engram is stored, at least in part, within subcortical formations of the rat brain comes from lesion studies on visually guided behaviors (Bauer & Cooper, 1964; Braun, Meyer, & Meyer, 1966; Breen & Thompson, 1966; LeVere & Morlock, 1973; Tryggvason & Tees, 1974). It is also conceivable that the engrams underlying odor discriminations (Swann, 1935) and Pavlovian conditioning (Oakley & Russell, 1977) are induced at subcortical levels.

Although the foregoing studies cast serious doubt on Lashley's claim that the engram is exclusively established within the neocortex, they do not provide information on either the precise locus of the memory trace or the extent to which the memory trace is localized. It is not very likely that either one of these issues will be resolved within the near future.

However, the findings related to the identification of the functional blocks underlying learned responses in the rat do have some bearing on the localization of the memory trace. It will be recalled that those learned habits requiring the subject to advance from one locus within the environment to another to obtain a reward depend on the integrity of the integrating block. Whether or not a second (visual), third (proprioceptive-kinesthetic), fourth (cognitive map), fifth (fear-initiating response), and/or sixth (skilled-response) functional block is engaged with the integrating block depends upon the sensory, motor, and motivational demands of the task itself. Granting the validity of the foregoing analysis, several alternative sites of the engram may be proposed.

First, it may be assumed that the engram develops at those sites that connect one functional block with another. With respect to simultaneous visual discrimi-

[4]Interestingly, Isaacson (1976) reports that Lashley's cortically damaged rats with invasion of the septo-hippocampal complex did indeed exhibit greater deterioration in maze performance than those without septo-hippocampal involvement

nation habits, for example, occipito-incertal, occipito-reticular, occipito-caudoputamenal, and reticulo-geniculate pathways unite the visual block with the integrating block. The engram would then be expected to be found within these subcortical sites. No direct evidence is available concerning the identity of those functional pathways uniting other blocks with the integrating block (or with each other), but it is reasonable to anticipate multiple interconnecting links. In any case, the trace would take on a localized character even though it would not be confined to a single brain region.

Second, it may be assumed that the engram is formed in neural circuits residing within functional blocks as well as between functional blocks. If this is indeed the case, then the engram would take on a diffuse character, particularly in relation to those habits supported by three or more functional blocks (successive visual discrimination, maze, avoidance conditioning, and latch-box problems).

Third, it may be assumed that the engram is stored only within the subcortical (or cortical) components of those functional blocks supporting the habit.

Finally, it may be assumed that the engram is established within one or more components of that block that participates in all goal-directed activities. In this case, the site of the engram would be found somewhere within the basal ganglia, brain stem reticular formation, and/or limbic midbrain area.

It may not be necessary to subscribe fully to any one of these alternatives. After all, learning is not a unitary phenomenon. In fact, I have recently published evidence favoring the notion that all goal-directed learned activities can be fractionated into three habits (Thompson, 1979a). One (incentive habit) would be related to the initiation of the learned response leading to the goal object; the second (location habit) would be related to the location of the goal object or the correct route to the goal object; and the third (response habit) would be related to the motor sequence necessary to gain access to the goal object. Conceivably, the engrams underlying each of these habits may have different loci within the brain. Thus the engram underlying one of these habits (location) may be stored at those sites that connect one functional block with another; that underlying a second habit (response) may reside within one or more functional blocks; and that underlying a third habit (incentive) may occupy the entire integrating block.

CONCLUDING REMARKS

There is little doubt that Lashley's research program was a fruitful one. Perhaps the main criticism of this program is that it excluded subcortical formations from consideration as possible sites in the elaboration of learned activities. This oversight, however, is excusable in light of the fact that the usefulness of stereotaxic techniques in producing accurately placed subcortical lesions was not fully realized until the latter years of Lashley's life.

Because of his focus on cortical systems and his emphasis on lesion data derived from the study of maze habits, Lashley was led to the conclusion that the cerebral cortex constituted the integrating mechanism of the brain concerned in large part with the complexities of adaptive behavior. This conclusion left little room for the parcellation of the brain's surface (or interior) into discrete functional units but could readily accommodate concepts such as mass action.

Neurobehavioral studies of more recent origin favor the doctrine of cerebral localization and the participation of subcortical formations in learned activities.

REFERENCES

Bauer, J. H., & Cooper, R. M. Effects of posterior cortical lesions on performance of a brightness-discrimination task. *Journal of Comparative and Physiological Psychology*, 1964, *58*, 84-92.

Berntson, G. G., & Micco, D. J. Organization of brainstem behavioral systems. *Brain Research Bulletin*, 1976, *1*, 471-483.

Bindra, D. *A theory of intelligent behavior*. New York: Wiley, 1976.

Bjursten, L. M., Norrsell, K., & Norrsell, U. Behavioral repertory of cats without cerebral cortex from infancy, *Experimental Brain Research*, 1976, *25*, 115-130.

Braun, J. J., Meyer, P. M., & Meyer, D. R. Sparing of a brightness habit in rats following visual decortication. *Journal of Comparative and Physiological Psychology*, 1966, *61*, 79-82.

Breen, T. E., & Thompson, R. Cortical and subcortical structures mediating a visual conditioned response motivated by thirst. *Journal of Comparative and Physiological Psychology*, 1966, *61*, 146-150.

Brodal, A. Anatomy of the vestibular nuclei and their connections. In H. H. Kornhuber (Ed.), *Handbook of sensory physiology. Vestibular systems: Basic mechanisms*. New York: Springer-Verlag, 1974.

Carey, R. J. Impairment of maze retention resulting from septal injury. *Physiology and Behavior*, 1968, *3*, 495-497.

Castro, A. J. The effects of cortical lesions on digital usage in the rat. *Brain Research*, 1972, *37*, 173-186.

Castro, A. J. Tongue usage as a measure of cerebral cortical localization in the rat. *Experimental Neurology*, 1975, *47*, 343-352.

Divac, I., Rosvold, H. E., & Schwarcbart, M. K. Behavioral effects of selective ablation of the caudate nucleus. *Journal of Comparative and Physiological Psychology*, 1967, *63*, 184-190.

Goodman, D. C., & Horel, J. A. Sprouting of optic tract projections in the brain stem of the rat. *Journal of Comparative Neurology*, 1966, *127*, 71-88.

Hernández-Peón, R., & Brust-Carmona, H. Functional role of subcortical structures in habituation and conditioning. In J. F. Delafresnaye (Ed.), *Brain mechanisms and learning*. Oxford: Blackwell, 1961.

Horvath, F. E. Effects of basolateral amygdalectomy on three types of avoidance behavior in cats. *Journal of Comparative and Physiological Psychology*, 1963, *56*, 380-389.

Isaacson, R. L. Experimental brain lesions and memory. In M. R. Rosenzweig & E. L. Bennett (Eds.), *Neural mechanisms of learning and memory*. Cambridge: MIT Press, 1976.

Kaada, B. R., Rasmussen, E. W., & Kveim, O. Effects of hippocampal lesions on maze learning and retention in rats. *Experimental Neurology*, 1961, *3*, 333-355.

Knook, H. L. *The fiber-connections of the forebrain*. Philadelphia: Davis, 1965.

Konorski, J. *Integrative activity of the brain*. Chicago: University of Chicago Press, 1967.

Kornhuber, H. H. Cerebral cortex, cerebellum, and basal ganglia: An introduction to their motor functions. In F. O. Schmitt & F. G. Warden (Eds.), *The neurosciences. Third study program.* Cambridge: MIT Press, 1974.

Krettek, J. E., & Price, J. L. The cortical projections of the mediodorsal nucleus and adjacent thalamic nuclei in the rat. *Journal of Comparative Neurology,* 1977, *171,* 157–192.

Lashley, K. S. Studies of cerebral function in learning. III. The motor areas. *Brain,* 1921, *44,* 255–286.

Lashley, K. S. Studies of cerebral function in learning. V. The retention of motor habits after destruction of the so-called motor area in primates. *Archives of Neurology and Psychiatry* (Chicago), 1924, *12,* 249–276.

Lashley, K. S. *Brain mechanisms and intelligence.* Chicago: University of Chicago Press, 1929.

Lashley, K. S. Studies of cerebral function in learning. XI. The behavior of the rat in latch box situations. *Comparative Psychological Monographs,* 1935, *11,* 1–42.

Lashley, K. S. Studies of cerebral function in learning. XII. Loss of the maze habit after occipital lesions in blind rats. *Journal of Comparative Neurology,* 1943, *79,* 431–462.

Lashley, K. S. In search of the engram. In *Symposia of the Society for Experimental Biology,* (No. 4) Cambridge: Cambridge University Press, 1950.

Lashley, K. S., & McCarthy, D. A. The survival of the maze habit after cerebellar injuries. *Journal of Comparative Psychology,* 1926, *6,* 423–433.

LeVere, T. E., & Morlock, G. W. Nature of visual recovery following posterior neodecortication in the hooded rat. *Journal of Comparative and Physiological Psychology,* 1973, *83,* 62–67.

Livesey, P. J., & Muter, V. Functional differentiation within the neostriatum of the rat using electrical (blocking) stimulation during discrimination learning. *Journal of Comparative and Physiological Psychology,* 1976, *90,* 203–211.

Lubar, J. F., & Middaugh, L. D. Avoidance conditioning in cats with striate and auditory cortex lesions and contrasting effects of peripheral blindness. *Journal of Comparative and Physiological Psychology,* 1971, *76,* 26–30.

Lubar, J. F., Schostal, C. J., & Perachio, A. A. Nonvisual functions of visual cortex in the cat. *Physiology and Behavior,* 1967, *2,* 179–184.

Luria, A. R. *Higher cortical functions in man.* New York: Basic Books, 1966.

Lynch, G., Smith, R. L., & Robertson, R. Direct projections from brainstem to telencephalon. *Experimental Brain Research,* 1973, *17,* 221–228.

McNew, J. J. Role of the red nucleus in visually guided behavior in the rat. *Journal of Comparative and Physiological Psychology,* 1968, *65,* 282–289.

Mehler, W. R. Some neurological species differences—a posteriori. *New York Academy of Sciences,* 1969, *167,* 424–468.

Meyer, P. M. Analysis of visual behavior in cats with extensive neocortical ablations. *Journal of Comparative and Physiological Psychology,* 1963, *56,* 397–401.

Miller, J. J., Richardson, T. L., Fibiger, H. C., & McLennan, H. Anatomical and electrophysiological identification of a projection from the mesencephalic-raphe to the caudate-putamen in the rat. *Brain Research,* 1975, *97,* 133–138.

Moruzzi, G., & Magoun, H. W. Brain stem reticular formation and activation of the EEG. *Electroencephalography and Clinical Neurophysiology,* 1949, *1,* 455–473.

Mowrer, O. H. *Learning theory and behavior.* New York: Wiley, 1960.

Myers, R. E. Visual deficits after lesions of brain stem tegmentum in cats. *Archives of Neurology,* 1964, *11,* 73–90.

Nadel, L., & O'Keefe, J. O. The hippocampus in pieces and patches: An essay on modes of explanation in physiological psychology. In R. Bellairs & E. G. Gray (Eds.), *Essays on the nervous system.* Oxford: Clarendon Press, 1974.

Nagel, J. A., & Kemble, E. D. Effects of amygdaloid lesions on the performance of rats in four passive avoidance tasks. *Physiology and Behavior,* 1976, *17,* 245–250.

Nauta, W. J. H. Hippocampal projections and related neural pathways to the mid-brain in the cat. *Brain,* 1958, *81,* 310–340.

Nauta, W. J. H., & Bucher, V. M. Efferent connections of the striate cortex in the albino rat. *Journal of Comparative Neurology*, 1954, *100*, 257-286.

Niki, H. The effects of hippocampal ablation on the behavior of the rat. *Japanese Psychological Research*, 1962, *4*, 139-153.

Norman, D. A. What have the animal experiments taught us about human memory? In J. A. Deutsch (Ed.), *The physiological basis of memory*. New York: Academic Press, 1973.

Oakley, D. A. Instrumental learning in neodecorticate rabbits. *Nature (New Biology)*, 1971, *233*, 185-187.

Oakley, D. A., & Russell, I. S. Subcortical storage of Pavlovian conditioning in the rabbit. *Physiology and Behavior*, 1977, *18*, 931-937.

O'Keefe, J., & Nadel, L. *The hippocampus as a cognitive map*. Oxford: Clarendon Press, 1978.

Olton, D. S. Spatial memory. *Scientific American*, 1977, *236*, 82-98.

Orbach, J. "Functions" of striate cortex and the problem of mass action. *Psychological Bulletin*, 1959, *56*, 271-292.

Reubi, J. C., & Emson, P. C. Release and distribution of endogenous 5-HT in rat substantia nigra. *Brain Research*, 1978, *139*, 164-168.

Routtenberg, A. Intracranial self-stimulation pathways as substrate for stimulus-response integration. In J. D. Maser (Ed.), *Efferent organization and the integration of behavior*. New York: Academic Press, 1973.

Russell, D. G. Spatial location cues and movement production. In G. E. Stelmach (Ed.), *Motor control*. New York: Academic Press, 1976.

Scheibel, M. E., & Scheibel, A. B. Structural substrates for integrative patterns in the brain stem reticular core. In H. H. Jasper (Ed.), *Reticular formation of the brain*. Boston: Little, Brown, 1958.

Shute, C. C. D., & Lewis, P. R. The ascending cholinergic reticular system: Neocortical, olfactory and subcortical projections. *Brain*, 1967, *90*, 497-520.

Smith, A. M. Deficits in conditioned movement and visual discrimination following rubral area lesions in the rat. *Physiology and Behavior*, 1970, *5*, 893-898.

Spiliotis, P. H., & Thompson, R. The "manipulative response memory system" in the white rat. *Physiological Psychology*, 1973, *1*, 101-114.

Sprague, J. M., Levitt, M., Robson, K., Liu, C., Stellar, E., & Chambers, W. W. A neuroanatomical and behavioral analysis of the syndromes resulting from midbrain lemniscal and reticular lesions in the cat. *Archives Italiennes de Biologie*, 1963, *101*, 225-295.

Swann, H. G. The function of the brain in olfaction. The effects of large cortical lesions on olfactory discrimination. *American Journal of Physiology*, 1935, *111*, 257-262.

Swanson, L. W. The anatomical organization of septo-hippocampal projections. In K. Elliott & J. Whelan (Eds.), *Functions of the septo-hippocampal system*. Oxford: Elsevier, 1978.

Swanson, L. W., & Cowan, W. M. A note on the connections and development of the nucleus accumbens. *Brain Research*, 1975, *92*, 324-330.

Thomas, G. J. Maze retention by rats with hippocampal lesions and with fornicotomies. *Journal of Comparative and Physiological Psychology*, 1971, *75*, 41-49.

Thompson, R. Learning in rats with extensive neocortical damage. *Science*, 1959, *129*, 1223-1224.

Thompson, R. Localization of the "visual memory system" in the white rat. *Journal of Comparative and Physiological Psychology Monograph*, 1969, *69*, Part 2, 1-29.

Thompson, R. Localization of the "maze memory system" in the white rat. *Physiological Psychology*, 1974, *1*, 1-17.

Thompson, R. Entorhino-subicular lesions: Amnestic effects on an assortment of learned responses in the white rat. *Bulletin of the Psychonomic Society*, 1976, *8*, 433-434. (a)

Thompson, R. Stereotaxic mapping of brainstem areas critical for memory of visual discrimination habits in the rat. *Physiological Psychology*, 1976, *4*, 1-10. (b)

Thompson, R. A possible nonvisual function of the lateral geniculate nuclei in the white rat. *Bulletin of the Psychonomic Society*, 1977, *9*, 45-46.

Thompson, R. *A behavioral atlas of the rat brain*. New York: Oxford University Press, 1978. (a)

Thompson, R. Localization of a "passive avoidance memory system" in the white rat. *Physiological Psychology*, 1978, *6*, 263-274. (b)

Thompson, R. Dissociation of a visual discrimination task into incentive, location and response habits. *Physiology and Behavior*, 1979, *23*, 63-68. (a)

Thompson, R. Hippocampal and cortical function in a maze devoid of left and right turns. *Physiology and Behavior*, 1979, *23*, 601-603. (b)

Thompson, R. Odor discrimination performance as affected by cortical, thalamic and cerebellar lesions in rats. *Physiology and Behavior*, 1980, *24*, 797-800.

Thompson, R., Arabie, G. J., & Sisk, G. B. Localization of the "incline plane discrimination memory system" in the white rat. *Physiological Psychology*, 1976, *4*, 311-324.

Thompson, R., & Bachman, M. K. The occipito-striate pathway and visual discrimination performance in the white rat. *Bulletin of the Psychonomic Society*, 1979, *14*, 433-434. (a)

Thompson, R., & Bachman, M. K. Zona incerta: A link between the visual cortical sensory system and the brainstem motor system. *Physiological Psychology*, 1979, *7*, 251-253. (b)

Thompson, R., Bernard, B. A., & Hale, D. B. *The successive visual discrimination habit has a proprioceptive-kinesthetic basis*. Manuscript in preparation, 1980.

Thompson, R., & Craddock, S. N. Lateral cerebral peduncle lesions: Amnestic effects on a visual habit in the rat. *Psychonomic Science*, 1972, *27*, 140-142.

Thompson, R., Gates, C. E., & Gross, S. A. Thalamic regions critical for retention of skilled movements in the rat. *Physiological Psychology*, 1979, *7*, 7-21.

Thompson, R., & Massopust, L. C. The effect of subcortical lesions on retention of a brightness discrimination in rats. *Journal of Comparative and Physiological Psychology*, 1960, *53*, 488-496.

Thompson, R., & Peddy, C. P. The lateral pedunculo-nigral area and visually guided behavior. *Physiology and Behavior*, 1979, *23*, 1049-1055.

Thompson, R., & Thorne, B. M. Brainstem reticular formation lesions: Amnestic effects on learned habits in the rat. *Physiological Psychology*, 1973, *1*, 61-70.

Tryggvason, S., & Tees, R. Retention of three brightness discriminations by rats following posterior cortical lesions. *Journal of Comparative and Physiological Psychology*, 1974, *86*, 637-647.

Ungerstedt, U. Adipsia and aphagia after 6-hydroxydopamine-induced degeneration of the nigro-striatal dopamine system. *Acta Physiologica Scandinavica*, 1971, Supplementum 367, 95-122.

Ursin, H. Effect of amygdaloid lesions on avoidance behavior and visual discrimination in cats. *Experimental Neurology*, 1965, *11*, 298-317.

Valverde, F. Reticular formation of the albino rat's brain stem cytoarchitecture and corticofugal connections. *Journal of Comparative Neurology*, 1962, *119*, 25-53.

Van Hoesen, G. W., Pandya, D. N., & Butters, N. Cortical afferents to the entorhinal cortex of the rhesus monkey. *Science*, 1972, *175*, 1471-1473.

Watson, J. B. Kinesthetic and organic sensations: Their role in the reactions of the white rat to the maze. *Psychological Monograph*, 1907, *8*, No. 2, 1-100.

Webster, K. E. Cortico-striate interrelations in the albino rat. *Journal of Anatomy* (London), 1961, *95*, 532-545.

Winer, J., & Lubar, J. F. Alternation behavior of cats with medial visual cortex ablation. *Physiology and Behavior*, 1976, *17*, 635-643.

Zeman, W., & Innes, J. R. M. *Craigie's neuroanatomy of the rat*. New York: Academic Press, 1963.

11 Lashley as Iconoclast in the Temple of Neuroscience: Some Thrusts He Would Have Enjoyed Today

Robert W. Doty
Center for Brain Research
University of Rochester Medical Center
Rochester, New York

I must confess to a certain degree of trepidation in choosing by this title to depict one of my major heroes of science as being an "iconoclast" of that science. Is my portrayal perhaps overdrawn? A chance conversation with Donald O. Hebb at Dalhousie this past summer, however, strengthened my perception that Lashley took exceptional delight in attacking overly simplistic concepts of neural function. Hebb charmingly related how he, as a very junior colleague, had invited Lashley to join him in coauthoring what was to become a classic essay in psychological theory, Hebb's justly famous *Organization of Behavior* (1949). This was a major constructive effort, but Lashley wished no part of it, preferring his experiments, instead, and his incomparable role as deflator of facile explanations.

The evidence is certainly at hand to convict Lashley of such continuing attack, from his early (1921) sally against the idea that "automatization" of a habit transfers its organization from cortical to subcortical levels, to his masterpiece, "In Search of the Engram" (1950), which—with its emphasis on the diffuseness of neural mnemonic processes—has in its own turn become something of gospel to neuroscientists. He disputed the Pavlovian theory of "stimulus generalization" (Lashley & Wade, 1946). This Pavlovian idea of "irradiation" of excitation over the cortex, together with the concept that "Gestalten" might be represented by cortical electrical fields (Köhler & Wallach, 1944), was challenged directly by Lashley and his colleagues, who showed that extensive interruption or distortion of intracortical paths or electrical fields was essentially without behavioral effect (e.g., Lashley, Chow, & Semmes, 1951; Sperry, Miner, & Myers, 1955). These experiments adumbrate the current thesis that the neocortex is vertically organized into functional units.

In historical perspective, another of Lashley's thrusts, against the cytoarchitectonic parcellation of the neocortex into numerous discrete areas (Lashley & Clark, 1946), has not fared so well (e.g., Powell & Mountcastle, 1959; Pubols & Pubols, 1979; Zeki, 1978).

It is interesting to speculate that some of the vigor of the Lashley and Clark (1946) criticism as to the reliability of putative cytoarchitectonic boundaries might owe something to an earlier experience of Lashley regarding the expertise of neuroanatomists. In replying to a lengthy, detailed letter I had written him only 15 days previously, he begins:

> October 25, 1957
>
> Dear Dr. Doty:
>
> Your letter raises many questions which have puzzled me. I have no data which certainly preclude your hypothesis concerning the role of the pulvinar system in pattern vision. Most of my work on the visual system of the rat was done before I had the technique of retrograde degeneration. As late as 1929 a group of the leading neuroanatomists in Chicago looked at my rat material and diagnosed the cell loss and gliosis in the thalamus as evidence of a low grade infection. Only when Polyak came was the nature of retrograde degeneration recognized. So I cannot say how complete my destructions of the striate cortex had been or what other areas were involved, in experiments before 1931.

(The letter continues for three pages, double-spaced and obviously typed by Lashley himself.) That neuroanatomists should be unaware of retrograde degeneration almost 50 years after von Monakow (1882) made and extensively published this fundamental discovery was not a fact to inspire confidence in their interpretative skills.

In any event, it is apparent that many of Lashley's arguments and experiments were directed against concepts that were basically naive. Indeed, he evolved a memorable dictum in this regard (Lashley, 1952): "The neurological activity in a psychological event cannot be simpler in structure or number of elements than the psychological activity which it constitutes [p. 535]." He forthrightly and brilliantly identified the shortcomings and problems in endeavors, including his own, that sought to explain behavioral and subjective events in terms of neural action. The overriding problem here, of course, is the unity and temporal orderliness achieved for the total outcome from the multimillioned spatially and temporally distributed bits of neuronal electrochemistry. That remains one of the central mysteries of neuroscience and, as Lashley so clearly foresaw, is not likely to be dispelled for many decades to come.

I was privileged to meet Lashley only once. It was a flying visit, on Saturday, 9 January 1954. I was returning from lavish surroundings at Boca Raton, where—thanks to my colleague James Bosma—I had participated in a conference on bulbar poliomyelitis. My fortune at being so near the Yerkes Laboratories at Orange Park was simply too good to miss. Lashley met me first at his home, most cordially and graciously, and then lavished much of his day showing me the famous laboratories and discussing our mutual interest in the visual system. I was deeply impressed with his kindness, generosity, and enthusiasm in receiving me. We parted after he confided his secret ambition, to sail his boat in the Java Sea and study the color vision of the spectral tarsier!

I suppose my heritage from Lashley and his astute skepticism may actually have begun when, as a student, I learned about the visual system from his close friend and colleague, Heinrich Klüver. In the letter quoted earlier, Lashley also mentioned that it was he and Paul Bucy who had performed the surgery on Klüver's famous monkeys lacking striate cortex. He and Klüver were thus very close. In this light, I find it a bit surprising that Klüver himself would not have pointed out to Lashley "von Monakow's phenomenon" of retrograde thalamic degeneration some time before the arrival of Stefan Polyak in Chicago. At least when I was his student, Klüver had an encyclopedic knowledge of the literature in German neuroscience, and I specifically remember his recommending to me a biography of Constantin von Monakow, *Begegnung am Abend*.

Be that as it may, I, too, acquired a certain skepticism for neuroanatomy when, as a student in one of the last courses that George Bartlemez must have taught (together with Roger Sperry), I had to submit drawings showing the cytoarchitectonic differences between Brodmann areas 1 and 6 in man. My eye for histological nuances was too inexperienced and my artistic ability much too meager to depict such details accurately. But Professor Bartlemez insisted I must complete my assignments if I was to pass the course. He was very kind but firm; and so one afternoon he guided my faltering hand and unseeing eye until I had produced the appropriate density of stippling in the appropriate cortical "layers" to satisfy his perception of the brain sections before us. I remained an unbeliever for many years thereafter and, of course, took Lashley and Clark (1946) to be kindred spirits and vindicators of my recalcitrance.

VISUAL SYSTEM

Perhaps this skepticism concerning the discreteness of functional and architectonic boundaries in neocortex played a significant role in the formulation of one of my major research endeavors. In any event, I had the simplistic notion that one might be able to remove the striate cortex in newborn kittens and thereby induce some degree of novel organization for visual function in surviving cortical areas, which would be developing as the kitten matured and endeavored to use its retinal input. The degree of such unusual organization might be gauged behaviorally, electrophysiologically, and—with a bit of luck—perhaps even anatomically. This otherwise wild idea was derived very directly from observations by Soltmann (1876), who, using puppies, found that Fritsch and Hitzig's (1870; see Doty, 1969, for historical note) newly discovered "motor" areas were largely dispensable if removed neonatally; and by Kennard and McCulloch (1943), who showed a somewhat similar situation for macaques, adding the important detail that some of the surviving areas of cortex became more excitable electrically for producing bodily movement. These results suggest that the function of at least some cortical area is mutable and, if so, that cytoarchitecture must either change in such instances or be of unreliable significance as to function.

Over the years, my experiments gradually came to fruition; the cat lacking striate cortex from infancy had remarkably good vision, and surrounding cortical areas gave unequivocal electrophysiological evidence of visual input without prima facie change in cytoarchitecture (Doty, 1961). As Lashley might have predicted, however, things were not that simple. Even adult cats (Doty, 1971) retained the ability to make refined discrimination of visual patterns in the absence of striate cortex (Fig. 11.1). Of course, it is not likely that one could remove cortex without producing a behavioral deficit, and recent studies of

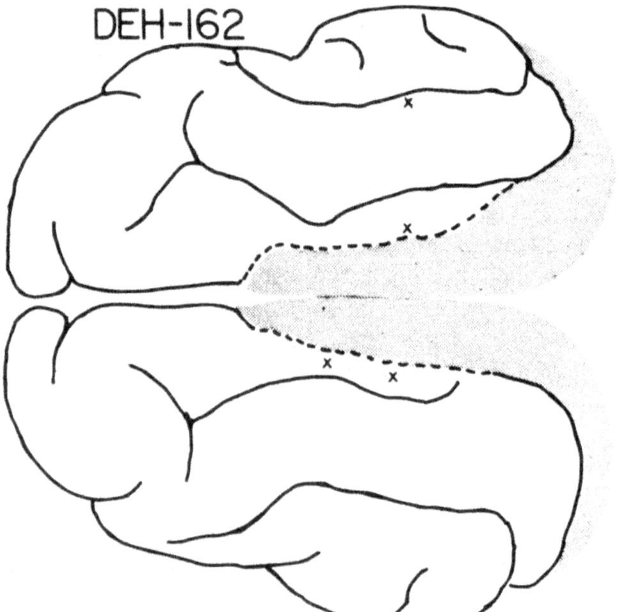

FIG. 11.1. Brain of cat from which area striata had been totally removed (stippled area). Not shown is the fact that the splenial gyrus had also been removed; laminae A, A_1, and B of the LGN were fully degenerated. Despite this, the cat was consistently able to discriminate various triangles from other variously sized geometric figures, averaging 82% correct over 200 trials. The Xs to the right (posterior) mark the points at which evoked potentials were maximal for photic stimulation; that to the left marks the rostral boundary from which such potentials could be recorded (Doty, 1971).

Berkley and Sprague (1979) begin the important work of defining just what this deficit may be. Nevertheless, the existence of pattern vision in the absence of striate cortex severely challenges interpretations commonly derived from the elegant studies of single-unit activity in that area (e.g., Bishop, 1979; Hubel & Wiesel, 1962; Lee, Cleland, & Creutzfeldt, 1977; Singer, Tretter, & Cynader, 1975).

For many years, again as a poor student of anatomy, I failed to appreciate (Doty, 1958) that the neurons surviving in the dorsal lateral geniculate nucleus (LGN) of many of the adult cats from whom I had endeavored to remove striate cortex (Doty, 1971) signified, not a lapse in the accuracy of my extirpation, but a strong projection of LGN into nonstriate areas. It remained for Sprague (1966), Garey and Powell (1967), and Niimi and Sprague (1970) to decipher this situation. It is now apparent that in the cat, the LGN distributes fibers to a puzzlingly large number of cortical areas; but even so, the electrophysiologically definable areas of neocortex having visual input (Doty, 1958; Palmer, Rosenquist, & Tusa, 1978) significantly exceed the anatomical and functional parceling of the cortex; and the same is now developing for macaques (e.g., Zeki, 1979). Most intriguing, however, is the possibility that the original, naive idea may have been correct—that is, that following neonatal removal of striate cortex, visual input may be enhanced to other areas, particularly to the lateral portion of the middle suprasylvian gyrus (Doty, 1961). Spear, Kalil, and Tong (1980) have found that visual properties of units in this area are preserved if studied at maturity after removal of striate cortex in infancy, but not when the removal occurs in the adult.

One has a certain confidence that Lashley would have welcomed these complications, this proliferation of "visual" areas, and the enigma that in cats, at least, the major cortical visual area can be removed without producing the anticipated drastic loss of vision. Certainly, simplistic views of the visual process as occurring mapwise in a single sheet of neurons, topographically representing little but the geometry of photic contrasts at the retina, are no longer credible. I have long felt that even the significance of the topographical projection is suspect (Doty, 1961), despite its undeniable prevalence (e.g., Tusa, Palmer, & Rosequist, 1978).

If one looks beyond the first-order effects, there are several instances in which it can be seen that electrically recorded responses to discrete visual stimuli considerably exceed what might be expected from a simple retinocortical topological mapping. Figure 11.2 is such a case. On two occasions about 100 min apart, a series of 16 lamps—each subtending 1° at positions indicated in the temporal and nasal fields, just below the horizontal meridian of the right eye—were individually illuminated for 180 msec at about 0.1 cd/m^2 while evoked potentials were recorded from a point estimated, from the data of Tusa et al. (1978), to lie over the position in left striate cortex representing the visual field very close to the center of gaze. The cat was anesthetized with sodium pentobarbital; the pupil had been dilated and the right optic tract cut. The ordinate (Fig.

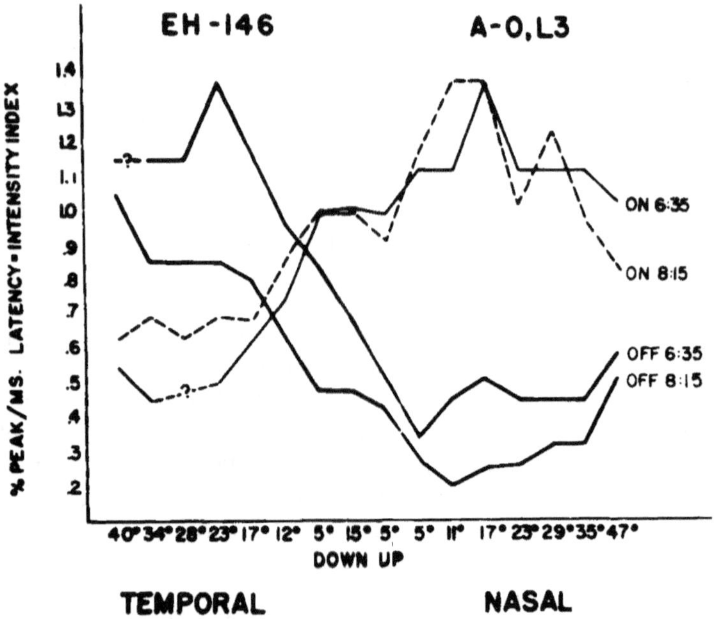

FIG. 11.2. Degree of responsiveness of a point on left striate cortex for 180-msec flashes, 0.1 cd/m², subtending 1° delivered at the designated points along the horizontal meridian of the visual field of the right eye in a cat anesthetized with pentobarbital. Since the apparatus was centered on the optic disc, the *area centralis* would lie at about 17° in the nasal field. Two sequences were run, at 6:35 P.M. and at 8:15 P.M. Responses to onset and cessation of the flash are plotted separately and are seen to be reciprocal; see text. (Doty, 1958.)

11.2) is scaled in relation to percentage of the maximum amplitude of potential elicited in this procedure, divided by the latency in milliseconds to onset of the response; that is, if the maximum response (100%) had a latency of 100 msec, it was scaled at 1.0. This was done to allow comparison of responses at different points (not relevant here) and on the supposition that the "best" response—that is, the largest and earliest—should result from stimulation at a locus most closely "represented" by the cortical point from which the recording was made.

It is obvious that whatever phenomena the data in Fig. 11.2 represent, they are stable and sufficiently reproducible over the 100-min interval. The data are, however, clearly paradoxical. The "best" response to the onset of the flash is for sites 11 and 17° in the nasal field, which—since the apparatus was centered on the optic disc—approximates the center of gaze at the *area centralis* and thus is concordant with subsequent findings (e.g., Tusa et al., 1978). However, responses of almost equal magnitude and latency arise from flashes directed at the deafferented temporal retina (e.g., 47° nasal field). Although this might very well represent merely scattered light or some degree of misalignment of the apparatus on the eye, the anomaly cannot be so readily dismissed. The "best" response for onset is reciprocal in position for offset. Furthermore, the latency for onset of illumination at 35° nasal was 15 to 20 msec earlier, and that to offset, 15 to 20 msec later, than the responses for 47° nasal, with both lamps directed far into that portion of the retina denervated by the optic tract transection. It thus seems most parsimonious to conclude that complex intraretinal processes are at play and that they, in effect, have the capability of placing every retinal point in potential communication with every point in striate cortex.

That this may indeed be the case is strongly supported by experiments in which the questions of light scattering and misalignment are wholly eliminated. This was accomplished by placing electrodes upon the exposed retina under direct vision (Doty & Grimm, 1962). With the application of electrical stimulating pulses (6 V, 1 msec) to the retina of the anesthetized cat, and with ipsilateral trigeminal nerve transected, responses are elicited over wide areas of visual cortex (Fig. 11.3). Most important is the fact that such stimulation of temporal

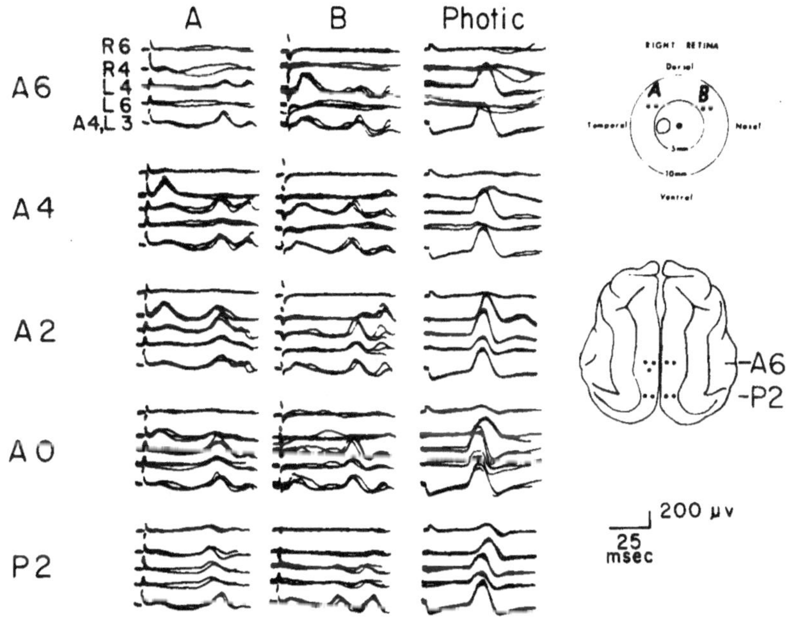

FIG. 11.3. Responses of a series of points in left and right striate cortex between anterior-posterior levels indicated and shown in diagram, for electrical stimuli (6 V, 1.0 msec) applied to temporal and nasal points A and B in exposed right retina, and to diffuse photic stimulation of that retina. The lower of the five traces in each set is from an electrode that remained fixed, whereas the other four electrodes were moved from anterior to posterior positions. Note that the electrical stimulation of right nasal retina A elicits late responses over a wide area of the left cortex (Doty & Grimm, 1962).

retina still commonly elicits ''late'' responses (ca. 35 msec) in contralateral cortex (L 3, 4, and 6 for stimulus location A in Fig. 11.3). The elaboration of this response, which is so unequivocally contradictory to predictions for a retinocortical topographic projection, very likely occurs within the retina. Such results, together with the responses elicited photically from the far nasal field in Fig. 11.2, could be explained if the cat had, as does the rat (Cowey & Perry, 1979), retinal ganglion cells projecting to the contralateral LGN from the far temporal retina. There are a substantial number of contralaterally projecting ganglion cells in the temporal retina of the cat (Stone, 1966). However, neither studies of single units in ''visual'' cortex nor of the electrophysiological characteristics of these ganglion cells (Kirk, Levick, & Cleland, 1976) encourage the idea that they might activate geniculocortical input to any significant degree. Neither could input from far temporal retina, were it to exist, be easily accomodated into present concepts of the retinocortical topographical projections.

These anomalous facts (Figs. 11.2 and 11.3) have made little impression on visual physiologists, but the corresponding phenomenon at the single-unit level is now very well documented (e.g., Derrington, Lennie, & Wright, 1979). This is McIlwain's ''periphery effect'' (1964), which can be obtained from the denervated eye and which shows that a substantial population of retinal ganglion cells are discharged or inhibited by stimuli extending at least 35° beyond their classically defined receptive fields (Derrington et al., 1979). Thus, just as for Figs. 11.2 and 11.3, it is again apparent that at the physiological level, the influence of the retina upon the cortex is not restricted to the narrow topographical arrangement suggested by anatomy. There are now indications that a form of McIlwain's effect may be particularly prominent in the magnocellular laminae of the primate LGN (Kruger, 1977), and that its presence may be demonstrable psychophysically (Breitmeyer & Valberg, 1979).

Finally, as if these assaults upon traditional, ''straightforward'' views of the organization and operation of the visual system were not enough, it is becoming apparent that the striate cortex in primates, so definitively the sole terminus of the geniculocalcarine projection, is also in receipt of substantial inputs from a half dozen other loci. Following massive injection of horseradish peroxidase (HRP) into the opercular area striata of macaques, I find—in addition to the expected labeling in the LGN (entirely ipsilateral, thus again failing to confirm the small contralateral projection claimed by Glickstein, King, Miller, & Berkley, 1967)—input from the ventral claustrum, nucleus basalis of Meynert, pyramidal cells in layer VI of an extensive region within the superior temporal sulcus, all ipsilateral; and a primarily ipsilateral projection from the locus coeruleus, raphe and deep pontine nuclei. Such projections to striate cortex have been described in fragmentary fashion for several species, including primates (e.g., Carey, Fitzpatrick, & Diamond, 1979; Kievit & Kuypers, 1974; Riche & Lanoir, 1978). There are also sparse connections from the intralaminar nuclei, medial hypothalamus, and hippocampal gyrus. Taken in sum, these heretofore unknown inputs to striate cortex probably rival numerically that from the LGN!

I had undertaken these experiments with HRP because of two sets of observations that suggested the existence of nongeniculate afferents to striate cortex. First, Sakakura and I had found (1976) that the EEG of striate cortex in the blind monkey was grossly disturbed (almost absent!) when the animal was awake, but that in either the slow-wave or rapid eye movement stage of sleep, it was essentially normal. Thus, during sleep, some nonretinal input, unlikely to be coming via the "degenerated" LGN, exerts a powerful control over the electrical activity of the striate cortex.

In the second instance, the LGN was essentially absent, having degenerated completely consequent to destruction of the retina within a few hours after the monkey's birth. The late John Bartlett and I (Bartlett, Doty, Kayama, & Riso, 1977) recorded single-unit activity in striate cortex from two such animals in the fully alert state when they were several years old. There were, of course, many units for which we could discern no relation between the animal's activity and the firing pattern of the unit. There were also rather frequently encountered units that appeared to fire in relation to movement of the eyes, but the poor quality of the electrooculogram from these blind animals and their almost ceaseless nystagmus made it difficult to establish this relation unequivocally for most such units. The most interesting result, however, was the discovery of units that increased their rate of discharge two- to threefold whenever the monkey manually explored the "extrapersonal" space around it. Such exploration was commonly elicited by gently touching the restrained, blind monkey, but the great increase in activity of units of this type also accompanied exploratory movements the monkey made without our provoking them. One now wonders, of course, whether activity of this type in striate cortex may not have something to do with the inputs from superior temporal cortex or the claustrum; and whether the units in parietal cortex, which Mountcastle and his colleagues (Mountcastle, Lynch, Georgopoulos, Sakata, & Acuna, 1975) have found to signal relations to extrapersonal visual space, may not also exist in striate cortex of the normal macaque.

The historically minded will quickly perceive the relation of these observations to those of Lashley, in which he (1929/1963, 1943) and his student Tsang (1936) showed that the striate cortex of the rat contributes to spatial analyses independent of vision. This was also true even of the rat blinded at birth so that maturation of neuronal circuitry, as with our two macaques, proceeded wholly in the absence of visual input. What should one expect here!? Does this great, intricate mass of neurons deprived of its primary input from the retina merely tick away idly and uselessly for the life of the animal (or man), or are there other, nonvisual functions performed in striate cortex? From the gross electrical abnormality of striate cortex in macaques losing all retinal input as adults (Sakakura & Doty, 1976), it might be surmised, prima facie, that most of the striate cortex has become useless in such cases. However, the existence of substantial nongeniculate input to striate cortex in primates, the presence of units there that can—at least in very special circumstances—discharge in relation to nonvisual activity (Bartlett et al., 1977), together with the demonstrations by Lashley (1943) and by Tsang (1936) that striate cortex in the rat contributes to the solution of maze problems even in the absence of vision, all suggest that striate cortex may serve important functions in addition to vision. The wide distribution of its output is certainly compatible with such a suggestion. Orbach (1959) endeavored, but with only marginal success, to extend to macaques the findings of Lashley and of Tsang on blind rats. There is also the work of Lubar, Schostal, and Perachio (1967), which hints at the possibility that striate cortex in cats may participate in analyzing the animal's orientation in space. They found that small lesions, limited to striate cortex and not interfering with visual pattern perception, produced a severe deficiency in the cat's ability to acquire an avoidance reaction when a buzzer was presented as a conditional stimulus in a shuttle box.

In sum, there is a strong case for the rat, a somewhat tentative one for macaques, and a hint for the cat that striate cortex provides an important substrate for orienting an animal in space even in the absence of vision. It would certainly seem appropriate that these clues receive more vigorous attention than they have in the past, particularly in view of the present strong evidence that the hippocampus (O'Keefe & Nadel, 1978; Olton, Branch, & Best, 1978) also plays a role in spatial orientation. Finally, the intriguing observations of Marczynski and his colleagues (Marczynski, Hackett, Sherry, & Allen, 1971; Rick & Marczynski, 1978) should not be overlooked. They have consistently found an interaction of visual input with food reward to produce unique electrical activity in striate cortex of cats—a further example, presumably, of the influence of the nongeniculate afferents described earlier. It may thus not be unrealistic to suppose that the parceling of functions among cortical areas may be neither as obvious nor as unimodal as it presently appears.

MEMORY

As summarized in his famous essay (1950), one of Lashley's lifelong endeavors was to understand the nature of the neural processes underlying mnemonic phenomena. He was not successful in his efforts to identify any combination of circumstances that would restrict these processes to a specifiable locus, and he therefore concluded that they were diffuse. His conclusions certainly still stand for the experiments he performed. However, it may yet be possible by surgical restriction of neural pathways, particularly the forebrain commissures (e.g., Doty, Overman, & Negrão, 1979), to constrain the critical mnemonic events to an identifiable set of neurons. On the other hand, it may well be that all neurons possess a rudimentary capability for at least an ephemeral retention of past activity; but memory that is truly, and surprisingly, permanent may possibly be a property only of special types of neurons (Doty, 1979).

Rather than deal here with these still speculative issues, I instead review some facts that, following Lashley's modus operandi, challenge a common conceptualization of mnemonic phenomena: "short-term memory." The first challenge is to the idea that a relatively prolonged period (15 to 20 min) of "fixation" or "consolidation" must ensue, in which it is variously envisioned that neuronal circuits are "reverberating," or producing certain critical molecular entities, before the memory trace is established in enduring form. The second challenge is the readiness with which a distinction is drawn between "short-term" and "long-term" memory, a body of fact and interpretation already subjected to much penetrating criticism by Weiskrantz (1970).

The observations that I think challenge the "consolidation" idea were made by Kesner, McDonough, and myself (1970) and are summarized in Figs. 11.4 and 11.5. Hungry cats were allowed to enter a compartment to obtain a savory morsel of food each time the door was opened. They ate the food from a metal dish while standing on a metal floor. After 10 such trials per day for 5 days, the

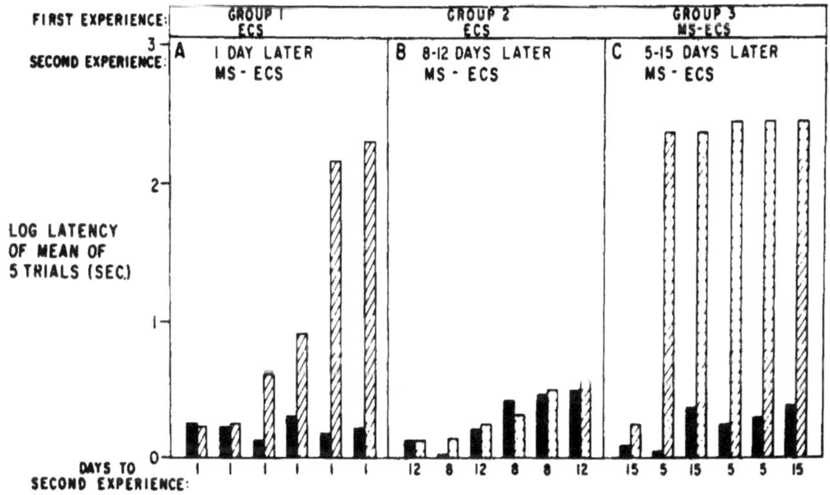

FIG. 11.4. Time, on logarithmic scale (ordinate) for cats to enter feeding compartment before (black bars) and after (hashed bars) treatments indicated. In Group 1 it is likely that the seizure (ECS) just 1 day before receipt of a combined mouth shock (MS) and a second ECS diminished the effectiveness of this second seizure, so that some cats remembered the aversive experience and failed to enter the compartment in the allotted 5 min (2.47 log sec). When the second seizure is given after a recovery period of 8 to 12 days (Group 2), amnesia for the MS occurs. However, if this second experience includes a second mouth shock (Group 3), five of six cats fail to enter—that is, remember the aversive experience (Kesner, McDonough, & Doty, 1970).

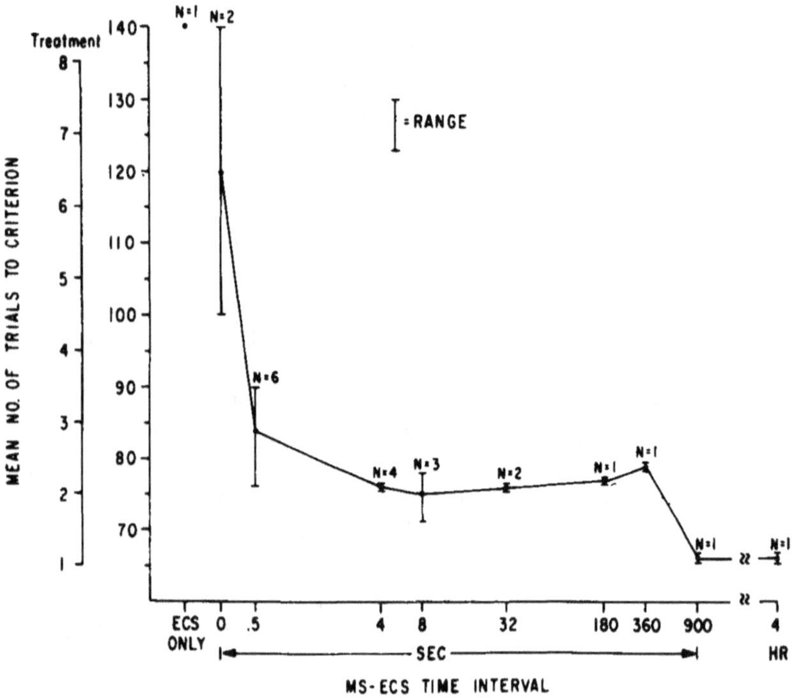

FIG. 11.5 Effect of intervals between mouth shock and ECS on the number of combinations needed to produce aversion—that is, failure to enter feeding compartment. The ECS alone produces aversion only after eight exposures, and this effect is probably also present in the two cats ($N = 2$) given concurrent mouth shock and ECS (0 interval). At 15 min and 4 h, the ECS has no effect, the memory is accessible; but at intervals from 0.5 to 360 sec (log scale), 3 or 2 mouth shocks are required for effective memory (Kesner, McDonough, & Doty, 1970).

cats were entering the compartment avidly, within 1 or 2 seconds after the door was opened. Then, without warning, they received a severely aversive electrical shock between mouth and feet as they endeavored to seize the food. Removed from the compartment and given the opportunity to enter it again 24 hours to 15 days later, the great majority of cats simply refuse to do so, and thus manifest a memory for the aversive event (mouth shock). If, on the other hand, they receive a mouth shock and 4 sec later experience an electroconvulsive fit consequent to electrical stimulation across electrodes implanted bilaterally over temporal cortex, they subsequently enter the compartment without hesitation, thus manifesting amnesia for the aversive event.

The prima facie interpretation of such results is simply that the convulsion has destroyed the incipient engram, which—not having yet been "consolidated" from a short-term mnemonic holding process—is vulnerable to such disruption by the chaotic activity of the fit. However, upon probing further, this turns out to be completely untrue; the incipient memory trace has survived the seizure activity, and a repetition of these events 5 to 15 days later—that is, a second mouth shock followed in 4 sec by a second fit—produced a robust memory for the mouth shock in five of six cats (Fig. 11.4C). In other words, two 4-sec periods of normal activity following aversive experiences occurring at an interval of 5 to 15 days is sufficient to "consolidate" the engram even though each period is followed by a severe electrical fit. Thus not only is it surprising that the memory trace survives the chaotic neuronal discharge but also that the "fixation time" is more than two orders of magnitude less than is usually claimed. That there is, however, a real "fixation time" and that the seizure, unlike those elicited from the frontal cortex or mesencephalic reticular formation (Kesner & Doty, 1968), does have a genuine amnestic effect in this situation is shown in Fig. 11.5, where it can be seen that an interval of only 0.5 sec between mouth shock and seizure requires a third experience before "fixation" (or the possibility of recall!?) occurs.

Further evidence for the rapid fixation and "nonerasability" of memory traces is provided by the observations that Overman and I (1979) made with tetanization of the anterior commissure in macaques performing a delayed matching-to-sample task. If the tetanization was administered while the monkey viewed the visual "sample" or when it was endeavoring to select a picture identical to the "sample" previously seen (i.e., to "match" it), its mnemonic performance was severely impaired. If, however, the monkey had seen and responded to the "sample," then tetanization of the commissure immediately thereafter had no significant effect upon its subsequent memory of that visual image.

Finally, as shown in Fig. 11.6, Overman and I (1980) demonstrated that macaques retain these somewhat fleeting visual images for many hours. The longer time intervals are logistically difficult to test with any assurance that an impatient monkey is paying attention, but one animal did achieve a level of 76% after 96 hours, correctly selecting 19 of the previously seen 25 images. Perhaps not surprising in themselves, beyond the technical achievement, these results differ dramatically from those obtained for many decades with this procedure, which had become known almost as the paradigmatic test for "short-term" memory in monkeys (Overman & Doty, 1980). The only thing done differently in these tests, as opposed to those preceding, was the use of a different visual image for each trial. Previous investigators had used the same pair of images over and over again, and in Fig. 11.6, "Repeated Stimuli" shows the devastating effect this has upon performance; monkeys that can retain visual images rather well for hours ("Novel Stimuli") are now unable to perform much above chance after a delay of only 15 sec! "Short-term" memory in this instance is thus nought but a procedural artifact. That is a result that Lashley would have warmed to; and it forces just a bit more clarity of fact into the convenient but deceptive terminology with which one is inevitably forced to describe that which is not understood.

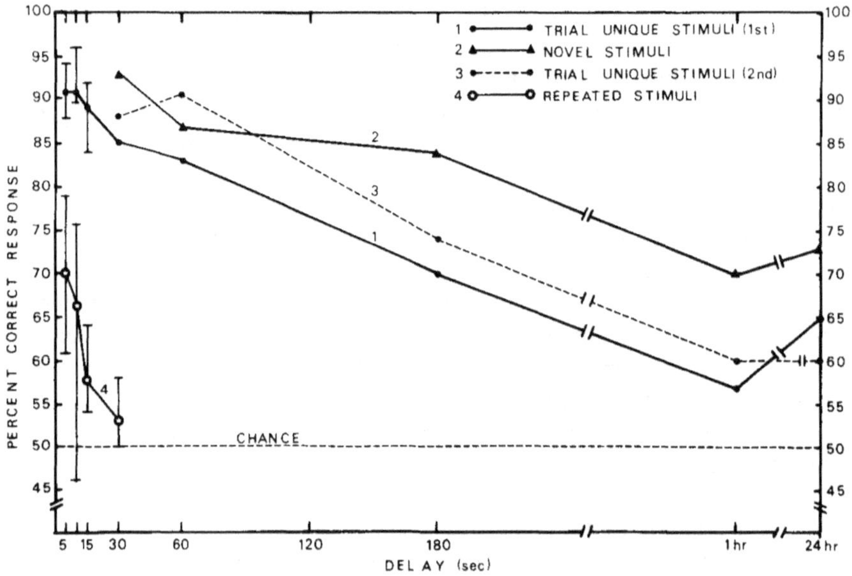

FIG. 11.6. Mean percent correct for six macaques performing a delayed matching-to-sample task at various delays between viewing the "sample" image and making the "match." "Trial unique" stimuli were unique pairings from 100 images shuffled daily to make 50 new pairings for each session. "Novel" stimuli were images the monkeys had never seen before. For all of these, performance was above chance even at an interval of 24 h (range 54% to 88% for "novel" stimuli). When the same pair of stimuli were used continually ("repeated" stimuli), the monkeys were little above chance for choices after only 30 sec (Overman & Doty, 1980).

SUMMARY

Lashley, as Einstein wrote of Ernst Mach, was possessed of an incorruptible skepticism. He vigorously attacked, experimentally and polemically, concepts that he considered to be overly facile, or simply wrong, in relating psychological to neural phenomena.

In addition to a historical footnote, I have here offered a number of observations that, in their turn, challenge certain widely accepted perspectives in neuroscience. These are:

1. That the striate cortex, endowed with such extensive and intricate visual input, can nevertheless be removed totally in cats without drastic effect upon their ability to discriminate visual patterns.
2. That the topological ordering of retinal projection to the cortex is deceptive

in its simplicity, since every retinal point may, potentially, be capable of influencing every cortical point.

3. That the nongeniculate afferents to striate cortex (in macaques) may be of the same order of magnitude as those from the lateral geniculate nucleus, and that this and other observations suggest participation of striate cortex in nonvisual activity.
4. That the "consolidation" period for permanent fixation of a memory trace may endure for only a second or two.
5. That what was thought to be "short-term memory" in monkeys was merely a procedural artifact, and that monkeys form essentially permanent visual memories upon viewing an image for only a few seconds.

I have some confidence that Lashley would have relished these challenges to current concepts; and I have no doubt that he would equally have enjoyed attacking them.

REFERENCES

Bartlett, J. R., Doty, R. W., Kayama, Y., & Riso, R. R. Responses of units in LGN and striate cortex of alert macaques in Ganzfeld, darkness or blindness. *Proceedings of the International Union of Physiological Sciences*, 1977, *13*, 55.

Berkley, M. A., & Sprague, J. M. Striate cortex and visual acuity functions in the cat. *Journal of Comparative Neurology*, 1979, *187*, 679–702.

Bishop, P. O. Stereopsis and the random element in the organization of the striate cortex. *Proceedings of the Royal Society of London Series B*, 1979, *204*, 415–434.

Breitmeyer, B. G., & Valberg, A. Local foveal inhibitory effects of global peripheral excitation. *Science*, 1979, *204*, 463–464.

Carey, R. G., Fitzpatrick, D., & Diamond, I. T. Layer I of striate cortex of *Tupaia glis* and *Galago senegalensis:* Projections from thalamus and claustrum revealed by retrograde transport of horseradish peroxidase. *Journal of Comparative Neurology*, 1979, *186*, 393–437.

Cowey, A., & Perry, V. H. The projection of the temporal retina in rats, studied by retrograde transport of horseradish peroxidase. *Experimental Brain Research*, 1979, *35*, 457–464.

Derrington, A. M., Lennie, P., & Wright, M. J. The mechanism of peripherally evoked responses in retinal ganglion cells. *Journal of Physiology (Lond.)*, 1979, *289*, 299–310.

Doty, R. W. Potentials evoked in cat cerebral cortex by diffuse and by punctiform photic stimuli. *Journal of Neurophysiology*, 1958, *21*, 437–464.

Doty, R. W. Functional significance of the topographical aspects of the retino-cortical projection. In R. Jung & H. Kornhuber (Eds.), *The visual system: Neurophysiology and psychophysics*. Berlin: Springer, 1961.

Doty, R. W. Electrical stimulation of the brain in behavioral context. *Annual Review of Psychology*, 1969, *20*, 289–320.

Doty, R. W. Survival of pattern vision after removal of striate cortex in the adult cat. *Journal of Comparative Neurology*, 1971, *143*, 341–356.

Doty, R. W. Neurons and memory: Some clues. In M. A. B. Brazier (Ed.), *Brain mechanisms and learning: From the single neuron to man* (IBRO Monograph Vol. 4). New York: Raven, 1979.

Doty, R. W., & Grimm, F. R. Cortical responses in local electrical stimulation of retina. *Experimental Neurology*, 1962, *5*, 319–334.

Doty, R. W., Overman, W. H., Jr., & Negrão, N. Role of forebrain commissures in hemispheric specialisation and memory in macaques. In I. Steele Russell, M. W. van Hof, & G. Berlucchi (Eds.), *Structure and function of cerebral commissures*. London: Macmillan, 1979.

Fritsch, G., & Hitzig, E. Ueber die elektrische Erregbarkeit des Grosshirns. *Archiv für Anatomie und Physiologie*, 1870, *37*, 300–332.

Garey, L. J., & Powell, T. P. S. The projection of the lateral geniculate nucleus upon the cortex in the cat. *Proceedings of the Royal Society of London*, 1967, *B 169*, 107–126.

Glickstein, M., King, R., Miller, J., & Berkley, M. Cortical projections from the dorsal lateral geniculate nucleus of cats. *Journal of Comparative Neurology*, 1967, *130*, 55–76.

Hebb, D. O. *The organization of behavior*. New York: Wiley, 1949.

Hubel, D. H., & Wiesel, T. N. Receptive fields, binocular interaction and functional architecture in the cat's visual cortex. *Journal of Physiology (Lond.)*, 1962, *160*, 106–154.

Kennard, M. A., & McCulloch, W. S. Motor response to stimulation of cerebral cortex in absence of areas 4 and 6 (*Macaca mulatta*). *Journal of Neurophysiology*, 1943, *6*, 181–189.

Kesner, R. P., & Doty, R. W. Amnesia produced in cats by local seizure activity initiated from the amygdala. *Experimental Neurology*, 1968, *21*, 58–68.

Kesner, R. P., McDonough, J. H., Jr., & Doty, R. W. Diminished amnestic effect of a second electroconvulsive seizure. *Experimental Neurology*, 1970, *27*, 527–533.

Kievit, J., & Kuypers, H. G. J. M. Basal forebrain and hypothalamic connections to frontal and parietal cortex in the rhesus monkey. *Science*, 1974, *187*, 660–662.

Kirk, D. L., Levick, W. R., & Cleland, B. G. The crossed and uncrossed destination of sluggish-concentric and non-concentric cat retinal ganglion cells, with an overall synthesis of the visual field representation. *Vision Research*, 1976, *16*, 233–236.

Köhler, W., & Wallach, H. Figural after-effects: An investigation of visual processes. *Proceedings of the American Philosophical Society*, 1944, *88*, 269–357.

Kruger, J. The shift-effect in the lateral geniculate body of the rhesus monkey. *Experimental Brain Research*, 1977, *29*, 387–392.

Lashley, K. S. Studies of cerebral function in learning. II. The effects of long-continued practice upon localization. *Journal of Comparative Psychology*, 1921, *1*, 453–468.

Lashley, K. S. *Brain mechanisms and intelligence*. Chicago: University of Chicago Press, 1929. (Reprinted by Dover, New York, 1963.)

Lashley, K. S. Studies of cerebral function in learning. XII. Loss of the maze habit after occipital lesions in blind rats. *Journal of Comparative Neurology*, 1943, *79*, 431–462.

Lashley, K. S. In search of the engram. In *Symposium of the Society for Experimental Biology, No. 4*. Cambridge: Cambridge University Press, 1950.

Lashley, K. S. Functional interpretation of anatomic patterns. *Proceedings of the Association for Research in Nervous and Mental Diseases*, 1952, *30*, 529–547.

Lashley, K. S., Chow, K. L., & Semmes, J. An examination of the electrical field theory of cerebral integration. *Psychological Review*, 1951, *58*, 123–136.

Lashley, K. S., & Clark, G. The cytoarchitecture of the cerebral cortex of *Ateles:* A critical examination of architectonic studies. *Journal of Comparative Neurology*, 1946, *85*, 223–306.

Lashley, K. S., & Wade, M. The Pavlovian theory of generalization. *Psychological Review*, 1946, *53*, 72–87.

Lee, B. B., Cleland, B. G., & Creutzfeldt, O. D. The retinal input to cells in area 17 of the cat's cortex. *Experimental Brain Research*, 1977, *30*, 527–538.

Lubar, J. F., Schostal, C. J., & Perachio, A. A. Non-visual functions of visual cortex in the cat. *Physiology and Behavior*, 1967, *2*, 179–184.

Marczynski, T. J., Hackett, J. T., Sherry, C. J., & Allen, S. Diffuse light input and quality of reward determine the occurrence of "reward contingent positive variation" (RCPV) in cat. *Brain Research*, 1971, *28*, 57–70.

McIlwain, J. T. Receptive fields of optic tract axons and lateral geniculate cells: Peripheral extent and barbiturate sensitivity. *Journal of Neurophysiology*, 1964, *27*, 1154-1173.

Mountcastle, V. B., Lynch, J. C., Georgopoulos, A., Sakata, H., & Acuna, C. Posterior parietal association cortex of the monkey: Command functions for operations within extrapersonal space. *Journal of Neurophysiology*, 1975, *38*, 871-908.

Niimi, K., & Sprague, J. M. Thalamo-cortical organization of the visual system in the cat. *Journal of Comparative Neurology*, 1970, *138*, 219-250.

O'Keefe, J., & Nadel, L. *The hippocampus as a cognitive map*. Oxford: Clarendon Press, 1978.

Olton, D. S., Branch, M., & Best, P. J. Spatial correlates of hippocampal unit activity. *Experimental Neurology*, 1978, *58*, 387-409.

Orbach, J. "Functions" of striate cortex and the problem of mass action. *Psychological Bulletin*, 1959, *56*, 271-292.

Overman, W. H., Jr., & Doty, R. W. Disturbance of delayed match-to-sample in macaques by tetanization of anterior commissure versus limbic system or basal ganglia. *Experimental Brain Research*, 1979, *37*, 511-524.

Overman, W. H., Jr., & Doty, R. W. Prolonged visual memory in macaques and man. *Neuroscience*, 1980, *5* (11), 1825-1831.

Palmer, L. A., Rosenquist, A. C., & Tusa, R. J. The retinotopic organization of lateral suprasylvian visual areas in the cat. *Journal of Comparative Neurology*, 1978, *177*, 237-256.

Powell, T. P. S., & Mountcastle, V. P. Some aspects of the functional organization of the cortex of the postcentral gyrus of the monkey: A correlation of findings obtained in a single unit analysis with cytoarchitecture. *Bulletin of Johns Hopkins Hospital*, 1959, *105*, 133-162.

Pubols, B. H., Jr., & Pubols, L. M. Variations in the fissural pattern of the cerebral neocortex of the monkey. *Brain, Behavior and Evolution*, 1979, *16*, 241-252.

Riche, D., & Lanoir, J. Some claustro-cortical connections in the cat and baboon as studied by retrograde horseradish peroxidase transport. *Journal of Comparative Neurology*, 1978, *177*, 435-555.

Rick, J. H., & Marczynski, T. J. Electrical activation of visual pathways substitutes for tonic light input in triggering EEG correlates of food reward during conditioned behavior in cat. *Brain Research*, 1978, *154*, 105-118.

Sakakura, H., & Doty, R. W. EEG of striate cortex in blind monkeys: Effects of eye movements and sleep. *Archives Italiennes de Biologie*, 1976, *114*, 23-48.

Sirger, W., Tretter, F., & Cynader, M. Organization of cat striate cortex: A correlation of receptive-field properties with afferent and efferent connections. *Journal of Neurophysiology*, 1975, *38*, 1082-1098.

Soltmann, O. Experimentelle Studien über die Functionen des Grosshirns der Neugeborenen. *Jahrbuch der Kinderheilkunde*, 1876, *9*, 106-146.

Spear, P. D., Kalil, R. E., & Tong, L. Functional compensation in the lateral suprasylvian visual area following neonatal visual cortex removal in cat. *Journal of Neurophysiology*, 1980, *43*, 851-869.

Sperry, R. W., Miner, N., & Myers, R. E. Visual pattern perception following subpial slicing and tantalum wire implantations in the visual cortex. *Journal of Comparative and Physiological Psychology*, 1955, *48*, 50-58.

Sprague, J. M. Visual acoustic and somesthetic deficits in the cat after cortical and midbrain lesions. In D. P. Purpura & M. D. Yahr (Eds.), *The thalamus*. New York: Columbia University Press, 1966.

Stone, J. The naso-temporal division of the cat's retina. *Journal of Comparative Neurology*, 1966, *126*, 585-600.

Tsang, Y. C. The functions of the visual areas of the cerebral cortex of the rat in the learning and retention of the maze II. *Comparative Psychology Monographs*, 1936, *12*, 1-41.

Tusa, R. J., Palmer, L. A., & Rosenquist, A. C. The retinotopic organization of area 17 (striate cortex) in the cat. *Journal of Comparative Neurology*, 1978, *177*, 213–236.

von Monakow, C. Über einige durch Exstirpation circumscripter Hirnrindenregionen bedingte Entwickelungshemmungen des Kaninchengehirns. *Archiv für Psychiatrie und Nervenkrankheiten*, 1882, *12*, 141–156.

Weiskrantz, L. A long-term view of short-term memory in psychology. In G. Horn & R. H. Hinde (Eds.), *Short-term changes in neural activity and behavior*. Cambridge: Cambridge University Press, 1970.

Zeki, S. M. Uniformity and diversity of structure and function in rhesus monkey prestriate visual cortex. *Journal of Physiology* (*Lond.*), 1978, *277*, 273–290.

Zeki, S. M. Functional specialization and binocular interaction in the visual areas of rhesus monkey prestriate cortex. *Proceedings of the Royal Society of London Series B*, 1979, *204*, 379–397.

12 Multipotentiality: A Theory of Recovery of Function After Brain Injury

E. Roy John, Ph.D.
Department of Psychiatry
New York University Medical Center

In this survey of neuropsychology 20 years after the death of Karl Lashley and 30 years after the appearance of "In Search of the Engram" (Lashley, 1950), it seems appropriate to examine our current understanding of the neurophysiology of memory and its resistance to brain injury. Contemporary theories of brain function, strongly influenced by anatomical tradition, conceive of relatively discrete localization of sensory and motor functions. Until fairly recently, with the emergence of cognitive psychology, most studies of the learning process have utilized conditioning methods. In conditioning, new movements constitute the responses learned to the conditioned stimuli. As a logical consequence of the assumption that sensory perception and the control of movements are mediated by localized neuronal circuits, most theories of learning are "connectionistic"; that is, they assume that the crucial event that takes place in learning is the establishment of a new pathway between selected sensory and motor circuits. The memory of what was learned is mediated by these newly established or facilitated connections; remembering consists of activity in these pathways; learned behaviors appear when such activity occurs.

SHORTCOMINGS OF LOCALIZATIONISTIC THEORIES

Many objections can be raised against such theories (for reviews, see John, 1967, 1972; John & Schwartz, 1978). From the psychological viewpoint, they emphasize stimulus-response learning of the sort epitomized by operant conditioning. They offer little insight into observation or imitation learning, gestalt process or insightful learning. They are unable to deal with cognitive processes, with thinking about possible solutions to problems. They treat learning as a type of reflex. Although there has been little or no direct support for the assumptions underlying these theories, their widespread acceptance has led to many adverse effects within psychology itself and in many educational and therapeutic practices adopted by society.

From the neuropsychological viewpoint, generations of physiological psychologists both before and after Lashley have tried and failed to prove the existence and to establish the location of these hypothetical connections by lesion experiments. Such experiments seek to abolish memories by destroying specific brain regions or sectioning selected pathways. As long as the sensory input pathways, motivational systems, and final motor output pathways are spared, such experiments have overwhelmingly been unsuccessful. Apparent successes abound in the literature, but careful analysis has usually indicated that the apparent memory deficit was in fact due to a loss of sensory acuity, a decrease in motivation, an inability to maintain attention, and similar unspecific causes rather than to destruction of a specific memory. Even in the few instances in which deficits could not be explained as unspecific effects, they appear to reflect loss of a *class* of response capabilities rather than loss of a specific learned *member* of the class. Although there are a few examples of the loss of a generic class of responses after localized brain injury, there is no convincing evidence that different members of the class are mediated by specific neuronal circuits, or *labeled lines*.

EQUIPOTENTIALITY AND FEATURE EXTRACTION

Impressed by the largely negative outcome of such experiments, various theorists in the past have proposed that brain functions, including memory, were not localized. Perhaps the best-known American theorist of this school was Lashley, whose law of equipotentiality expressed his belief that many different cortical regions could mediate the same learned functions, and whose law of mass action expressed his belief that the amount of functional deficit after brain injury was dependent on the volume of brain tissue damaged rather than its specific locus (Lashley, 1931, 1933, 1938). A fundamental tenet of the law of mass action is that the participation of any part of the brain, especially the cortex, in the acquisition, retention, and performance of complex integrative functions is conditioned by interactions with many other regions. Lashley's views, although provocative and still controversial, have not prevailed for several reasons. One reason that has influenced the thinking of many critics is that Lashley focused on the retention of learned responses after lesions and ignored the *quality* of the motor movements. Detailed examination of the motor performance reveals marked alterations in how the response is performed (Goldberger, 1974). In my opinion, the fact that a learned behavior is accomplished is a *new* way, rather than being abolished after brain injury, emphasizes even more the goal-directed, cognitive nature of the systems established by learning and constitutes strong refutation of connectionistic assumptions, in favor of Lashley's beliefs.

Especially influential in the recent decline of acceptance of such beliefs were certain neurophysiological experiments showing great precision in the extraction of certain types of information about the external environment by apparently specific "feature extractor" cells (Hubel & Wiesel, 1962) or about the position of certain muscles by cells in the motor system (Mountcastle, 1967; Mountcastle & Powell, 1959). For slightly longer than a decade after these seminal papers, an enthusiastic series of studies of the receptive fields of cells in different sensory systems constructed a picture of sets of sensory analyzers that decomposed the environment into unitary elements and then combined these unitary elements into complex compounds. Activity of cells receiving converging inputs from unitary feature extractors was interpreted to reflect coding of increasingly more integrated representations of holistic environmental events. These impressive demonstrations of apparent encoding of specific environmental events as activity in selected cells led some theorists to construct models of perception as mediated by forests of neuronal trees, with the neuron at the apex of each tree mediating a single percept. Such data also tended to reinforce beliefs in localization and discreteness of the representation of information in the brain, whether that information reflected the action of a present stimulus or the memory of a past event.

Flaws in Feature Extraction Theory

Gradually, however, flaws began to appear in the feature extraction theories. A major defect in the logic became evident with the observation that the latencies of the responses of so-called complex cells, upon which the outputs of simple-cell feature detectors supposedly converged, were often shorter than the latencies of the simple cells. A fundamental further flaw became apparent with demonstrations that the observed properties of supposed feature extractor cells could be explained as arising from the analysis of spatial frequencies. At different levels of the visual system, single cells respond preferentially to certain spatial frequencies. Critical experiments compared the responses of the same cells to isolated features in local receptive fields and to grids of different spatial frequencies. The outcome of these evaluations makes it appear that the correlation between cellular activity and stimulus characteristics is better explained by assuming that many cells have a finite receptive field size and can be described as "medium band with spatial filters" than by using feature extractor theory (for review, see deValois & deValois, 1980).

Spatial frequency models have become a popular alternative to feature extractor theories, although few explicit spatial frequency theories have been published. It should be pointed out that the problems inherent to single-cell feature extractor models, reviewed by John and Schwartz (1978), are not circumvented by making the feature detector a spatial frequency detector. Further, such findings have led many workers to believe that the encoding of visual information may be accomplished by a sort of Fourier analysis. Physiological and psychological evidence that spatial frequency filtering takes place merely supports the statement that some aspects of the processing of visual information may be represented in linear system terms, for which spatial frequency is a natural and convenient language. However, no direct evidence supports the suggestion that the brain actually computes a Fourier transform. In fact, the existence of retinotopic structure excludes the possibility of the computation of global Fourier transforms. Recognition of this fact has led some to coin the phrase "piece-wise Fourier transform." Further areas of visual cortex that do not display retinotopic mapping show little preference for spatial frequencies.

The arguments against spatial frequency as well as feature extractor models have been reviewed in detail by Schwartz (1980). He concludes that the evidence is most compatible with a *configuration* model, in which the formation is encoded by the actual spatiotemporal configuration of neuronal activity in anatomically extensive ensembles.

Other neurophysiological studies (for review, see John, 1972; John & Schwartz, 1978; Thatcher & John, 1977), especially those involving activity of single nerve cells in brains of behaving animals, show that the responses of a neuron to a specified sensory stimulus are extremely variable and unreliable, that many different neurons respond to any specific stimulus, that many different stimuli can affect any neuron, and that neurons often discharge "spontaneously" for no apparent cause. If remembering consists of firing in some "labeled line," some pathway that stands for a memory, how is firing due to a familiar event distinguished from firing due to spontaneous discharge? How is firing from a familiar event presumed to have a higher probability of eliciting discharge distinguished from that due to a novel event presumed to have a lower probability of eliciting discharge, once such firing has occurred? Neurons are effusively responsive, often unresponsive or refractory, noisy, unreliable reporters. These facts pose further obstacles for connectionistic theories of information coding and functional mediation.

In view of these psychological, neuropsychological, and neurophysiological limitations, the theory of extreme localization of memory seems suspect. It is highly unlikely that memory consists of the establishment or facilitation of a specific neuronal circuit in which firing constitutes remembering.

RECOVERY OF FUNCTION AFTER BRAIN INJURY

The search for the locus of a memory is really a search for a localized function. Recovery of memory after brain lesions or ablations can be considered a special case of the recovery of function after brain injury. The topic of recovery of function is currently having a resurgence of interest. The striking feature, common to a wide variety of types of damage, is the extent to which functional recovery is eventually almost complete. Studies of residual impairment after traumatic head injury show a high incidence of posttraumatic amnesia. Memories and skills return at a rapid rate during the first 6 months, with recovery sustained at a lower rate for up to 24 months (Bond, 1975). Defects in sensory, motor, and cognitive functions caused by brain injury due to penetrating wounds are characterized by an enormous resiliency of function in the great majority of cases, ultimately leading to little or no detectable deficit. Certain exceptions do exist, however. For example, visual field defects involving damage to central visual pathways can remain unchanged for as much as 30 years. Nevertheless, even in these cases there is a marked recession of symptoms during the first 2 years. There appears to be an initial "overshoot" of defects, with a subsequent shrinkage and partial recovery. Even the aftereffects of damage that initially caused total blindness can diminish to a partial hemianopsia (Teuber, 1975). Similarly, the effects of cerebrovascular accidents that initially cause dyslexia, aphasia, or hemiparesis often evolve to little or no permanent residual defects (Matthews & Onbury, 1975). In all of these examples, it must be recognized that the brain tissue destroyed by an injury remains destroyed and occluded blood vessels remain blocked.

Factors Influencing Recovery of Function

A crucial factor in the extent of recovery appears to be what is sometimes referred to as "the momentum of the lesion"; that is, an important factor influencing outcome is how fast the damage occurs. Innumerable experiments show that massive brain damage, if inflicted in a single stage, normally causes a severe loss of some functional capacity that is reversed only with great difficulty; if inflicted in serial stages, on the other hand, the injury often results in little or no functional loss (for review, see Stein, Rosen, & Butters, 1974). Such paradoxical and contradictory sparing of functions after multiple- but not single-stage lesions has long been known. Certain experiments strongly suggest that a critical parameter in the survival or recovery of function after serial lesions may be the nature of pre-, inter-, and postlesion experience (for review, see Goldman & Lewis, 1978). Just as experience is important in the maturation of the brain, it may play an equally important role in the evolution of deficits after brain injury.

The recovery of function soon after damage need not occur spontaneously but depends upon the quality and quantity of postoperative stimulation. This is dramatically illustrated by the observation that the recovery of pattern vision after complete, two-stage removal of striate cortex in rats does not occur if the animals are deprived of visual experience or are given unpatterned visual experience or even passive, patterned visual experience between lesions; but it does occur if the animals are permitted to execute visually guided behaviors during the interlesion interval (Dru, Walker, & Walker, 1975). Although the effects of interlesion stimulation were not explored, an equally dramatic example of functional recovery after serial lesions was long ago provided by the demonstration that massive bilateral destruction of the brain stem reticular formation resulted in long-term loss of consciousness when performed in a single stage but rapid recovery when inflicted in multiple stages (Adametz, 1959).

In a recent demonstration of the remarkable influence of the momentum of a lesion in human beings, neither hemiplegia nor hemianopsia resulted after complete hemispherectomy was performed in an adult patient years after a childhood head injury (Damásio, Lima, & Damásio, 1975). This is reminiscent of other findings that animals receiving lesions early in life often escape functional deficits usually seen when similar damage is inflicted in adulthood, or the so-called escape of language function after left-hemisphere damage early in life. Such early damage seems to lead to "derepression" of functional capabilities elsewhere in the brain (Teuber, 1975).

Possible Mechanisms Underlying Recovery of Function

Experimental studies of recovery after brain injury indicate that at least five major processes may be involved. A detailed review of the relevant literature can be found in Cotman (1978).

1. *Substitution of function*. Brain-damaged organisms may learn alternate strategies that permit the same goals to be attained via different behaviors.
2. *Diaschisis*. Damage to particular brain regions often results in depressed function of intact regions because of metabolic or neuroelectrical consequences of the damage. The behavioral effects of the injury may reflect both the primary and secondary consequences. As the secondary consequences are ameliorated and intact regions regain their normal capability, substantial behavioral recovery may ensue.
3. *Denervation supersensitivity*. Deafferentation is sometimes followed by increased sensitivity to remaining afferent inputs or neurochemical influences on certain brain regions. This gradual increase in reactivity might compensate for the loss of a proportion of afferent input that was large enough to produce an initial functional deficit.
4. *Receptive field shifts*. When cells lose their normal afferent input, they may begin to respond to a previously ineffective input. Apparently, many neurons in structures with detailed somatotopic maps have a diversity of afferent inputs. Under normal circumstances, one or a few of these inputs dominate the response characteristics of the cell, with concomitant inhibition of less effective inputs. However, should damage result in loss of the dominant afferentation, disinhibition occurs, and new, unusual receptive fields or reactivities appear.

These functional changes reflect the emergence of new capabilities arising from the dynamic reorganization of effectiveness of previously existing afferents. This has been beautifully demonstrated by Sherrill and Wall (1978), who discuss six classes of neuronal mechanisms that might mediate such a functional shift.

In this context, Goldberger and Murray (1978) have reported that after a lesion, previously silent synapses may become effective in driving cells. Their evidence suggests that there is a subliminal fringe of excitatory inputs that converge on a cell from regions far away from the naturally evoked receptive field. Under usual conditions, such afferents produce too small a depolarization to reach firing thresholds unless artificially synchronized by direct electrical stimulation. These effects may normally be selectively inhibited. Deafferentation of other input may cause these remote afferents to become dramatically more effective, leading to powerful synaptic drives not seen in the intact animal.

5. *Reafferentation*. Destruction of presynaptic fibers due to brain injury may eventually lead to reinnervation of denervated neurons by regenerating axons or by the sprouting of collaterals. This reafferentation might eventually lead to behavioral recovery. A special case of this effect is the spread of the axonal field of residual afferent fibers occupying portions of the presynaptic volume.

Crucial Role of Trophic Influences

Goldman and Lewis (1978) have gathered a body of evidence to support their suggestion that loss of trophic influences may play a crucial role in diaschisis. A variety of biochemical and structural changes are known to result from prolonged neurological arousal, whether due to massed sensory stimulation or enriched experience. The evidence indicates that arousal stimulates a wide range of metabolic processes, leading to increased neuronal content of ribonucleic acid and higher levels of protein synthesis. This may reflect the greater release of neurotransmitters, especially acetylcholine. Afferent input, especially in cholinergic pathways, may lead to transsynaptic induction of enzymes that are needed for neurotransmitter synthesis in the postsynaptic cells (Chuang & Costa, 1976). The long-term effect of afferent input to regulate metabolic activity in the postsynaptic target cells is referred to as *trophic influence*.

The loss of trophic influences could obviously depress postsynaptic neuronal metabolism and excitability. Evidence exists that, conversely, loss of postsynaptic contacts can block presynaptic cells from effective interaction with other postsynaptic cells with which they remain in contact. Thus, diaschisis can be considered the result of removal of transsynaptic trophic influences. Plausibly, the effects of diaschisis might be reversed by the restoration of trophic influences by sensory stimulation, direct brain stimulation, or pharmacologic interventions that might enhance diminished neurotransmitter synthesis rates. Further, it seems possible that cells unresponsive to a subset of their afferent inputs may be so because of "hypotrophism." Blockade of certain inhibitory influences might release trophic activity and cause responsivity to previously ineffective inputs—a sort of inhibitory deafferentation.

In this context, it is interesting to realize that there is evidence that environmental enrichment or sustained stimulation by noise or light promotes more rapid behavioral recovery after brain lesions, that recovery of visuomotor functions can be enhanced by centrally active drugs such as d-amphetamine or cholinergic substances between serial lesions or even postoperatively, and that direct electrical stimulation of the brain can prevent loss of apical dendrite spines and other degenerative changes after cortical lesions and can lead to more rapid behavioral recovery after hypothalamic lesions (Goldman & Lewis, 1978; Harrell, Raubeson, & Balagura, 1974; Rutledge, 1978). Perhaps even more interesting are reports that direct electrical stimulation of unspecific projection systems or treatment with drugs can produce behavioral and EEG arousal in patients in long-term coma after brain injury (Hassler, 1979; Hassler, Dalle Ore, Dieckmann, Bricolo, & Dolce, 1969; Sturm, Kuhner, Schmitt, Assmus, & Stock, 1979; Wild & Dolce, 1976).

Reactive Synaptogenesis

Abundant evidence shows that neuronal systems often reorganize by forming new synapses after external perturbations, such as altered environments, as well as internal perturbations, such as lesions. Since such changes are reactions to unusual stimuli rather than a part of the normal developmental process, Cotman and Nadler described them with the term *reactive synaptogenesis* in their recent review of this topic (1978). Reactive synaptogenesis subsumes diverse processes such as reafferentation by axon growth or collateral sprouting and receptive field shifts. The precise mechanism may vary from brain region to region or with different types of perturbation but underlies recovery of function after lesions of the spinal cord, hippocampus, and other brain regions. There is no reason to preclude these processes from possible mediation of some of the adaptive properties of the brain displayed to environmental challenges that result in learning, but not in the sense of establishing new discrete pathways. We return to this issue later.

Cotman and Nadler have examined a variety of different interventions that can induce reactive synaptogenesis. Their results suggest that the growth of fibers may be initiated by the action of some humoral substance, such as *nerve growth factor*. Substances released by normal neuronal activity may inhibit the action of this growth factor. In other words, mature axons might have the potentiality for continuous growth but are inhibited by the release of growth retardants from other axons. Thus, functional denervation or inhibition might initiate axon growth. Lesions can therefore initiate the events leading to subsequent growth.

A voluminous literature, reviewed in Stein et al. (1974), shows that lesions inflicted in several stages often cause little or no lasting functional deficit, although long-lasting, severe deficits occur when the same injury is incurred in a single stage. In this context, it is especially interesting to note that serial lesions seem to enhance reactive synaptogenesis. Cotman and Nadler (1978) report studies in which a small primary lesion was followed several days later by a large second lesion. The first lesion induced little axon growth. However, the second lesion produced greatly accelerated reactive processes, with more abundant as well as more rapid fiber growth. The amount of increased reactivity depended upon several factors, including time between lesions and relative size of the lesions. Such effects can be observed in regions quite distant from the site of the primary lesion and suggest that they may be mediated by humoral factors. The onset of behavioral and physiological recovery coincides with the onset of anatomically detectable growth, which seemed to occur at newly created, rather than newly vacated, sites.

Neurochemistry of Learning and of Recovery after Injury

Analogous effects of a priming or "conditioning" lesion have also been described by Grafstein and McQuarrie (1978), who have studied some of the neurochemical mechanisms involved in such processes. Although no clear answer is yet available as to what the stimulus may be that facilitates axonal regeneration, it is clear that shortly after injury, RNA and protein synthesis are markedly increased. These changes seem to be dependent upon several factors, including the relative concentrations of inorganic electrolytes, especially Ca^{++}.

It is of interest to consider the present status of the neurochemistry of learning and memory (for a recent review, see Dunn, 1976, 1980). There is general agreement that there are several temporal stages in the formation of a memory. Most workers agree that there probably exist at least three stages: a very brief or "iconic" stage, a short-term memory, and a long-term memory. There is abundant evidence that the brain is altered metabolically during learning. It is unlikely that any of the observed changes represent stored information as specific molecular configurations. Rather, these changes probably reflect the cellular processes necessary for learning to occur. Neurochemical changes correlated with learning have been reported in numerous direct studies of RNA and protein synthesis. Similar conclusions can be drawn from interventive approaches, which study the disruption of memory as various metabolic processes are blocked. A substantial body of opinion indicates that the inhibitors of protein synthesis might act by impairing catecholaminergic functions. Direct antagonists of catecholamine metabolism usually interfere with learning and memory, whereas agonists such as amphetamine, epinephrine, norepinephrine, and dopamine all facilitate performance in learning tasks. Similar results also implicate serotonin and the pituitary hormones such as ACTH, whose effects resemble those of the catecholaminergic agonists.

In the context of this cursory overview of current beliefs about the neurochemistry of learning, the findings of Grafstein and McQuarrie (1978) already cited are especially intriguing in that the increases in RNA and protein synthesis that they reported after brain lesions are reminiscent of those found in learning situations. Similarly, there is evidence that behavioral recovery after brain injury can be enhanced by catecholaminergic or cholinergic agonists, just as these substances facilitate performance on learning tasks (Beck & Chambers, 1970; Braun, Meyer, & Meyer, 1966; Luria, Naydin, Tsvetskova, & Vinarskaya, 1969; Macht, 1950; Meyer, Horel, & Meyer, 1963; Ward & Kennard, 1942). These similarities may be fortuitous or may reflect the fact that the brain mechanisms that mediate behavioral recovery after internal perturbations and those that mediate behavioral adaptation after external perturbations share certain fundamental processes.

STATISTICAL CONFIGURATION THEORY

During the last 20 years, my colleagues and I have carried out a series of electrophysiological studies of brain mechanisms of learning and memory (for reviews, see John, 1967; Thatcher & John, 1977). Those studies led me to propose what I call statistical configuration theory (John, 1972). This theory proposes that neurons in most brain regions receive diffuse afferent inputs reflecting not only every modality of sensory information but also the dominant processes being performed in many other regions. Movements can be initiated from a wide variety of regions, whose efferent outflows converge upon the final common pathways of the motor system. The information in the system is represented, not by activity in a specific neuron or a selected pathway, but by the spatiotemporal pattern of nonrandom or coherent activity in anatomically extensive ensembles of neurons. The activity of any neuron is significant only insofar as it contributes to the statistical behavior of the ensemble. The difference between brain regions is not "*qualitative all-or-none mediation*" of sensory, motor, or other functions specifically localized to discrete regions. Rather, each region is involved in the "*quantitative graded mediation*" of a wide variety of functions, each with its characteristic, local "*signal-to-noise ratio.*"

EEG Evidence

Statistical configuration theory rested upon a number of experimental observations. In our initial studies (John & Killam, 1959, 1960) a flash or click at a specified repetition rate was defined as the conditioned stimulus for a new behavioral response. Chronically implanted electrodes allowed us to monitor the electrical rhythms appearing in numerous brain regions as cats learned and performed conditioned approach and avoidance responses. Electrical waves at the *frequency* of the repetitive conditioned stimulus were called "labeled rhythms" and were considered to reflect neuronal responses to the "tracer-conditioned stimulus," or TCS.

In the naive animal, labeled rhythms appeared in only a few brain regions when a visual TCS was presented. These regions primarily corresponded to the classical notions of the visual system. As conditioning continued and a new behavioral response became established to the TCS, the labeled rhythms became far more widespread, appearing in many brain regions where they were previously absent or faint. When cats were trained to make two differentiated behavioral responses, CR_1 and CR_2, to two discriminated frequencies of tracer stimuli (for example, a light flickering at 1/sec [TCS_1] versus 5/sec [TCS_2]), an intriguing fact was noted. If the cat committed an error and performed CR_2 to TCS_1, some brain regions displayed 5/sec rhythms as if TCS_2 were present. Conversely, if CR_1 was performed to TCS_2, electrical waves appeared at the frequency of TCS_1. Further, if a neutral test stimulus midway between the two conditioned stimulus frequencies was occasionally introduced into a random sequence of TCS_1 and TCS_2, generalization often occurred. The frequency of the electrical waves in some brain regions during generalization corresponded to that of TCS_1 or TCS_2, and the behavioral response appropriate to that signal frequency was then performed. Since these incongruous rhythms disagreed with the actual frequency of the generalization stimulus but corresponded to the frequency of an absent conditioned stimulus appropriate to the behavior subsequently displayed, it became apparent that part of the electrical activity recorded from the brain while an animal evaluated sensory information must be released from memory systems activated during such information processing. These released electrical processes were termed *endogenous* or *readout* activity.

Evoked Response Evidence

Similar results were obtained in studies of the anatomical distributions and waveshapes of average evoked responses (AERs) computed as differentiated conditioned responses were elaborated to discriminative stimuli. Such studies showed that as learning proceeded, AERs appeared in regions that showed little response to the stimuli before training began. As signals acquired meaning, new long-latency components appeared in the AER waveshape from most structures. The waveshape of these long-latency components differed for stimuli with different meanings (Bartlett, John, Shimokochi, & Kleinman, 1975; John, 1963, 1967, 1972; John, Bartlett, Shimokochi, & Kleinman, 1973; Thompson, Patterson, & Teyler, 1972).

Analogous to our earlier findings with the frequencies of labeled rhythms, we found that during behavioral errors to one TCS, the AER waveshapes from many regions resembled the waveshapes normally elicited by the other TCS, which would have been the appropriate cue for that behavior (John, Ruchkin, Leiman, Sachs, & Ahn, 1965). In studies of generalization or of differential generalization, when the cat performed one or another CR to neutral test stimuli, the AER to the test stimuli displayed the waveshape characteristic of the response to the cue appropriate for that behavioral performance, as seen in Fig. 12.1 (John,

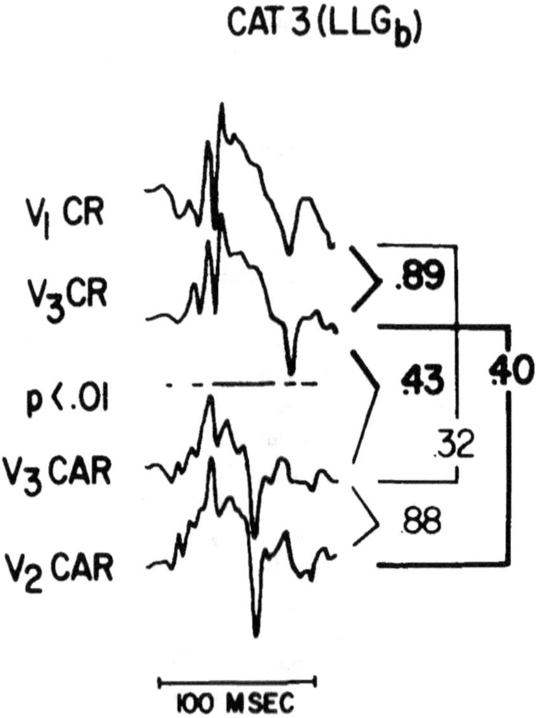

FIG. 12.1. *Top:* Waveshape elicited by TCS_1 in trial resulting in correct performance of CR_1. *Bottom:* EP waveshape elicited by TCS_2 in trial resulting in correct performance of CR_2. Second and third waveshapes both elicited by neutral test stimulus TCS_3. *Second* waveshape is average response to TCS_3 from trials in which differential generalization resulted in CR_1. Note similarity to *upper* waveshape. *Third* waveshape is average response to TCS_3 from differential generalization trials resulting in CR_2. Note similarity to *lower* waveshape. Numbers at right are correlation coefficients between indicated waves. (Data from John, Shimokochi, & Bartlett, 1969.)

Shimokochi, & Bartlett, 1969; Ruchkin & John, 1966). Pattern recognition programs were written that enabled a computer to analyze the evoked response waveshape elicited by each presentation of a test stimulus and to predict with very high accuracy which behavioral response would be forthcoming in every trial (Bartlett et al., 1975; John, 1972; John et al., 1973). Thus, it became apparent that the AER actually contained two different processes: a relatively short-latency ("exogenous") process reflecting the arrival of afferent information about the actual physical stimulus, and a relatively long-latency ("endogenous") process reflecting the release of stored information from memory that was the interpretation of the meaning attributed to the incoming information. These experiments showed that the system established in the brain could produce an accurate facsimile of a previous event released from storage in memory. These released facsimiles could be observed in many different brain regions.

Related human studies show that when an expected event does *not* occur, a cerebral potential appears at a latency similar to that of potentials usually evoked by the expected stimulus (Barlow, Morrell, & Morrell, 1967; Klinke, Fruhstorfer, & Finkenzeller, 1968; Picton, Hillyard, & Galambos, 1973; Riggs & Whittle, 1967; Rusinov, 1959; Sutton, Tueting, Zubin, & John, 1967; Weinberg, Grey-Walter, Cooper, & Aldridge, 1974; Weinberg, Grey-Walter, & Crow, 1970). Similar findings in the cat were reported by John (1963). These cerebral events, termed *readout* or *emitted* potentials, have been interpreted by Weinberg et al. (1970, 1974) to reflect the activation of memories about past or imaginary stimuli, and such experiments establish that there is a subjective correlate to their appearance.

Single-Unit Evidence

It was necessary to rule out the possibility that these widely distributed AER phenomena arose from the electrical fields generated by distant, localized neuronal activity. In order to examine the actual neuronal activity associated with these processes, we developed a chronically implanted, movable microelectrode that could be moved at will along long traverses through the brain of a cat performing behavioral responses. This method permitted long-term observation of the effects of stimuli on single neurons and small groups (multiunit activity). After sufficient study of a particular group of cells, the electrode could be moved slightly deeper, to an adjacent group of cells. Thus, maps of the correlation of the activity of many neurons with AERs could be constructed for many electrode positions in each cat.

These direct observations showed that stimulus-driven neural activity was indeed widespread, confirming the AER findings. Every cell we observed showed highly variable responses to single presentations of the same stimulus, highly reproducible average temporal firing patterns (poststimulus histograms) to repeated presentations of the same stimulus, different average temporal firing patterns to different stimuli, and a high level of spontaneous activity. In trained cats, cells in different brain regions displayed highly similar and closely synchronized average temporal firing patterns to the same stimulus. A few cells were found that displayed a facsimile property, producing the same average firing patterns during generalization to a novel stimulus as was shown during normal correct response to the conditioned stimulus (John & Morgades, 1969a, 1969b; Ramos, Schwartz, & John, 1976c).

Our initial studies largely recorded multiunit activity. Those observations showed excellent correlation between the contour of the multiunit poststimulus histogram (temporal firing probability of the ensemble) and the waveshape of the AER, in agreement with the results of other workers (for review, see John, 1967;

Thatcher & John, 1977). In subsequent work using electrodes that provided better resolution of single cells, we found that the firing patterns of different single cells often correlated well with the AER in a particular latency band after the stimulus. *No cells* were found that responded to only one type of stimulus or during only one of the different CRs. There seemed to be two different classes of cells: "stable" cells, which primarily participated in all exogenous processes, and "plastic" cells, which participated in all exogenous processes. These two kinds of cells were found intimately related in every region we studied (Ramos, Schwartz, & John, 1976a, 1976b, 1976c).

Thus, the results of our studies of single and multiple units supported and extended the AER evidence, providing more direct support for statistical theory. Many of these observations have been confirmed by other workers (Shvyrkov, 1975, 1977; Shvyrkov & Aleksandrov, 1973; Shvyrkov & Bezdenezhnykh, 1977; Shvyrkova & Shvyrkov, 1975).

These observations support the conclusion that information is represented by the average temporal pattern of firing in the ensembles of neurons (spatiotemporal coherence, or departure from random probability). Neither we nor other students of relationships between neuronal activity and learned behavior in mammals have found evidence of reliable, all-or-none firing restricted to single neurons or specific pathways established by learning and unique to some particular past experience.

SEPARABILITY OF EXOGENOUS AND ENDOGENOUS PROCESSES

Once it appeared probable that both exogenous and endogenous processes were reflected in the evoked response, we devised methods to separate and quantify the relative amounts of each of these processes that contributed to the AERs recorded from different brain structures (Bartlett & John, 1973). Sets of simultaneous equations were constructed in which AERs obtained from the same brain structure—when one or another CR was performed to TCS_1, TCS_2 and a neutral test stimulus—were added or subtracted like terms in algebraic equations. By performing these simple operations in a computer, it was possible to "solve" the sets of equations to isolate the waveshapes corresponding to the endogenous processes representing the different stimuli and the exogenous processes representing the different meanings attributed to them in trials with differing outcomes. These solutions consisted of pictures of waveshapes that were the residuals obtained when the algebraic procedures were carried out on the AERs. Since each stimulus and each response could be included in several different, independent equations, these manipulations yielded several independent examples of each residual. The accuracy of the computation could then be checked by quantifying the similarity between several residuals representing independent estimates of the same process. Similarity was assessed by computing the correlation coefficients between residuals. This technique revealed the existence of processes within the AER that could be separated to provide reproducible examples of relatively "pure" endogenous and exogenous processes. An example of these residuals is shown in Fig. 12.2.

Once we had established that replicable exogenous and endogenous processes could be extracted from the AERs recorded in complex decision-making tasks, these operations were carried out on thousands of AERs computed from many different anatomical structures in dozens of cats. The contributions of the separated exogenous and endogenous processes to the AERs in any particular anatom-

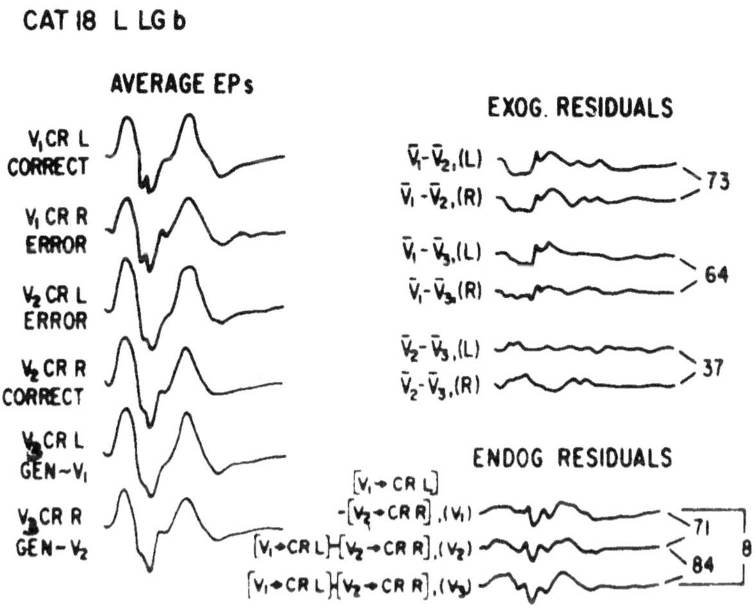

FIG. 12.2. *Left:* Average evoked potentials obtained from the left lateral geniculate body (bipolar derivation) of a cat subjected to differential behavioral generalization during trials in which six different stimulus-response contingencies were represented: V_1CR L, the cat pressed the left lever in correct response to stimulus V_1; V_1CR R, the cat pressed the right lever in erroneous response to V_1; V_2CR L, the cat pressed the left lever in erroneous response to V_2; V_2CR R, the cat pressed the right lever in correct response to V_2; V_3CR L, the cat pressed the left lever in response to the novel stimulus V_3 during test of differential generalization; V_3CR R, the cat pressed the right lever in response to V_3. *Top right:* Waveshapes representing pairs of exogenous residuals obtained by manipulating the appropriate averages as described in the text. *Bottom right:* Waveshapes representing independent estimates of endogenous residuals obtained by subtraction of the appropriate average response waveshapes. Numbers at the right refer to Pearson product moment correlation coefficients between the bracketed waves. (Data from Bartlett & John, 1973.)

ical region were averaged across all the examples computed from that region in the different cats in our study to obtain as accurate an estimate as possible for that brain region. In general, the values found for different anatomical structures belonging to the same functional system were closely similar. In order to simplify presentation of the data, a grand average was computed across the groups of structures belonging to different major functional systems. The average contribution of endogenous processes to the AERs within a given system was then plotted versus the average contribution of the exogenous processes for the same region, separately for data from visual and auditory conditioned stimuli. The final results of these computations are shown in Fig. 12.3 (Bartlett & John, 1973; Bartlett, John, Shimokochi, & Kleinman, 1975).

It was remarkable that the resulting points showed a lawful relationship. The endogenous contribution ("readout from memory") was logarithmically proportional to the exogenous contribution ("sensation") to the electrical activity observed in any brain region or functional system. The aspect of brain activity on which these measures were based—average evoked potentials recorded from closely spaced implanted electrodes—can be considered an epiphenomenon. It does not reflect the firing of any neuron in the region. It does, however, reflect the integrated postsynaptic potentials of a huge pool of neurons around the electrode tips and gives an estimate of the *probability of firing in that ensemble* as a function of time after presentation of a given stimulus. This point is further discussed later.

MULTIPOTENTIALITY

Viewed in this way, these results help us to evaluate both localizationistic and equipotential theories of information processing and memory functions in the brain. Inspection of the data make it clear that localizationistic theories are not consistent with the results. Were they accurate, exogenous and/or endogenous processes would only be present in a few structures in a single functional system. In trained cats, all regions studied displayed measurable contributions from *both* exogenous and endogenous processes. This establishes that the probabilities of firing in neuronal ensembles were influenced by information about different sensory stimuli and by memories about the meaning of those stimuli in all these functional systems and their constituent anatomical structures. In addition, the data demonstrate that the theory of equipotentiality is also not accurate. Were it accurate, all or most brain regions and functional systems would display the same exogenous and/or endogenous influences. This is obviously far from the case.

These findings demonstrate that *both* localizationist and equipotential theories are qualitatively correct but quantitatively wrong. Information about sensory events is very widely distributed throughout the brain, but the signal-to-noise ratio varies by more than a factor of 20. Memories about previous sensory

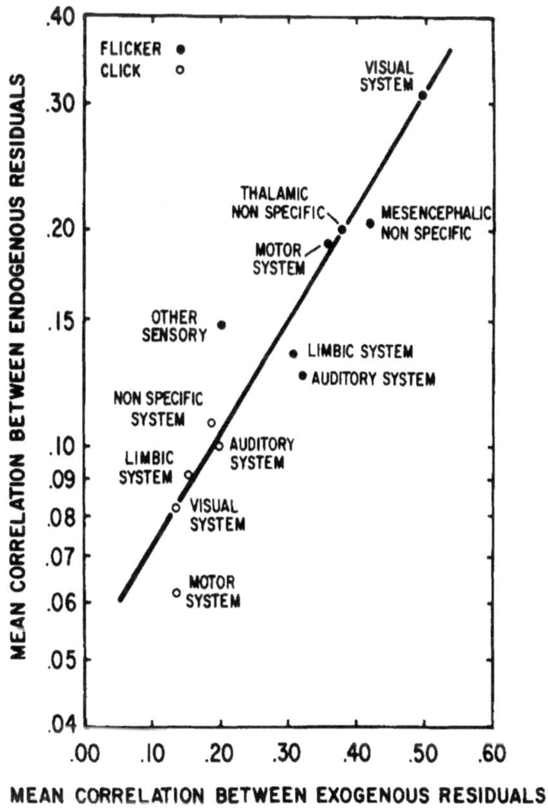

FIG. 12.3. Plot of mean correlation coefficients between exogenous residuals versus endogenous residuals for different neural systems and for different cue modalities.

Closed circles: flicker frequencies as stimuli. Auditory system: N = 305; Aud. CX (16 cats), Med. Genic. (16), Brach. Inf. Coll. (1). Limbic system; N = 303; Hippocampus (16), Dentate (5), Cingulate (5), Septum (5), Prepyriform (6), Med. Forebrain Bundle (6), Mamm. Bodies (5), Hypothalamus (7). Mesencephalic nonspecific: N = 158; Retic. Form. (18), Cent. Gray (1), Cent. Teg. Tract (1). Motor system: N = 146; Motor Cx. (4), Subs. Nigra (10), Nuc. Ruber (4), Nuc. Vent. Ant. (9), Subthal. (5). Other sensory: N = 54; Sensorimotor Cx. (4), Nuc. Post. Lat. (1), Nuc. Vent. Post. Lat. (5), Nuc. Vent. Post. Med. (1). Thalamic nonspecific: N = 139; Cent. Lat. (13), Nuc. Retic. (6), Nuc. Reuniens (1), Med. Dors. (5), Pulvinar (1). Visual system: N = 394; Visual Cx. (18), Lat. Genic. (18), Sup. Coll. (2).

Open circles: click frequencies as stimuli. Auditory system: N = 48; Aud. Cx. (5 cats), Med. Genic. (5). Limbic system: N = 69; Hippocampus (5), Dentate (3), Cingulate (3), Septum (3), Prepyriform (2), Med. Forebrain Bundle (3), Mamm. Bodies (3), Hypothalamus (2). Motor System: N = 37; Motor Cx. (1), Subs. Nigra (4), Nuc. Ruber (1), Nuc. Vent. Ant. (5), Subthal. (2). Nonspecific system: N = 50; Mesen. Retic. Form. (6), Cent. Gray (1), Cent. Teg. Tract (1), Cent. Lat. (3), Nuc. Retic. (3). Visual system: N = 55; Visual Cx. (6), Lat. Genic. (6), Sup. Coll. (1).

N denotes the number of independent measurements within the designated system. Data from monopolar and bipolar derivations were combined. Replications varied across cats and structures. (Data from Bartlett, John, Shimokochi, & Kleinman, 1975.)

experiences are also very widely distributed, but the signal-to-noise ratio varies by about a factor of 10.

Presumably, under normal circumstances, the brain relies primarily on the information available from regions with the highest signal-to-noise ratio and does not make use of the same information available elsewhere with poorer reliability. The term *multipotentiality* is a good way to describe this property of the brain. It suggests that any region may contribute to the mediation of a diversity of functions and that many systems contribute to every function, but it does not imply that different regions are functionally equivalent or that different functions depend equally on diverse regions.

It is noteworthy that the slope of the line, reflecting the constant of proportionality between the involvement of a region in representing a sensory event and in representing the memory of that event, is the same whether the event be in the visual or the auditory modality. This finding makes excellent intuitive sense. For neurons to participate in the memory of an event, they must be influenced by the occurrence of the event. Most theories of the chemistry of memory agree that there must be an early phase, possibly mediated by reverberatory activity in neuronal networks, and that this phase is somehow coupled to a later stable phase by means of the consolidation process (John, 1970). In some fashion, the afferent activity in the early phase (produced by exogenous processes) must influence the production of the chemical compounds mediating long-term storage (and responsible for endogenous processes). The logarithmic relation reflected in the slope of the line in Fig. 12.3 must be related to the nature of the coupling between the early labile and long-term stable memory storage mechanisms.

Multipotentiality, Learning, and Recovery of Function after Brain Injury

In a learning situation, information about a multidimensional event is widely distributed throughout anatomically extensive brain regions. This includes information about the external and internal environment, motivation levels, and motor movements. Each brain region sends outputs to and receives inputs from many or most other regions, via indirect as well as direct pathways. Transactions within and between these regions establish a *common mode of coherence* shared by many different neuronal ensembles, analogous to the interference pattern produced by interactions between the initial local coherence patterns. The set of neuronal ensembles, linked in that characteristic common mode, constitutes a *functional representational system* for that particular event. A different event might be represented by the same set of neuronal ensembles, but with a different common mode of coherence. The system thus possesses *multipotentiality*. These shared average temporal patterns of coherence constitute departures from baseline or random probabilities of simultaneous or phase-locked discharges between the neural elements within each ensemble and between ensembles.

Common modes of coherence can be discerned both in the similar poststimulus time histograms computed from multiunit recordings and in the similar waveshapes of average evoked responses that have been observed simultaneously in different brain regions. Coherence patterns involve periods of simultaneous inhibition as well as excitation within the elements of an ensemble.

When a portion of the functional representational system is activated in the common mode characteristic of some particular event, and when that portion is sufficiently large to influence a substantial proportion of the entire system, the functional representational system *as a whole* is activated in that common mode. This process corresponds to the *activation of the memory* of the corresponding event. The potentiality for the functional representational system to enter that common mode constitutes the *engram*. An engram can be activated in a large number of ways, and the same neuronal ensembles can mediate a large number of engrams. The activity of a single cell is important only insofar as it contributes to the statistical behavior of the ensemble to which it belongs.

A MODEL FOR CONSTRUCTION OF AN ENGRAM

At this stage in our understanding, we can only speculate about possible ways that the probability of certain firing patterns can be modulated in the set of neurons constituting an ensemble. Although one must acknowledge, on one hand, that no direct evidence yet exists at the synaptic or cellular level to support or refute such speculations, there exists, on the other hand, the set of electrophysiological and behavioral phenomena that have already been described and a variety of neuroanatomical, neurophysiological, and neurochemical findings that permit tentative models to be proposed. Imagine an ensemble of neurons, each receiving hundreds or thousands of synaptic terminals from afferent fibers, local circuit neurons, and recurrent collaterals. Homeostatic mechanisms regulate the membrane potentials of each cell, so that the probability of discharge depends upon summation of a large number of afferent inputs within a relatively short period. This condition requires a reasonably high level of coherence in the afferent inputs converging upon the neuron from many other cells. Depending upon the spatial and temporal distribution of such inputs, each cell can fire with a great variety of temporal patterns and for a vast number of antecedent conditions.

Assume, further, that the chemical consequences of such discharge tend to be rapidly dissipated by intra- and extracellular, homeostatic mechanisms. In order for these chemical consequences to exceed some critical threshold, it is necessary for weak cooperative influences to take place among a large number of cells in close proximity. These cooperative influences can only become substantial when the level of coherence in ensemble activity exceeds an improbable level.

Perhaps at that level, activation of inhibitory local circuits decreases noncoherent neuronal activity in the ensemble, leading to decreased local release of a growth-retarding substance. This decreased local concentration of growth retardant would permit shifts of the active presynaptic fields so that afferent inputs that were subliminal in the absence of the cooperative effects of coherence might become potentiated. This might lead to a sort of reactive synaptogenesis due to environmental stimulation.

The result of this potentiation of previously subliminal fields would *not* be to establish new specific connections, but to increase the probability of new modes of responses in the ensembles of neurons subjected to these common influences. Since similar cooperative processes are assumed to be taking place in all of the interconnected ensembles in the functional representational system, the neuronal populations in the multiple ensembles become selectively tuned to the corresponding common mode of coherence. The signal-to-noise ratios for that common mode will vary from ensemble to ensemble, depending on the proportion of the total afferentation that enters the coherent pattern.

One can further imagine the influence of these potentiated presynaptic fields on the postsynaptic membranes as including certain trophic effects, leading to cytoplasmic changes that might feed back upon the nucleus of the neuron to initiate derepression of deoxyribonucleic acid. The resulting RNA and protein syntheses might stabilize the increased sensitivity of the postsynaptic neuron to the particular spatiotemporal pattern of the coherent afferent barrage. An earlier version of this derepressor hypothesis was presented in John (1967). This hypothesis does not envisage synthesis of a different protein for each memory, but rather synthesis of a class of substances capable of *tuning* neuronal membranes to preferred spatiotemporal distributions of afferent input. How this tuning requirement of the model is actually accomplished is admittedly vague.

This model assumes no inherent difference between the mechanisms subserving innate and acquired behavior, save that the protein synthesis for innate behavior mediations are part of the genetic capability of all neuronal DNA, whereas the synthesis for acquired behavior mediations require derepression of reactions that are usually inhibited.

RECOVERY FROM BRAIN INJURY

A brain injury can cause deafferentation of mode-specific afferent input from the damaged region into the remainder of the functional representational system. Whether the behavior in question is innate or acquired, if that afferentation is critical for nonrandom levels of spatiotemporal coherence to be attained, a behavioral deficit must ensue. Nonetheless, activation of substantial portions of the intact remainder of the functional representational system must continue to achieve a nonrandom signal-to-noise ratio in extensive undamaged ensembles. Conceivably, the temporal pattern of coherence in the remainder of the functional system might also be sufficiently altered so as to disturb the tuning of the neuronal membranes. Studies of altered poststimulus time histograms and average evoked response waveshapes elicited by sensory cues after brain lesions causing behavioral deficits could cast crucial light on this issue.

Judging by the pervasiveness of behavioral recovery after extensive brain lesions, changes in trophic influences and reactive synaptogenesis gradually cause shifts in synaptic fields to occur with respect to the remaining afferentation from the functional representational system. The result of these changes is to expand and potentiate the afferent drives impinging on the surviving ensembles, causing them to respond more strongly to mode-specific inputs from the remainder of the functional representational system. Eventually, the signal-to-noise ratio achieved by the residual afferentation becomes sufficient to exceed the system threshold, or the system threshold is reset to accept a lower signal-to-noise ratio, and recovery of behavioral function emerges.

The sequence of events can be summarized as follows:

1. An injury destroys the brain region with the highest signal-to-noise ratio to a particular functional representational system. (If this lesion is in the primary sensory pathways, the effect might be irreversible since no alternative signal inputs remain.
2. This injury deprives the system of trophic influences as well as dominant afferents to regions dependent for coherence upon that high signal-to-noise ratio, as well as the secondary outputs from such regions to the remainder of the system.
3. This change causes diaschisis, followed by structural deafferentation, followed by functional deafferentation. The result is to disrupt a statistical mechanism as effectively as if it were based upon discrete connections.
4. Especially in gradual or serial lesions, continued activity reverses diaschisis and gradually restores trophic influences, now somewhat altered.
5. This leads to reactive synaptogenesis and shifts of synaptic fields.
6. The preceding item leads to increased effectiveness of remaining afferent inputs to cells at a distance from the lesion that were structurally or functionally denervated in part but that are part of the original functional representational system.
7. Previous subliminal fringes of synaptic fields impinging on these cells are now disinhibited or potentiated in the system common mode.
8. This increased residual synaptic drive increases the common mode signal to-noise ratio leading to functional recovery.

This theoretical picture argues the following:

1. In the absence of conclusive data, no brain lesion should be assumed to cause irreversible loss of innate or acquired functions, provided that unique sensory input or motor output pathways remain intact.

2. Stimulation per se, whether via direct electrical stimulation, behavioral inputs, or pharmacological intervention, may have a beneficial effect in reversing loss of trophic influences.

3. Systematic exploration of pharmacological agents, especially catecholaminergic and cholinergic substances, is highly desirable to ascertaining whether essential trophic influences may be restored in a nonspecific manner.

4. In some cases, training on new tasks might facilitate the recovery of functional capacity for tasks disrupted by a lesion.

5. In some cases, retraining on previously learned tasks might be necessary to provide the required stimulation to overcome the loss of essential trophic influences.

CONCLUSION

Acceptance of theories of localization of function may well lead to a self-fulfilling prophecy: Since functions are anatomically localized, brain damage creates a deficit that the patient must learn to accept rather than to overcome. In many cases this may be true, but in many others it may be false. At present, our knowledge is insufficient to classify remediable and nonremediable injuries accurately. Multipotentiality theory challenges these prophecies, arguing that only intensive remedial explorations can establish the nature of irreversible functional deficit. Aggressive, optimistic intervention techniques may well lead to functional recovery in many cases now assumed to be hopeless. Such interventions must combine pharmacological, electrophysiological, biofeedback, and behavioral techniques with quantitative evaluations not only of behavioral capacity but of brain state. This philosophy is beginning to be incorporated in rehabilitation medicine (Bach-y-Rita, 1979; Brudny & Korein 1976). This positive approach to remediation after brain injury may be the most important practical heritage of Karl Lashley's life work.

REFERENCES

Adametz, J. H. Rate of recovery of functioning in cats with rostral reticular lesions. *Journal of Neurosurgery,* 1959, *16,* 85–97.

Bach-Y-Rita, P. Brain plasticity: Basis for therapeutic procedures. *Sensory World,* December 1979, 15–18.

Barlow, J. S., Morrell, L., & Morrell, F. Some observations on evoked responses in relation to temporal conditioning to paired stimuli in man. *Proceedings International Colloquium on Mechanisms of Orienting Reactions in Man.* Bratislava-Smolenice: Slovak Academy of Sciences, 1967.

Bartlett, F., & John, E. R. Equipotentiality quantified: The anatomical distribution of the engram. *Science,* 1973, *181,* 764–767.

Bartlett, F., John, E. R., Shimokochi, M., & Kleinman, D. Electrophysiological signs of readout from memory. II: Computer classification of single evoked potential waveshapes. *Behavioral Biology,* 1975, *14,* 409–449.

Beck, C. H., & Chambers, W. W. Speed, accuracy and strength of forelimb movements after unilateral pyramidectomy in rhesus monkeys. *Journal of Comparative and Physiological Psychology,* 1970, *70,* 1–22.

Berger, B. D., Wise, C. D., & Stein, L. Nerve growth factor: Enhanced recovery of feeding after lateral hypothalamic damage. *Science,* 1973, *180,* 506–508.

Bond, M. R., Psychosocial outcome after severe head injury. In *Outcome of severe damage to the central nervous system* (Ciba Foundation Symposium 34, new series). New York: Elsevier, 1975.

Braun, J. J., Meyer, P. M., & Meyer, D. R. Sparing of a brightness habit in rats following visual decortication. *Journal of Comparative and Physiological Psychology,* 1966, *61,* 79–82.

Brudny, J. & Korein, J. EMG feedback therapy: review of treatment of 114 patients. *Archives of Physiology, Medicine and Rehabilitation.* 1976, *57,* 55–61.

Chuang, D. M., & Costa, E. Trans-synaptic regulation of ribonucleic acid biosynthesis in rat adrenal medulla. *Molecular Pharmacology,* 1976, *12,* 514–518.

Cotman, C. W. (Ed.). *Neuronal plasticity.* New York: Raven Press, 1978.

Cotman, C. W., & Nadler, J. V. Reactive synaptogenesis in the hippocampus. In C. W. Cotman (Ed.), *Neuronal plasticity.* New York: Raven Press, 1978.

Damásio, A. R., Lima, A., & Damásio, H. Nervous function after right hemispherectomy. *Neurology,* 1975, *24,* 89–93.

deValois, R. L., & deValois, K. K. Spatial vision. *Annual Reviews in Psychology,* 1980, *31,* 309–341.

Dru, D., Walker, J. P., & Walker, J. B. Self-produced locomotion restores visual capacity after striate lesions. *Science,* 1975, *187,* 265–266.

Dunn, A. J. The chemistry of learning and the formation of memory. In W. H. Gispen (Ed.), *Molecular and functional neurobiology.* Amsterdam: Elsevier, 1976.

Dunn, A. J. Neurochemistry of learning and memory: An evaluation of recent data. *Annual Reviews in Psychology,* 1980, *31,* 343–390.

Goldberger, M. E. Recovery of function after CNS lesions in monkeys. In D. G. Stein, J. J. Rosen, & N. Butters (Eds.), *Plasticity and recovery of function in the central nervous system.* New York: Academic Press, 1974.

Goldberger, M. E., & Murray, M. Recovery of movement and axonal sprouting may obey some of the same laws. In C. W. Cotman (Ed.), *Neuronal plasticity.* New York: Raven Press, 1978.

Goldman, P. S., & Lewis, M. E. Developmental biology of brain damage and experience. In C. W. Cotman (Ed.), *Neuronal plasticity.* New York: Raven Press, 1978.

Grafstein, B., & McQuarrie, I. G. Role of the nerve cell body in axonal regeneration. In C. W. Cotman (Ed.), *Neuronal plasticity.* New York: Raven Press, 1978.

Harrell, L. E., Raubeson, R., & Balagura, S. Acceleration of functional recovery following lateral hypothalamic damage by means of electrical stimulation in the lesioned area. *Physiology and Behavior,* 1974, *12,* 897–899.

Hassler, R. Striatal regulation of adverting and attention directing induced by pallidal stimulation. *Applied Neurophysiology,* 1979, *42,* 98–102.

Hassler, R., Dalle Ore, G., Dieckmann, G., Bricolo, A., & Dolce, G. Behavioral and EEG arousal induced by stimulation of unspecific projection systems in a patient with post-traumatic apallic syndrome. *Electroencephalography and Clinical Neurophysiology,* 1969, *27,* 306–310.

Hubel, D. H., & Wiesel, T. N. Receptive fields, binocular interaction and functional architecture in the cat's visual cortex. *Journal of Physiology (London),* 1962, *160,* 106–154.

John, E. R. Neural mechanisms of decision making. In W. S. Fields & W. Abbot (Eds.), *Information storage and neural control.* Springfield, Ill.: Charles C. Thomas, 1963.

John, E. R. *Mechanisms of memory.* New York: Academic Press, 1967.

John, E. R. Summary: Symposium on memory transfer AAAS. In W. L. Byrne (Ed.), *Molecular approaches to learning and memory*. New York: Academic Press, 1970.

John, E. R. Switchboard versus statistical theories of learning and memory. *Science*, 1972, *177*, 850-864.

John, E. R., Bartlett, F., Shimokochi, M., & Kleinman, D. Neural readout from memory. *Journal of Neurophysiology*, 1973, *36*, 893-924.

John, E. R., & Killam, K. F. Electrophysiological correlates of avoidance conditioning in the cat. *Journal of Pharmacology and Experimental Therapy*, 1959, *125*, 252.

John, E. R., & Killam, K. F. Electrophysiological correlates of differential approach-avoidance conditioning in the cat. *Journal of Nervous and Mental Disease*, 1960, *131*, 183.

John, E. R., & Morgades, P. P. Neural correlates of conditioned responses studied with multiple chronically implanted moving microelectrodes. *Experimental Neurology*, 1969, *23*, 412-425. (a)

John, E. R., & Morgades, P. P. Patterns and anatomical distribution of evoked potentials and multiple unit activity elicited by conditioned stimuli in trained cats. *Communications in Behavioral Biology*, 1969, *3*, 181-207. (b)

John, E. R., & Morgades, P. P. A technique for the chronic implantation of multiple movable micro-electrodes. *Electroencephalography and Clinical Neurophysiology*, 1969, *27*, 204-208. (c)

John, E. R., Ruchkin, D. S., Leiman, A., Sachs, E., & Ahn, H. Electrophysiological studies of generalization using both peripheral and central conditioned stimuli. *Proceedings of 23rd International Congress of Physiologic Sciences* (Tokyo), 1965, *4*, 618-627.

John, E. R., & Schwartz, E. L. The neurophysiology of information processing and cognition. *Annual Reviews in Psychology*, 1978, *29*, 1-29.

John, E. R., Shimokochi, M., & Bartlett, F. Neural readout from memory during generalization. *Science*, 1969, *164*, 1519-1521.

Klinke, R., Fruhstorfer, H., & Finkenzeller, P. Evoked responses as a function of external and stored information. *Electroencephalography and Clinical Neurophysiology*, 1968, *26*, 216-219.

Lashley, K. S. Mass action in cerebral function. *Science*, 1931, *73*, 245-254.

Lashley, K. S. Integrative functions of cerebral cortex. *Physiology Review*, 1933, *13*, 1-42.

Lashley, K. S. Factors limiting recovery after central nervous system lesions. *Journal of Nervous System and Mental Disorders*, 1938, *88*, 733-755.

Lashley, K. S. In search of the engram. *Symposium of the Society of Experimental Biology*, 1950, *4*, 454-482.

Luria, A. R., Naydin, V. L., Tsvetskova, L. S., & Vinarskaya, E. N. Restoration of higher cortical function following local brain damage. In R. J. Vinken & G. W. Brujn (Eds.), *Handbook of clinical neurology* (Vol. 3). Amsterdam: North Holland, 1969.

Macht, M. B. Effects of d-amphetamine on hemidecorticate, decorticate and decerebrate cats. *Federation Proceedings*, 1950, *63*, 731-732.

Matthews, W. B., & Onbury, J. M. Prognostic factors in stroke. In *Outcome of severe damage to the central nervous system* (Ciba Foundation Symposium 34, new series). New York: Elsevier, 1975.

Meyer, P. M., Horel, J. A., & Meyer, D. R. Effects of Dl-amphetamine upon placing responses in neodecorticate cats. *Journal of Comparative and Physiological Psychology*, 1963, *56*, 402-404.

Mountcastle, V. B. The problem of sensing and the neural coding of sensory events. In G. C. Quarton, T. Melnechuk, & F. O. Schmitt (Eds.), *The Neurosciences*. New York: The Rockefeller University Press, 1967.

Mountcastle, V. B., & Powell, T. P. S. Neural mechanisms subserving cutaneous sensibility, with special reference to the role of afferent inhibition in sensory perception and discrimination. *Bulletin Johns Hopkins Hospital*, 1959, *105*, 201-202.

Picton, T. W., Hillyard, S. A., & Galambos, R. Cortical evoked responses to omitted stimuli. In M. N. Livanov (Ed.), *Major problems of brain electrophysiology*. Moscow: USSR Academy of Sciences, 1973.

Ramos, A., Schwartz, E., & John, E. R. Evoked potential-unit relationships in behaving cats. *Brain Research Bulletin,* 1976, *1,* 69-75. (a)

Ramos, A., Schwartz, E., & John, E. R. An examination of the participation of neurons in readout from memory. *Brain Research Bulletin,* 1976, *1,* 77-86. (b)

Ramos, A., Schwartz, E., & John, E. R. Stable and plastic unit discharge patterns during behavioral generalization. *Science,* 1976, *192,* 393-396. (c)

Riggs, L. A., & Whittle, P. Human occipital and retinal potentials evoked by subjectively faded visual stimuli. *Vision Research,* 1967, *7,* 441-451.

Ruchkin, D. S., & John, E. R. Evoked potential correlates of generalization. *Science,* 1966, *153,* 209-211.

Rusinov, V. S. Electroencephalographic studies in conditioned reflex formation in man. In M. A. Brazier (Ed.), *The central nervous system and behavior.* New York: Josiah Macy, Jr., Foundation, 1959.

Rutledge, L. J. Effects of cortical denervation and stimulation on axons, dendrites and synapses. In C. W. Cotman (Ed.), *Neuronal plasticity.* New York: Raven Press, 1978.

Schwartz, E. Computational anatomy and functional architecture of striate cortex: a spatial mapping approach to perceptual coding. *Vision Research,* 1980, *20,* 645-669.

Sherrill, E. G., & Wall, P. D. Plasticity of connections in the adult nervous system. In C. W. Cotman (Ed.), *Neuronal plasticity.* New York: Raven Press, 1978.

Shvyrkov, V. B. Mechanisms in conditioning. *XXVI International Congress of Physiological Sciences* (Brain Information Service), 1975, pp. 5-15.

Shvyrkov, V. B. On the relationship between physiological and psychological processes in the functional system of the behavioral cat. *Studia Psychologica,* 1977, *19* (2), 82-96.

Shvyrkov, V. B., & Aleksandrov, Yu. I. Data processing, behavior act and cortical neurons. *Records of USSR Academy of Sciences,* 1973, *212,* 1021-1024.

Shvyrkov, V. B., & Bezdenezhnykh, B. N. On the relationship of neurophysiological and neurochemical mechanisms of memory. *Studia Psychologica,* 1977, *19* (3), 207-210.

Shvyrkova, N. A., & Shvyrkov, V. B. Activity of neurons of the optical cortex in eating and defense. *Neurophysiology,* 1975, *1,* 100-102.

Stein, D. G., Rosen, J. J., & Butters, N. (Eds.). *Plasticity and recovery of function in the central nervous system.* New York: Academic Press, 1974.

Sturm, V., Kuhner, A., Schmitt, H. P., Assmus, H., & Stock, G. Chronic electrical stimulation of the thalamic unspecific activating system in a patient with coma due to midbrain and upper brain stem infarction. *Acta Neurochirurgia,* 1979, *47,* 235-244.

Sutton, S., Tueting, P., Zubin, J., & John, E. R. Information delivery and the sensory evoked potential. *Science,* 1967, *155,* 1436-1439.

Teuber, H. L. Recovery of function after brain injury in man. In *Outcome of severe damage to the central nervous system* (Ciba Foundation Symposium 34, new series). New York: Elsevier, 1975.

Thatcher, R. W., & John, E. R. *Functional neuroscience: Volume 1: Foundations of Cognitive Processes.* Hillsdale, N.J.: Lawrence Erlbaum Associates, 1977.

Thompson, R. F., Patterson, M. M., & Teyler, T. J. The neurophysiology of learning. *Annual Reviews in Psychology,* 1972, *23,* 73-104.

Ward, A. A., & Kennard, M. A. Effects of cholinergic drugs on recovery of function following lesions of the central nervous system. *Yale Journal of Biology and Medicine,* 1942, *15,* 189-228.

Weinberg, H., Grey-Walter, W., Cooper, R., & Aldridge, V. J. Emitted cerebral events. *Electroencephalography and Clinical Neurophysiology,* 1974, *36,* 449-456.

Weinberg, H., Grey-Walter, W., & Crow, H. H. Intracerebral events in humans related to real and imaginary stimuli. *Electroencephalography and Clinical Neurophysiology,* 1970, *29,* 1-9.

Wild, K. V., & Dolce, G. Pathophysiological aspects concerning the treatment of the apallic syndrome. *Journal of Neurology,* 1976, *213,* 143-148.

13 Localization and Distribution of Function in the Brain

Karl H. Pribram
Departments of Psychiatry and Psychology
Stanford University School of Medicine

INTRODUCTION

Throughout his research career, Karl Lashley remained puzzled by the relationship between brain, behavior, and experience. On one hand, his experiments showed the brain to be put together with exquisite anatomical precision, which was to some degree reflected in the separation by behavioral function of the several sensorimotor systems and even regional differences within the so-called association areas. On the other hand, results of other experiments and observations made it clear that engrams, memory traces, could not be localized and that perceptual images and motor patterns displayed constancies and equivalences for which it was difficult to conceive *any* permanent "wiring diagram." Lashley is best known for his continuing attention to these nonlocalizable aspects of brain function that he formalized in the laws of mass action and equipotentiality. But it should be remembered that these aspects were puzzling to Lashley in large part because he was so keenly aware of the anatomical precision of the connectivity that gave rise to nonlocal characteristics in function. Had the brain been shown to be essentially a randomly connected network (as was so often assumed by those then working in the field of artificial intelligence), the problem might not have loomed so insurmountable.

In this chapter I present data that fill out a theoretical frame that was proposed by Lashley as a possible resolution of the localization/nonlocalization puzzle. These data have accumulated during the quarter century that has intervened since his last paper. The data have been gathered without reference to the frame, and the frame itself was derived, not from brain-behavior studies, but from the problems posed by morphogenesis during embryological development: Structural theories based on the principle of chemical gradients and resonances that "tune" specific locations in cytoplasm as inductors for organelles have been influential in embryology since before the turn of the century (see, e.g., Jacques Loeb, 1907; and Paul Weiss, 1939). In 1906, Goldscheider suggested that the structures of perception and memory might be similarly constructed by resonances among wave fronts created by sensory inputs in brain, especially cortical, tissue. In 1942, Lashley adopted this view as an alternative both to Köhler's field theory and to a localizationist view in which one percept or engram is matched to one neuron or neuron assembly. Lashley was never satisfied with this adoption because he could not envision the specific mechanisms that would give rise to resonant (and interfering) wave fronts in brain tissue and, equally important, how these, in turn, might be responsible for the structures that comprise perception and engram. He nonetheless held to the view that neither field nor localization (as, e.g., in the sophisticated development of Hebb, 1949) could account for the complex relationship between brain anatomy and phenomenal experience or could deal adequately with the encoding of memory.

Today a resonance theory *can* be detailed with high precision. Such a theory is thoroughly grounded in the structures and functions of the microanatomical connectivity of the nervous system and provides a mathematically sophisticated formulation of the relationship between anatomy and the images of perception, and also between anatomy and memory structure. Further, instantiations of this mathematical formulation in hardware have made possible in vitro observations that allow the exploration of the range and limits of the formulation. Finally, in vivo experimentation has provided a wealth of neurophysiological data that can be used to test the theory against alternative formulations.

THE NEURAL MICROSTRUCTURE

A fundamental observation concerning the structure and function of the nervous system is the fact that the relationship between locations that characterize peripheral receptors and effectors is reflected in the organization of the input to and output from the brain cortex. The peripheral relationship may become distorted through convergence in the pathways to synaptic way stations that are intercalated between periphery and cortex and by divergence from those way stations, but enough of the relationship is maintained to be recognizable as a mapping of periphery onto cortex. In order for such cortical mapping to be possible, signals must be transmitted from and to specific locations in the periphery by way of pathways of nerve axon systems in which impulses are generated and propagated.

A second fundamental fact about the organization of the nervous system is that these peripheral-cortical axonal pathways are interlaced at every station—that is, in the periphery (e.g., in the retina), in central nuclei (e.g., in the lateral geniculate nucleus), and at the cortex (e.g., in the striate cortex)—with cells that possess either very short, fine-fibered axons or no axons at all. Such cells, called "local circuit neurons" (Rakic, 1976), are incapable of maintaining and transmitting action potentials, the nerve impulses, that convey signals over distances. Instead, these local circuit neurons are characterized by profusely branching dendrites that intersect with others from adjacent neurons. The electrical potential changes in such dendritic structures tend to be graded rather than impulsive, and when impulses are generated they are small in amplitude, decay rapidly, and thus are not conducted over any considerable distance (Rall, 1970; Shepherd, 1974). In sum, the potential changes in these dendritic arborizations are most often hyperpolarizing and thus inhibitory (e.g., Benevento, Creutzfeldt, & Kuhnt, 1972; Creutzfeldt, Kuhnt, & Benevento, 1974).

The interaction between vertical (i.e., periphery to cortex) axonal transmission pathways and the interlaced horizontal dendritic networks has been worked out in several sensory systems by extracellular recordings made from the separate neurons composing the axonal transmission pathways. In essence, the interaction leads to a center-surround organization when a discrete stimulus excites the neuron. A center-surround organization is one in which the spatial extent of the signals transmitted becomes enveloped in a penumbra of signals of opposite sign. This center-surround organization often displays the characteristics of a waveform in that several excitatory and inhibitory bands surround the center much as ripples are formed in a pond when the surface is excited by a pebble. Precise mathematical descriptions of such center-surround organizations have been given by Bekesy for the auditory and somatosensory systems (1959) and Hartline (1940) and by Rodieck and Stone (1965) for the visual system (see also the review of early formulations by Ratliff, 1961). The data oblained from the olfactory system appears somewhat more complicated (Shepherd, 1974), but mathematical treatment has been successfully achieved by Freeman (1975).

The results of these studies have in common the finding that whatever the nature of the inciting stimulus to receptor excitation, such excitation and its subsequent processing can be readily formulated in terms of a calculus describing the microstructure of a network of hyper- and depolarizations. This formulation shows that the principle of superposition applies to the local spatial interactions between excitation (depolarizations) and inhibition (hyperpolarizations). Superposition indicates that the system is linear within the ranges examined and that a waveform interpretation of the data is useful. This does not necessarily mean that the dendritic potentials actually make up discernible wave fronts; what it does mean, at the minimum, is that the center-surround data describe transfer functions by which a matrix of discrete polarizations is related to an exciting input, functions that can readily be treated by linear wave equations.

Holography

These mathematical treatments of the data obtained from recordings of potentials of single neurons in the nervous system are akin to those that spawned holography. In 1948 Dennis Gabor devised a mathematics showing that image reconstruction might attain greater resolution if, instead of intensity, the pattern of wave fronts generated on a photographic film by an exciting electron or photon were recorded. Gabor addressed his mathematics to electron microscopy, but in the early 1960s optical holography succeeded in implementing this image-processing technique in such a way that the properties of holograms became readily demonstrated (Leith & Upatnicks, 1965). The essential properties are as follows: (1) The holographic store is distributed; (2) vast amounts of storage can be concentrated in a small holographic space; (3) image reconstruction is three-dimensional, displaying constancies and parallax, and is highly textured; (4) images do not appear coextensive with the holographic store; they are projected away from the film surface; (5) the hologram has associative properties; when it is made by the reflected light of two objects, subsequent illumination of the stored hologram by light reflected from only one object will reconstruct a ghost image of the missing object.

These properties of holograms are so similar to the elusive properties that Lashley sought in brain tissue to explain perceptual imaging and engram encodings that the holographic process must be seriously considered as an explanatory device. In doing this, however, it must constantly be remembered that it is the mathematics of holography and brain function that needs to be compared and tested, not the optical holograms or computer instantiations of holography.

The essentials of this mathematics can best be summarized by reference to a particular form of holography—the construction of a Fourier hologram. The Fourier theorem states that any pattern, no matter how complex, can be decomposed into a set of component, completely regular, sine waves. The Fourier transform of an image is formed by encoding these component waveforms. Thus, in the transformed record, each point indicates the presence of a particular component waveform rather than the corresponding local intensity, as in an ordinary record. Take for comparison an ordinary photograph and a Fourier-transformed record. The ordinary photograph is made up of a mosaic of points of varying intensities, the intensity of each point corresponding to the intensity of a point of light reflected from a specific location on the object being photographed. In the Fourier-transformed record, by contrast, each point represents the amount of energy present in a waveform component of the entire array of light reflected from the object. The bandwidth of that component may vary; the resolving power of the transform is in part dependent on this bandwidth.

To make a (Fourier) hologram, two such Fourier-transformed records must be linearly superposed. Mathematically, this is performed by the transfer function in which one record is convolved with the other and then the resultant complex conjugate stored. In essence, convolving consists of "adding" the waveforms together. Now each point in the record contains this "addition"—that is, the resultant of superposing the energy contained in two waveform components derived from the entire array of reflected light. A holographic record can be made by superposing the Fourier transform of the light reflected from two (or more) objects or by using the transform of a nonreflected reference. When two or more objects are used, the light reflected from each serves as a reference for the other(s). This accounts for the property of associative recall already noted. In addition, since parts of objects as well as whole objects serve as sources of reflection and thus as references for other parts, constancies are generated when images are (re)constructed. Constancies are therefore the result of the fact that the transformed "view" of any part of the objects acts as a reference for every other part.

It is these enfolding properties of holograms that make them so counterintuitive. Within the holographic domain, geometry as we sense it disappears and is replaced by an order in which the whole becomes enfolded and distributed into every part—thus the term *hologram*—but from each part, the whole can again be reconstituted. This is due to another property of the Fourier theorem: Applying the identical transform inverts the waveform domain back into the image! The process (the Fourier transfer function) that converts images into waveforms can therefore also accomplish the inverse and convert waveforms into images.

This parsimony in processing raises the question of utility. If image and waveform domain are so readily transformed into each other, why bother? The answer to this question is that correlations are much simpler to accomplish in the waveform domain; they essentially entail superposition, addition. That is why the Fast Fourier Transform (FFT) has proved so useful in computer programming—for instance, when image reconstruction by CAT scan in X-ray tomography is desired. It is this power of the Fourier domain that the brain can exploit.

In the introduction it was noted that there really have been only three classes of neural mechanisms proposed to explain the properties of perception. The three may, for convenience, be labeled: field theoretic, feature correspondent, and holographic. A review of currently available data regarding each of these classes follows:

DEFINITION AND EVIDENCE: FIELD THEORY

Wolfgang Köhler proposed that direct current (DC) fields were set up in the brain cortex by sensory stimulation and that these fields were isomorphic with—that is, had the same shape as—the phenomenally perceived stimulus. Köhler showed that, in fact, sensory stimulation did result in DC shifts (Köhler & Wegener, 1955), and in our laboratory we showed that such shifts were accompanied by desynchronization of the electrocorticogram (Gumnit, 1960). However, several experiments that throw doubt on the relationship between such shifts and perceptual performance were performed by Lashley, Sperry, and Pribram. In these experiments gold foil was placed over the surface of the cortex (Lashley, Chow, & Semmes, 1951); the cortex crosshatched the mica insulating strips inserted (Sperry, Miner, & Myers, 1955); and aluminum hydroxide cream injected in minute amounts into the cortex to produce gross abnormalities (Kraft, Obrist, & Pribram, 1960; Pribram, 1951; Stamm & Knight, 1963; Stamm & Pribram, 1960, 1961). See Figs. 13.1 and 13.2.

In none of these experiments did the animals show any change in their ability to discriminate among cues; gross alteration of the cortical DC field was not accompanied by any gross change in perceptual performance. These findings take additional meaning from the fact that the aluminum hydroxide cream implantation produced a fivefold retardation of learning and that imposing direct currents across cortex impairs (when cathodal) and enhances (when anodal from surface to depth) learning (Stamm & Rosen, 1972). Direct current fields are thus shown capable of biasing learning rate; and at the same time such fields seem to be unrelated to the structuring of percepts.

DEFINITION AND EVIDENCE: FEATURE CORRESPONDENCE THEORY

Field theory and feature correspondence concepts either explicitly or implicitly imply a brain–perceptual isomorphism. In the case of feature correspondence, isomorphism is thought to be established when a particular cell or cell assembly responds uniquely to a feature of the phenomenally experienced image; that is, a

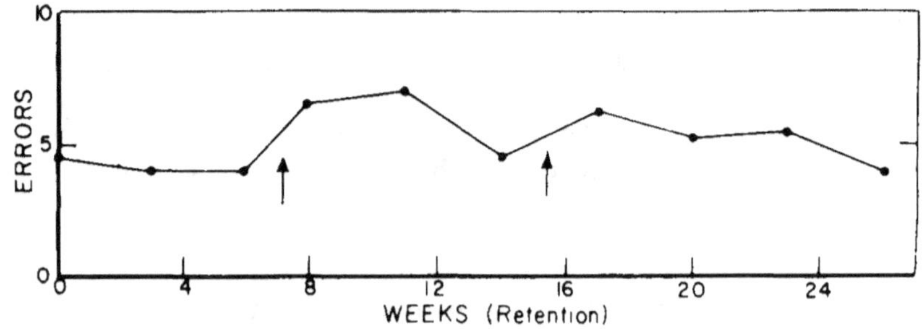

FIG. 13.1. Record of *retention* of a visual discrimination performance (+ vs. □) *before and after* implantation of aluminum hydroxide cream (first arrow) in primary visual cortex and the subsequent development of electrical seizure patterns (second arrow). Note that no deficit has occurred. The same result was obtained when the implantations were performed in inferotemporal, parietal, and frontal cortex.

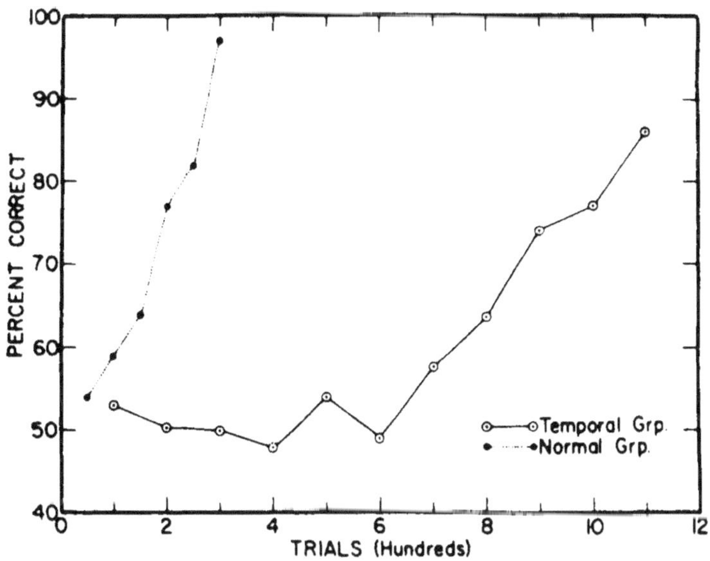

FIG. 13.2. Record of *learning* the same visual discrimination *after* the development of electrical seizure patterns. Note the prolongation of the "period of stationarity"—the flat part of the learning curve prior to its rise.

feature of the imaged object is detected. It is then assumed that the organism's response to the total object is composed by convergence of the outputs from a set of feature selective elements onto a higher-level neuroperceptual unit—a "pontifical" cell or cell assembly (Hebb, 1949) composed of like elements ("cardinal" cells; Barlow, 1972).

In the late 1950s and early 1960s, Hubel and Wiesel (e.g., 1962) discovered that the center-surround organization of the dendritic microstructure of cells (their receptive fields) in the peripheral visual system became elongated at the cortex. Further, they presented indirect evidence that this enlongation might be due to convergence onto the cortical cells of fibers from cells with center-surround receptive fields. Their demonstration emphasized that cells in the visual cortex responded best to bars of light presented in specific orientations. It was easy to generalize these findings into a Euclidean geometry of brain function—points to oriented lines, to curves and planes, to complex figures of all sorts. The search for feature detectors was on.

The results of the search were by no means meager. For instance, one cell in monkey cortex was found to respond maximally to a monkey's hand (Gross, Bender, & Rocha-Miranda, 1969); another cell was shown to respond best when a stimulus was repeated six times (Groves & Thompson, 1970); still others appeared to be activated largely by vocalizations of their own species (Maurus & Ploog, 1971).

Such specific selectivities can be misleading, however, if they are interpreted as showing that the cells in question function as feature detectors. To serve as a detector, the output of the cell must uniquely reflect the input feature, and this is only occasionally the case. More often a cell responds to a variety of feature triggers. In the visual system, for example, a cell that responds selectively to a bar in a specific orientation will modify that response with a change in luminance, with the direction of movement of that bar and the velocity of such movement (Pribram, Lassonde, & Ptito, 1981; Spinelli, Pribram, & Bridgeman, 1970). Furthermore, that very same cell may show a differential response to color and even be tuned to a specific auditory frequency (Spinelli, Starr, & Barrett, 1968). Finally, the number of bars, their widths, and spacings also influence the response of the cell, which suggests that "stripes" rather than "bars" form the critical stimulus dimension for their orientation selectivity (DeValois, Albrecht, & Thorell, 1978; Glezer, Ivanoff, & Tscherbach, 1973; Movshon, Thompson, & Tolhurst, 1978; Pollen & Taylor, 1974; Schiller, Finlay, & Volman, 1976). More of this in a moment.

Findings such as these, and they are equally true of other systems (e.g., see Evans, 1966, for cells in the auditory cortex), make untenable the view that these cortical cells are simple detectors of features. Nonetheless, each cell is selectively responsive to a variety of highly specific stimulus dimensions, the "feature triggers." Some of these dimensions appear to be mapped into recognizable patterns in adjacent cells; for example, orientation selectivity has been related to the columnar structure of cortex (Hubel & Wiesel, 1977), and selectivity to bar width and spacing has been reported to be a function of cortical layers (Maffei & Fiorentini, 1973). Other stimulus dimensions, such as the tuning of cells in the visual cortex to auditory frequencies, are distributed without any apparent regularity over much wider expanses of cortex. These distributed forms of organization become especially evident when recordings are made from groups of neurons when problem solving is being investigated (Gross, Bender, & Gerstein, 1979; John, Bartlett, Shimokochi, & Kleinman, 1973; Pribram, Spinelli, & Kamback, 1967).

The view obtained from the results of these studies is that rather than feature detection by single neurons, some sort of feature selection is effected by neuron networks. Some features seem to relate a structured network response; these same features and others may, however, under other conditions, elicit a more widely dispersed response. Furthermore, features are not always what they initially seem to be, and little attempt has yet been made to classify features systematically in such a way as to relate their phenomenal to their neural response characteristics. An exception to this has been the experiments of DeValois on the color system of primates, which can serve as a model for studies of feature analysis by neural networks (DeValois, 1960).

Feature selection by neural networks may be considered a form of feature correspondence. As noted in the previous paragraphs, however, the nature of the features responded to by a neural network property is often considerably different from their perceived phenomenal nature. Perception is only under very restricted circumstances limited to bars of certain width and spacings, or to a limited range of tonal frequency. With the exceptions of color and species-specific vocalizations, the phenomenal-neural correspondence seems at best strained in view of the multiple selectivities of most cells and the fact that these multiple selectivities fail, for the most part, in any cell or cell assembly to map coherently phenomenally experienced psychophysical characteristics. In the case of color and that of species-specific vocalizations, however, such mappings show that feature correspondence can be abstracted from the multiple selectivities of neurons and neuron assemblies. The question of how this abstraction is accomplished remains.

DEFINITION AND EVIDENCE: HOLOGRAPHIC THEORY

One possibility for abstraction lies in the powerful correlational facility of holographic transformations. The idea that the neural network performs holographic transformations on sensory input must be clearly distinguished from both field theory and feature correspondence theory. In a holographic transformation, the various stimulus dimensions become enfolded into every part of the transform domain; a set of neural signals is transformed, and transfer functions, often readily dealt with by waveform mathematics, describe the transformation. However, statistical mathematical procedures have proved equally useful, and a combination of waveform and statistical approaches has been found to be most powerful (e.g., see Julesz, 1971, for the visual system; Flanagan, 1972, for the auditory system). Transformation of a set of signals into an enfolded order is very different from simply generating a DC field in cortex by the arrival of neural signals. Holographic theory is therefore not a field theory, although it is related to field theory in that wave mechanical descriptions are relevant and holistic, rather than point-to-point, analysis is emphasized.

Holographic transformations also resemble feature correspondence theory to some extent, although once again they can be sharply distinguished. The similarity comes from the fact that, as already noted, performing a transform a second time will reinstate the image (with all its features) from the transform domain. The difference between holographic transformation and feature correspondence is that the transform domain is recognized and, in the strongest form of the theory, is recognized as *the* domain in which neural networks operate. The finding of multiple feature selectivities of most brain cells and cell assemblies is compatible with such a view. As we shall see, however, this strongest form of the theory does not account for all the available data, thus necessitating some specifiable modifications. In either the strongest or modified version, *features are generated, constructed, when the encoded transform domain is addressed* through additional sensory input or by "reference" from other neural processes such as sensitivities to internally produced stimulation.

There is thus no brain-perceptual isomorphism in the holographic theory as there is in the field and the feature correspondence theories. Rather, phenomenal experience is generated when sensory or internally derived inputs activate a holographic process or store. There is therefore no necessary identity between brain structure and phenomenal experience, just as in an optical hologram there is no identity between the structure of the photographic film and the image produced when that film is properly illuminated. Even a functional identity between phenomenal experience and brain processes becomes suspect if this means ignoring the input to senses from the world outside the organism and the input to other receptors from within the body.

What, then, are the transfer functions that describe the transformations of sensory and bodily inputs into a brain holographic process? And what are the limits of explanatory power of such transfer functions with respect to the data at hand? The first suggestion that brain processing might involve a Fourier analysis was made a century ago for the auditory system by Ohm, the same Ohm who formulated Ohm's law of electricity. This suggestion was adopted by Herman von Helmholtz, who performed a series of experiments that led to the place theory of hearing—essentially a view of the cochlea as a piano keyboard whose keys, when struck by acoustic waves, would initiate nerve impulses to the brain, where resonant neurons were activated. This view was modified in this century by Georg v. Bekesy (1959), whose experiments showed the cochlea and peripheral neurosensory mechanism to operate more like a stringed instrument, sensitive to superposition of acoustic waveforms. Good evidence has accrued to the effect that a major effect of initial auditory processing can be described in terms of a Fourier transform of the acoustic input (Evans, 1974).

Bekesy (1959) then went on to make a large-scale model of the cochlea composed of a set of five vibrators arranged in a row. The model could be placed on the forearm and the phase of the vibrators adjusted. At particular adjustments the phenomenal perception produced by the model was that of a point source of stimulation. When two such model "cochleas" were properly adjusted and applied, one to each forearm, the point source appeared, at first, to jump alternately from one forearm to the other, then suddenly to stabilize in the space just forward and between the two arms. In short, the stimulus was "projected" away from the stimulating source and receptive surface into the external world.

Both macro- and microelectrode studies have shown that multiple vibratory stimulations of the skin also evoke unitary responses in cortex (Dewson, 1964; Lynch, 1971). The electrical potentials evoked fail, therefore, to reflect the actual physical dimensions of the stimulus. Instead, they reflect the fact that the sensory process has transformed the physical stimulus according to some transfer functions. Bekesy noted that sensory inhibition, effected by lateral inhibitory dendritic networks of neurons, might be the responsible agent in the transformations.

Evidence is therefore at hand to indicate that the input to the ear and skin becomes transformed into neural patterns that can be described by sets of convolutional integrals of the type that Gabor (1969) has suggested as stages in achieving a fully developed Fourier holographic process. In the olfactory (Freeman, 1975) and visual systems, as well, such transformations have been described by Rodieck (1965) as convolving input with retinal receptive field properties as recorded from units in the optic nerve. See Figures 13-3a and 13-3b.

The manner in which such a stepwise process occurs is best worked out for the visual system. A second step in the process occurs at the lateral geniculate nucleus, where each geniculate cell acts as a peephole, "viewing" a part of the retinal mosaic. This is due to the fact that each geniculate cell has converging

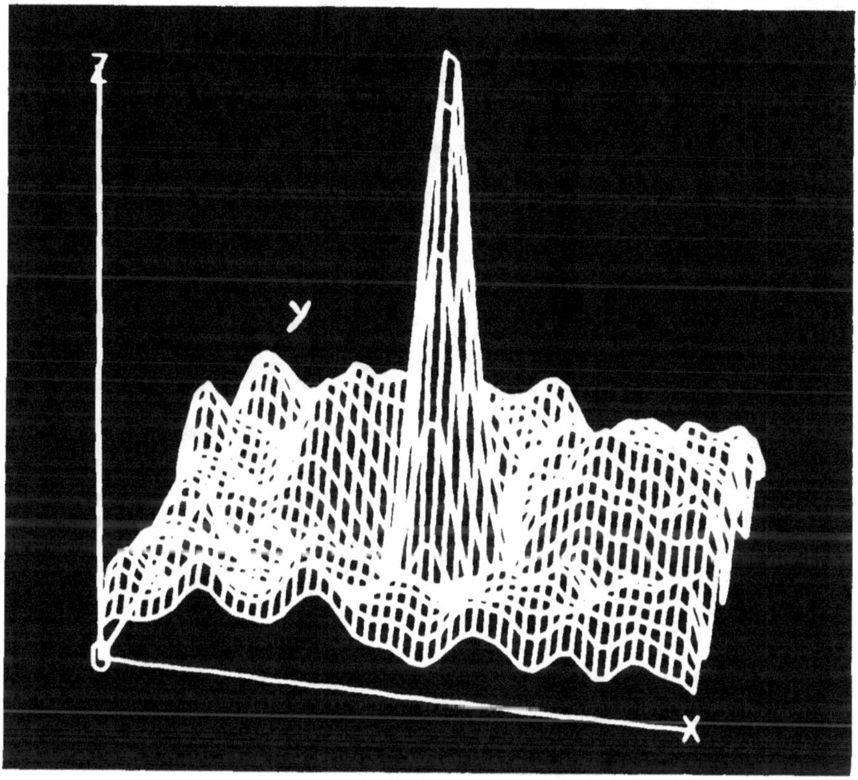

FIG. 13.3a. Three-dimensional computer-generated reconstruction of the receptive field of a neuron in the lateral geniculate nucleus. Note the "Mexican hat" configuration where the height of the crown (z axis) reflects the number of impulses generated by the cell in response to a moving light displayed over the reach of the x-y plane represented as the brim of the hat. A similar, though not as completely regular, receptive field configuration is found when cells in the optic nerve are plotted.

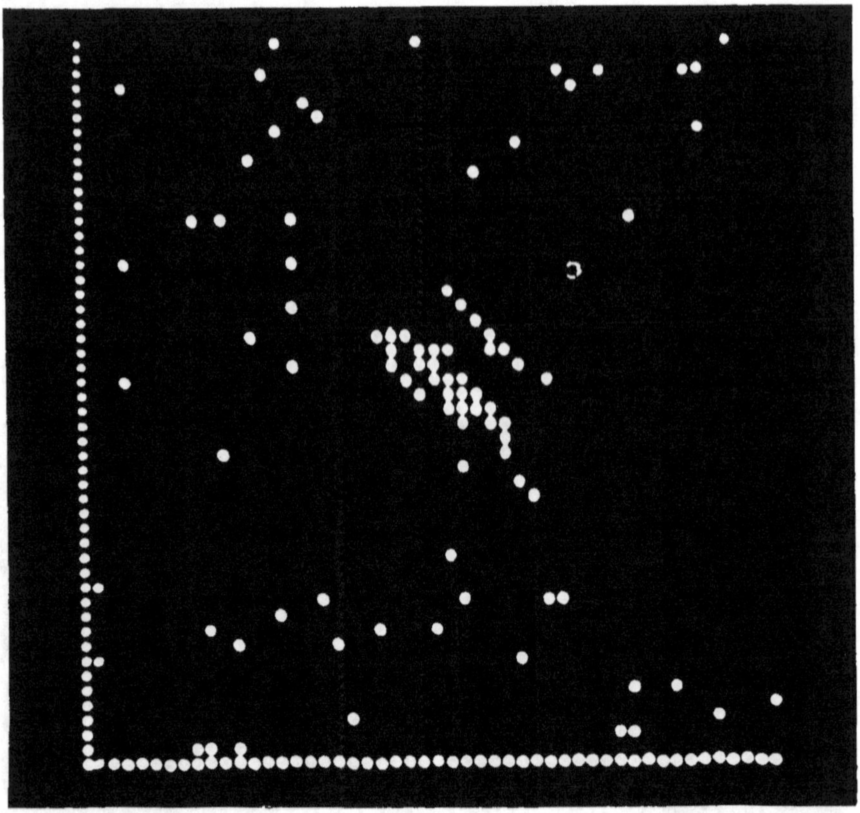

FIG. 13.3b. Cross section of a receptive field of a cell in the visual cortex. Now the three-dimensional reconstruction would resemble a homburg rather than a Mexican hat because the receptive field has become elongated. Note the sidebands (inhibitory and excitatory) which suggest that the cell's best response might not be produced by a single line but rather by multiple lines (gratings). Note also the orientation selectivity of the receptive field which is a consequence of its elongation.

upon it some 10,000 optic nerve fibers originating in the ganglion cells of the retina. The receptive field of the geniculate neuron is composed of a center surrounded by concentric rings, each consecutive ring of sharply diminishing intensity and of sign opposite that of its neighbors (Hammond, 1972). This type of organization is characteristic of units composing a near-field Fresnel hologram (Pribram, Nuwer, & Baron, 1974).

At the cortex the transformation into the Fourier domain becomes complete. Beginning with the work of Campbell and Robson (1968); Pollen, Lee, and Taylor (1971); Maffei and Fiorentini (1973); and Glezer, Ivanoff, and Tscher-

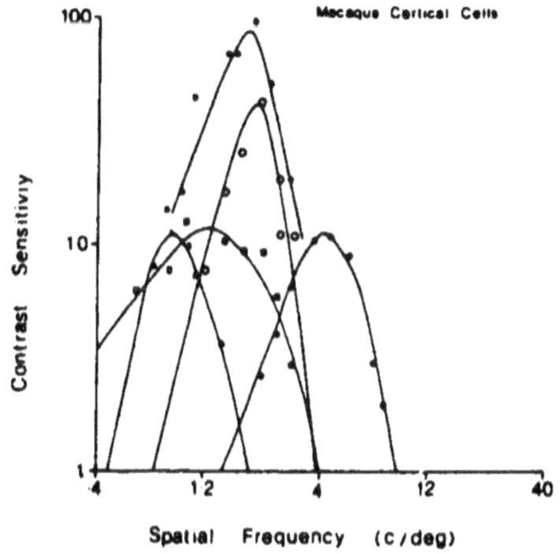

FIG. 13.4. Graph of tuning curves of five individual adjacent neurons in the vivisual cortex of a rhesus macaque monkey exposed to a range of gratings of various spatial frequencies (widths and spacings). These tuning curves were obtained at threshold (when the grating contrast was just sufficient to elicit a constant response). Results such as these are interpreted to indicate that the visual system performs a spectral analysis on the patterns of light and dark distributed across space that make up the visual scene. In a very basic sense, therefore, the visual system can be said to operate somewhat like the auditory and somatosensory systems where spectral analyses of sound patterns and vibratory patterns are performed. (From "Cortical Cells: Bar and Edge Detectors, or Spatial Frequency Filters?" by R. L. De Valois, D. G. Albrecht, & L. G. Thorell. In S. J. Cool & E. L. Smith (Eds.), *Frontiers in Visual Science*. New York: Springer-Verlag, 1978, p. 548.)

bach (1973), investigators using gratings as stimuli (e.g., Pribram et al., 1981; Schiller et al., 1976) have repeatedly confirmed that the cells in visual cortex are selectively tuned to a limited bandwidth of spatial frequency of approximately an octave (½ to 1½ octaves). The spatial frequency (or wave number) of a grating reflects the widths and spacings of the bars making up the grating. When such widths and spacings are narrow, the spatial frequency is high; when widths and spacings are broad, the spatial frequency is low. See Fig. 4. Ordinarily the term *frequency* implies a temporal dimension; in the case of spatial frequency, this temporal dimension can be evoked by successively scanning across the grating (e.g., by walking across the path of illumination of a projection of a slide of such a grating). Conversion to the temporal dimension is, however, not necessary. The grating is a filter whose characteristics can be expressed either as spatial or temporal or both.

The difference between a feature correspondence and a holographic transform approach has recently been brought into sharp focus by tests of hypotheses devised to contrast the two. In the visual cortex the center-surround orgainzation

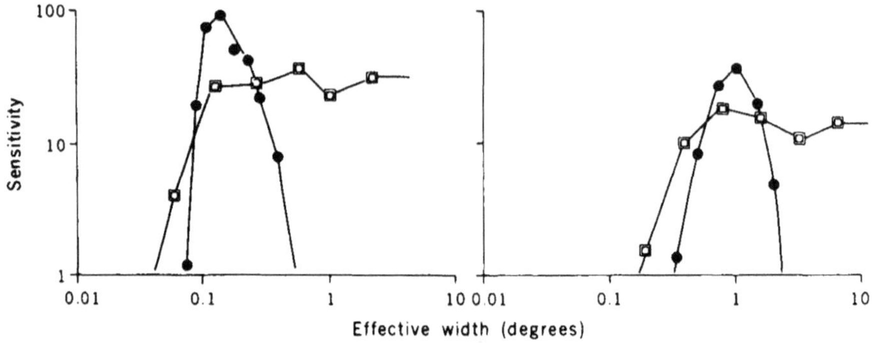

FIG. 13.5. Selectivity functions for bars (squares) and gratings (circles) of two striate neurons: (Left) macaque monkey simple cell; (Right) cat complex cell. There is little selectivity for bars and essentially no drop in the sensitivity as bar width increases. In contrast, the cells are sensitive to only a limited range of spatial frequencies and are therefore selective for gratings. (From "Visual Cortical Neurons: Are Bars or Gratings the Optimal Stimuli?" by D. G. Albrecht, R. L. De Valois, & L. G. Thorell. *Science*, 1980, *207*, 88.)

of visual receptive fields that obtains in the geniculale nucleus gives way to an elongated receptive field with sidebands of opposite sign. In their original discovery of this change, Hubel and Wiesel (1959) emphasized that lines presented at specific orientations were the most effective stimuli to activate units with such receptive fields. They also presented evidence that the elongated fields might be composed by convergence from geniculate cells with spotlike concentric fields. The feature hierarchy Euclidean view of feature correspondence grew naturally from these early results and their interpretation. More recently it has been shown, as noted earlier, that these cells with orientation-selective, elongated receptive fields also vary their output with changes in luminance, movement of lines across the receptive field, the direction of that movement, its velocity, and the number and spacings of such lines (gratings of various spatial frequencies). In addition, it has been shown that changes in the width of single lines have little effect on the responses of these cells (DeValois et al., 1978; Henry & Bishop, 1971). See Fig. 5. Finally, in a direct confrontation of feature correspondence theory, DeValois, DeValois, and Yund (1979) showed that the complex stimulus such as a plaid or checkerboard had to be rotated in such a way that the axes of the Fourier transform, rather than the edges per se of the stimulus pattern, would engage the orientation selectivity of the cell. Every cell examined responded maximally when the plaid or checkerboard pattern was rolated to the degree and minute of visual angle predicted by the Fourier (and no other) transform of the pattern as determined by computer (using the Fast Fourier Transform—FFT). See Fig. 6. the cortical cells were thus shown to respond holistically (i.e., to the Fourier transform of the entire pattern) rather than feature by feature. In another elegant

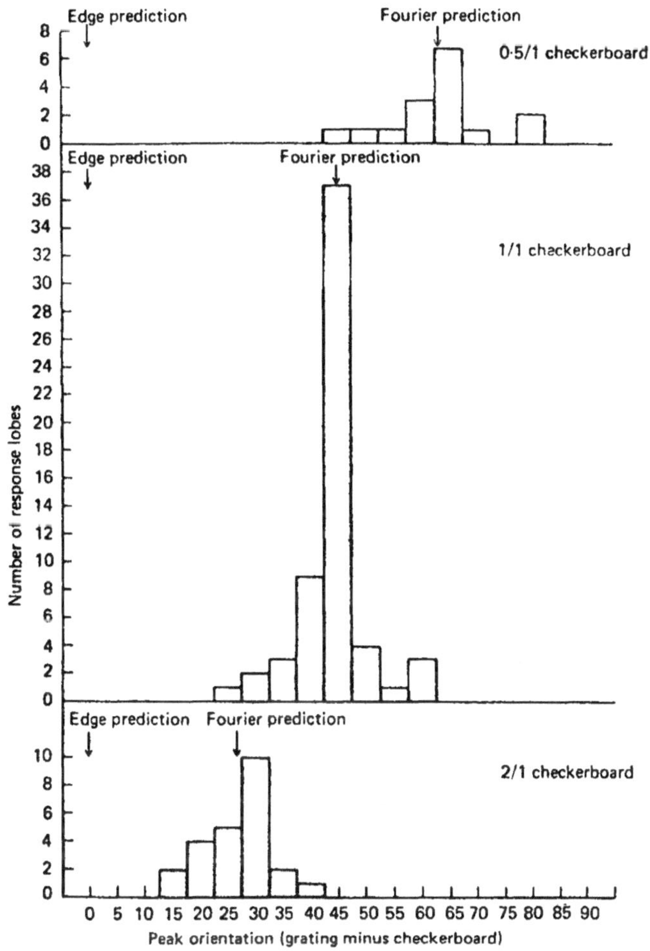

FIG. 13.0. Histograms of the differences between optimum orientations for gratings and for the various checkerboards. Our entire cell sample from cat and monkey is included. The arrows indicate the difference predicted on the basis of the orientation of the edges of the checks in the patterns (edge precipitation) and the difference predicted on the basis of the orientations of the patterns' fundamental Fourier components (Fourier prediction). The mean orientation shifts, compared with the Fourier prediction, for each of these patterns are as follows: 2/1 checkerboard 26.9° (Fourier prediction 26.6°); 1/1 checkerboard 44.3° (predicted 45°); 0.5/1 checkerboard 63.9 (predicted 63.4°). (From "Responses of Striate Cortex Cells to Grating and Checkerboard Patterns" by K. K. De Valois, R. L. De Valois, & E. W. Yund, 1979.)

experiment, Movshon et al. (1978) has detailed the complementarity between the spatial profile of the receptive fields of these cells and the Fourier transform of the stimulus giving rise to that profile. That cells in the visual cortex encode in the Fourier domain is thus an established fact.

These findings do not, however, mean that the visual system performs a global Fourier transform on the input to the retina (see also Julesz & Caelli, 1979). The moving retina decomposes the image produced by the lens of the eye into a ''Mexican hat'' receptive field organization that can be described as convolving retinal organization with sensory input (Rodieck, 1965). But the spread function, as such convolutions are called, does not encompass the entire retina; rather, it is limited to the receptive field of a retinal ganglion cell. Similarly at the cortex, full-fledged encoding in the Fourier domain is restricted to the receptive field of the cortical neuron. This patchy organization of the Fourier domain (Robson, 1975) does not impair its holographic characteristics. The technique of patching or stripping together Fourier-transformed images has been utilized in radio astronomy by Bracewell (1965) to cover expanses that cannot be viewed with any single telescopic exposure. The technique has been further developed by Ross (see Leith, 1976) into a multiplex hologram to produce three-dimensional *moving* images when the inverse transform is effected. Movement is produced when the Fourier-encoded strips capture slightly different images—for instance, when adjacent frames of a motion picture are used as the image base for the Fourier transformation.

In the multiplex hologram, spatial relationships among the Fourier-transformed patches or strips become important. Thus, this form of hologram is a hybrid from which movement can be derived. Recall that a simple hologram is characterized by translational *invariance;* that is, the image that results from inversion is essentially stationary and appears the same from different vantages except for changes in perspective (object constancy). The hybrid multiplex form has therefore considerable advantage for moving organisms.

Suggestions have been made that the orientation-selective, elongated receptive fields that compose the visual cortex are arranged in Fibonacci spirals along the axes of cortical columns (Schwartz, 1977). Such an arrangement of the spatial relationships among the Fourier-transformed patches of receptive field would enhance still further the power of the transform domain in that three-dimensional movement (and therefore the resultant space-time relationship) would be readily explained. At present evidence for this sort of helical arrangement is not firmly established; on the other hand, the suggestion is consonant with what is already known.

Perhaps more important is the well-established fact that there is a topographic correspondence between receptor surface and its cortical representation in cortical columns (Edelman & Mountcastle, 1978; Hubel & Wiesel, 1977). Thus, the holographic patches have an overall arrangement that corresponds to the sensory surface of the organism. Therefore in coarse grain (i.e., between receptive fields), the sensory mechanism is represented; in fine grain (i.e., within receptive fields), a holographic representation becomes manifest. The situation is not altogether different from that in physics. At a certain grain of analysis—the ordinary—the principles of mechanics operate. At a finer grain (where electrons and photons come into focus) quantum principles come into operation with their complementarities, such as between locus and moment and between wave and particle.

David Bohm (1971, 1973) has pointed out that we can begin to conceptualize these complementarities in quantum physics if we realize that concepts about particles devolve from the use of lenses. Lenses built into the objectives of our telescopes (to deal with photons) and microscopes (to deal with photons and electrons) objectify by *focusing* electromagnetic energy. The result is that we experience objects, particles, things. If, on the other hand, we should peer at the universe through gratings of various spatial frequencies, Bohm suggests, we would experience a holographlike universe of interfering waveforms (which, in physics, is what results in double-slit experiments and the like).

Take this formulation and apply it to the brain. The ordinary coarse-grained representation of receptor surfaces provides a lenslike mechanism for processing input. With this mechanism we can ''make sense'' of the universe in terms of images of objects because we sense it through lenses and lenslike structures (the cochlea, the skin, as in Bekesy's experiments). But at the same time, a finer-grained—quantum level—process operates to provide a different sort of order, a holographlike, distributed, and enfolded order superior in correlating and in storing and in computing. Is this order best described in wave or in statistical terms or both? The Fourier approach has been extremely successful; but are we in the brain sciences about where physics was when Schrödinger proposed his encompassing wave equation?

COUNTERPOINT

The multiplex hybrid nature of cortical holographic organization serves as a warning that any simply conceived ''global- Fourier- transform- of- input- into-cortical-organization'' is untenable. Furthermore, the multiple selectivities of cortical cells in the visual (Morrell, 1972; Spinelli, Pribram, & Bridgeman, 1970; Spinelli, Starr, & Barrett, 1968), auditory (e.g., Evans, 1974), and somatosensorimotor (e.g., Bach-y-Rita, 1972) projection areas clearly indicate that such cells serve as nodes in neural networks in which the Fourier transform is only one, albeit an important, process. Several attempts have been made therefore to characterize more fully such cortical networks in terms of their essential properties. Thus, Longuet-Higgins (see Willshaw, Buneman, & Longuet-Higgins, 1969) proposed an associative-net model, and Leon Cooper (1973) has developed this model into a self-organizing distributed net whose mathematical description contains as a special case the Fourier transform hologram. Julesz (1971), Uttal (1978), Borsellino and Poggio (1973), Poggio and Torre (in press), and (in our laboratories) Sutter (1976) have taken a more statistical stance. Thus, for instance, Uttal emphasizes spatial autocorrelation functions, whereas Poggio and Sutter rely on Wiener polynomial expansions. In addition, Poggio treats the dendritic potential microstructure in terms of the Volterra solution of cable equations. His carefully worked out proposal includes a stage of Fourier analysis and another in which the Laplace transform occurs. David Marr, Tomaso Poggio, and Whitman Richards (Marr, 1976a, 1976b; Marr & Poggio, 1977; Richards, 1977; Richards & Polit, 1974) are developing a model based on repetitive convolving of Laplacians of a Gaussian distribution. E. Roy John speaks of "hyperneurons" constituted of the distributed system of graded potentials he records from the brains of problem-solving animals. Such organizations have been described in terms of Lie groups by Hoffman (1970), vector matrices by Stuart, Takahashi, and Umezawa (1978), and tensor matrices by Finkelstein (1976) in which the tensors represent multidimensional Fourier transforms. Finally, Edelman & Mouuncastle (1978) have proposed a degenerative group model, also based on an essentially random connectivity.

On looking over these various proposals, one finds commonalities and distinctions that can be summarized as problem areas that need further inquiry: (1) To what extent is the idealization warranted that the brain cortical connectivity is essentially random? This issue was discussed earlier in this chapter. In addition, the models proposed by Hoffman and by Poggio clearly opt for nonrandomness, whereas the others are either explicitly or implicitly based on the assumption that an idealized random connectivity is not too far from actuality. (2) To what extent can brain systems be treated with linear (and reversible) equations, and to what extent must nonlinearities be introduced to explain the available data? Good evidence is at hand that the primary sensory systems (as discussed throughout this chapter) and primary motor systems (see, e.g., Granit, 1970) are essentially linear in most of their overall operations despite many local nonlinearities. Overall nonlinearities are apparently introduced into the system when decisions have to be made—decisions involved in discriminating between inputs, in performing this rather than that action. Decisional operations have been shown to be local functions of the intrinsic (association) systems of the brain (Pribram, 1972a, 1972b, 1974, 1977a, 1977b). Thus, the question is raised as to how these nonlinearities relate to the essentially linear sensorimotor functions. (3) Nonlinear decisional operators can enter the system in two ways: They can be imposed by a parallel corticifugal process upon the sensorimotor systems (Christensen & Pribram, 1979; Pribram, 1971a, 1974; Pribram, Spinelli, & Reitz, 1969; Ungerleider & Pribram, 1977), or the decisions can be attained by a serial processing hierarchical abstraction of the relevant variables (see, e.g., Gross, 1973; Mishkin, 1973; Weiskrantz, 1974). It is, of course, also possible that the hierarchical serial process operates during learning (as, e.g., suggested by Hebb,

1949) while parallel corticifugal operators determine momentary perceptions and performances. (4) These nonlinear decisional operators are localized to one or another brain system. Two major classes of such operators can be distinguished. One is a set of sensory-specific processes that involve the posterior cerebral convexity (inferotemporal cortex for vision; superior temporal for audition; anterior temporal for taste; posterior parietal for somesthesis). In addition, a set of higher-order, executive—that is, context-sensitive—processes has been identified to involve the frontolimbic portions of the forebrain (see, e.g., reviews by Pribram, 1954, 1969, 1973).

When these decisional processes operate on the distributed memory store, they re-member an input that had on earlier occasions become dismembered. The sensory-specific operators deal with recognition and with the processing of referentially meaningful information. The frontal lobe executive operators deal with recall and with the pragmatics of processing context-sensitive, episode-related instances (for review, see, e.g., Pribram, 1971a, 1977a).

The persistent puzzle that brain functions appear to be both localized and distributed is thus resolved. Memory storage is shown to be distributed; decisional operators involved in coding and retrieval are localized. These operators can be conceived as separate brain systems, genetically inherent in their function but dependent on sensory input from the environment to trigger and shape their development (see, e.g., Chomsky, 1980; Pribram, 1971b). In short, there are "boxes in the brain," each "box" corresponding to a "faculty of mind." But these "boxes" operate on a distributed matrix that is nonlocal and therefore available to all.

Perhaps the easiest way to conceptualize this "model" of brain function is in terms of states and operators on those states. At present it appears reasonable to continue to search for linearities in the state descriptions of sensory perception, highly practiced skilled action, and memory storage processes. The greater part of this manuscript has been devoted to detailing problems inherent in such state descriptions. Only in this final section have we briefly dealt with the abundant evidence that these states come under the control of localized nonlinear operators whenever discriminate decisions (e.g., recognition) or selective (planned) actions are involved. Whether these nonlinearities are abstracted serially and hierarchically from the states or whether they are imposed corticifugally by a parallel process—or both—continues to be an active area of investigation.

CONCLUSION

There is a considerable intellectual distance between Lashley's despair in finding a localized engram in 1950 and the richness of data and theory on cerebral localization and distribution in 1980. To his credit, Lashley recognized the problem and specified it in sufficient detail so the generation of investigators standing on his shoulders could deal effectively with it. That so much progress has been made reflects the support given by society to the brain and behavioral sciences during this 30-year period. Should this support continue, the issue of localization-distribution that has mobilized such differing views over the past two centuries may yet be resolved before the end of the twentieth.

REFERENCES

Albrecht, D. G., de Valois, R. L. & Thorell, L. G. Visual cortical neurons: are bars or gratings the optimal stimuli? *Science*, 1980, *207*, 88-90.

Bach-Y-Rita, P. *Brain mechanisms in sensory substitution*. New York: Academic Press, 1972.

Barlow, H. B. Single units and sensation: A neuron doctrine for perceptual psychology? *Perception*, 1972, *1*, 371-394.

Bekesy, G. v. Synchronism of neural discharges and their demultiplication in pitch perception on the skin and in hearing. *Journal of the Acoustical Society of America*, 1959, *31*, 338-349.

Benevento, L. A., Creutzfeldt, O. D., & Kuhnt, U. Significance of intracortical inhibition in the visual cortex: Data and model. *Nature New Biology*, 1972, *238*, 124-126.

Bohm, D. Quantum theory as an indication of a new order in physics. Part A. The development of new orders as shown through the history of physics. *Foundations of Physics*, 1971, *1*(4), 359-381.

Bohm, D. Quantum theory as an indication of a new order in physics. Part B. Implicate and explicate order in physial law. *Foundations of Physics*, 1973, *3*(2), 139-168.

Borsellino, A., & Poggio, T. Convolution and correlation algebras. *Kybernetik*, 1973, *13*, 113-122.

Bracewell, R. *The Fourier transform and its applications*. New York: McGraw-Hill, 1965.

Campbell, F. W., & Robson, J. G. Application of Fourier analysis to the visibility of gratings. *Journal of Physiology*, 1968, *197*, 551-566.

Chomsky, N. *Rules and representations*. New York: Columbia University Press, 1980.

Christensen, C. A., & Pribram, K. H. The effect of inferotemporal or foveal prestriate ablation on serial reversal learning in monkeys. *Neuropsychologia*, 1979, *17*(1), 1-10.

Cooper, L. N. A possible organization of animal memory and learning. In F. Lindquist & S. Lindquist (Eds.), *Proceedings of the Nobel symposium on collective properties of physical systems*. New York: Academic Press, 1973.

Creutzfeldt, O.D., Kuhnt, U., & Benevento, L. A. An intracellular analysis of visual cortical neurones to moving stimuli: Responses in a cooperative neuronal network. *Experimental Brain Research*, 1974, *21*, 251-272.

DeValois K. K., DeValois, R. L. & Yund, E. W. Responses of striate cortex cells to grating and checkerboard patterns. *Journal of Physiology*, 1979, *291*, 483-505.

DeValois, R. L. Color vision mechanisms in monkey. *Journal of General Physiology*, 1960, *43*, 115-128.

DeValois, R. L., Albrecht, D. G., — Thorell, L. G. Cortical cells: Line and edge detectors, or spatial frequency filters? In S. J. Cool and E. L. Smith (Eds.), *Frontiers in visual science*. New York: Springer-Verlag, 1978.

Dewson, J. H., III. Cortical responses to patterns of two-point cutaneous stimulation. *Journal of Comparative and Physiological Psychology*, 1964, *58*, 387-389.

Edelman, G. M., & Mountcastle, V. B. *The mindful brain*. Cambridge, Mass.: MIT Press, 1978.

Evans, D. C. Computer logic and memory. *Scientific American*, 1966, *215*, 74-85.

Evans, E. F. Neural processes for the detection of acoustic patterns and for sound localization. In F.

O. Schmitt & F. G. Worden (Eds.), *The neurosciences third study program*. Cambridge, Mass.: MIT Press, 1974.

Finkelstein, D. Classical and quantum probability and set theory. In Harper W. L. & Hooker C. A. (Eds.), *Foundations of probability theory, statistical inference, and statistical theories of science* (Vol. III). Dordrecht, Holland: D. Reidel, 1976.

Flanagan, J. L. *Speech analysis, synthesis and perception*. Berlin: Springer-Verlag, 1972.

Freeman, W. *Mass action in the nervous system*. New York: Academic Press, 1975.

Gabor, D. A new microscopic principle. *Nature*, 1948, *161*, 777–778.

Gabor, D. Information processing with coherent light. *Optica. Acta*, 1969, *16*, 519–533.

Glezer, V. D., Ivanoff, V. A., & Tscherbach, T. A. Investigation of complex and hypercomplex receptive fields of visual cortex of the cat as spatial frequency filters. *Vision Research*, 1973, *13*, 1875–1904.

Goldscheider, A. Uber die materiellen veranderungen bei der assoziationsbildung. *Neurologische Zentralblatt.*, 1906, *25*, 146.

Granit, R. *The basis of motor control*. New York: Academic Press, 1970.

Gross, C. G. Inferotemporal cortex and vision. In E. Stellas & J. M. Sprague (Eds.), *Progress in physiological psychology*. New York: Academic Press, 1973.

Gross, C. G., Bender, D. B., & Gerstein, G. L. Activity of inferior temporal neurons in behaving monkeys. *Neuropsychologia*, 1979, *17*, 215–229.

Gross, C. G., Bender, D. B., & Rocha-Miranda, C. E. Visual receptive fields of neurons in inferotemporal cortex of the monkey. *Science*, 1969, *166*, 1303–1305.

Groves, P. M., & Thompson, R. F. Habituation: A dual-process theory. *Psychological Review*, 1970, *77*, 419–450.

Gumnit, R. J. DC potential changes from auditory cortex of cat. *Journal of Neurophysiology*, 1960, *6*, 667–675.

Hammond, P. Spatial organization of receptive fields of LGN neurons. *Journal of Physiology*, 1972, *222*, 53–54.

Hartline, H. K. The nerve messages in the fibres of the visual pathway. *Journal of the Optical Society of America*, 1940, *30*, 239–247.

Hebb, D. O. *The organization of behavior: A neuropsychological theory*. New York: Wiley, 1949.

Henry, G. H., & Bishop, P. O. Simple cells of the striate cortex. In W. D. Neff (Ed.), *Contributions to sensory physiology*. New York: Academic Press, 1971.

Hoffman, W. C. Higher visual perception as prolongation of the basic lie transformation group. *Mathematical Biosciences*, 1970, *6*, 437–471.

Hubel, D. H., & Wiesel, T. N. Receptive fields of single neurones in the cat's striate cortex. *Journal of Physiology*, 1959, *148*, 574–591.

Hubel, D. H., — Wiesel, T. N. Receptive fields, binocular interaction and functional architecture in the cat's visual cortex. *Journal of Physiology*, 1962, *160*, 106–154.

Hubel, D. H., & Wiesel, T. N. Functional architecture of macaque monkey cortex. *Proceedings of the Royal Society of London Series B* 1977, *198*, 1–59.

John, E. R., Bartlett, F., Shimokochi, M., & Kleinman, D. Neural readout from memory. *Journal of Neurophysiology*, 1973, *36*(5), 893–924.

John, E. R., & Morgades, P. P. The pattern and anatomical distribution of evoked potentials and multiple unit activity elicited by conditioned stimuli in trained cats. *Communications in behavioral biology*, 1969, *3*(4), 181–207.

Julesz, B. *Foundations of cyclopean perception*. Chicago: University of Chicago Press, 1971.

Julesz, B. & Caelli, T. On the limits of Fourier decompositions in visual texture perception. *Perception*, 1979, *8*(1), 69–73.

Köhler, W., & Wegener, J. Currents of the human auditory complex. *Journal of Cellular and Comparative Physiology*, 1955, *45*, 25–54.

Kraft, M. S., Obrist, W. D., & Pribram, K. H. The effect of irritative lesions of the striate cortex on learning of visual discriminations in monkeys. *Journal of Comparative and Physiological Psychology,* 1960, *53,* 17–22.

Lashley, K., Chow, K. L., & Semmes, J. An examination of the electrical field theory of cerebral integration. *Psychological Review,* 1951, *58,* 123–136.

Leith, E. N. White-light holograms. *Scientific American,* 1976, *235*(4), 80.

Leith, E. N., & Upatnicks, J. Photography by laser. *Scientific American,* 1965, *212*(6), 24–35.

Loeb, J. *Comparative physiology of the brain and comparative psychology.* New York: Putnam, 1907.

Lynch, J. C. *A single unit analysis of contour enhancement in the somesthetic system of the cat.* Ph.D. dissertation, Stanford University, May 1971.

Maffei, L., & Fiorentini, A. The visual cortex as a spatial frequency analyzer. *Vision Research,* 1973, *13,* 1255–1267.

Marr, D. Analyzing natural images: A computational theory of texture vision. *Cold Spring Harbor Symposium Quant. Biol.,* 1976, *40,* 647–662. (a)

Marr, D. Early processing of visual information. *Philosophical Transactions of the Royal Society of London Series B,* 1976, *275,* 483–524. (b)

Marr, D., & Poggio, T. From understanding computation to understanding neural circuitry. *Neurosciences Research Program Bulletin,* 1977, *15,* 470–488.

Maurus, M., & Ploog, D. Social signals in squirrel monkeys: Analysis by cerebral radio stimulation. *Brain Research,* 1971, *12,* 171–183.

Mishkin, M. Cortical visual areas and their interaction. In A. G. Karczmar & J. C. Eccles (Eds.), *The brain and human behavior.* Berlin: Springer-Verlag, 1973.

Morrell, F. Visual system's view of acoustic space. *Nature* (London), 1972, *238,* 44–46.

Movshon, J. A., Thompson, I. D., & Tolhurst, D. J. Receptive field organization of complex cells in the cat's striate cortex. *Journal of Physiology,* 1978, *283,* 79.

Poggio, T., & Torre, V. A new approach to synaptic interactions. In H. Palm (Ed.), *Approaches in complex systems.* Berlin: Springer-Verlag, in press.

Pollen, D. A., Lee, J. R., & Taylor, J. H. How does the striate cortex begin the reconstruction of the visual world? *Science,* 1971, *173,* 74–77.

Pollen, D. A., & Taylor, J. H. The striate cortex and the spatial analysis of visual space. In F. O. Schmitt & F. G. Worden (Eds.), *The neurosciences third study program.* Cambridge, Mass.: MIT Press, 1974.

Pribram, K. H. Some aspects of experimental psychosurgery: The effect of scarring frontal cortex on complex behavior. *Surgical Forum,* 1951, *36,* 315–318.

Pribram, K. H. Toward a science of neuropsychology: Method and data. In R. A. Patton (Ed.), *Current trends in psychology and the behavioral sciences.* Pittsburgh: University of Pittsburgh Press, 1954.

Pribram, K. H. The amnestic syndromes: Disturbances in coding? In G. A. Talland & M. Waugh (Eds.), *The psychopathology of memory.* New York: Academic Press, 1969.

Pribram, K. H. *Languages of the brain: Experimental paradoxes and principles in neuropsychology.* Englewood Cliffs, N.J.: Prentice-Hall, 1971. (a)

Pribram, K. H. *What makes man human.* James Arthur Lecture, New York American Museum of Natural History Monograph, 1971. (b)

Pribram, K. H. Association: Cortico-cortical and/or cortico-subcortical. In T. Frigyesi, E. Rinvik, & M. D. Yahr (Eds.), *Corticothalamic projections and sensorimotor activities.* New York: Raven Press, 1972. (a)

Pribram, K. H. Neurological notes on knowing. In J. R. Royce & W. W. Rozeboom (Eds.), *The second Banff conference on theoretical psychology.* New York: Gordon & Breach, 1972. (b)

Pribram, K. H. The primate frontal cortex-executive of the brain. In A. R. Luria & K. H. Pribram (Eds.), *Psychophysiology of the frontal lobes.* New York: Academic Press, 1973.

Pribram, K. H. How is it that sensing so much we can do so little? In F. O. Schmitt & F. G. Worden (Eds.), *The neurosciences third study program*. Cambridge, Mass.: MIT Press, 1974.
Pribram, K. H. Modes of central processing in human learning and remembering. In T. J. Teyler (Ed.), *Brain and learning*. Stamford, Conn: Greylock Press, 1977. (a)
Pribram, K. H. New dimensions in the functions of the basal ganglia. In C. Shagass, S. Gershon, & A. J. Friedhoff (Eds.), *Psychopathology and brain dysfunction*. New York: Raven Press, 1977. (b)
Pribram, K. H., Lassonde, M., & Ptito, M. *Intracerebral influences on the microstructure of visual cortex: I. Classification of receptive field properties. Experimental Brain Research,* 1981 (in press).
Pribram K. H., Lassonde, M. & Ptito, M. Classification of receptive field properties in cat visual cortex. *Experimental Brain Research*, 1981, *43*, 119-130.
Pribram, K. H., Nuwer, M., & Baron, R. The holographic hypothesis of memory structure in brain function and perception. In R. C. Atkinson, D. H. Krantz, R. C. Luce, & P. Suppes (Eds.), *Contemporary developments in mathematical psychology*. San Francisco: Freeman, 1974.
Pribram, K. H., Spinelli, D. N., & Kamback, M. C. Electrocortical correlates of stimulus response and reinforcement. *Science*, 1967, *157*, 94-96.
Pribram, K. H., Spinelli, D. N. & Reitz, S. L. The effect of radical disconnexion of occipital and temporal cortex on visual behaviour of monkeys. *Brain: A Journal of Neurology*, 1969, *92*(2), 301-312.
Rakic, P. *Local circuit neurons*. Cambridge, Mass.: MIT Press, 1976.
Rall, W. Dendritic neuron theory and dendro-dendritic synapses in a simple cortical system. In F. O. Schmitt (Ed.), *The neurosciences second study program*. New York: Rockefeller, 1970.
Ratliff, F. Inhibitory interaction and the detection and enhancement of contours. In W. A. Rosenblith (Ed.), *Sensory communication*. New York: Wiley, 1961.
Richards, W. Stereopsis with and without monocular cues. *Vision Research*, 1977, *17*, 967-969.
Richards, W., & Polit, A. Texture matching. *Kybernetick*, 1974, *16*, 155-162.
Robson, J. G. Receptive fields, neural representation of the spatial and intensive attributes of the visual image. In E. C. Carterette (Ed.), *Handbook of perception, Vol. V: Seeing*. New York: Academic Press, 1975.
Rodieck, R. W. Quantitative analysis of cat retinal ganglion cell response to visual stimuli. *Vision Research*, 1965, *5*, 583-601.
Rodieck, R. W., & Stone, J. Response of cat retinal ganglion cells to moving visual patterns. *Journal of Neurophysiology*, 1965, *28*, 833-850.
Schiller, P. H., Finlay, B. L., & Volman, S. F. Quantitative studies of single-cell properties in monkey striate cortex. *Journal of Neurophysiology*, 1976, *39*, 1288-1374.
Schwartz, E. L. Spatial mapping in the primate sensory projection: Analytic structure and relevance to perception. *Biological Cybernetics*, 1977, *25*, 181-194.
Shepherd, G. *The synaptic organization of the brain—An introduction*. New York: Oxford University Press, 1974.
Sperry, R. W., Miner, N., & Meyers, R. E. Visual pattern perception following subpial slicing and tantalum wire implantations in the visual cortex. *Journal of Comparative and Physiological Psychology*, 1955, *48*, 50-58.
Spinelli, D. N., Pribram, K. H., & Bridgeman, B. Visual receptive field organization of single units in the visual cortex of monkey. *International Journal of Neuroscience*, 1970, *1*, 67-74.
Spinelli, D. N., Starr, A., & Barrett, T. W. Auditory specificity in unit recordings from cat's visual cortex. *Experimental Neurology*, 1968, *22*, 75-84.
Stamm, J. S., & Knight, M. Learning of visual tasks by monkeys with epileptogenic implants in temporal cortex. *Journal of Comparative and Physiological Psychology*, 1963, *56*, 254-260.
Stamm, J. S., & Pribram, K. H. Effects of epileptogenic lesions in frontal cortex on learning and retention in monkeys. *Journal of Neurophysiology*, 1960, *23*, 552-563

Stamm, J. S., & Pribram, K. H. Effects of epileptogenic lesions in inferotemporal cortex on learning and retention in monkeys. *Journal of Comparative and Physiological Psychology,* 1961, *54,* 614–618.

Stamm, J. S., & Rosen, S. C. Cortical steady potential shifts and anodal polarization during delayed response performance. *Acta Neurobiologiae Experimentalis,* 1972, *32*(2), 193–209.

Stuart, C. I., Takahashi, Y., & Umezawa, H. On the stability and non-local properties of memory. *Journal of Theoretical Biology,* 1978, *71,* 605–618.

Sutter, E. A revised conception of visual receptive fields based on pseudorandom spatio-temporal pattern stimuli. In P. Z. Marmarelis & G. D. McCann (Eds.), *Proceedings 1st Symposium on Testing and Identification of Nonlinear Systems.* Pasadena, Calif.: California Institute of Technology, 1976.

Ungerleider, L. G. & Pribram, K. H. Inferotemporal versus combined pulvinar-prestriate lesions in the rhesus monkey: Effects on color, object and pattern discrimination. *Neuropsychologia,* 1977, *15,* 481–498.

Uttal, W. R. *The psychobiology of mind.* Hillsdale, N.J.: Lawrence Erlbaum Associates, 1978.

Weiskrantz, L. The interaction between occipital and temporal cortex in vision: An overview. In F. O. Schmitt & F. G. Worden (Eds.), *The neurosciences third study program.* Cambridge, Mass.: MIT Press, 1974.

Weiss, P. *Principles of development: A text in experimental Embryology.* New York: 1939.

Willshaw, D. J., Buneman, O. P., & Longuet-Higgins, H. C. Non-holographic associative memory. *Nature,* 1969, *222,* 960–962.

14 Some Aspects of the Neuropsychology of Memory in Humans and Animals

L. Weiskrantz
Department of Experimental Psychology
University of Oxford, England

It is difficult to know how a neuropsychologist could be more honored than to be asked to honor Karl Lashley. By now, in this volume, you will have read many eulogies and know why he has had such a lasting impact. There are certain difficulties, to be sure, for the eulogist. Lashley was sometimes gloriously wrong, and not only about questions of detail. But I say "gloriously" wrong because he was the first to tell us how to find out. More than that, he was the first to tell us *what* to find out. He was vigorous in attack on humbug; stubborn in defense, and ingenious in his analysis of the complexity and richness of psychological phenomena; and insistent on the need for a direct and final appeal to empirical evidence. Very few of his predecessors in neuropsychology could have been shown to be right *or* wrong, although Lashley did not shirk from trying to do so. Above all, he was the first to give psychology primacy in the brain and behavior courtship, and was insistent about the proper form in which a successful proposal for the marriage had to be put.

My own personal contact with Lashley started when I was a graduate student at Harvard, to which once a year he would rise up with lanky discomfiture from a mysterious and murky place known as the Yerkes Laboratory, which was then in Orange Park, Florida, to fulfill his duties as a member of the department. To some of us, he made it clear that he found these trying; he finished his teaching obligations as rapidly as possible, leaving us all, after some weeks, in a numbed, even shocked, state of breathlessness and postexhilaration collapse. He himself conducted his teaching at rapid pace, delivered in a thick cloud of smoke produced by an obscure brand of Russian cigarettes, the rich aroma of which permeated Memorial Hall and probably far beyond and which lingered after he happily headed south again. When forced to venture into the cold Cambridge air, he enveloped himself in a heavy fur coat that formed a huge, bristly cocoon from which would issue, however, excited and rapid conversation and more Russian smoke. He was a true original, one of the most formidable and inspiring teachers with which our field has been blessed.

In anticipation of this occasion, I thought it would be instructive to go over my notes from his Harvard seminars. They suffer somewhat from illegibility because I well remember the great difficulty in keeping up with his rapid delivery. And although I found my notes intact, alas I cannot locate his reading lists. It is even possible that I later deliberately destroyed them, perhaps even with relish, because we all received them in utter disbelief. How could anyone expect us to read thousands of pages of most difficult material in time for next week! And the next week—a new, equally impossible assignment. And so on.

Now, in retrospect, his seminars are perhaps even more remarkable than they were to me as a student. We all knew of his important contributions. We knew about mass action, of course, and continuity-discontinuity theory, of his jumping stand and the Lashley mazes, his classic paper on instinct, his gold foil experiments attacking the gestalt theory of DC field potentials, his attack on cytoarchitectonics with Clark, and so forth. His paper on serial order was not yet out, but we were given a preview of that remarkable paper. What was extraordinary in his teaching was the enormous variety of his interests, his depth of knowledge, and the freshness and originality of his approach. In his first seminar he told us why he had been forced to change his views on imagery, then turned to insect learning, telling us why field studies were more successful than laboratory studies. And so the topics rolled off: Schiller and the two-stick problem with chimps, immediate versus retentive memory, "dating" of memories, contrasts between the visual and auditory systems in retrograde degeneration, why the effects of motor cortex lesions in humans are probably reversible, masses of material on neuroembryology, experiments on nerve crossing (including in the monkey), reverberating circuits, why Lorenté de No worked only with adult brains, what was wrong with strychnine neuronography, why cutting the corpus callosum was not an effective treatment for epilepsy, the effects of removal of Broca's area bilaterally on mute catatonia, how Hebb had shown that normal hospital staff had performed poorly on Weisenburg and McBridge's aphasia tests, why the Montreal evidence was hardly conclusive for the demonstration of left-hemisphere dominance, why the hypothalamus was not the center of emotion, the importance of mirror foci in epilepsy, the nerve-muscle junction, how figural aftereffects are altered by attention, and so forth. He was a polymath who thought deeply and widely, and was utterly generous in sharing his knowledge and enthusiasm, and indeed his skepticism. I saw him once or twice a year after I finished at Harvard in 1952 until I went abroad in 1955, and they were all unforgettable occasions. I also witnessed some unforgettable exchanges—between him and Penfield, for example, and between him and Skinner—the first time, I suppose, that I saw Skinner box—so to speak. But enough of reminiscences.

In going over my seminar notes again, I discovered something else: namely, an opinion about the nature of amnesia that I thought we had reached only gradually some years later and therefore, I thought, with originality. There it was in my seminar notes: "In man accessibility can sometimes be destroyed without traces themselves being destroyed." And in his paper, "In Search of the Engram," he says (Beach, Hebb, Morgan, & Nissen, 1960): "I believe the evidence strongly favours the view that amnesia from brain injury rarely, if ever, is due to the destruction of specific memory traces. Rather, the amnesias represent a lowered level of vigilance, a greater difficulty in activating the organised pattern of traces, or a disturbance of some broader system of organised functions [p. 495]." (All references to Lashley's papers will be to the Selected Papers, edited by Beach, Hebb, Morgan and Nissen, 1960.)

I am entirely amnesic for having listened to or read these statements. Therefore, my claim to originality must be unlike that made by one well-known neuropsychologist when he defended himself against his rather common habit of citing 19th-century German neurology in his discussion of practically any neuropsychological issue. Why, he was asked once in exasperation, did he do that when there was much better modern neurological evidence? "How else," was the reply, "can I be original?" If Lashley affected my approach, I am only too pleased to acknowledge it and to join him in his conclusion about amnesia, although I must say, in passing, it is difficult to find any evidence that he provided to help support his assertion. There was also another comment I found in my notes that may well have affected my attitude. In discussing a case of Brickner of a frontal lobe patient in which a large, unsuspected tumor was found at autopsy in the occipital lobe, Lashley commented to us how extremely rare it is to have *both* psychological and pathological investigation of brain injury. That observation is similar to one made in his book, the 50th anniversary of which this volume commemorates (Beach et al., 1960):

> I know of no attempt in the whole literature of neurology to determine what proportion of any anatomical area was destroyed by a lesion, and in many cases which are cited as evidence on the localization question, the delineation of the lesions is woefully inexact. In recent studies, where exact methods of measuring behavior have been introduced, it has for the most part been impossible to determine the exact position of the lesions because of the survival of the patients [pp. 151–152].

What I want to tell you about today is how Elizabeth Warrington and I came to agree with Lashley about the importance of inaccessibility in amnesia, but also how neuropathological evidence from two of our long-studied amnesic patients, though filling a lack that he would have approved of, produced a conclusion that he probably would have found uncongenial.

My starting point was from a basic premise that perhaps I had also acquired implicitly from Lashley; at any rate, I am certain it is one that he embraced—

namely, that the same laws of cerebral organization apply equally to humans as to other vertebrates. Indeed, he wrote (Beach et al., 1960): "If there exist, in *human* cerebral action, processes which seem fundamentally different or inexplicable in terms of our present construct of the elementary physiology of integration, then it is probable that the *construct* is incomplete or mistaken [p. 526; my italics]." For some years I have tried to understand why there are certain apparent discrepancies between the results of animal research and of human research on the same regions or systems of the brain. One such discrepancy concerns the effects of lesions of the medial temporal lobe, and especially of the hippocampus and fornix, which in patients such as H. M. are said to cause a severe and crippling amnesic state. This state is the most severe pure form of a retrograde plus anterograde memory failure known, and therefore its mechanism is of direct relevance to the theme that so exercised Lashley—the neural mechanisms of learning and memory. Neurologists had known of patients with very similar, severe memory impairments for many years, especially alcoholic Korsakoff psychosis patients and others with herpes simplex encephalitis, but the dramatic findings with the patient H. M. (Scoville & Milner, 1957) reawakened interest in the critical anatomical pathways. Needless to say, after 1957 there was a rash of animal experiments directed to just that end.

And that is where the difficulty began. Even those experiments modeled directly on Scoville's surgery on H. M. produced findings in animals that were apparently different from the memory impairment in humans—for example, in the study by Orbach, Milner, and Rasmussen (1960). They found no deficit in medial bitemporal monkeys on a discrimination task in which widely spaced trials were filled with massed trials in irrelevant discriminations, which would certainly be expected to reveal a severe impairment in a human amnesic. Nor could they even find more than a mild impairment on the retention of postoperatively acquired tasks. The result is that the question of critical anatomical pathways is still unsettled and, indeed, has become rather controversial. The Montreal workers have tended to focus upon the hippocampus as the critical structure, given the correlation between the degree of specific memory impairments in unilateral temporal lobectomies and the extent of hippocampal involvement (evidence by Corsi, reviewed by Milner, 1970, 1971). But, of course, this correlation is only an indirect and rough indication of precise pathology, and structures near the hippocampus would also correlate as highly as hippocampus itself. Horel (1978), in fact, has taken up this point and has suggested that the fibers in the "temporal stem" may be crucial, not the hippocampal tissue at all. And it is of interest to recall that even before H. M. appeared on the scene, the discovery had been made that lesions of inferotemporal neocortex in monkeys severely retarded visual discrimination learning (Mishkin, 1954; Mishkin & Pribram, 1954). It is often forgotten that one of the control lesions in that early research was a bilateral hippocampectomy—which produced little if any impairment! Iversen and I (1970) thought that the inferotemporal focus might, in fact, be an important homologue of the critical site in humans, or that a cortical lesion *plus* a hippocampal lesion might be such a homologue; even Scoville's drawings show neocortical as well as hippocampal involvement in H. M., although H. M. is still very much alive, and therefore the only information available comes from the drawings and surgical notes. Iversen and I obtained quite impressive long-term retention deficits in baboons with such a combined lesion, quite independent of any short-term learning incapacity. But I abandoned that approach (perhaps foolishly, in retrospect) because on further analysis, the deficits turned out to be due to enhanced interference among our tasks rather than a failure of storage as such (Iversen, 1970). At the time, as you will see, it seemed obvious that the human amnesic deficit was one of long-term storage. Meanwhile, Gaffan has returned to the hippocampal-fornix hypothesis and has generated some ingenious animal experiments suggesting that lesions produce a specific deficit in recognition but not in associative memory (1972, 1974). Concentrating on the fact that Scoville's lesions included both hippocampus and amygdala, Mishkin has reported (1978) a severe deficit in a Gaffan-type recognition task in monkeys with combined hippocampal and amygdala lesions, much more severe than is produced by either lesion alone.

The difficulty is that we still do not know whether any of these deficits is, indeed, functionally homologous to the human amnesic deficit. It is even quite possible—I would say likely—that a more severe learning or retention deficit in animals will emerge from lesions that are quite irrelevant to the amnesic deficit than from other lesions that ultimately turn out to be directly relevant. The same difficulty resides in the impressive work on radial maze learning by Olton and his colleagues, which they have shown to be impaired by hippocampal lesions in the rat (Olton, 1978; Olton & Papas, 1979). Is this the kind of deficit we would expect to be the model for human amnesia? After all, neurological patients with documented spatial disorders are by no means clinically amnesic, and topographical amnesia is found in isolation from global amnesia (De Renzi, Faglioni, & Villa, 1977). Various other workers have drawn parallels between their findings with animals with hippocampal lesions and the human amnesic syndrome—for example, Winocur and the importance of contextual cues (Winocur, 1978; Winocur & Olds, 1978), Jarrard on the exaggerated effects of between-task interference (1975), and O'Keefe and Nadel (1978) on "cognitive maps." All this work is of great interest in its own right, but will it help us to solve the problem of the critical pathways for the human amnesic syndrome? I believe the answer to be no—not until we know what the correct behavioral homologue is in animals. As you shall see, in pursuing that tack, some intriguing and difficult methodological puzzles arise for comparative neuropsychologists.

The clinical description of amnesic patients is so graphic and clear that it is not surprising that animal workers felt they could extrapolate directly from that description to the laboratory. The patients appear to be unable to learn new material, to store new experiences, even though they need not have any intellectual impairment in tasks not requiring the bridging by memory of more than a minute or two. They are, or at least can be, normal in short-term memory tasks such as digit span or the Brown–Peterson test (Baddeley & Warrington, 1970). There is also a retrograde amnesia extending back over a varying period that is difficult to measure. So, in a word, the deficit looks like one of failure of consolidation or, which is not quite the same thing, a blockage of transfer from short-term to long-term memory. This description applies not only to H. M. but, in its salient features, to amnesic patients of varying etiologies.

After the disappointing and uncertain results of animal experiments, some 13 years or so ago, Elizabeth Warrington of the National Hospital, London, and I decided to have a fresh look at amnesic patients. We had the opportunity to study one surgical case and a number of other cases, including Korsakoff patients and encephalitics. They all presented the clinical appearance that I have just described, and they performed hopelessly on conventional verbal memory tests. But what we found experimentally surprised us deeply: The patients did far too well in certain special tests of learning and retention. Our earlier evidence has been reviewed (Warrington & Weiskrantz, 1973; Weiskrantz, 1978; Weiskrantz & Warrington, 1975a), so it is not necessary to go over all the details here. What I would like to do, instead, is concentrate on the evidence that seems to us to suggest that the amnesic patient suffers from what Lashley called a difficulty of "accessibility" of memory traces, rather than their destruction or their failure to consolidate.

If one wants to demonstrate a retrieval failure, one has to be lucky. One has to find either the right conditions or the right material with which to demonstrate that the patient can, after all—despite his or her apparent amnesia—remember. On the other hand, whereas one needs luck to demonstrate a retrieval failure, one needs an eternity to prove a storage failure. It is as impossible to demonstrate that a failure to remember is one of storage as it is to demonstrate the universal negative: There might always be *some* condition, if one searched long and hard enough for it, that would reverse the amnesia and so reveal adequate retention of apparently forgotten material. The breakthrough for us came when Dr. Warrington suggested using a test that did not require asking patients *what* they remember or *whether* they recognize a word or a picture or a story or a face. Many amnesic patients can remember that they have very poor memory, and it is not a kindness to keep asking them questions about their memory. So instead, the patient was shown some material—say, a series of words or pictures—and then later was simply given a cue that matched each item and was asked to say what the cue stood for. If the earlier exposure to the material had some benefit, the cue would be more likely to elicit the correct answer than if there had been no prior exposure. We have used this method with a wide variety of cues and material. Good retention can be demonstrated over intervals generally accepted as belonging to long-term memory; indeed, using this type of method, Milner found retention of pictures by H. M. over 1 hour and also over 4 months (Milner, 1970;

Milner, Corkin, & Teuber, 1968). Our findings were not the first examples of long-term retention by amnesic patients. Milner (1962) and Corkin (1968) had shown that motor skill learning could be retained, but motor skills were taken to be an exception to the general rule. What surprised us was that we found reasonable retention with verbal material, for which amnesic patients were indeed supposed to be amnesic.

One possible comment on our findings would make them trivial if we had fallen into a familiar trap (Weiskrantz, 1968). Perhaps the neuropsychological deficit was not absolute, and perhaps we hit on a task that was especially easy, so that even in an amnesic subject, some retention could be demonstrated. But apparently what makes a task easy for an amnesic patient does so differentially; control subjects are not helped by the cued-recall method to the same extent. There is an interaction between type of method (conventional memory tests vs. cued recall) and groups (controls vs. amnesics) (Warrington & Weiskrantz, 1970, 1974), so it is not merely a question of task sensitivity. Even this type of result has been challenged, however, by those who would prefer to adhere to the older view of a storage or input difficulty; it has been suggested that perhaps forgetting occurs more rapidly when measured by recognition than by cuing, so that all we demonstrated was weaker memory traces in the amnesic subjects than in controls. An attempt was made to simulate our findings in control subjects using very long retention intervals, thereby yielding weaker memories (Woods & Piercy, 1974). Questionable logic and methodology aside (and our own failure to replicate when the methodology was corrected; Weiskrantz & Warrington, 1975b), and aside from the fact that under certain conditions, retention—as demonstrated by cued recall—is quite as good in amnesic subjects as it is in controls, there are three other lines that suggest a retrieval rather than a storage failure.

The first is that the amnesic subject, far from showing more rapid "forgetting," can, under certain appropriate conditions, display slower "forgetting"; and the persistence of the unforgotten material in turn leads directly to an interference with new learning. This condition is akin to one in which hippocampectomized animals also show slower "forgetting"—namely, in extinction and reversal tasks. Even though such animals can learn a task at normal speed, they are apt to take longer to extinguish, or they may be impaired in reversing a discrimination even though their initial learning was normal. We deliberately designed our task with patients to be a verbal analogue of a discrimination reversal task. A set of cues was made to match the first set of items to be learned, and then later the same cues matched a second different set of items to be learned. We found that the amnesic patients went on giving the first-learned item to each cue far longer than did controls, thereby holding up learning of the second item. A feature of this experiment was that each cue (which was the first three letters of a word) matched *only* the two items in question; we chose our words deliberately so that they were the only two common words in English that started with the same three letters. This meant that any error of commission in the second list had, by definition, to be false positive intrusion from the first list; and such intrusions were, in fact, common (Warrington & Weiskrantz, 1974, 1978). A closely related result, using rule-governed paired-associate learning, was produced by Winocur and Weiskrantz (1976). So the difficulty for the amnesic subject is the proper access to the particular item out of the pair of items when both are matched by the same cue. Incidentally, this study also demonstrates that the cues do not work merely as "reminders" or that we are dealing with a "tip of the tongue" phenomenon; whether cues help or not depends on the precise conditions of the experiment and the cues' prior history.

The second line of evidence stems from the evidence on retrograde amnesia. It is easy to ask how far back it extends but very difficult in practice to find out. Sanders and Warrington (1971) constructed questionnaires about public events and photographs of faces that had been topical at different times. With these tests, our amnesic subjects have a retrograde amnesia going back at least 25 years—which is as far back as the questionnaires themselves reach. It is important, as this has become a somewhat controversial area, to stress that the tests must be designed so that they are genuinely topical. If you ask any schoolboy to identify a picture of George Washington, he will probably get the correct answer—and so may an amnesic subject—without being entitled to a memory going back 200 years. That way you could easily demonstrate the preservation of "old" memories. George Washington is part of semantic memory, part of the culture, and often rehearsed publicly. Such items are relatively impervious to amnesia, as is memory for one's language, one's own name, and so forth. Warrington and Sanders rejected such culturally rehearsed items by a very simple device—they gave the items to schoolchildren, and if they "remembered" an item they were not entitled to remember within their lifetime, it was not included in the questionnaire. If the questionnaire is designed to test *topical* events or personalities, then the retrograde amnesia seems to extend very far back in the life of our patients. One might nevertheless assume that old episodic traces continue to consolidate even more throughout life, and that the extensive retrograde amnesia still reflects interference with consolidation. I believe that this assumption is not parsimonious; there is no suggestion of a gradient in our subjects favoring older topical memories. The alternative is to assume that the extensive retrograde amnesia reflects a difficulty with accessibility. This assumption is bolstered by evidence that cuing also helps with the retrieval of apparently forgotten items in the retrograde amnesia questionnaires (Marslen-Wilson & Teuber, 1975; Sanders & Warrington, 1975).

The literature on the amnesic syndrome has now become so voluminous and the protagonists so skilled at defending their own interpretations that you might well be skeptical about any evidence supporting an interpretation of inaccessibility, or indeed any other interpretation. William James was right not only for his time when he commented in 1890 that "the subject of localization of functions in the brain seems to have a peculiar effect on the temper of those who cultivate it experimentally [p. 46].''

But there is a third line of evidence, one of quite old vintage, that I find difficult to describe in any other way except in terms of accessibility. Korsakoff himself drew attention to a number of examples of acquired memories without awareness in his amnesic patients. For example, one of his patients always showed apprehension in front of the ''faradization'' apparatus after it was used to treat her polyneuritis, but she said she had never seen the apparatus before and did not know what it was used for (cited by Delay & Brion, 1969, p. 17).

An anecdote of a milder aversive experience was given by Claparède (1911; quoted by MacCurdy, 1928):

> I tried the following experiment . . . to see if she would better retain an intense impression that set affectivity into play. I pricked her hand forcibly with a pin hidden between my fingers. This little pain was as quickly forgotten as indifferent perceptions and, shortly after the pricking, she remembered no more of it. However, when I moved my hand near hers again, she pulled her hand back in a reflex way and without knowing why. If, in fact, I demanded the reason for the withdrawal of her hand, she answered in a flurried way, ''Isn't it allowed to withdraw one's hand?'' . . . If I insisted, she would say to me, ''Perhaps there is a pin hidden in your hand.'' To my question, ''What can make you suspect that I would like to prick you,'' she would take up her refrain, ''It is an idea which came into my head'', or sometimes she would try to justify herself with ''Sometimes pins are hidden in hands.'' But she never recognised this idea of pricking as a memory [pp. 115].

As this is an anecdotal example of classical avoidance conditioning, apparently without awareness, Warrington and I tried formally to establish classical conditioning of the eyelid response in two Korsakoff patients, questioning them during the frequent breaks for their comments on the experiment while they continued to sit in front of the unusual-looking apparatus, which had been delivering highly memorable air puffs to the eye. The conditioned stimulus was a combined light and tone. We measured the conditioned eyelid response. Clear evidence of conditioning was obtained, with good retention over 24 hours. Neither subject offered any comment, even of the air puff itself, that revealed any memory for the situation; yet when the conditioning trials started once again, the conditioned responses promptly appeared (Weiskrantz & Warrington, 1979).

There are other incidental reports of such an inaccessibility in the face of objective evidence of acquired memories. Sidman, Stoddard, and Mohr (1968), for example, reported a striking disparity in H. M. between his visual discrimination learning achievement and his lack of awareness of having learned. Milner (1962) also reported that H. M. was able to learn mirror drawing, showing good savings from day to day; yet on each day he was completely unaware that he had done the task before.

Each time I give you an example of failure of access, I give you yet another example of learning and retention by the amnesic subject. Given the logic of an argument of inaccessibility, that is inevitable. But there are still further examples, many of them, of adequate learning and memory in addition to those I have given so far that have emerged from recent research. Do all of these various tasks have anything in common? Here is a list of tasks that amnesic subjects can learn: (1) motor skills (Corkin, 1968; Milner, 1962); (2) visual discriminations (Sidman et al., 1968); (3) cued recall of pictures and words, using a variety of cues (Warrington & Weiskrantz, 1968, 1974, 1978; Weiskrantz & Warrington, 1970); (4) retention of learning of anomalous pictures in the McGill Anomalies Test (Baddeley & Brooks, personal communication, 1979; Warrington & Weiskrantz, 1973); (5) rule-governed paired-associate learning and retention (Winocur & Weiskrantz, 1976); (6) retention of facilitation of stereoscopic perception of random dot stereograms (Ramachandran, 1976, personal communication); (7) retention of the McCulloch color-grating illusion over 24 hours (Warrington & Weiskrantz, unpublished observations, 1979); (8) retention of facilitation of solving jigsaw puzzles and for arranging words into sentences (Baddeley & Brooks, personal communication, 1979).

There may be other examples, but the great variety of these tasks makes it impossible to characterize them as a particular *kind* of learning, such as verbal, visual, motor, or the like. But all the tasks *do* have one feature in common: It is not necessary to say to the patients, "Tell me what you remember" or "Do you recognize this?" as a practical requirement in order for their memories to be tested and demonstrated objectively. In all cases a cue or a signal is given and the subject responds, or the individual is asked to perform a certain act, as in mirror drawing, and does it. Not only is it unnecessary to ask the patient a memory-type question, but if you do ask, he or she is likely to be the only one in the experiment who does not know that it is memory being demonstrated. But there is a more subtle aspect as well of the tasks on which the patients succeed: The cue or signal provides an *unambiguous* route to the answer, given that the answer was established by learning. That is what distinguishes rule-determined paired-associate learning (Winocur & Weiskrantz, 1976) from ordinary paired-associate learning, at which amnesic patients are unsuccessful. To be certain about some memories, one has to think, to order, to choose; other memories can be rolled out acognitively. The crux of the theoretical question is to determine what allows some memories to be accessed objectively by amnesic patients and what prevents others from being accessed objectively, and how the dissociation between objective performance and the subjects' commentaries fits into the answer, as I feel sure it must. That is what Dr. Warrington and I are pursuing at the moment, but conventional learning theory does not offer very much help; in fact, the study of amnesia may well suggest new types of theories.

Be that as it may, at the descriptive level there is ample justification for Lashley's statement that amnesia is (at least in the types of cases we have studied) a question of inaccessibility. And he offers an interesting and pertinent theoretical comment (Beach *et al.*, 1960): "Apparent loss of memory is secondary to a disorder in the structuring of concepts. Some physiological mode of organising or integrating activity is affected rather than specific associative bonds [p. 496]."

I trust you can see the dilemma for the comparative neuropsychologist. Given the characteristics of the human amnesic subject—whatever the theoretical explanation of them may be—how do you design an animal model of them in practical terms? How do you design an animal test, for example, of a dissociation between the objective demonstration of an acquired memory and an acknowledgment of that memory? How, in other words, do you decide whether an animal knows that it remembers? Our conventional tests of learning and savings are patently inadequate for that, and indeed might yield normal scores even if the animal were behaving like a human amnesic. Therefore the lack of a deficit in a hippocampectomized animal could even be taken as positive, not negative, evidence. And if we cannot design a proper animal model, how do we determine the critical anatomical circuits for this most devastating of memory disorders known to us?

There is a way around, although it depends on fortuitous circumstances. Patients eventually die, and one may be lucky enough to study their brains, and even luckier if one has studied their psychological state first. Given that we are approaching a century since the syndrome was first described, one might have thought that the question of neuropathology would have been settled by now. It has not. Indeed, it has become more controversial with time. But as Brierley points out (1977): "The length of retrograde amnesia and the severity of the disorder of memory for recent events cannot be set beside the neuropathological findings in any one case [p. 206]." And in 1969 Adams commented: "Unfortunately not a single human example has been adequately studied by clinical and anatomical methods. . . . Thus one can see the need for a collaborative effort between clinicians and neuropathologists if our knowledge of the precise anatomy of the memory and learning process is to be consolidated [p. 105]."

One classical site of Korsakoff pathology is the mammillary body. But Victor, Adams, and Collins (1971) have emphasized the medial dorsal nucleus of the thalamus as being critical, largely on the grounds that they found lesions of the mammillary bodies in five patients who were not amnesic, and these five patients were also the only ones in which the thalamic nucleus was spared among those brains in which it was available for study. From these facts, however, it does not follow either that the mammillary body pathology is not necessary for the amnesic state or that the medial dorsal pathology is sufficient for the amnesic state.

There is a major source of difficulty in all neuropathological studies, whether of groups or of single cases, if the neuropsychological assessment has not been detailed fully and deeply. It has become patently clear over the past few years that one research group's amnesics are not another group's amnesics. Unfortunately, there has been no common, adequate scale on which to place them. Many amnesic subjects suffer from cognitive defects outside the mnemonic realm. Many are diagnosed clinically as amnesic who are not, on testing, globally amnesic; in particular, many tend to have verbal memory difficulties but much less severe nonverbal memory defects. Clinical neurologists often, quite reasonably, base their diagnosis on verbal interchange with the patient. Other patients may not be especially densely amnesic but are confused or demented during clinical assessment. Dr. Warrington has developed an anterograde memory battery of six components with which to assess both verbal and nonverbal memory, a battery that also makes use of our findings with cued recall (Warrington, in preparation). Independently an assessment can be made of retrograde amnesia, as well as the standard assessment measures. From the memory battery one can derive an age-corrected memory quotient. We reject any patient who falls less than two standard deviations below his or her age norm on both verbal and nonverbal measures. And of course we also reject patients who fall significantly below their estimated premorbid IQ level.

Two of our Korsakoff patients recently died. Both had been extensively and repeatedly tested—one for over 9 years and one over 3—so Warrington and I had full information about the extent of retrograde amnesia (at least 25 years); on the anterograde memory battery both scored off the bottom of the scale (less than 60, whereas the normal mean is 100 with an SD of ± 75) for both verbal and nonverbal memory. Both also showed the characteristic normal performance with cued recall. Dr. Mair carried out a thorough neuropathological examination. The concordance of the neuropathology in both patients was very close. Both had severe bilateral degeneration in the medial nucleus of the mammillary bodies, and both had a thin band of gliosis in the thalamus—not, we judge, in the medial dorsal nucleus but somewhat anterior and medial to that nucleus extending ventrally from the region of the paratenial nucleus. (Dr. T. P. S. Powell gave us expert advice and confirmation regarding the thalamic locus.) This is not the time to offer a full psychological and pathological account, which has been published (Mair, Warrington, & Weiskrantz, 1979), or to review various possible anatomical mechanisms of amnesia. All that need be said here is that I believe Lashley would have been surprised to find such a devastating and global amnesia associated with such restricted anatomical damage. The fact that the amnesia can be characterized, as he himself proposed, as a matter of inaccessibility, would have made the surprise that much greater to him, because he argued that amnesia neglected a widespread disturbance of organization and integration.

It may be worth dwelling, just for a moment, on the fact that we found a *double* lesion in our two amnesic patients. I believe Lashley would have had something to say about that because he argued (Beach et al., 1960) that "many activities seem to require for their performance *both* a specific patterning and also a general facilitation. . . . In many of the organic amnesias the pattern of integration seems to be retained but can be reactivated only by an abnormally intense sensory or central reinforcement [p. 514; my italics]." The midline thalamic subependymal region probably has a diffuse cortical projection (Jones & Leavitt, 1974) and might therefore be involved in general facilitation. Mishkin (1978), as we have noted, also has argued for a double lesion—hippocampus (which would lead to mammillary degeneration) and amygdala. We now know (Aggleton, personal communication, 1980) that this thalamic region projects to the amygdala in the monkey. But I would not think that the arguments in favor of a double lesion being *necessary* are strong. The classical literature sometimes records just a single lesion—that is, the mammillary bodies (cf. Brierley, 1977; Delay & Brion, 1969)—and where there are other lesions in addition to the mammillary bodies, they tend to be variable and may spare the amygdala altogether. The mammillary bodies are a funnel through which the midbrain as well as the neocortex of the temporal lobe and the limbic system can communicate with the frontal lobes. Lesions in the mammillary bodies must cause a major disconnection, but there are still circuitous routes around it in which the midline thalamus might be involved. So another possibility is that the mammillary body lesions, if severe enough, can be sufficient to produce amnesia but that if they are incomplete (and typically there is more fiber than cell loss in many of the classical reports), an additional lesion may make the disconnection more complete and the amnesia more profound and enduring.

Of course, it is possible that there are hidden neurochemical lesions in these patients that would, because of the generous distribution of some of the neurotransmitter systems, provide closer confirmation of Lashley's original ideas about widespread involvement. No matter how one approaches the question of the critical lesion—through neuropathology or neurochemistry—the field will not be advanced; rather, it will be obstructed, given the variety and complexity of cognitive disorders, if it is not combined with searching psychological analysis of the behavioral defect itself. In this, Lashley was surely correct in giving behavioral analysis primacy. There is no point in having a neuropathology or a neurochemistry of this or that if you do not know, as precisely as possible, what the this or that is.

At least there is neuropathological evidence now at hand, and we might use this information in animal research to explore all sorts of questions. Above all, one might think, it would provide a way of discovering just what the correct animal model actually is: Just make a bilateral mammillary body plus midline thalamic lesion, and see what happens. That is one approach that will undoubtedly be followed. But there will be a lingering dissatisfaction and superficiality with it, at least to me; and worse, it might even lead to a waste of time and animals if one merely studies the behavior on a hit-or-miss basis. As we have seen, the human deficit can be considered to be a disconnection between acquired memories and a system that monitors them. The monitoring is not merely providing amusement for another homunculus (or even just a monkulus); it allows past experience to be ordered and operated upon, and without this the patient is indeed crippled. The study of disconnections is not foreign to animal research, as in the work of Mishkin and Horel—not to mention the large literature on commissurotomies. But these are, so to speak, disconnections made in the vertical plane. Functionally, the amnesic syndrome—and other neuropsychological phenomena as well (for example, "blind-sight")—is a disconnection between levels; it is a horizontal disconnection. It inevitably reintroduces concepts such as *higher* and *lower* into the analysis. It is wasteful to monitor information that leads to an unambiguous outcome—like the pupillary reflex, or foveation, or cognitive skills that become routine. It is equally disastrous not to monitor those that are not routine.

It is perhaps ironic that Lashley followed one great tradition that flowed from 19th-century neurology—the concept that the cerebral cortex was not only the great pinnacle of evolutionary achievement but that it also took over many of the functions that were assigned to lower centers in lower creatures, including consciousness itself. Read William James in 1890 on the visual system: "If our lower optical centres, the corpora quadrigemina, and thalami, do have any consciousness, it is at all events a consciousness which does not mix with that which accompanies the cortical activities, and which has nothing to do with our personal Self. In lower animals this may not be so much the case [Vol. 1, p. 66]." Lashley went for the biggest game and made all question their localizationistic assumptions about it. Lashley strenuously resisted any dualistic notion that would give a special status to consciousness or experience even though, historically, that notion is what was assumed to elevate the cortex to its special status.

The other great tradition that stemmed from Hughlings Jackson and led to work, for example, such as Bard and Mountcastle's, seems to have been ignored by Lashley. Lashley was not deeply concerned with neural levels or with hierarchies. Even when he dealt with the thalamus (1938/1960), for example, it was to consider a specific hypothesis concerning emotion. He showed with remarkable insight in his paper, "The Problem of Serial Order" (Beach et al, 1960), that a purely associative theory could not handle the questions of the syntax of language or of behavior, but his answer was to delve more deeply into complex networks of cells of short axons producing waves of activity, using the metaphor of the brain as "the surface of a lake" (Beach et al., 1960, p. 525). The release from the associationist grip on syntax in language came when the emphasis shifted to hierarchical levels of organization, and it is possible that a similar release must occur in our study of the neurology of memory and its organization.

I do not pretend to know how to tell whether an animal knows that it remembers, but I believe it must involve giving it a response possibility in parallel to the discriminative responses—if you will, a "commentary" key. The recent approach by Beninger, Kendall, and Vanderwolf (1974) seems to me very promising in a related context: Rats were allowed to carry out any one of a number of response patterns, such as freezing, grooming, etc., but their subsequent reward was made contingent on the animal making a further particular lever press depending on what it had just done. Roughly speaking, the animal indicated that it knew what it had just done. If you were to give amnesic subjects a set of discriminative choices, as in a simple maze they had learned, they would get them correct. If, in parallel, they had to press a "yes" or "no" button indicating whether they had carried out the task before, they would press the "no" button (or perhaps the "yes" button when they had no right to do so). The same dissociation would apply to patients with "blind-sight." They will perform well above chance if they have to make a reaching response toward a stimulus in their "blind" visual field, but they will press the "no" button if asked whether they see the stimulus. The problem of mind and awareness, as I see it, is a problem of monitoring, and the practical problem is one of separating the monitoring response from the responses or the information being monitored.

Let me try, by way of summary, to retrace our steps. The most devastating form of a pure memory failure known to us occurs after certain surgical operations or disease states. The question of the critical anatomical locus was tackled in animal research, but lesions in animals in what is thought to be the same neural system produce a variety of deficits that do not appear to be purely or even mainly amnesic. The question of the correct animal model to the human amnesic state remains unresolved. A reexamination of the human amnesic deficit confirms Lashley's assertion that it is a failure of accessibility, but one that appears to involve a disconnection between acquired memories and the subject's awareness of them. That makes it necessary to invent quite new paradigms in animals if we wish to use them as models. Meanwhile, neuropathological evidence has become available that helps to narrow down the circuits to be explored in animals in order to investigate both the nature of the deficit and its possible treatment more fully. But to tell us just how to design the behavioral analysis at the animal level so that it properly reflects an inaccessibility due to a functional disconnection, we need, I am afraid, some new Lashleys.

Lashley would not, I hope, have objected. In his last paper, reprinted in Beach et al (1960), he states: "Psychological analysis reveals nothing but varying organisation or structure. Studies of the physiology of the nervous system and analysis of behaviour reveal the same principles of organisation as are discovered by subjective analysis [p. 457]." "I have . . . tried to show," he says later, "that the organisation of mental states does not reveal any operations which cannot be accounted for in principle by the mechanisms of the brain [p. 539]." "Mind," said Lashley in the last paragraph of his last paper, "has no distinguishing features other than its organisation [p. 542]." It is precisely this that has been revealed in the neuropsychology since Lashley—an astonishing richness of dissociations, both horizontal and vertical, that cast new light on the *organization* of the mind, both animal and human, and therefore on the organization of the brain.

REFERENCES

Adams, R. D. The anatomy of memory mechanisms in the human brain. In G. A. Talland & N. C. Waugh (Eds.), *The pathology of memory*. New York and London: Academic Press, 1969.

Aggleton, J. Personal communication, 1980.

Baddeley A. D. & Brooks, N. Personal communications, 1979.

Baddeley, A. D., & Warrington, E. K. Amnesia and the distinction between long- and short-term memory. *Journal of Verbal Learning and Verbal Behaviour*, 1970, *9*, 176-189.

Beach, F. A., Hebb, D. O., Morgan, C. T., & Nissen, H. W. *The neuropsychology of Lashley*. New York: McGraw-Hill, 1960.

Beninger, R. J., Kendall, S. B., & Vanderwolf, C. H. The ability of rats to discriminate their own behaviours. *Canadian Journal of Psychology*, 1974, *28*(1), 79-91.

Brierley, J. B. Neuropathology of amnesic states. In C. W. M. Whitty & O. L. Zangwill (Eds.), *Amnesia*. London: Butterworths, 1977.

Claparède, E. Récognition et moiïte. *Arch. Psychol. Genève*, 1911, *11*, 79-90.

Corkin, S. Acquisition of motor skill after bilateral medial temporal-lobe excision. *Neuropsychologia, 1968*, *6*, 225-265.

Delay, J., & Brion, S. *Le syndrome de Korsakoff*. Paris: Masson, 1969.

De Renzi, E., Faglioni, P., & Villa, P. Topographical amnesia. *Journal of Neurology, Neurosurgery and Psychiatry*, 1977, *40*, 498-505.

Gaffan, D. Loss of recognition memory in rats with lesions of the fornix. *Neuropsychologia*, 1972, *10*, 327-341.

Gaffan, D. Recognition impaired and association intact in the memory of monkeys after transection of the fornix. *Journal of Comparative and Physiological Psychology*, 1974, *86*, 1100-1109.

Horel, J. A. The neuroanatomy of amnesia: A critique of the hippocampal memory hypothesis. *Brain*, 1978, *101*, 403-445.

Iversen, S. D. Interference and inferotemporal memory deficits. *Brain Research*, 1970, *19*, 277-289.

Iversen, S. D., & Weiskrantz, L. An investigation of a possible memory defect produced by inferotemporal lesions in the baboon. *Neuropsychologia*, 1970, *8*, 21-36.

James, W. *Principles of psychology*. London: Macmillan, 1890.

Jarrard, L. E. Role of interference in retention by rats with hippocampal lesions. *Journal of Comparative and Physiological Psychology*, 1975, *89*, 400-408.

Jones, E. G., & Leavitt, R. Y. Retrograde axonal transport and the demonstration of non-specific projections to the cerebral cortex and striatum from thalamic intralaminar nuclei in the rat, cat, and monkey. *Journal of Comparative Neurology*, 1974, *154*, 349-378.

MacCurdy, J. T. *Common principles in psychology and physiology*. London: Cambridge University Press, 1928.

Mair, W. G. P., Warrington, E. K., & Weiskrantz, L. Memory disorder in Korsakoff's psychosis: A neuropathological and neuropsychological investigation of two cases. *Brain*, 1979, *102*, 749-783.

Marslen-Wilson, W. D., & Teuber, H.-L. Memory for remote events in anterograde amnesia: Recognition of public figures from newsphotographs. *Neuropsychologia*, 1975, *13*, 353-364.

Milner, B. Les troubles de la mémoire accompagnant des lésions hippocampiques bilatérales. In *Physiologie de l'hippocampe*. Paris: Centre National de la Récherche Scientifique, No. 107, 1962.

Milner, B. Memory and the medial temporal regions of the brain. In K. H. Pribram & D. E. Broadbent (Eds.), *Biology of memory*. New York: Academic Press, 1970.

Milner, B. Interhemispheric differences and psychological processes. *British Medical Bulletin*, 1971, *27*, 272-277.

Milner, B., Corkin, S., & Teuber, H.-L. Further analysis of hippocampal amnesic syndrome: 14 year follow-up study of H. M. *Neuropsychologia*, 1968, *6*, 215-234.

Mishkin, M. Visual discrimination performance following partial ablations of the temporal lobe. II. Ventral surface vs. hippocampus. *Journal of Comparative and Physiological Psychology*, 1954, *47*, 187-193.

Mishkin, M. Memory in monkeys severely impaired by combined but not by separate removal of amygdala and hippocampus. *Nature, London*, 1978, *273*, 297-298.

Mishkin, M., & Pribram, K. H. Visual discrimination performance following partial ablations of the temporal lobe. I. Ventral vs. lateral. *Journal of Comparative and Physiological Psychology*, 1954, *47*, 14-20.

O'Keefe, J., & Nadel, L. *The hippocampus as a cognitive map*. Oxford: Oxford University Press, 1978.

Olton, D. S. The function of septo-hippocampal connections in spatially organized behaviour. In *Functions of the septo-hippocampal system (Ciba Foundation Symposium 58)*. New York: Elsevier, 1978.

Olton, D. S., & Papas, B. C. Spatial memory and hippocampal function. *Neuropsychologia*, 1979, *17*, 669-682.

Orbach, J., Milner, B., & Rasmussen, T. Learning and retention in monkeys after amygdala-hippocampus resection. *Archives of Neurology*, 1960, *3*, 230-251.

Ramachandran, V. S. Learning-like phenomena in stereopsis. *Nature, London*, 1976, *262*, 382-384.

Ramachandran, V. S. Personal communication, 1979.

Sanders, H. I., & Warrington, E. K. Memory for remote events in amnesic patients. *Brain*, 1971, *94*, 661-668.

Sanders, H. I., & Warrington, E. K. Retrograde amnesia in organic amnesic patients. *Cortex*, 1975, *11*, 397-400.

Scoville, W. B., & Milner, B. Loss of recent memory after bilateral hippocampal lesions. *Journal of Neurology, Neurosurgery and Psychiatry*, 1957, *20*, 11-21.

Sidman, M., Stoddard, L. T., & Mohr, J. P. Some additional quantitative observations of immediate memory in a patient with bilateral hippocampal lesions. *Neuropsychologia*, 1968, *6*, 245-254.

Victor, M., Adams, R. D., & Collins, G. H. *The Wernicke-Korsakoff syndrome*. Oxford: Blackwells, 1971.

Warrington, E. K., & Weiskrantz, L. New method of testing long-term retention with special reference to amnesic patients. *Nature, London*, 1968, *217*, 972-974.

Warrington, E. K., & Weiskrantz, L. Amnesic syndrome: Consolidation or retrieval? *Nature, London*, 1970, *228*, 628-630.

Warrington, E. K., & Weiskrantz, L. An analysis of short-term and long-term memory defects in man. In J. A. Deutsch (Ed.), *The psychology of memory*. New York and London: Academic Press, 1973.

Warrington, E. K., & Weiskrantz, L. The effects of prior learning on subsequent retention in amnesic patients. *Neuropsychologia*, 1974, *12*, 419-428.

Warrington, E. K., & Weiskrantz, L. Further analysis of the prior learning effect in amnesic patients. *Neuropsychologia*, 1978, *16*, 169-176.

Warrington E. K. & Weiskrantz, L. Unpublished observations, 1979.

Weiskrantz, L. *Analysis of behavioral change*. New York and London: Harper & Row, 1968.

Weiskrantz, L. A comparison of hippocampal pathology in man and other animals. In *Functions of the septo-hippocampal system (Ciba Foundation Symposium 58)*. New York: Elsevier, 1978.

Weiskrantz, L. & Warrington, E. K. Verbal learning and retention by amnesic patients using partial information. *Psychonomic Science*, 1970, *20*, 210-211.

Weiskrantz, L., & Warrington, E. K. The problem of the amnesic syndrome in man and animals. In R. L. Isaacson & K. H. Pribram (Eds.), *The hippocampus (Vol. 2): Neurophysiology and behavior*. New York and London: Plenum Press, 1975. (a)

Weiskrantz, L., & Warrington, E. K. Some comments on Woods' and Piercy's claim of a similarity between amnesic memory and normal forgetting. *Neuropsychologia*, 1975, *13*, 365-367. (b)

Weiskrantz, L., & Warrington, E. K. Conditioning in amnesic patients. *Neuropsychologia*, 1979, *17*, 187-194.

Winocur, G. Discussion. In *Functions of the septo-hippocampal system (Ciba Foundation Symposium 58)*. New York: Elsevier, 1978.

Winocur, G., & Olds, J. Effects of context manipulation on memory and reversal learning in rats with hippocampal lesions. *Journal of Comparative and Physiological Psychology,* 1978, *92,* 312-321.

Winocur, G., & Weiskrantz, L. An investigation of paired-associate learning in amnesic patients. *Neuropsychologia,* 1976, *14,* 97-110.

Woods, R. T., & Piercy, M. A similarity between amnesic memory and normal forgetting. *Neuropsychologia*, 1974, *12*, 437-445.

15 Neural Mechanisms of Arousal, Attention, and Information Processing

Donald B. Lindsley
University of California, Los Angeles

PART 1

I feel highly honored to be a participant in this series of lectures honoring Karl S. Lashley and celebrating the 50th anniversary of the publication of his book, *Brain Mechanisms and Intelligence* (Lashley, 1929). I began my graduate studies in Physiological Psychology at the University of Iowa in 1929 under the sponsorship of Professor Lee Edward Travis, and the appearance of Lashley's book that year was a highly stimulating and motivating event for all of us. Lashley, more than anyone else up to that time, sought to combine behavioral studies of animals with operative manipulations of their brains by both specific lesions and mass ablations. He developed unique methods for observing and quantifying behavior, including discrimination, learning, and memory. He perfected operative and histological techniques for making precise lesions, and for assessing and mapping them quantitatively. Much of his early work was with the rat but in later years he turned to the more highly organized nervous system and the more complex behavior of the monkey. The mechanism of vision played a prominent role in his thinking, theorizing, and speculating about how the brain mediates and integrates the sensory information essential to the higher-level functions of humans, such as perception, concept formation, thinking, and the utilization of speech and language.

The serial order of behavior as in speech and language fascinated Lashley and he was always ready and eager to discuss it and the problems it presented in attempting to unravel the mechanisms of the brain. He was widely read and knowledgeable about basic psychological and neurological data and with the mental phenomena associated with various states of consciousness in normal and pathological conditions. In the course of a discussion or argument, it was often amazing and exciting to hear him cite reference after reference and even specific case histories to bring forth relevant data to his argument. One could not help but be impressed by the brilliance and scintillating verbal expression of his ideas and the basis for them. He was thin, tall, and of rather nervous temperament. He talked very fast but clearly and precisely, and one had to keep alert and attentive in order to get the full import of what he said.

I was not a student of Lashley's except in an indirect way, through the reading of his research articles and his brain mechanisms book. Also, I never missed an opportunity to hear him speak at the scientific meetings that I attended, and on a few occasions I was drawn into small groups for lunch with Lashley on a quite informal basis. Physiological psychologists were few in number during the 1930's and so tended to fraternize at meetings. Later, I had more extensive contacts and relations with Lashley. In 1943 I was called from Brown University to direct a radar-operation project sponsored by the Army Signal Corps and the Navy Bureau of Ships. A group of about 20 psychologists and I operated as civilians under the Office of Scientific Research and Development. The contract for our work was held by Yale University. Initially our project was located in the Army's Southern Signal Corps School in Hobe Sound, Florida, about 25 miles north of Palm Beach. Later, we were shifted to the U.S. Air Force Base at Boca Raton, Florida. It was felt that some representative of Yale should monitor our project, at least financially, and because Lashley was Director of the Yerkes Laboratories of Primate Biology at Orange Park, Florida, jointly coordinated by Yale and Harvard, it fell to him to become our "monitor." Actually, Lashley knew nothing about radar and could not have cared less about our activities, especially the financial matters, for as was pointed out by Frank A. Beach (1961) in the Biographical Memoir reprinted in this volume, Lashley was "completely impractical with respect to financial matters [p. 187]" and the family finances were handled by his wife. Fortunately, Henry W. Nissen, a colleague on Lashley's staff, had been trained as a Certified Public Accountant before becoming a psychologist and Lashley gladly turned over the financial monitoring of my project to him. Lashley, however, was most cordial and willing to discuss scientific matters each time I visited with them, and these discussions were a real joy and satisfaction to me as well as a diversion from the frenetic rush of our war-time research activities. On one occasion Lashley invited several members of my project to visit the Yerkes Laboratories and we drove up in my project's battered Pontiac station wagon and had a marvelous tour conducted by Lashley and Nissen, with lunch and a discussion afterwards. It was on this occasion that Lashley and Nissen warned our group not to get too close to the big outdoor cage in which one of their favorite big chimpanzees was kept, for he had a reputation of throwing things at visitors. He would get to the far end of the runway and then make a rapid, scaring, run and jump forcefully on the bars at the front of the cage. One of my group did not heed their warning and on one of the chimp's runs he scooped up a fistful of excrement and let it fly at our friend, soiling badly his white linen suit and causing him some chagrin and loss of interest!

My next opportunity to associate with Lashley came in the fall of 1948 when I was invited to participate in the Hixon Symposium on Cerebral Mechanisms in Behavior held at the California Institute of Technology. Dr. Lloyd A. Jeffress of the University of Texas was a visiting professor at Cal Tech in 1947-1948 and had planned and organized this conference. It was a very timely event, putting into focus many of the psychological and behavioral issues that a postwar impetus and new technologies for studying the brain and nervous system were once again beginning to stimulate. Also, the interdisciplinary character and approach of this conference as represented by its participants (see Fig. 15.1) signaled the beginning of widespread interest among those whose varied disciplines touched upon neuroscience in trying to understand behavior and psychological phenomena not only in terms of the structural organization (morphology and hodology) of the brain and nervous system but in terms of its functional organization and dynamics as well. The appearance of Hebb's (1949) book, *The Organization of Behavior,* the following year, and the extent to which it was found on the shelves of varied scientists ranging from anatomists to zoologists was probably a further indication of the increasing interdisciplinary character of brain research and the feeling on the part of many that there was a need for a "conceptual nervous system" that could speculatively go beyond the range of the empirical of that time. Along these lines, Lashley's chapter, "The Problem of Serial Order in Behavior," which appeared in the Hixon Symposium volume, is indeed a classic and one of his finest and most stimulating papers. It certainly elicited extensive discussion on the part of the participants. In his inimitable way Lashley drew from real-life situations, as well as from classical studies, examples of behavior and psychological phenomena that offered formidable challenges to brain and neural theory, including various hypotheses and theories of his own.

Fig. 15.2 shows Lashley in animated discussion with Wolfgang Köhler, the famous Gestalt psychologist, at a Society of Experimental Psychologists meeting in Princeton in 1947. In the movie from which this frame is taken, Lashley's repeated, rapid hand gestures, together with his typical staccato speech pattern, tend to illustrate his usual tense and involved manner. Whatever the issue, or stage of the argument being put forth by Lashley, Köhler did not appear to be impressed or convinced, for in this stretch of movie, he maintains a stolid, unexpressive downward gaze throughout!

Another frame from the movie (Fig. 15.3) shows Lashley in a more relaxed mood at the Princeton meeting while in friendly discussion with Frank A. Beach, then professor of comparative psychology at Yale but a former graduate assistant in neuropsychology with Lashley at Harvard in 1935-1936, and Henry W. Nissen, his Assistant Director at the Yerkes Laboratories.

My most extensive association with Lashley came in 1952 when we had several exchanges of correspondence. One such exchange seems worth recording

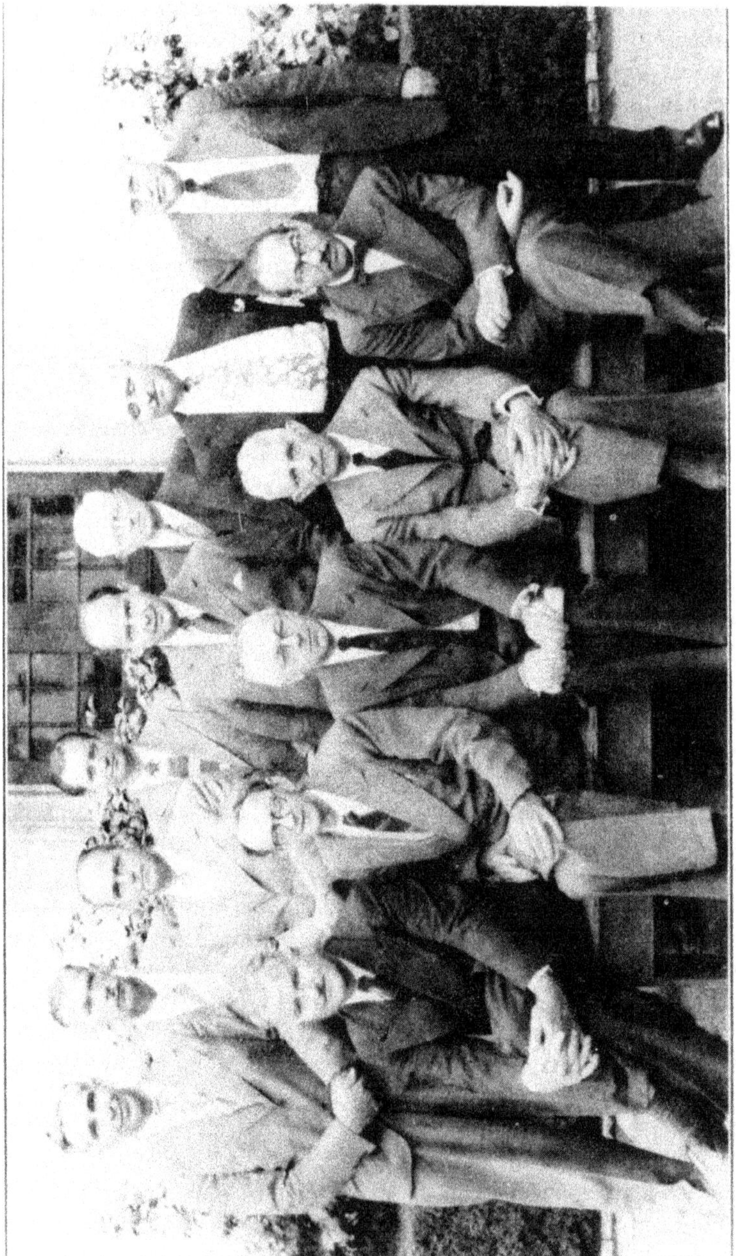

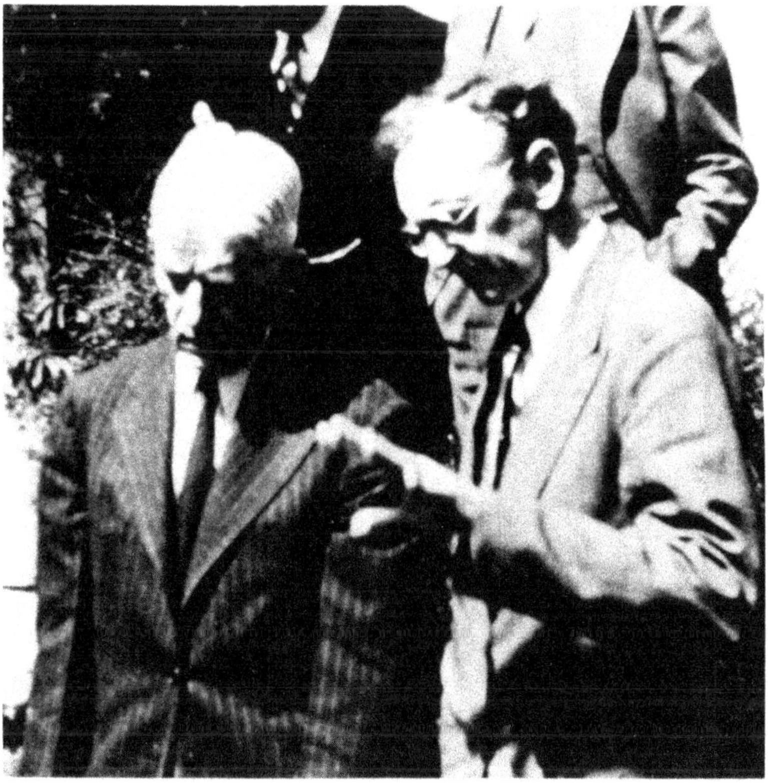

FIG. 15.2. Karl S. Lashley (gesturing) attempting to drive home a point with Wolfgang Köhler, German Gestalt psychologist, then at Swarthmore College. Köhler does not appear to be convinced! Discussion took place at the Princeton meeting of the Society of Experimental Psychologists, April, 1947. This frame is from the Donald B. Lindsley historical film, "Psychologists Here, There, and Everywhere." By permission.

FIG. 15.1. Members of the Hixon Symposium on Cerebral Mechanisms in Behavior held at the California Institute of Technology, from September 20-25, 1948. Identification of the members reflects the interdisciplinary character of the meeting. *Left to right:* (seated) Ward C. Halstead, *neuropsychologist,* U. of Chicago; Karl S. Lashley, *neuropsychologist,* Harvard and Yerkes Laboratories; Heinrich Klüver, *neuropsychologist,* U. of Chicago; Wolfgang Köhler, *Gestalt psychologist,* Swarthmore College; Rafael Lorente de No, *neuroanatomist,* Rockefeller Institute for Medical Research; (standing) Henry W. Brosin, *psychiatrist,* U. of Pittsburgh; Lloyd A. Jeffress, *experimental psychologist,* U. of Texas; Paul Weiss, *zoologist,* U. of Chicago; Donald B. Lindsley, *physiological psychologist,* Northwestern University; John von Neumann, *mathematician,* Institute for Advanced Study, Princeton University; J. M. Nielsen, *neurologist-psychiatrist,* U. of Southern California; Ralph W. Gerard, *physiologist,* U. of Chicago; Howard S. Liddell, *Pavlovian physiologist-psychologist,* Cornell University; Warren S. McCulloch, *neurophysiologist-psychiatrist,* U. of Illinois College of Medicine and Illinois Neuropsychiatric Institute (McCulloch absent from photo). This photo from frontispiece of L. A. Jeffress (Ed.), *Cerebral Mechanisms in Behavior: The Hixon Symposium,* New York: Wiley, 1951, is reproduced here by permission of the publisher.

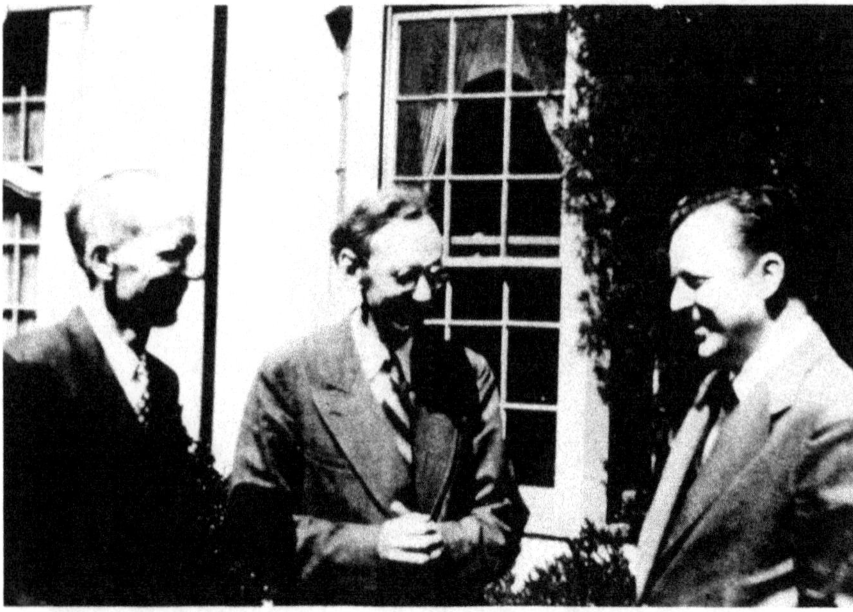

FIG. 15.3. *Left to right:* Henry W. Nissen, Assistant Director, Yerkes Laboratories, Orange Park, Florida; Karl S. Lashley, Director; Frank A. Beach, Yale University. Photo taken at the Princeton meeting of the Society of Experimental Psychologists, April, 1947. Printed from the Donald B. Lindsley historical film, "Psychologists Here, There, and Everywhere." By permission.

here in full for two reasons. First, having elected in the early days to pursue the relationships between brain and behavior by the lesion and ablation method, Lashley had apparently neglected to follow closely the initially primitive methods of electrophysiology, the development of the electroencephalogram, and the more intensive electrophysiological studies of the late 1930's and 1940's. His letter reflects his wish to try out some of his concepts about basic neurophysiology and electrophysiology and try to understand the possible role of brain waves in relation to *attention* and *vigilance*. Secondly, his letter and mine in reply provide some insight into the zeitgeist in neuroscience and behavior in the early 1950's.

YERKES LABORATORIES OF PRIMATE BIOLOGY, INC.
ORANGE PARK, FLORIDA
Conducted by Yale University and Harvard University

July 1, 1952

Dr. Donald B. Lindsley
Department of Psychology
University of California
Los Angeles, 24 California

Dear Dr. Lindsley:

I have been speculating a good bit of late about the significance of brain waves, especially in relation to the problems of attention, and was on the point of writing to you when I received your letter. The interpretations that you suggest are so different from mine that I should like to compare impressions and get your criticisms of my concepts. I have no first hand knowledge of electrical techniques (a year with the string galvanometer cured me of ambition in that direction), and I may be missing important material.

In attempting to understand the brain wave picture, I have made the following assumptions.

1. Neurons which are not stimulated or are stimulated at low intensity tend to build up excitability and fire "spontaneously," their activities becoming synchronized as a result of spreading electric current (Weiss, motor cells implanted in tail fin).
2. Groups of cortical cells firing synchronously block their own transmission at synapses. (Strong stimulation of the cortex does not spread; strychnine spikes do not cross synapses.) The mechanism of blocking might fit with the Pitts-McCulloch theory of inhibition.
3. The associative cortex is a homogeneous band extending from the parietal lobe to the frontal pole. The median dorsal nucleus and pulvinar form a similar thalamic band projecting to the cortical. Different parts of the band are not specialized for function, except as they differ in input from adjacent areas or thalamic nuclei.
4. Under conditions of low sensory input and low associative activity, parts of the cortex develop spontaneous rhythmic firing which is blocked from conduction and incapable of arousing any organized activity. The frequencies are determined by the inherent character of the tissue. (I was led to this view by the fortification figures of migraine, which I take to be the wave of excitation preceding a spreading depression (Jasper) and which seem to have the alpha frequency.)
5. This non-functional rhythmic activity is detected as the alpha and other rhythms. When attention develops the rhythmic activity is destroyed. It perhaps develops in the associative cortex where there is little spread from sensory areas.
6. Different types of attention involve different mechanisms.
    a. Sensory. Strong input to a sensory area dominates its activity, spreads to other areas and arouses associative patterns. No extraneous facilitation is required.
    b. Sensory reinforcement. I am set to cancel all the "A's" on a page of advertisements. The associative process sets up some sort of generalized pattern of facilitation. This is perhaps somehow tied up with the space-coordinate system (perhaps a sort of central postural tonus representing the sequence of directions of the lines of the "A." My present speculations concerning stimulus equivalence are emphasizing relations to a sort of premotor organization).
    c. Vigilance. This concept of Head's may represent some sort of general level of reinforcement. One is tempted to look to the reticular complex for it, but I am suspicious of a multiplicity of functions always ascribed to newly discovered systems. It may be metabolic.

All this sounds pretty wild, but I feel that there are serious objections to other interpretations also. First with regard to speculations concerning a scanning mechanism. The theory of Pitts-McCulloch, as applied to the problem of transposition, seems to me to be absolutely ruled out by considerations of anatomy and comparative psychology. They postulate transcortical connections of different lengths producing duplicate patterns at different cortical levels, with scanning in depth. I am positive that there are no such connections. In the auditory cortex their theory of chord transposition demands that the diagonal fibers extend throughout the auditory range. In the much touted Cajal picture, the fibers actually cover only a few cell diameters—a minute distance compared with the extent of the auditory cortex. Similarly in the striate cortex the horizontal fibers of their diagram would have to extend over the full area in which size transposition occurs (2 or 3 cm in the rhesus brain). My own Marchi work on the rat and Clark's on the monkey have not shown intracortical fibers in the visual area longer than a few cell diameters.

All of the sensory phenomena in vision and audition of mammals are also present in birds. The talking shell-parakeet imitates human intonation at a quite different pitch level with its soft whispering voice. The visual organization of birds is not demonstrably different from the human. The mechanisms of these sensory organizations are therefore probably more primitive than those of thalamo-cortical organization. Electrical studies of birds should be of great value in giving a basis for interpreting the mammalian picture.

The scanning theory of P-M overlooks the essential point of the problem of visual recognition. You will recall in Descartes' theory of scanning by the pineal body the statement, "it is thus that the soul knows that it is this which it wishes to remember." The P-M theory provides for reduplicated patterns but does not provide for the set which selects the recorded pattern. The scanning beams must be set to reinforce a particular pattern, wherever and in whatever size it occurs on the striate cortex. The theory provides no mechanism for this and with a different mechanism to set the pattern, there is no need for scanning.

These considerations make me feel that the concept of scanning, such as might be represented by the alpha wave, is not a profitable hypothesis. There is another set of phenomena which does seem to call for some scanning mechanism but this is a relatively slow process. It is the translation of a spatial pattern into a temporal series—for example, describing from memory a complicated piece of apparatus, where one can start at any point and survey the parts successively.

I also doubt that the alpha cycle is facilitative. I am not sure that I understand aright your comment on lack of smearing during eye-movements. A small neon lamp on 60 cycle AC in a dark room describes clear arcs of dots or dashes with eye movements, showing that there is no discontinuity of vision while the eye moves. The apparent suppression of vision during movement seems to occur only when the pattern is complex.

Brightness enhancement might be due, not to reinforcement by the alpha wave as such but to the fact that the frequency coincides with the natural frequency of the tissue. This possibility would have to be considered, I think, in all attempts to correlate functions with the alpha rhythm.

We have not confirmed Kennard on area 8. I have gone over her protocols and her results were very erratic. George Clark got the temporary amblyopia from removal of the entire lateral surface of the prefrontal lobe but not from destroying the eye field alone. I have seen an apraxia from the removal of area 8, without the visual symptoms. Removal of area 8 combined with 18 and 19 does not produce any permanent detectable disturbance of visual attention or perception in monkeys.

I should appreciate your reactions to all this and a reprint of your discussion when it appears. I am working over my Vanuxem lectures, in which I attempted unsuccessfully to tell how the brain thinks, and am thoroughly stymied with the problem of attention.

Sincerely yours,

Lashley

K. S. Lashley
Director

KSL:beb

UNIVERSITY OF CALIFORNIA

Department of Psychology
Los Angeles 24, California

July 24, 1952

Dr. K. S. Lashley
Director, Yerkes Laboratories
of Primate Biology
Orange Park, Fla.

Dear Dr. Lashley:

I am very sorry that your most interesting and thought-provoking letter has gone unanswered for so long. I have been working pretty steadily for the past two or three weeks with Dr. Magoun in the laboratories at Long Beach, and am in the midst of many details in getting my laboratory set up here in the psychology department. I hope you will pardon my delay in sitting down to answer your challenging questions.

The questions you raise are all very good ones and I am not sure I am up to the task of giving very adequate answers, but I will try to comment on each of the points you raise, taking them in order.

1. I do not agree with your first assumption as it stands, because I do not believe that the "spontaneous" electrical activity (alpha and other rhythms) of aggregates of nerve cells provides any indication that the individual cell "fires" or discharges a nerve impulse. Rather I am inclined to believe, and I think there is both older and newer evidence to support it, that nerve cells wherever they are found, but especially in aggregates, are constantly giving rise to an electrical change on or near the surface of the cell body. This I believe is a function of the intrinsic metabolic activity of the cell, which in a resting state is somewhere around 10 alternations of positivity to negativity per second. This varies somewhat for the different species, as it does also in man whose alpha rhythm ranges from

8 to 12 or 13 per second. One of the fundamental questions is whether the alpha wave of approximately 1/10 second in duration is composed of similar slow electrical changes in the individual cells which somehow come to ''beat'' more or less in unison, or whether there are short bursts of faster potentials which form a kind of envelope with the slow alpha wave as the total summation of such rapid discharges in aggregates of cells. There is some evidence that both processes may occur. Adrian and Matthews (1934) attempted to record cortical response from individual neurons and concluded that cortical waves are summations of temporally dispersed faster components in individual neurons. Renshaw et al. (1940) using microelectrodes in the hippocampal region of the cat found both slow and rapid potential fluctuations. More recently Thomas (Seattle) presented a paper at the spring Atlantic City meeting of the EEG Society which showed both slow and fast components, and Jasper in March at the Macy Conference on the Nerve Impulse reported a similar thing, with some slow components of about 10 per second and some faster spike-like waves.

If the myriads of individual nerve cells actually discharged an impulse (accompanied by an axonal spike-discharge) with each alpha wave it would seem that the nervous system (and behavior) would be in an extremely chaotic state.

My own thoughts on this matter are that the alpha rhythm of about 10/sec in human adults represents the synchronized waxing and waning of thousands of cells in some kind of chemical or metabolic process which gives rise to a minute potential in the individual cell, but a recordable rhythmically oscillating potential when thousands are in synchrony. This state seems to exist only when a person is relaxed and in the presence of minimal stimuli to which he is presumably adapted. The slightest change in environmental stimuli (especially if an appropriate ''set'' is present, but also often if no ''set'' has been established and the new stimulus is unexpected) may then disrupt the synchrony of the alpha beat, destroying the alpha rhythm as such, by virtue of desynchronization. But, not destroying the basic 10 per second alpha activity of the individual cell or smaller aggregates of these cells which may still beat in unison. The result of this desynchronization is to block or reduce the large alpha rhythm of the resting state, and because the myriads of cells in such a state of ''alertness'' or ''attention'' or possibly a new or directed ''set'' are now waxing and waning more or less at random or in smaller aggregates, it seems to me that it means that incoming stimuli via classical sensory pathways now find a greater range of associative possibilities. In order to explain this last statement, I must now make an assumption, which I believe has some evidence in its support. This is that with each waxing and waning of the metabolic or cellular potential there is a corresponding waxing and waning of *excitability* of the individual cell. Therefore the timing of incoming impulses must jibe with the particular phase of the excitability cycle of a given cell (and its aggregates or associates if some kind of previous conditioning or habit association has been built up) if it is to excite that cell and its associates. This does not imply a simple switchboard arrangement of cells but probably some kind of ''cell assembly'' arrangement (Hebb). Furthermore it seems to me that in the initial establishment of habit formation and subsequent reinforcement of the learning that many aggregates of cells (or assemblies) may become alternative links in this particular behavior, since their excitability cycles might with each successive stimulation represent favorably disposed aggregates for response at that given moment, rather than a previous aggregate which responded earlier. This would represent a statistical sampling of aggregates during the establishment of any habit pattern. This is why I believe that when the resting alpha rhythm is blocked and desynchronization of the individual cellular rhythms occurs, there is a much greater possibility of incoming impulses to find a given aggregate of cells in a suitable excitability phase (or to put it another way, a much wider range of associative possibilities). However, once a continuing stimulus makes this coincidence with the excitability phase of an aggregate of cells it presumably continues to remain "locked-in" with it and one might say that this represents the focussing of attention to the exclusion of other sensory avenues, except when they succeed in breaking through. This breaking through, I believe may be accomplished through activation of the reticular system, which seems to have the power to disrupt tendencies to synchronism of cells (especially in associative areas—see Moruzzi and Magoun and Starzl and Magoun). A new sensory influx via the reticular activating system may thus reset excitability cycles or so modify them as to break any previous "locking-in" and make available new channels of excitation.

Moruzzi and Magoun demonstrated that stimulation of the brain stem reticular formation electrically will produce an "activated" cortex, i.e., a desynchronized, fast picture of the electrocortical activities, even though a highly synchronized state existed in a nebutalized animal up to time of stimulation, or a less synchronized state in an unanesthetized animal existed previously. Lindsley, Bowden and Magoun showed in acute preparations (encephale isole) the significance of the reticular system to this "activation" or desynchronizing process, for with its gradual elimination by successively higher or more rostral sections activation of the cortex became less possible even though the lateral (classical) afferent pathways in the midbrain region were left intact and only the tegmental region was interrupted. When the tegmental interruption (in cat) was at the rostral end of the midbrain, only synchronized waves resembling those of sleep existed. Upon stimulation through the remaining afferent pathways desynchronization occurred but only momentarily; it was not persisting activation of the cortex. Lindsley, Schreiner, Knowles and Magoun demonstrated the same thing in chronic, unanesthetized preparations. And French and Magoun have shown this also in the monkey. French has also assembled data upon human patients with lesions in the midbrain tegmentum and hypothalamus which bear this out in terms of their behavioral symptoms, namely comatose states etc. The work of Starzl, Magoun, et al. have further defined the relations of sensory stimulation (sciatic, auditory etc.) to activation via the reticular system when the lateral afferent pathways are interrupted. All the evidence (and there is a good deal more than I have cited here) indicates that the afferent pathways by means of collaterals in the brain stem region excite the reticular system, so that even with the afferent pathways interrupted rostrally to these collaterals the cortex can be "activated" (this is probably not a good term since the actual result seems to be desynchronization of cortical potentials). Starzl and Magoun have shown that the recruiting response (Morison and Dempsey) elicited from certain thalamic areas seems to be limited to the associative cortex, plus the motor region, but not primary sensory areas. However, activation via reticular formation seems to be more widespread, although there may be something in common between these two types of phenomena since at least in the thalamic area they may involve common anatomical structures. (Perhaps I should not have introduced the "recruiting phenomena" here, for its mechanism and functions have not been resolved and certainly do not clarify our concept of the activation system at the moment.)

Under separate cover I have sent a batch of reprints which furnish some of the documentation by Dr. Magoun and his group. However, he should not be held responsible for all I have said here, for I am not sure he agrees with all I read into the basic results in terms of explanation of psychological phenomena. I keep struggling with these problems, as you do, and I am sure you appreciate the difficulties involved of attempting to bring two or more areas of data together. I am also sending a reprint of my chapter on Emotions in the Hdbk of Exp'l, since some discussion of the "activation" concept was brought in there toward the end of the chapter.

2. Your point about cortical cells firing synchronously block their own transmission at synapses (strong stim. of cortex doesn't spread, strychnine spikes do not cross synapses). This does not appear to be true, certainly epileptic discharges spread, whether they are naturally aroused or by electrical stimulation from a focal point. Also the strychnine story is only partly true—McCulloch and D de B. did their work under Dial; under chlorolasane the story is different, or in an unanesthetized cortex. Furthermore, there is spreading of the effect, though not the spike per se—there is diffusion at the synapses rather than blocking, and the diffuse responses are much smaller and not registered as large spikes.

3. I don't understand this statement completely. However I think the work of Starzl and Magoun on the recruiting mechanism, and also that of Dempsey and Morison, have a distinct bearing on what I believe to be the concept you are expressing here. The fact that the recruiting responses initiated by electrical stimulation in the intralaminar and other portions of the thalamus have been delimited to the various associative cortices plus the motor region, but exclusive of the primary sensory areas, would seem to be consistent with your concept of homogeneity, apparently arrived at from quite different data. Also Verzeano, Lindsley and Magoun (in press J. Neurophysiol.) have found quite similar latencies of the recruiting effect in these various cortical areas.

4. This I believe I answered under 1. Again you seem to have a quite different concept than I do of the spontaneous, or autonomous activities of the cortex. I do not believe they lead to conduction or firing of the neuron at all, they simply reflect its waxing and waning excitability and availability to serve as a conducting unit. The whole concept of spreading depression seems to be so confused that I believe most people are ready to write it off—Marshall thinks it mainly a physiological condition of the cortex (drying etc.), others seem to be in very big disagreement about its existence and/or function.

5. This again has been covered under 1. Distraction or selective focussing of attention certainly seems to disrupt the alpha rhythm, but again I do not believe it disturbs the basic alpha activity cycle of the individual cell other than to break up its synchronous beat with other large aggregates of cells. The result of this on the record is of course a reduction or complete abolition of the *alpha rhythm* as such, and the picture is always one of reduced

amplitude, sometimes as if two or more groups of cells at 10/sec were beating with phase relationships which make possible a multiple of the original alpha rhythm, at other times just low level fast activity as if many cells were beating at random. With cessation of light as a stimulus for blocking there is a gradual recovery of the alpha rhythm in about 1 second and then a rebound lasting perhaps a second, as if an optimum state of synchronization occurred but did not hold indefinitely.

6a. This I believe is true, but I would not say with no extraneous facilitation required, if we consider the reticular system as extraneous. The effect of direct sensory stimulation via thalamic relays is to produce at the primary sensory cortex an evoked potential, often both "on" and "off". However, the influences of the same stimulus via the brain stem collaterals and the reticular system is more pervasive and may outlast the stimulus by many seconds—keeping cortical areas desynchronized much longer than the sensory influx via direct pathways.

6b. Sensory reinforcement. I agree in part, but I wonder if this central "set" to cancel "A's" although necessarily specific to some space coordinate system which permits identification of the task, may not also play back upon the reticular system in order to maintain the basic state of "vigilance" or attention necessary to the task. At least Magoun and I believe that other influences than peripheral sensory influx play a role in the reticular activating system. Alertness or set or attention may certainly be aroused by central as well as peripheral "stimuli"—that is ideas, instructions, etc. as well as actual physical stimuli.

6c. Vigilance. I am not too familiar with this concept of Head's, but I believe I understand what is meant. It is more of a "state" of readiness or attention which persists over a period of time or which may be characteristic of one individual rather than another. Certainly the individual differences in brain wave patterns ranging from desynchronized to highly synchronized, almost sinusoidal alphas, would suggest this. It does not suggest a general tone of alertness or attention maintained either by metabolic factors, or by autonomic and somatic sensory levels of influx to the reticular system.

The remainder of your letter is extremely interesting and valuable to me but it almost defies any very comprehensive discussion of it in a letter such as this. There are just too many facets to be discussed. I can only make a few scattered remarks now, and hope that we may have time to sit down informally and really hash it over. I have thought many times that it would be a valuable thing to get two or three people who are sincerely interested in these problems for informal and prolonged discussions of the problems from their different points of view and approaches. One gets so inevitably bound to the particular approach he has been limited to, that unless he can be faced with the challenges of others who are looking in at the same thing from a different angle he is apt to miss the really significant problems, or spend his time seeking the wrong kind of information. I hope we can get together sometime. I personally feel overwhelmed with the amount of data there are to be integrated into this tremendous picture, and from time to time would greatly welcome the additional assurance and security one gets from an opportunity to talk it over with someone else, regardless of whether there is agreement on all points. I also constantly feel so ignorant of the many facts, both psychological and neurophysiological, which have to be considered.

I think your point about electrical studies in birds is very well taken. I am currently working with the cat on the visual mechanism, recording simultaneously from the optic tract, lateral geniculate and cortex, the response to repetitive photic stimulation. The preliminary results are very interesting in that the cortex does not seem to be able to follow everything that the optic tract and lateral geniculates do. The number of parameters to be investigated, intensity, duration, frequency, l-d ratio, area of cortex, region of thalamus and midbrain etc. is going to make it a long study. I feel sure, however, it can be broken up considerably by taking one parameter at a time. I am also planning some similar studies in the human, but not of course with probing electrodes in the depth of the brain—in the human I will have the advantage at least of the subjective report and will be able to investigate what is perceived when the brain is functioning differently than in the non-stimulated resting state. I may want to try something with birds later, after this mechanism becomes a little clearer to me in cats and monkeys.

The scanning concept of McC and P. is not essential to my view, although a scanning concept (not necessarily that which they propose) may be useful. I think we need much more information about the individual cell's response by microelectrode technique which several laboratories are now using and which we expect to be using here soon. Also we need much more information about the limits, and extent of spread of influence from one aggregate of autonomously beating cells to another. That is, how cells become synchronized into smaller or larger groups so far as these alpha activities (excitability cycles) are concerned. The problem of how much they are controlled by thalamic pacemakers, or thalamo-cortical loops, or what not is still very much unsettled. There does seem to be evidence that isolated cortex can develop a rhythmic beat independent of connections with the thalamus or other subcortical regions, but likewise there is evidence that synchrony of activity in cortex and thalamus is the rule when the connections are intact (see Lindsley, Bowden and Magoun).

You present very telling arguments against the McC.-P. concepts. Likewise your other arguments are all very well taken. My lack of comment about them is more one of ignorance than lack of appreciation; also, I have been stimulated to harrangue at such great length about some of my views.

I am enclosing my only copy of the ms. submitted to Jasper for publication in the EEG Clin. Neurophysiol. journal as part of the Atlantic City Symposium. Will you kindly return it and the figures after you have had a chance to read it.

Sincerely yours,

Donald B. Lindsley

P.S. Under separate cover I have already sent a group of reprints from Dr. Magoun's laboratory.

Note: For those interested, an attempt has been made to identify work referred to in these two letters. These references are included among others at the end of the chapter.

In 1952, when these letters were written, there was a considerable state of confusion with respect to the understanding of behavior and psychological processes in terms of neuroanatomy and neurophysiology. Neuroanatomy had gradually become less morphological and more functional in emphasis; neurophysiology had become more electrophysiological and less dependent upon gross ablation procedures. Technical developments emerging from World War II led to refinements in electronic equipment for stimulating local structures deep in the brain and for recording locally from them without disturbing overlying brain tissue. Microelectrodes capable of isolating the electrical response of single cells in the brain and DC amplifiers introduced before the war were both further refined and gradually coming into use. Electronic computers, in somewhat primitive forms, were beginning to be adapted for use in neuroscience. These and other advances, plus educational and scientific support via government agencies themselves newly established in the 1950's, were beginning to make it possible to develop laboratories and research teams for undertaking more difficult problems and research programs. Furthermore, the inevitable aftermath of war left many veterans with brain injuries, which caused investigators and clinicians to think more broadly about brain and behavior correlations, as was the case after World War I some 30 years earlier. But let us turn the clock back a little to see how we got where we were in the early post-World War II period.

Historical Introduction

In the second decade of the 20th century, when Lashley got his training and began to strike out on an independent research career, there was a considerable body of knowledge about the brain and nervous system that had accumulated mainly during the period from 1850 to 1900, but that came to a focus during the decades immediately before and after the turn of the century. There was a linking of neuroanatomy and neuropathology with clinical neurology by the famous neurologist, John Hughlings Jackson (1835–1911), of the National Hospital for Nervous Diseases in Queen Square, London. Also, the work on cerebral anatomy of the well-known Scottish neurologist-neuropathologist David Ferrier (1843–1928) contributed much to an understanding of the functions of the brain and to cerebral localization of function, which led to advances in neurosurgery. Ferrier held professorships in medicine and neuropathology at King's College, London.

There was a linking of neuroanatomy and neurophysiology, and the development of a concept of integration in the nervous system, by the highly esteemed physiologist, Charles Scott Sherrington (1856–1952). His famous book, *The Integrative Action of the Nervous System* (1906), was reprinted many times and the second edition published in 1947 had a second printing in 1948. Sherrington spent the first half of his career at the University of Liverpool where he collaborated with H. E. Hering, A. S. F. Grünbaum, A. Frölich, E. E. Laslett, T. Graham Brown, and others. The latter half of his long and distinguished scientific career was at Oxford University where he had many students and collaborators, among them E. G. T. Liddell, D. E. Denny-Brown, Sybil Cooper, R. S. Creed, J. C. Eccles, and John F. Fulton.

The neurologist-neurosurgeon Otfrid Foerster (1873–1941) of the University of Breslau contributed importantly to the structure and function of the nervous system, and especially to neurosurgery. Many others, of course, made contributions during the latter half of the 19th century and the early part of the 20th century that led to a better understanding of the structure and function of the brain, the peripheral nervous system, the sense organs, and the effectors; included among these are Johannes Müller, Du Bois-Reymond, Helmholtz, Sechenov, Wundt, E. H. Weber, Golgi, Ramon y Cajal, von Economo, Brodmann, and others. Pavlov (1849–1936) was awarded a Nobel Prize in Physiology and Medicine in 1904 for his earlier work on the neural mechanisms of digestive functions. Thereafter he began a whole new career in research and writing on conditioned reflexes, for which he is even better known. In this work his approach was behavioral and physiological with respect to the sensory and effector systems involved in conditioned responses, but largely inferential so far as brain function was concerned.

Missing, to a large extent, in the foregoing was the linking of neuroanatomy and neurophysiology with behavior and the higher cognitive functions of humans. The psychologist Edward Lee Thorndike (1876–1949), although not especially interested in or knowledgeable about the brain and nervous system per se, was involved in the careful qualitative and quantitative study of behavior in chicks, cats, dogs, monkeys, and humans, thus being a true comparative psychologist. Later, he became completely fixed in his interests upon the theory and measurement of learning and intelligence in humans. Thorndike, in his early studies of the behavior of animals, and Shepherd Ivory Franz (1874–1933), a neuropsychologist who studied behavior and cognitive functions in rats, monkeys, and humans where ablations or brain lesions were involved, were probably the principal influences upon Lashley that eventually directed him into brain and behavior research studies in animals. He was also aided in his studies and interest in behavior by the behavioral psychologist John Broadus Watson (1878–1958), who was professor of experimental and comparative psychology and director of the laboratory at Johns Hopkins from 1908 to 1920. Franz held positions as professor of physiology and psychology at George Washington University and at St. Elizabeth's Hospital in Washington, D.C. He worked with human patients with mental and neural disorders and he did brain ablations in monkeys and chimpanzees in order to determine their behavioral deficits. In this work he was certainly a pioneer. Although Lashley took his Ph.D. in genetics in the Zoology Department at Johns Hopkins, and published a few studies with S. O. Mast and H. S. Jennings on paramecia, he also published with Watson, indicating that he had divided interests between zoology and psychology. In 1917 he began work with Franz at St. Elizabeth's Hospital, while holding a fellowship at Johns Hopkins. It was from Franz that Lashley learned operative technique and histological procedures in vertebrates, especially the rat, on which they published two studies in 1917 dealing with learning and memory and the effect of brain ablations (Franz & Lashley, 1917; Lashley & Franz, 1917). Lashley, however, was his own man, and began his subsequent studies quite independently and set his own goals, one of which was the subject of the 1929 book that these lectures memorialize.

It was during this second decade of the 20th century, when Lashley was getting his start in research, that electrophysiology was coming into prominence. In 1903, Willem Einthoven, a Dutch physiologist, devised and adapted the string galvanometer for registering the electrical activity of the heart (elektrokardiogramm or EKG). This instrument was quickly put to use by other physiologists to study the electrical activity of muscles and nerves, among them Alexander Forbes of the Harvard Medical School, with whom I had the privilege of working in 1933-1935. Others engaged in this type of work were Keith Lucas and his student, E. D. Adrian of Cambridge University. In their recording they used the capillary electrometer rather than the string galvanometer.

Initially, the string galvanometer and other sensitive recording instruments such as the electrometer were used without amplification, but when made sensitive enough, the fine quartz string of the galvanometer tended to break with each surge of current, thus making its use often a frustrating experience. As an outcome of the development and use of radio communication during World War I, Forbes and Thacher (1920) applied electron tube amplification to the string galvanometer. This permitted the use of less sensitive and more durable quartz strings and allowed recording of nerve and muscle potentials of moderate frequency. Gasser and Erlanger (1922), at Washington University in St. Louis, soon discovered that the cathode ray tube (invented by Karl F. Braun, physicist of Tübingen, and then known as the Braun tube) could be adapted, with suitable amplification, to recording the rapid variations of potential that accompany transmission of the nerve impulse. Their subsequent analysis of the compound potential of the nerve trunk won for them the Nobel Award in Physiology and Medicine in 1944. Prior to that, in 1932, Sherrington and Adrian shared the Nobel Award in Physiology and Medicine for their respective studies of reflexes and electrical activity of neurons. (Also included was Thomas Hunt Morgan in genetics.)

It is interesting that Hans Berger, a German neuropsychiatrist at the University of Jena, was the first to record human brain potentials from electrodes on the surface of the scalp and publish his results in 1929. He had been struggling with various physiological measures of brain state (brain circulation by plethysmography and electrical activity) in the hope of finding physiological correlates of psychological states and functions, during the period from 1910–1914 but with little success. Using the Lippmann capillary electrometer and the Edelmann string galvanometer, as early as 1910 Berger attempted to record brain potentials through trepanations of the skull of humans and dogs. Later, in 1924, he began again to try to record potentials from the brain of humans, but now using a more sensitive string galvanometer, though still without amplification. Finally, he was successful and published his results before anyone else had done so. When they learned about Berger's publication the electrophysiologists of that time were incredulous and believed the phenomena he described were artifactual! However, their attitudes changed when they learned that Adrian and Matthews (1934) had published confirmation of Berger's results. Soon thereafter, Jasper and Carmichael (1935) of Brown University and Bradley Hospital in Providence and Gibbs, Davis, and Lennox (1935) of Boston City Hospital and the Harvard Medical School added their confirmations of Berger's articles, which now began to appear in a steady stream, mainly in the *Archiv für Psychiatrie und Nervenkrankheiten* (e.g. 1932, 1938), until he was forced out of his laboratory by the Nazis in 1938. Thereafter he became increasingly depressed and despondent over his incredible mistreatment at the hands of the Hitler government then in control of the university, and he took his own life in June of 1941 at the age of 68 (see Gloor, 1969).

It is small wonder that Lashley, struggling in post-World War I days to establish a research program and to try to study behavior and psychological functions in terms of the brain and nervous system, elected not to go in the direction of the string galvanometer, which, without amplification, could scarcely record muscle and nerve potentials and offered at the time little hope of utilization in connection with brain and behavior study in animals. Instead, he chose to attack the brain directly and delimit its behavioral and psychological functions by operative procedures, making ablations in various regions of the brain of the rat. In relation to this work, in which he was encouraged and instructed by Franz, nearly 100 years after the French physiologist Flourens (1824) had used a similar ablation approach in birds and various animals in successfully disproving the hypotheses of Gall and Spurzheim with regard to phrenology and the strict localization of function it required in the brain.

Considering the conflict of opinions among American psychologists and educators about the nature, definition, and measurement of intelligence, it is surprising that in summarizing his studies of the 1920's Lashley (1929) used the word "intelligence" in the title of his monograph. In part this may have been due to the influence of Thorndike, who initially was motivated to do animal behavioral studies of learning and intelligence, and who subsequently did much theorizing and investigation of human learning with the goal of understanding intelligence and its measurement. Also, the period of World War I was one of challenge to psychologists of that day to demonstrate that they could develop tests of intelligence and performance that might be used for the selection and employment of men in various military tasks. After the war they were expected to develop tests for the assessment of brain injury, the selection and placement of students in schools, and use in industry. There was markedly increased development and use of intelligence and achievement tests during the 1920's and 1930's, but the vigorous argument about the nature of intelligence and its measurement persisted, even as it does today! Lashley was no doubt caught up in this problem of the theory of intelligence and may have sought to help clarify the issue by the results of his studies of maze and discrimination learning and memory in rats.

Despite the stock market crash of 1929 and the severe economic depression that followed during the 1930's, electrophysiology continued to grow and thrive along with the further developments in electronics that accompanied the growth of radio broadcasting and other applications. At that time there were no suppliers of ready-made equipment. Each laboratory had to develop its own resources and it was customary at the start to publish a description of one's amplifiers and recording equipment in some detail and to provide a graph of the overall frequency-response curves of the amplifier-recorder system. Usually the equipment had been made and assembled by the investigator or someone in the laboratory, or by local electrical engineers or physicists who were willing to help.

The main applications of electrophysiological recording of that era were to try to understand the nature of the nerve impulse in simple and compound nerves, the manner in which physical energy applied to various receptors gets transduced into excitations that generate nerve impulses, how these impulses are conducted over sensory nerves to the spinal cord or brain stem, and how reflexes at various levels result in motor discharges that in turn excite muscles to contract and elicit electrical responses of their own (electromyogram or EMG). For the first time the recording of sensory-nerve responses in single fibers afforded an exciting opportunity to try to understand the manner in which stimulus properties could be coded and transmitted to the central nervous system.

Adrian's (1928) little book, *The Basis of Sensation: The Action of Sense Organs,* was an important starting point, and was soon followed by *The Mechanism of Nervous Action: Electrical Studies of the Neurone* (Adrian, 1932), which dealt with the action of various sense receptors, pain, sensory- and motor-nerve discharges, and even suggested a new type of nonspike activity—that is, slow waves recorded in the abdominal ganglia of the water beetle (Adrian, 1931) and in the isolated brain stem of the goldfish (Adrian & Buytendijk, 1931). Curiously, at the time of the publication of these latter two studies as reported in this book (Adrian, 1932), no mention was made of the similar slow waves (alpha waves) reported by Berger (1929) as recorded from the human brain in the EEG, which suggests that Berger's publication was not known to them. Indeed, up to that time, Berger's work had not been acknowledged by any electrophysiologists, either because they were not accustomed to reading the journal in which it was published, or because they felt it could not be "true" and probably had to be an artifact mistaken by an investigator inexperienced in electrophysiology. The attitude then was that everyone "knew" that potentials in the nervous system occurred only in the form of brief, discrete spikes, such as were observed in sensory and motor nerves, and not slow waves of longer duration. Fortunately, Berger lived long enough to see his original findings confirmed by Adrian and Matthews in 1934, and subsequently by many others. His long series of papers continuing up to 1938 made numerous other contributions, particularly with regard to the EEG patterns of epilepsy and other neurological disorders. Berger, being a psychiatrist, was disappointed that in two major areas of psychiatric disorder, manic-depressive psychosis and schizophrenia, in the absence of complicating factors, the EEG often showed essentially normal tracings. Similar results were obtained later by others.

While many things were happening in neurophysiology during the 1930's and 1940's, electrophysiology continued to play a leading role. (For a review of electroencephalography during this era, see Lindsley, 1944.) The EEG took two principal directions of expansion, one along normative lines, the other along clinical and abnormal lines. The normative line utilized the EEG as an index and correlate of physiological and psychological changes related to cortical development, as an index of changes related to consciousness ranging from sleep to arousal and to alertness and attention, and as a monitor of changes in electrical activity (synchrony-desynchrony, activation-deactivation, etc.) induced by drugs, shifts in constancy of physiological state or homeostasis, and by affective and emotional arousal. The second direction was an applied one related to clinical conditions of abnormality, particularly neurological disorders involving interruption or loss of consciousness due to epileptic seizures, encephalitis, intracerebral pressure, trauma to the brain, and cerebrovascular inadequacies. A great variety of slow and fast activity outside the normal range often accompanied various neurological conditions. Such abnormal activity might be diffuse or localized, unilateral or bilateral, continuous or episodic. Along with several other methods of evaluating neurological state or condition of the brain, the EEG has taken its place as a diagnostic and evaluative procedure. Furthermore, it has made possible the experimental study of various clinical conditions in which monitoring devices such as the EEG, EMG, and EKG are applicable and valuable. It has also been found useful during neurological surgery where anesthetic state and level are important to the viability of the patient.

Thus electrophysiology generally, and the EEG specifically, became important methods for the investigation of brain and behavior relationships. Berger (1929, 1930, 1931, 1932), Adrian and Matthews (1934), Jasper and Carmichael (1935) and Gibbs, Davis, and Lennox (1935) set the stage for the use of the EEG and thus focused renewed attention upon the brain as the organ of the mind and consciousness, and the EEG as an important correlate and monitor of brain activity associated with behavioral state and psychological processes such as arousal, alertness, and attention.

Bremer (1935, 1936, 1938) demonstrated that contrasting behavioral and electrocortical effects could be obtained in the cat by transection of the neuraxis at the junction of the spinal cord and medulla (encephale isolé) or at the junction of the midbrain and hypothalamus (cerveau isolé). The former preparation manifested essentially normal waking and sleeping behavior and appropriately corresponding electrocortical activity, whereas the latter preparation was continually in a deep-sleep phase behaviorally and electrocortically and could only momentarily be aroused and activated slightly by cortical or diencephalic stimulation. Bremer's initial interpretation was that the interruption of flow of sensory impulses through classical sensory pathways to cerebral neural networks was responsible for the decrease of wakefulness to sleep with loss of consciousness, and therefore only the more rostral transection ahead of cranial sensory-nerve influx could effectively induce sleep and maintain it. The more caudal transection (encephale isolé) would eliminate spinal sensory influx but not that from the cranial nerves. Although Bremer's initial interpretation of these experiments was not entirely correct, the experiments themselves and the results were very important in stimulating more investigations and in engendering more thought about the neural mechanisms of sleep and wakefulness.

About this time Kleitman (1939) published an extensive book on *Sleep and Wakefulness* (revised in 1963) in which he reviewed old and new theories of sleep and summarized much empirical and clinical data, including some of his own studies with regard to the pattern and duration of sleep cycles. Prominent in Kleitman's position was the concept of sleep as a passive process and of wakefulness as an active process dependent on afferent impulses affecting a surmised diencephalic wakefulness center. This all fitted in well with his evolutionary concept of sleep and wakefulness and with the notion that there is a "wakefulness of necessity" associated with an increase in internal (visceral) and external (sensory) influx, and a "wakefulness of choice" associated with habit, learning, conditioning, and memory of past experience when higher cognitive functions are strongly motivated and stimulated. These were thought to facilitate or inhibit hypothalamic activities that enhance or diminish wakefulness. Such speculation, although not based strongly upon experimental data, has turned out to be not too far off the mark!

An interesting set of studies involving electrophysiological stimulation of thalamic nuclei and recording from the cortex (Dempsey & Morison, 1942a, 1942b; Morison & Dempsey, 1942) occurred shortly after our entry into World War II and no doubt these studies were curtailed or prematurely terminated as a consequence. The studies demonstrated that stimulation of midline and intralaminar thalamic nuclei electrically at a frequency corresponding more or less with the frequency of the alpha-like waves that can be recorded from a relaxed cat will cause a series of rhythmic waves over widespread areas of the cortex. These induced rhythmic waves were called "recruiting responses" because they gradually built up to a uniform amplitude and continued more or less indefinitely if stimulation was continued, but often with some waxing and waning of amplitude. These waves could be elicited in certain regions of the cortex (mainly in associational or nonspecific sensory areas) by stimulation of associational or nonspecific nuclei, sometimes referred to as "diffuse" thalamic nuclei because of their diffuse stimulation effects upon the cortex. Starzl and Magoun (1951) showed that several associational nuclei of the thalamus were involved in the recruiting as well as the areas of the cortex to which they project. Starzl and Whitlock (1952) confirmed this in the monkey and pointed out that the thalamic origins of the diffuse thalamic projection system include centre median, intralaminar, inferior medial, ventralis anterior, and anterior reticular nuclei. They also determined that intrathalamic connections from these sources of origin involved the association nuclei of the thalamus—medial, anterior, lateralis complex, and pulvinar—and that both the ascending reticular activating system and corticofugal discharges are received in the thalamic origins of the diffuse thalamic system. In the monkey, Starzl and Whitlock found a strong frontal lobe influence from stimulation of the diffuse thalamic recruiting system and came to believe that the system was involved in integration and synthesis of diffuse sensory and affective influences. In this context one might speculate that these influences might be part of a motivational system (Verzeano, Lindsley & Magoun, 1953).

In contrast to the effects of stimulation of diffuse thalamic nuclei, Dempsey & Morison (1942a, 1942b) found that stimulation of specific sensory thalamic relay nuclei gave rise to a different type of activity, which they called "augmenting responses." It thus began to appear that there were both primary and secondary pathways of sensory influence upon the cortex, and that perhaps the diffuse, nonspecific, midline thalamic nuclei might be responsible for the regulation and timing of cortical spontaneous rhythms such as the alpha rhythm discovered by Berger (1929). Furthermore, it suggested that ascending pathways from the level of the brain stem might have quite different functions concerning their influence upon the cortex. The classical or specific sensory pathways carry specific kinds of information to be processed and the nonspecific (or unspecific) system transmits impulses that "condition" or heighten the excitability or responsivity of cortical areas into which partially processed information must pass enroute from receptor to primary cortical areas and that must undergo further processing of an integrative sort—that is, achieve selectively differential status, be subjected to cross-modality comparison, activate past experience and undergo memory indexing, and cause preparatory storage or activation state. To accomplish these and other elaboration steps such as are obviously involved in the higher cognitive functions of humans, a spatial and temporal patterning system must be involved.

In their studies of thalamo-cortical relationships Morison and Dempsey saw a kind of pacemaker activity centered in the thalamus, especially in the nonspecific nuclei. Twenty-six years later, in their book *Physiological Basis of the Alpha Rhythm*, Andersen and Andersson (1968) bring forth a great deal of detailed data on thalamic and cortical rhythmicity, recruiting responses and the like, and a proposal that rhythmicity of discharge is due to a mechanism of recurrent inhibition that is intrinsic to both nonspecific and specific thalamic nuclei. They believe that their analysis of unit responses in thalamic nuclei demonstrate that any thalamic nucleus is capable of producing spindle waves and rhythmic bursting responses as a result of a single afferent volley from a receptor source. They refer to this property of any thalamic nucleus and its mechanism as a *facultative pacemaker theory*. Unfortunately, it does not yet explain the role of the rhythmicity generated or triggered in the cortex by thalamic pacemakers.

Towards the end of the 1940's three closely related studies (Moruzzi & Magoun, 1949; Lindsley, Bowden, & Magoun, 1949; Lindsley, Schreiner, Knowles, & Magoun, 1950) threw considerable light upon the neural mechanism underlying sleep and wakefulness and the behavioral and electrocortical aspects of arousal, orienting, alerting, and attention. These studies related closely to those of Bremer cited earlier (1935–1938), to the concepts of sleep and wakefulness put forward by Kleitman in 1939, to the nonspecific pacemaker concepts of Morison and Dempsey of the early 1940's, and to the earlier studies by Hess (1929a, 1929b, 1944, 1954) on induction of sleep by low-frequency stimulation (4–12 Hz), with asymmetric pulses of slow rising phase, in certain localized diencephalic structures.

The Lindsley et al. (1949, 1950) studies showed that Bremer's results demonstrating sleep by a cerveau isolé neuraxis transection were not due, as he supposed, to interruption of lemniscal pathways and the cutting off of primary sources of sensory input to the cortex but instead to the transection of the central reticular core (reticular formation) into which a multisensory influx flows and generates diffuse and nonspecific excitations that ascend to higher levels, including thalamus and cortex, thus keeping the brain activated and awake. A lesion of this ascending reticular activating system at the junction of the midbrain and hypothalamus, but without transection of the lemniscal or other sensory pathways, will cause sleep and profound somnolence, whereas with the reticular core left intact and only the lateral pathways severed, cats show a waking-type EEG pattern and behavioral evidence of wakefulness (Lindsley et al., 1950).

It seems clear that Magoun had well in mind what to look for because of his extensive experience in stimulating various parts of the brain stem and because of his background in neuroanatomy of the brain stem acquired through his work and training with Stephen Walter Ranson (1880–1942), his mentor through much of the 1930's. Ranson was Professor of Neurology and Director of the Neurological Research Institute of Northwestern University Medical School from 1928 until his death in 1942. Ranson, his students, and his colleagues were the first in the United States to use the Horsley-Clarke stereotaxic instrument extensively in their research beginning in 1930. The fascinating history of the Horsley-Clarke instrument has recently been assembled by Magoun and Fisher (1980) and the following has been abstracted from it with the kind permission of Dr. Magoun:

Apparently sensing the need for accurately pinpointing regions in the interior of the brain in connection with work they were doing on the cerebellum, Sir Victor Horsley, a distinguished pioneer neurosurgeon, and his colleague, Dr. Robert H. Clarke, a physiologist, conceived of a device using rectangular coordinates. Dr. Clarke designed this instrument and it was built by Mr. J. Swift of Palmer and Company, London, in 1905. Horsley and Clarke (1908) described this instrument and the method of examining the cerebellum with it, but their studies of the cerebellum were not completed due, apparently, to other pressing matters. The method, the instrument, and its use apparently lay fallow for some years and the instrument passing from one person to another was "lost" for a period of time. In 1907, Dr. Ernest Sachs, a budding neurosurgeon, was accepted for training with Horsley and soon became instructed in the use of the stereotaxic instrument. Sachs was impressed with the instrument and arranged to have a second one built which he could take back to America. This second one, a replica of the first, was made by Mr. Goodwin of the Palmer company, and was brought back to Washington University in St. Louis, where Sachs became the first professor of neurological surgery in the United States. Later Sachs continued the uncompleted work of Horsley and Clarke on the cerebellum and was joined in this during 1926–27 by Dr. Edgar Fincher. Sachs reported the preliminary results of this study at the joint meeting of the Royal Society of Medicine and the American Neurological Association in July of 1927. It occurred to Drs. J. C. Hinsey and Ranson as they observed Dr. Fincher at work with the stereotaxic instrument that it would be of great help to them in their studies of brain stem structures controlling postural contraction. Ranson then had an exact copy of this instrument made in Chicago and they began using it in 1930. Interestingly, in 1956, Dr. Sachs, then retired as a neurosurgeon but working on historical matters in Dr. John F. Fulton's library at Yale had arranged a surprise. At the conclusion of an invited lecture at Yale University by Professor H. W. Magoun, Dr. Sachs bestowed upon him the gift of this second-made Horsley–Clarke instrument produced by the Palmer Instrument Company of London. Dr. Magoun has since made the instrument the initial contribution to the Archives for the History of Neurosciences at UCLA where it resides in the Biomedical Library.

Throughout the 1930's Ranson and his various students and associates, and especially Magoun who continued the work into the 1940's after Ranson's death, used the stereotaxic instrument Ranson had commissioned to be built in Chicago after the exact design of the original Horsley–Clarke instrument. They used the instrument in systematic exploration and detailed study of the lower brain stem and diencephalon by electrical stimulation. In an extensive review of such work on the hypothalamus, Ranson and Magoun (1939) emphasized the role of the brain-stem reticular formation and its descending influences upon spinal motor outflows, a subject further elaborated upon by Rhines and Magoun (1946), Magoun and Rhines (1946), and later by Lindsley, Schreiner, and Magoun (1949), Schreiner, Lindsley, and Magoun (1949), and Lindsley (1952a) employing lesions, electrical stimulation, and the electromyogram.

In their 1939 review, Ranson and Magoun commented, "It is probable that the active hypothalamus not only discharges downward through the brain stem, spinal cord and peripheral nervous system into the body but also upward into the thalamus and cerebral cortex [p. 119]." Thus, they had anticipated the ascending reticular activating system (ARAS), which Moruzzi and Magoun (1949) were the first to identify in its functional role as a waking or arousal system stretched out more or less through the length of the brain stem. Electrical stimulation of it almost anywhere in its course, but particularly in the pontine and midbrain regions, awakened a sleeping cat, aroused a lightly anesthetized one, and activated or desynchronized the EEG.

Lashley's experimental work throughout the 1930's and into the 1940's was dominated by his interest in the neural mechanism of vision in the rat, especially the learning of pattern discriminations and the amount and locus of intact visual cortical tissue that made these functions possible. After his appointment as Director of the Yerkes Laboratories of Primate Biology in 1942, his interests turned to the visual mechanisms in the monkey and chimpanzee. Lashley never used electrical recording techniques in his work, and in only one study did he use electrical stimulation.

Ranson and his colleagues, including Magoun who took his Ph.D. under Ranson in 1934 and became his successor in brain-stem investigations after Ranson's death in 1942, relied solely upon electrical stimulation by stereotaxic control, histological confirmation of locus of stimulation, and physiological or behavioral response. They also employed electrolytic lesions, transections, and ablations when necessary. They did not use or have facilities for electrical recording of potentials from muscle or brain. My coming as a Professor of Psychology to Northwestern University in 1946, and my research association with Magoun from 1947 on, led to the incorporation of electrical recording (both EMG and EEG) with equipment that I brought with me from Bradley Hospital and Brown University in Providence. Later Magoun obtained such equipment from small grants by the Commonwealth Fund and the Office of Naval Research, which enabled us to have a Grass Model III Electroencephalograph suitable for both brain and muscle potential work. In the late 1940's, NIH and NSF granting sources were not yet in existence.

My experiences had been in electromyography and electroencephalography, along with behavioral and autonomic nervous system study in humans and animals. Such activities and perspectives complemented nicely, and fitted in well, with the extensive neuroanatomical and neurophysiological background of Magoun. He had a phenomenal grasp of the morphology and functioning of the brain stem, and a powerful conceptual framework for neurological and behavioral understanding. This situation was further augmented by Moruzzi's coming for the 1948-1949 year and participating with those of us working in Magoun's group in the Department of Anatomy of Northwestern University Medical

School. Moruzzi had spent time in 1937–1939 with Bremer in Brussels and Adrian in Cambridge and had just been appointed Professor of Physiology at the University of Pisa. He was already deeply involved in electrophysiology of the nervous system. At about that time Magoun and I were also collaborating in some experimental studies with Warren S. McCulloch, then head of neurophysiology at the Illinois Neuropsychiatric Institute of the University of Illinois College of Medicine in Chicago (Peterson, Magoun, McCulloch, & Lindsley, 1949).

In 1950 Professor Magoun was called to the University of California at Los Angeles (UCLA) to establish and head up the Anatomy Department of the new School of Medicine. He attracted an excellent staff, many of whom had vital interests in functional neuroanatomy and neurophysiology. He was also influential in attracting people interested in neuroscience to other departments of the medical school and soon there was a sizable interdisciplinary brain-research group, including both basic and clinical neuroscientists. Initially, classes and laboratories were conducted in temporary and inadequate buildings because the medical school and hospital buildings were under construction. But even when these were completed there was still inadequate space for the numerous research activities and the brain-research group found it necessary to use the facilities in the Veterans Administration hospitals in the region, but mainly at the Long Beach facility, where the VA Hospital had been a U.S. Navy Hospital during World War II. There were a number of barracks-like buildings of temporary nature behind the main hospital building where relatives of Navy men incarcerated in the hospital could stay while visiting. Some of these were made available to the brain-research group from UCLA at the instigation of John D. French, Chief of Neurosurgery at the VA Hospital and holding an appointment in surgery at UCLA. Both E. V. Edwards, Superintendent, and French were anxious to establish a research unit there and made space available to us.

Initially, there were only two small laboratory rooms and a shop and one set of equipment items (Grass EEG, DuMont Oscilloscope, Fairchild camera, Goodwin stimulator, Labtronics stereotaxic instrument, etc.) so that those of us from the UCLA campus had to take turns using the equipment and/or collaborate with others, signing up in advance for all hours of the day and night. This space was 35 miles from the campus and some 120 stop-lights enroute! At that time there was no freeway or turnpike for high-speed travel and it required about 1½ hours to make the trip, but once there one was free for uninterrupted research. Fortunately, the space and equipment limitations were soon remedied and additional investigators from UCLA, as well as visiting scientists from around the world, found accommodation there amidst rich and exciting stimulation in an always crowded but cooperative environment, and with eager and enthusiastic investigators engaged in zealous research!

These conditions prevailed for 10 years from 1951 to 1961, when the 11-storied Brain Research Institute was completed and occupied on the UCLA campus, adjacent to the Medical School and Hospital and the Neuropsychiatric Institute, and later the Reed Neurological Institute. John French became its first director and held that position for some 17 years and was then succeeded by Carmine Clemente, who is the present director. Magoun's persistent efforts to build a brain-research and interdisciplinary neuroscience group of worldwide distinction had succeeded and his efforts to secure funding and permission of the Regents of the University to build a Brain Research Institute ceased to be only a dream and became a reality. The period of 1961-1971 was one of intensive activity and growth for the Brain Research Institute and one we can look upon with great pride. In 1972 we held a 10th Anniversary Celebration of scientific nature and we took a census of the total number and distribution of trainees, visiting scientists, and members of the BRI. I was given the responsibility and privilege of writing a brief history of the Brain Research Institute for this 10th Anniversary, which appeared in the front of a sizable Brain Research Institute, UCLA, DIRECTORY (From origin to 1972). Origin was taken to mean the beginning of the brain-research group initiated by H. W. Magoun in 1951, so the history covered the 1951-1961 preinstitute period at the Long Beach VA Hospital, and the 1961-1971 period. During this period the membership in the BRI nearly doubled, increasing from 67 members in 1961 to 125, and the number of disciplines represented increased from 14 to 24. Research productivity, measured in terms of number of publications per year, increased from 286 in 1961 to 772 in 1971. Predoctoral trainees increased from 51 to 132 per year; postdoctoral fellows and trainees from 44 to 140 per year. The number of visiting scientists working in laboratories of BRI members, including both U.S. (185) and foreign visitors (316), averaged 50 per year. The total number of students, both pre- and postdoctoral and visiting scientists from all countries, including the U.S. was 1376. The foreign students and visiting scientists came from 41 countries. The chronology of various innovative programs and landmarks of progress include: Interdisciplinary Mental Health Training Program—1957; The Space Biology Laboratory—1959; The Data Processing Laboratory—1960; The Clinical Neurophysiology Program—1960; Bioengineering Laboratory—1964; Brain Information Service—1964; International Brain Research Institute in Yugoslavia—1964; Neuroscience Degree Programs (Ph.D. and M.D.-Ph.D.)—1968. Elsewhere in the United States, the growth of neuroscience and special programs also began to evolve, and the period of the 1960's with its post-Sputnik emphasis upon the training of scientists and engineers and the availability of funds from both NIH and NSF government agencies, as well as from NASA and from the various military branches supporting research on the nervous system and behavior, greatly facilitated this growth of the neurosciences. The Society for Neuroscience in the United States has grown from its origin several years ago to a membership approaching 7000.

Lashley would have been extremely proud to have known of this development of a strong and large neuroscience society, for he as much as or more than anyone kept alive the interest in brain and behavior research through the first half of the 20th century, and the value of his work lives on in his publications. His wisdom and his conceptions and interpretations of his findings will long be appreciated even though some of them may be proven wrong. They served the purpose of stimulating thought on the part of many of my generation and even succeeding generations, and that is what the march of science is all about!

As anyone who lived through the Depression years of the 1930's and the World War II years of the 1940's is apt to know, academic and research positions were very scarce and support for research was at best miniscule! One had to take work where one was lucky enough to find it and adapt one's research interests to whatever facilities were available. Although Lashley apparently faced similar problems early in his career, before and after World War I (that is, the 1917–1918 period of U.S. participation), and during the 1920's, nevertheless, thereafter, beginning in the late 1920's, his academic and research needs seem to have been adequately fulfilled in successive appointments at the University of Chicago, at Harvard, and at the Yerkes Laboratories for Primate Biology.

PART 2: RESEARCH REVIEW

Like Lashley, I too became interested in the neural mechanisms of vision and the modality of vision as one of the most prominent and accessible avenues for tracing sensory input and information processing to the higher levels of cognitive functioning. Combining this interest and my experiences with Magoun in relation to the role of the ascending reticular activating system in arousal behaviorally and activation electrocortically, I sought to find ways to study the neural mechanisms of attention and perception.

I would like to tell briefly about some of the approaches that my graduate students, postdoctoral visitors, and I have found stimulating and promising, in attempting to understand how the nervous system of complex organisms (cat, monkey, and human) mediates the behavior and psychological processes that they exhibit. As a rule we have deliberately chosen the simpler processes and behavior to study. We have also attempted, by what I call a "systems approach," to isolate in functional terms, as far as possible, the various neural pathways or systems that we know to exist and to be interactive. Often it has been necessary to start with acute animal preparations, stimulating and recording electrically in order to identify pathways, nuclei, and other structures involved in a particular action. However, once a system has been identified and suitably reduced or isolated by lesion, by cooling, by local anesthetic, or differentiated by electrical stimulation and recording, we identify the loci where we wish to implant electrodes for stimulating and others for recording, and where we wish to implant cryoprobes for temporarily blocking certain pathways or nuclei. The ultimate goal was always first to be able to make chronic behaving preparations with implanted electrodes and cryoprobes, and to train animals to make discriminations, and to learn, remember, and perform, and then, by stimulation, by cooling, by electrolytic lesion, or by differential and counteractive training, to determine how a particular system (or systems) might be involved in the behavioral processes concerned.

Thus, in chronic animal preparations, we may have stimulating electrodes implanted in certain crucial areas where we know we can reliably produce an effect elsewhere in the central nervous system that can be detected by electrical recording, and perhaps also in the spontaneous behavior of the animal or in a modification of its trained behavior. If two or more pathways are involved, the implantation of cryoprobes for cooling pathways or nuclei and blocking function reversibly without damage to the neural tissue may enable us to determine which pathways or nuclei are crucial to the particular electrophysiological and/or behavioral processes under study. Electrical recording tells us where in the brain both spontaneous and induced activity is going on. Unit cellular activities can be recorded, even during some limited behavioral functions, either extracellularly or intracellularly, as the case may warrant. We must always be aware, however, that electrical recordings are mainly ''signs'' of activity going on in a nerve, in a cell body, and in an aggregate or nucleus of cell bodies, and are not the primary action itself, which is usually a physico-chemical change that can only be inferred or possibly determined by more elaborate analytical methods. The recorded electrical response, though often complex and prolonged, can be analyzed in various ways, separating the various components that may have contributed to the overall waveform. An electrical response latency may be of tremendous value in identifying functional systems and their responses, and in determining whether a given transmission or discharge could have utilized one or another circuit. Electrically recorded responses can tell us much about what is happening in a given pathway, nucleus, receptor, or effector.

Now let me turn to my topic in this important series honoring Lashley and commemorating his landmark contribution 50 years ago! There are four experimental areas about which I wish to speak. They are interrelated to each other and they are all related in some way to the studies of the ascending reticular activating system of the late 1940's and early 1950's, which I have discussed earlier. Several studies were involved in each of these areas and I am only able to refer to them briefly, provide references to the primary studies, and attempt to make some integrative remarks. The four topics are: (1) the role of thalamo-cortical extensions of the ascending reticular activating system revealed by lesions and/or reversible cryogenic blockade: electrophysiological and behavioral effects; (2) brain stem-hypothalamic-hippocampal systems and their contrasting electrophysiological and behavioral effects; (3) role of the pulvinar in a secondary visual system: eye movements, attention, and information processing; (4) human-evoked potentials and information processing.

How did we get started on such an array of studies predominantly in the visual domain but with emphasis upon the arousing, orienting, alerting, attending, and motivating influences of the reticular formation and the ascending reticular activating system? How were we led to investigate the potential integrative roles of thalamo-cortical systems, particularly the midline and intralaminar nonspecific or unspecific thalamic nuclei, and the thalamic association nuclei, especially the large pulvinar nucleus of monkeys and humans? How did we come to utilize the human EEG, including average evoked potentials (AEPs) or as now frequently called, event-related potentials (ERPs), and the contingent negative variation (CNV), to investigate information processing and cognitive functions in humans? Once again, I revert to history to provide some answers to these questions.

On moving from Northwestern to UCLA in 1951, I decided to study the central neural mechanisms of vision electrophysiologically and psychologically or psychophysically in an effort to understand neurophysiologically more about the nature of visual experience and behavior. In 1952, I was invited to participate, along with George H. Bishop and others, in a symposium organized by the American Electroencephalographic Society on current issues in EEG. For my topic, I chose *Psychological Phenomena and the Electroencephalogram* (Lindsley, 1952b). Using largely the data of others, I attempted to show how the EEG in humans and animals might be related to psychological phenomena of vision, and how such electrophysiological methods might be of use in securing data to explain the neural basis of psychological processes and events (see also Lindsley, 1950, 1951, 1957, 1969, 1970).

Up to that time, incidentally, about the only electrophysiological studies of the central neural mechanisms of vision had been done in the rabbit and cat in the laboratory of George H. Bishop, a physiologist working in the Department of Ophthalmology of the Washington University Medical School in St. Louis. Bishop, with collaborators S. Howard Bartley, psychologist, and James L. O'Leary, neurologist, explored extensively the visual pathways and visual cortical areas by electrical recording (Bartley & Bishop, 1933a, 1933b: Bishop, 1933, 1935, 1936; Bishop & O'Leary, 1935, 1936, 1940). Others pioneering in the electrophysiological study of central neural pathways were Saul and Davis (1932, 1933) at Harvard, Gerard, Marshall, and Saul (1936) at the University of Chicago, Jasper (1936) and Rheinberger & Jasper (1937) in Providence, Talbot and Marshall (1941) and Marshall and Talbot (1942) at Johns Hopkins, and Chang and Kaada (1950) and Chang (1950, 1951, 1952) at Yale.

Much of the other work in vision of the 1930's and 1940's was confined to the bulbus of the eye and was concerned mainly with retinal chemistry, but also included recording of the electroretinogram (Granit, 1947, 1955) and the electrooculogram (Lindsley & Hunter, 1939; Mowrer, Ruch, & Miller, 1936). Of course, there was the monumental work of H. Keffer Hartline and collaborators on the lateral eye of the horseshoe crab (Limulus) in which they were able to tease out and record from single fibers in the optic nerve the responses of a single ommatidium and even from the several single sense cells within it (Hartline, 1934; Hartline & Graham, 1932; Hartline, Wagner, & MacNichol, 1952; see also Ratliff, 1974).

For some reason, during the 1930's and 1940's, investigators in the field of vision were reluctant to explore the electrical activity of central neural visual structures. Perhaps this was because stereotaxic instruments for guiding electrode probes accurately were not generally available and consequently depth recording was not common. There was, of course, following Lashley's lead, considerable effort to study the behavioral and perceptual effects of lesions of the visual cortex in animals ranging from rats to humans, but particularly in dogs, monkeys, and humans (Brouwer, 1930; Fox & German, 1936; Halstead, Walker, & Bucy, 1940; Marquis, 1934; Marquis & Hilgard, 1937).

With the aid of a small grant from the National Institute of Mental Health in 1952 (NIH and NSF were just getting started as granting agencies of the government), I was able to equip a small laboratory for human EEG and visual perceptual studies in the Department of Psychology at UCLA. There was no provision there for space in which to carry on my planned use of cats and monkeys so I established a laboratory with the brain-research group in the space becoming available in the laboratories of the Long Beach VA Hospital. When the Brain Research Institute building was completed in 1961, I was assigned four animal laboratories there, in addition to the Human Laboratory in the Department of Psychology.

During the 1950's we were struggling with a variety of ways to record evoked potentials through the intact scalp and skull of humans, but we were not very successful until Dawson (1950, 1954) described a computer summation technique, and then not until we obtained a Mnemotron Computer of Average Transients (CAT) in about 1962. From then on our work in humans increased very rapidly and included studies of AEPs to paired flashes (Donchin, Wicke, & Lindsley, 1963), the effects of stimulus parameters such as luminance and duration of flashes on AEPs (Wicke, Donchin, & Lindsley, 1964), the effects of attention and vigilance upon AEPs and performance (Haider, Spong, & Lindsley, 1964; Spong, Haider, & Lindsley, 1965), retroactive masking and brightness enhancement (Donchin & Lindsley, 1965a), relation of AEPs to reaction time (Donchin & Lindsley, 1966), and many subsequent studies on perception, attention, and information processing (for other early developments in the use of averaged evoked potentials, see Donchin and Lindsley, 1969).

Our work with animals proceeded very nicely during the 1950's for in most instances we could record potentials from the neural structures we were interested in without computer averaging. We investigated electrical responses from eye to visual cortex, testing the effects of various stimulus parameters such as luminance, wave length, duration, frequency of flashes, light-dark ratio, and so forth. We determined that the visual pathways (optic nerve, optic tract, lateral geniculate nucleus, optic radiations) would respond discretely to each and every flash of light upon the retina at frequencies over 100 per second, but the visual cortex, which followed repetitive flashes well at low frequencies, began to fail at or near fusion frequency, determined by behavioral methods (Lindsley, 1961a,

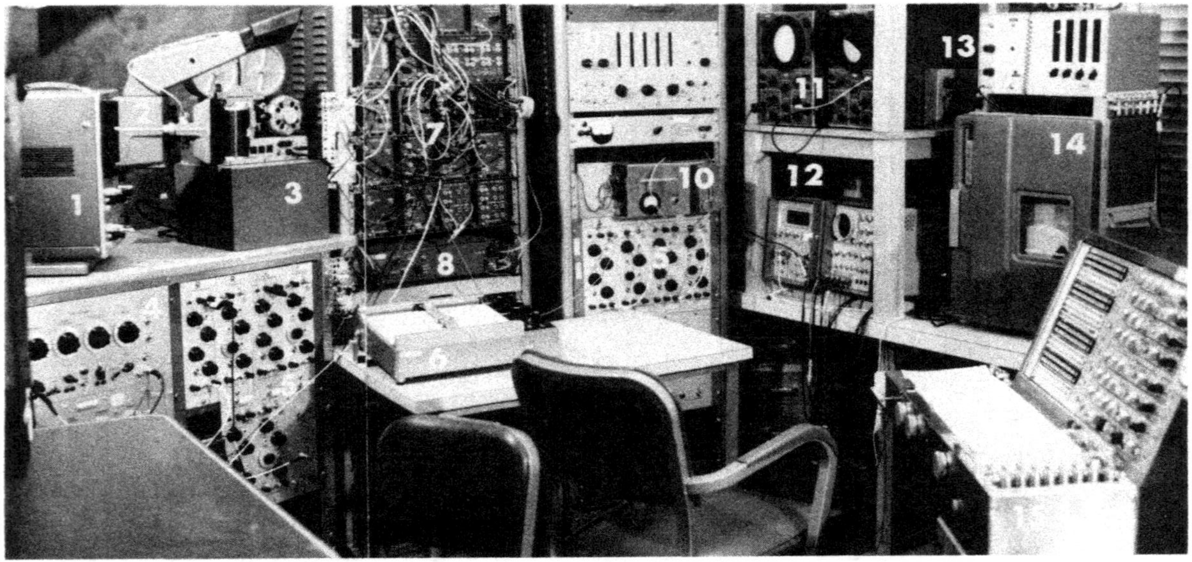

FIG. 15.4. Lindsley human psychophysiology laboratory at UCLA, 1962–1969. Subsequently revised and a PDP-12 computer added. Early average evoked potential studies were carried out here. This equipment represents stimulating, program controlling, recording, and analyzing of data. Items shown: (1) Tektronix oscilloscope; (2) Tektronix Scope Camera; (3) Grass Oscilloscope Camera; (4) Grass Stimulators; (5) Tektronix Power Supply and Waveform and Pulse Generators for stimulus control; (6) Moseley X–Y Plotter; (7) Massey Dickinson Control and Programming Equipment; (8) Massey Dickinson Power Supply; (9) Hewlett-Packard Electronic Counter for reaction time, etc.; (10) Tape-reader; (11) Oscilloscope stimulus Control Monitors; (12) Mnemotron (CAT) Computer of Average Transients (replaced by DEC PDP-12 Computer); (13) Computer Measurements, Inc. Preset Controller and Tape Coder; (14) Ampex FR-1300 7-channel FM Tape Recorder; (15) Grass Model VI Electroencephalograph. (Much more compact, efficient, and elaborate equipment is available today.)

1961b, & 1961c; Schwartz & Lindsley, 1964). Earlier, Lindsley and Griffiths (1955) studied differential responses of the eye and optic pathways to intensity and wave length and also determined that reticular stimulation in the cat facilitated the visual cortical response to brief, paired flashes (Lindsley, 1953, 1954, 1956, 1958a, 1958b, & Lindsley & Emmons, 1958). Pairs of flashes separated by only 50 msec were recorded as a single response at the visual cortex, whereas the same flashes after or during reticular stimulation resulted in two distinct visual cortical responses, thus apparently enhancing visual resolution. Similar facilitation effects from stimulation of the reticular formation were observed by Dumont and Dell (1958, 1960) and by Bremer and Stoupel (1958, 1959). These results of reticular stimulation were consistent with the important findings of Fuster (1958) in monkeys in whom stimulation of the reticular formation concurrent with discrimination of a learned tachistoscopically presented visual task produced significantly better and faster performance than in monkeys not so stimulated.

Another example of facilitation and enhanced excitation of the cerebral cortex presumably via activation of the reticular formation was found in a reaction-time study in humans. Lansing, Schwartz, and Lindsley (1959) found that the alerting and activation (alpha desynchronization) in a forewarned reaction-time task was most effective when the warning signal came at least 300 msec before the imperative or reaction-time signal. The shortest reaction times were obtained when the warning was 300 msec or longer and it was obvious that blocking of the alpha rhythm was complete. If activation and desynchronization were only partial after a 100- or 200-msec forewarning period, the reaction time was considerably longer. The latency of this activation, together with the reduction in reaction time that it effected, suggest that facilitation by reticular-formation excitation and activation was responsible. Because of this result we have, in our subsequent visual-pattern discrimination studies in monkeys, allowed an interval of 300 to 500 msec between a monkey's lever press to initiate a tachistoscopic presentation of visual patterns and the actual presentation of the patterns on the screen. Thus we felt that the monkey would be fully alert and attentive to the brief (10 msec) presentation of the stimuli and this appears to have been the case. This apparatus and the procedure with monkeys are described later in connection with pulvinar studies.

Fig. 15.4 shows the arrangement of our equipment in the human laboratory from about 1962 to 1969. The principal items, included the all-important CAT for computer averaging of evoked potentials. In 1969 the CAT was replaced by a Digital Equipment Corporation (DEC) PDP-12 computer and the CAT was then employed in the animal laboratories when evoked potential averaging was required. From time to time, the human laboratory facilities and equipment have been further updated to meet new requirements, so the present human laboratory is completely different from that shown in Fig. 15.4 and provides input arrangements from two subject rooms. One of these is equipped with a DEC VR-12 display oscilloscope upon which stimuli may be presented under control of the PDP-12 laboratory computer. The other room contains a three-field tachistoscope and other means of presenting visual stimuli in Maxwellian view and under programmed stimulus control.

The animal laboratories in the Brain Research Institute and those I had later in the Department of Psychology were all equipped with the latest apparatus and facilities. The most recent equipment units in each lab consisted of Grass Model 78 polygraphs with eight channels of AC recording and four of DC. Ampex SP-300 tape recorders permitted storage of experimental data for later analysis by means of the computer. Stereotaxic instruments, stimulators, split-screen TV monitoring of electrical recording simultaneously with videotaped behavior, and physiological maintenance and monitoring equipment was available. Both ink-writing records on the polygraph and Tektronix oscilloscope records by means of Grass or Polaroid cameras, simultaneously, were possible.

The Role of Thalamo-Cortical Extensions of the Ascending Reticular Activating System Revealed by Lesions and/or Reversible Cryogenic Blockade: Electrophysiological and Behavioral Effects

Some of the concepts of the functioning of the brain-stem reticular formation are illustrated in Fig. 15.5. Here we see it schematically illustrated in solid black, a central core structure extending from the medulla, caudally, to the diencephalon, rostrally. Alongside it are shown a somatosensory pathway from the periphery with synaptic junctions in the dorsal column nuclei and in the thalamic relay nuclei on its way to somatosensory cortex in the postcentral gyrus, and opposite, a somatomotor pathway, from motor or premotor cortex extending downward to form a synaptic junction with an anterior horn cell of the spinal cord. Collaterals from each of these pathways are also shown to illustrate their influence upon the reticular formation of the lower brain stem (small arrows). At the caudal end of the reticular formation, an arrow symbolizes the descending influences of the reticular formation; these have both inhibitory and facilitatory effects on spinal motor outflows and together help maintain normal reflexes, posture, and muscle tone (Lindsley, Schreiner, & Magoun, 1949; Schreiner, Lindsley, & Magoun, 1949; see also Magoun & Rhines, 1946, and Rhines & Magoun, 1946). Rostrally, there are several arrows extending diffusely over the cortical hemispheres symbolizing the diffuse influence of the ascending reticular activating system (ARAS). When the ARAS is excited by normal sensory means, or by electrical stimulation of the reticular formation, it tends to desynchronize on-going alpha-wave activity all over the cerebrum leaving mainly low amplitude fast activity sometimes referred to as beta waves. If instead of alpha waves of the waking state there are large, slow, billowy waves characteristic of sleep, these will be abolished or blocked and the low-level fast activity substituted as arousal and

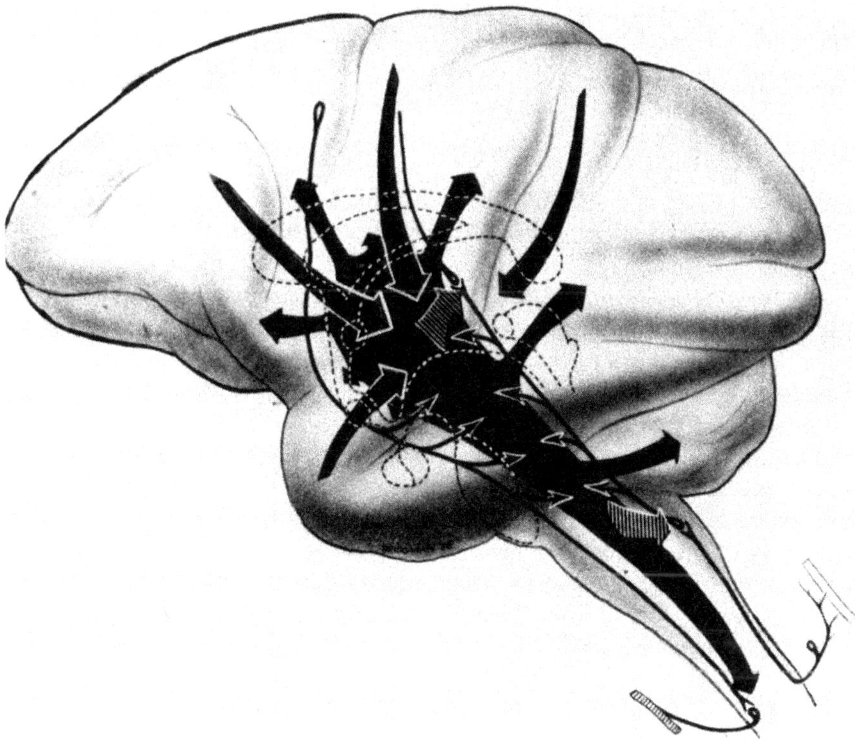

FIG. 15.5. Schematic representation of ascending reticular activating system from reticular formation with inputs to it and outputs from it illustrated against a background phantom monkey brain. See text for details. From Worden and Livingston, 1961. By permission.

awakening take place. Several large black arrows are shown originating from different cortical regions with the reticular formation as their destination (French, Hernandez-Peon, & Livingston, 1955). These indicate that reticular excitation may be initiated from central cerebral sources as well as from external and internal sensory sources. (For more detailed information, see Lindsley, 1960.)

Just as distracting, annoying, and discomforting stimuli (lights, sounds, odors, tastes, temperatures, pains, etc.) may, through the impulses they contribute via collaterals to the reticular formation, prevent one from getting to sleep, so also may distracting thoughts, worries, and anxieties. These latter activities of cerebral origin may, via corticofugal pathways, transmit impulses to the reticular formation, thus enhancing its excitatory state and causing its upward discharge to increase cerebral activity, thereby creating a circular effect. In addition, such central effects may contribute to muscular tension and restlessness, which in turn, through propriocetive feedback, influence the reticular formation and may initiate activation and arousal effects at the cerebral level.

The cross-hatched arrows emanating from the reticular formation symbolize inhibitory influences upon synaptic relays in classical sensory pathways, which tend to suppress and regulate the influx of sensory impulses by negative feedback very much as such circuits built into a radio adjust for sudden surges and persistent increases in loudness.

These characteristics of the reticular formation and the ARAS were already well known in the mid-1950's (Brodal, 1958; O'Leary & Cohen, 1958; Rossi & Zanchetti, 1957; Segundo, 1956). Much has been learned in the meantime about the detailed morphology of the reticular formation, including its many nuclei and the sources and destination of their impulses and their interactions; and also about the neuropharmacological make-up of the cells comprising these nuclei and the nature of their terminal transmitting substances and effective loci (Dahlström & Fuxe, 1965; Fuxe, Hökfelt, & Ungerstedt, 1970; Jouvet, 1972a, 1972b; Moore, 1975; and others).

Despite a great many studies carried out during the period 1955–1965 relating to the reticular formation and its influences upon thalamic and neocortical activity, and upon behavior when chronic animal preparations were used, the basic principles of the influence of the ARAS upon electrocortical activity and behavior has remained essentially unchanged from those described in the 1949 and 1950 studies of Moruzzi and Magoun, Lindsley, Bowden, and Magoun, and Lindsley, Schreiner, Knowles, and Magoun—that is, electrical stimulation of the reticular formation causes activation and desynchronization of the electrical activity of the cortex if the synchronized waves of waking or sleep are present. Furthermore, in chronic animal preparations, arousal or awakening and orienting tend to accompany the shift from synchronized slow waves of sleep to a desynchronized, low-level, fast-activity pattern when an animal is aroused from sleep by stimulation through normal sensory channels or by artificial, electrical stimulation to the reticular formation. In a series of studies in animals and humans carried out during this period, we attempted to gain more information about the behavioral and psychological processes affected by reticular activation.

After the foregoing and other studies aimed at learning more about the effects of reticular formation activation upon the on-going electrical activity of the brain, the behavioral effects, and the psychological processes influenced in humans, we turned our attention to the effects of lesions in the thalamus, orbitofrontal cortex, and elsewhere in the brain. The goal was to determine the pathways by means of which reticular activation was brought to bear upon the more diffuse and more specific areas of the forebrain. Four kinds of electrical phenomena of the cortex were available to us as indices of change due to the lesions. One was the *on-going electrocortical activity* manifesting some degree of synchrony and rhythmicity, such as the alpha-like waves of relaxed waking, and the large billowy slow waves of deep sleep. Another was the periodic bursts of rhythmic waves, called *spindle bursts,* which often characterize the onset of sleep as irregular slow waves begin to appear. A transection of the central reticular core at the level of the midbrain and hypothalamus caused persistent, rhythmic, spindle bursts over most of the cerebrum, and this constituted a constant and reliable background of electrical activity against which to test the effects of various lesions, stimulations, behavioral conditioning and learning (Velasco & Lindsley 1965, see also the various articles authored by Velasco and colleagues, 1968a, 1968b, 1975 and 1976 as well as those by Weinberger and his colleagues, 1965a, 1965b, 1967, 1968). Another electrocortical effect against which to test lesions and stimulation effects were *recruiting responses,* which could be reliably elicited by stimulation of intralaminar and midline thalamic nuclei of the nonspecific, diffusely projecting type. Still another possibility to be tested against lesion effects were the *augmenting responses* elicited by electrical stimulation of thalamic sensory relay nuclei more laterally placed than the nuclei whose stimulation produces the recruiting responses. In the cat, the frequency of stimulation for eliciting both recruiting and augmenting responses was usually optimal at about 7 to 8 per second.

Weinberger, Velasco, and Lindsley (1965b) demonstrated that thalamic lesions rostral to midline or intralaminar sites altered, reduced, or blocked the recruiting responses of the cortex elicited by low-frequency stimulation (7-8 per second). Lesions of the rostral nucleus reticularis or nucleus ventralis anterior abolished recruiting responses most effectively. High-frequency stimulation (100 per second) of the same sites was not affected by the same lesions. Only lesions caudal to the site of stimulation, near the posterior commissure, were effective in blocking the desynchronization of cortical electrical activity induced by high-frequency stimulation at recruiting sites in the thalamus. The effectiveness of such desynchronizing stimulation seemed to depend on pathways to, rather than from, the reticular formation, which would then influence the cortex by desynchronization. The pathways for recruiting and desynchronization appeared not to be the same.

Weinberger and Lindsley (1964) studied the effects of two contrasting novel stimuli upon arousal and electrocortical desynchronization and found that the *offset* of a continuous tone would awaken a sleeping cat as effectively as the *onset* of the same tone after complete silence, and the arousal or awakening was accompanied by electrocortical desynchronization. Weinberger, Velasco, and Lindsley (1965a) studied cats trained in classical differential conditioning and found that the same EEG desynchronization occurred during reinforced (CS) and nonreinforced (DS) stimulation, although the cats responded only to the CS. Thalamically initiated recruiting responses evoked prior to the CS or DS were differentially affected, being reduced by the CS but not by the DS.

In a series of experiments, we have attempted to gain an understanding of the mechanism by which excitation of the reticular formation, either by natural sensory stimulation or by direct electrical stimulation, causes, via the ARAS, its effects upon electrocortical activity (blocking or desynchronization of alpha waves of the waking state, abolition or desynchronization of the slow waves of sleep and induction of activation in the form of fast rhythmic waves, abolition of spindle bursts characteristic of the onset of sleep, interference or blocking of recruiting responses elicited by stimulation of nonspecific thalamic nuclei, and failure to block augmenting responses elicited from specific sensory thalamic nuclei, selective activity of which may be enhanced or depressed). Velasco and Lindsley (1965) found that lesions of various regions of the neocortex of the cat, even in large amount or area, had little or no effect, except in a comparatively limited region of the orbitofrontal cortex that appeared to be essential to the occurrence of spontaneous spindle bursts and thalamically induced recruiting responses, observed in both cortex and thalamus. It was concluded that orbitofrontal cortex played a crucial role in the regulation of thalamo-cortical synchronizing and integrating functions and that these functions may be associated with a nonspecific system governing internal inhibition manifesting itself by inattention, drowsiness, and sleep. The first of a series of experiments (Velasco, Weinberger, and Lindsley, 1968) on the effect of thalamo-cortical activation on recruiting responses by reticular stimulation showed that the waxing and waning modulation of recruiting responses was blocked by reticular stimulation as well as the incrementing process of the recruiting response. These features may be associated with regulatory aspects of inhibition and excitation in the cortex. A second set of studies (Velasco & Lindsley, 1968a) compared reticular activation with that induced by peripheral and central neural stimulation. It was found that activation appears to be the same whether induced by central neural stimulation (telencephalic, rhinencephalic, diencephalic, mesencephalic, or rhombencephalic structures) or by peripheral sensory stimulation (visual, auditory, olfactory, nociceptive, or proprioceptive). Thus it appears that a common mechanism, perhaps a reticulo-thalamo-orbitofrontal cortex system, produces a somewhat stereotyped cortical reaction even though the exciting sources of stimulation are varied. Even though the nature of the effects electrocortically may be similar, the variance in degree may reflect differences in the degree of behavioral arousal, alertness, and attentiveness. A third set of experiments (Velasco & Lindsley, 1968b) investigated effects of lesions of the reticular formation on thalamo-cortical activation induced by central and peripheral stimulation. Such stimulation capable of blocking recruiting responses in the intact animal failed to do so after lesions of the mesencephalic reticular formation at the level of the superior colliculi, indicating that this region of the reticular formation is a critical one for thalamo-cortical activation. There were further indications that a tonic influence of the reticular formation may have an inhibitory and regulatory effect upon the synchronizing properties of a thalamo-orbitofrontal system, which participates in amplitude modulation of cortical potentials (see also Skinner & Lindsley, 1969, 1971).

In another series of experiments, attempts were made to delimit the thalamo-cortical system regulating spindle bursts and recruiting responses (Velasco, Skinner, Asaro, & Lindsley, 1968, 1975; Velasco, Skinner, & Lindsley, 1976) by lesions of the cortex, thalamus, rostral diencephalon, and preoptic region of the forebrain. Extensive lesions of the dorsolateral convexity of the cortex, including primary sensory cortical areas (visual, auditory, and somatic), motor cortex, and association areas did not affect recruiting responses elicited by low-frequency stimulation of the midline thalamic nuclear complex or spindle bursts produced by mesencephalic lesions. Only orbitofrontal cortex ablations abolished recruiting responses and spindle bursts recorded at the cortex, in subcortical white matter, and in the thalamus. In the second study of this series involving thalamic lesions, it was found that only lesions limited to the frontal pole of the thalamus (N. ventralis anterior and N. reticularis) block spindle bursts and recruiting responses in both cortex and thalamus. In a third study (Velasco, Skinner, & Lindsley, 1976), it was found that small lesions limited to the inferior thalamic peduncle (ITP) abolished cortical and thalamic spindle bursts and recruiting responses, whereas control lesions surrounding this critical region were ineffective. Massive electrolytic lesions in the caudate nucleus, septum, diagonal band of Broca, preoptic region, hypothalamus, and internal capsule did not eliminate cortical and thalamic recruiting responses or spindle bursts.

The just-described experiments seem to indicate quite clearly that the reticular formation of the lower brain stem maintains a tonic influence upward and that its fluctuating activation influences via the ARAS, due to fluctuation of internal and external sensory influences upon the reticular formation as well as corticofugal influences, is mediated thalamically via the so-called nonspecific nuclei of the midline and intralaminar regions. The funnel-like pathway through which these activation influences ascend further is mainly by the ITP, which projects to the orbitofrontal cortex and then diffusely affects the cortical mantle, but is also subject to further influences and modulation in the regulation of electrocortical activity, both spontaneous and induced. All of these studies were performed in acute preparations. Operations were done under deep anesthesia, but then animals were maintained under local anesthesia and immobilized by gallamine triethiodide. Thus, we are dealing with an unanesthetized brain in an animal deprived of much of its proprioceptive feedback due to paralyzed musculature.

We now turn to experiments in chronic, behaving cats with implanted stimulating electrodes and cryoprobes for cooling and blocking, and then warming and unblocking, transmission in the funnel-like ITP pathway linking the ascending reticular activating system with the orbitofrontal cortex. These experiments by Skinner and Lindsley (1967; see also 1973) showed that blocking transmission in the ITP abolished spindle bursts and recruiting responses in the cortex of the cat. Warming the cryoprobe in the left ITP brought back the spindle bursts and the recruiting responses to precooling status on the left cortex. Augmenting responses, presumably mediated by the internal capsule, were not affected by the cooling and no change occurred after cooling. Fig. 15.6 shows these effects in a cat with bilateral mesencephalic reticular formation lesions to produce continuous, periodic spindle bursting bilaterally (A) against which to

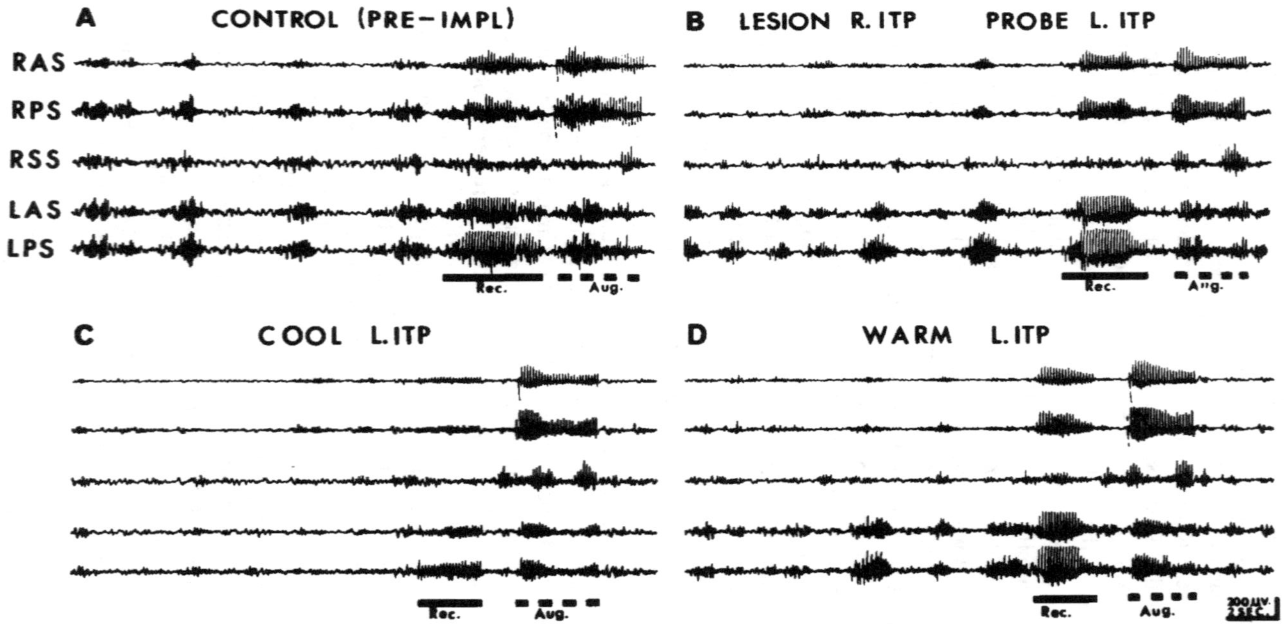

FIG. 15.6. The effect of blocking the inferior thalamic peduncle (ITP), a pathway of the ascending reticular activating system, at the thalamic level in the cat. In A, bilateral midbrain reticular formation lesions furnish rhythmic spindle burst background; also in A, recruiting responses (Rec.) elicited by stimulation of left nucleus centralis medialis, and augmenting responses (Aug.) by stimulation of nucleus ventralis lateralis (LNC) may be seen. Lesion of right ITP in B, with cryoprobe in place in left ITP but not cooled, blocks spindle bursts and recruiting on right (RAS, RPS, RSS—right anterior and posterior sigmoid, and right suprasylvian gyri), but not augmenting. In C, cooling the left ITP to 10°C blocks spindle bursts and recruiting on left, but not augmenting. In D, warming left ITP to normal temperature reversibly reinstates left anterior and posterior spindle bursts and recruiting. See text for further comment. From Skinner and Lindsley, 1967. By permission.

test the effects of lesion of the right ITP (B), which abolished the spindle bursts of the right cortex but not the left; recruiting elicited from left thalamic stimulation remains the same on the left. Cooling of the left ITP (C) to 10°C abolished the spindle bursts over the left cortex and also the recruiting response on the left. Finally, allowing the cryoprobe in the left ITP to return to normal temperature by warming it with the heater wire around its shaft (D) brought the spindles back in left cortex and also the recruiting response. Thus, blockade of ITP by either electrolytic lesion, as on the right side, or by cooling on the left blocked spindle bursts and recruiting response in the cortex.

In a cat with chronically implanted cryoprobes in ITP and trained to bar press repeatedly for a milk reward (Skinner & Lindsley, 1967), we see that with the cryoprobes in place but not yet cooled the cat's bar pressing shows a steady upward trend (bottom of Fig. 15.7) but when the ITP is cooled bilaterally to 10°C the cat stopped pressing and turned away from the lever and milk-delivery recess

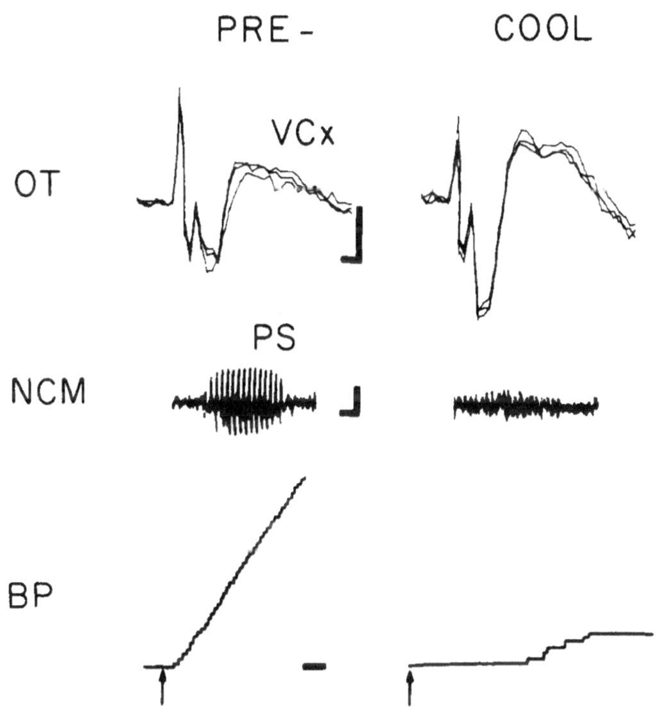

FIG. 15.7. Three effects of cryogenic blockade of inferior thalamic peduncle (ITP) in cat: Visual cortex (VCx) evoked response to optic tract (OT) stimulation (a specific sensory system effect) is enhanced in amplitude; recruiting response at posterior sigmoid (PS) is blocked to nucleus centralis medialis stimulation; cumulative bar-pressing response for milk reward is blocked. See text for further comment. From Skinner and Lindsley, 1967. By permission.

as if no longer interested, or perhaps inattentive and no longer remembering the meaning of the learned habit of bar pressing for milk. The stopping was not due to satiation or loss of drive for as soon as the cryoprobe in ITP returned to normal (37°C), the pressing was resumed at the precooling rate. Also shown in Fig. 15.7 are two other effects of ITP cooling. The middle portion shows the precooling recruiting response to stimulation of N. centralis medialis (NCM) when recorded on posterior sigmoid gyrus (PS). This is the classical recruiting-type response with each stimulus of an 8 per sec train giving rise to a surface negative potential of uniform amplitude except during the first four or five shocks when each one shows incrementation after the first ineffective shock. Recruiting gets its name from this progressive incrementation at the start as if more and more cellular units are brought into the discharge as stimulation continues. On the right during cooling of ITP to a reversible blocking level (10°C) the recruiting is all but blocked completely. In the top of Fig. 15.7 the optic tract (OT) was stimulated and the response at the visual cortex (VCx) was recorded before cooling. There is a sharp negative and positive-negative complex followed by a positive slow wave and a much longer duration negative return to baseline. The same optic-tract stimulation during the period of cooling shows that this specific visual-cortex response was enhanced in amplitude in its late components as if released from some tonic inhibition. In summary, we see that blockade of the ITP, thus interrupting the flow of reticular activation impulses enroute to cortex via an orbitofrontal cortex distribution center, may have at least three effects: enhancing stimulation effects in visual cortex, abolishing recruiting responses initiated from medio-thalamic nonspecific nuclei and recorded on the surface of the cortex, and inhibiting the pressing of a bar for a reward previously learned. We believe the latter effect to be an interference with, or inhibition of, an attentive set learned with respect to the pressing of the bar to satisfy a food-deprived state.

My former student, James E. Skinner, and his now former student, Charles D. Yingling, have gone on brilliantly to analyze the thalamic regulating mechanisms, especially nucleus reticularis, coupled with reticular formation and frontal cortex influences in the governance, they believe, of selective attention and general arousal effects (Skinner & Yingling, 1976, 1977; Yingling & Skinner, 1975, 1976).

Brain Stem–Hypothalamic–Hippocampal Systems and Their Contrasting Electrophysiological and Behavioral Effects

The period of the 1950's and 1960's was one of intensive investigation of the electrical activity of the hippocampus, triggered in large measure by the classic study of Green and Arduini (1954). They studied the rabbit and cat, but made additional observations in the monkey. Three main types of activity were recorded from the hippocampus, especially in the rabbit and cat. They called one of these, a synchronous, rhythmic series of waves of about 3-7 Hz, "*theta rhythm*" (after W. Grey Walter [1950, 1953], who had so labeled similar rhythms in humans). They identified this ubiquitous and prominent rhythm associated with sensory, alerting, and emotional stimuli as an hippocampal "arousal" reaction and noted that it diminished or habituated with repetition of the same stimulus. They called marked amplitude attentuation or abolition of the theta rhythm, often associated with onset or enhancement of low to medium amplitude rhythmic or arrythmic fast waves, a *desynchronization pattern*. A third type of activity consisted of high-voltage, irregular slow waves and fast waves mixed in an *irregular pattern*.

Green and Arduini observed that arousal or alerting stimuli that produced the theta rhythm in the hippocampus had an inverse effect upon the alpha-wave activity of the neocortex causing instead a desynchronization or blocking of the alpha rhythm. They repeatedly remarked about this apparent reciprocal relationship between the electrical activities of hippocampus and neocortex and commented that (Green & Arduini, 1954), "Such strikingly inverse patterns of activity are also evoked simultaneously in these two parts of the forebrain by direct excitation of the arousal mechanism in the brain stem described by Moruzzi and Magoun [p.552]." Others have observed this reversal of the arousal effect on hippocampal and neocortical electrical activity. Our studies in the cat (Coleman & Lindsley, 1975) have shown it, but as is illustrated shortly, the relationship is not inviolate because in some instances in which electrical stimulation of brain-stem sites produced hippocampal theta rhythm, sometimes a rhythmic activity in the cortex was also induced, usually only in certain areas of the cortex, but not all (Macadar, Chalupa, & Lindsley, 1974). However, as a general rule, the reciprocal relationship seems to hold.

Green and Arduini found that the theta rhythm could be induced in the hippocampus by high-frequency stimulation (100 Hz) in a variety of sites such as the reticular formation, hypothalamus, septum, preoptic region, and in the intralaminar nuclei of the thalamus. A number of other investigators have confirmed and extended such observations (Kawamura, Nakamura, & Tokizane, 1961; Stumpf, Petsche & Gogolak, 1965; Tokizane, Kawamura, & Imamura, 1960), and have sought to identify the nature, source, and role of the synchronizing and desynchronizing electrical activities of the hippocampus.

Because of our involvement with the features of the ascending reticular activating system and the thalamo-cortical mechanisms regulating neocortical electrical activity associated with arousal, alerting, and attention, I became interested in hippocampal electrical activity and its association with behavior. In particular, I was curious to know whether the various functions attributed to the hippocampus, for the most part rather speculatively, might be correlated with changes in the electrical activity of the hippocampus. In addition, I was interested in the potential of a thalamic pacemaker to govern or regulate cortical alpha rhythm, and the possibility as suggested by Petsche, Stumpf, and Gogolak

(1962) that the septum might be a pacemaker for hippocampal theta rhythm.

About this time, in September of 1966, I received a letter from Harvey Anchel, a graduate student in psychology at McMaster University, who expressed an interest in joining my group as a postdoctoral visitor. Anchel had been working with Woodburn Heron on the effects of strong sensory bombardment from birth on the development of the EEG rhythms in rats (Heron & Anchel, 1964) and as a result had become interested in ''neurological mechanisms and behavioral correlates of so-called 'synchronizing systems,' '' and felt that our investigations of the reticular activating system were along such lines. He obtained his degree and a postdoctoral fellowship from the National Research Council of Canada and joined us in my laboratories in the Brain Research Institute in the summer of 1968.

After some indoctrination in our methods and procedures, and in my concept of an isolated functional systems approach in the study of brain and behavior, Anchel began exploring various regions of the hypothalamus with high-frequency stimulation while recording from the hippocampus and neocortex. The result was a publication by Anchel and Lindsley (1972) on ''Differentiation of two reticulo-hypothalamic systems regulating hippocampal activity.''

Anchel's explorations soon confirmed the observations of others mentioned earlier, but more importantly his systematic and painstaking effort soon enabled us to identify two closely adjacent pathways in the posterior hypothalamus where stimulation at 100 Hz produced distinctly opposite effects in the hippocampus. Stimulation medially, near the midline, induced hippocampal theta waves, whereas stimulation 1 or 2 millimeters laterally desynchronized or blocked hippocampal theta rhythms and induced low-voltage fast waves. After many checks and careful mapping or the regions surrounding these apparently diverse functional pathways where stimulation had a contrasting influence upon hippocampal electrical activity, we concluded that we were dealing with two adjacent functionally balancing systems. The medial region close to the midline seemed to correspond to the dorsal longitudinal fasciculus of Schütz and the lateral one to the medial forebrain bundle.

A localized lesion in the medial hypothalamus (MH), anterior to the site where stimulation elicited theta rhythm in the hippocampus, blocked this effect. Similarly, a localized lesion anterior to the stimulating site in the lateral hypothalamus (LH), which caused desynchronization of hippocampal electrical activity, blocked or greatly attenuated this effect. Localized cooling to 10°C at the tip of a cryoprobe located anterior to MH and LH stimulating sites blocked their respective influences upon hippocampal activity. These effects of cooling in the two pathways of contrasting function are illustrated in Fig. 15.8.

With stimulating electrodes in the appropriate site in the medial hypothalamus (MH) where stimulation typically produces hippocampal theta rhythm and with the tip of a cryoprobe appropriately located anterior to it but not yet cooled, we see in the PRECOOL record (top left) that stimulation at 100 Hz and 5 volts

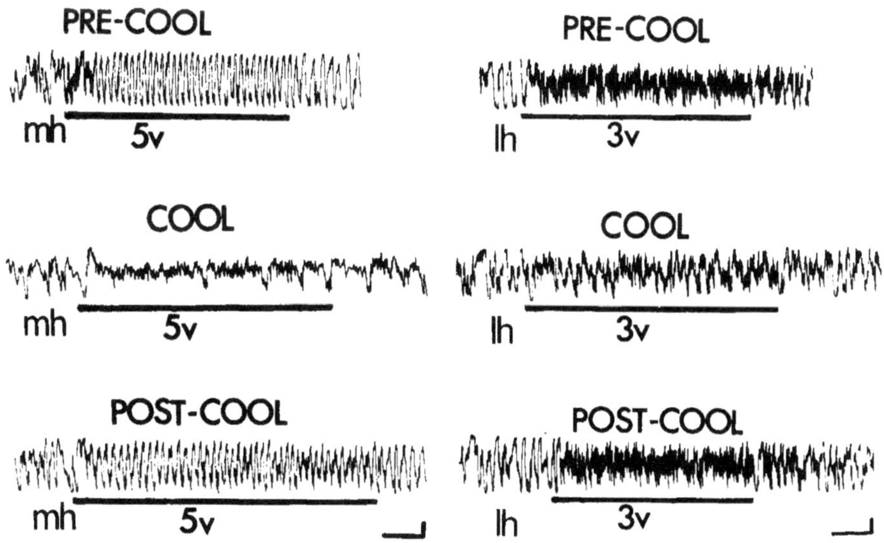

FIG. 15.8. Contrasting effects in the cat of stimulating two brain-stem-hypothalamic-hippocampal systems; stimulation of a medial hypothalamic (MH) pathway (on left) causes hippocampal theta rhythm, cooling MH anterior to stimulating site blocks the induction of theta waves, rewarming cryoprobes restores theta rhythm; stimulation of lateral hypothalamic (LH) pathway causes desynchronization of hippocampal theta activity, cooling makes little change (MH cooling, not LH cooling, hence LH effect not blocked), rewarming cryoprobes has nothing to restore—there is desynchronization from LH stimulation throughout. See text for additional comment. Calibrations: 100 uV; 1 sec. Adapted from Anchel and Lindsley, 1972. By permission.

produced a strong and rhythmic theta activity. In the record below it, the same MH stimulation did not produce hippocampal theta waves during the COOL period. Instead there is a low-amplitude, fast-activity pattern and desynchronization of the on-going irregular slow waves visible before stimulation began. These latter effects are apparently due to tonic activity in the LH pathway, which is now unopposed by the MH theta synchronizing system, which is temporarily blocked by the cooling. In the bottom POSTCOOL record, the theta rhythm is restored when the temperature of the tip of the cryoprobe is returned to normal level. The records on the right illustrate the same procedure when the stimulating electrodes and the cryoprobe are in the lateral hypothalamus (LH). In the PRECOOL period, LH stimulation has a strong desynchronizing and activating (high-amplitude, fast-activity) effect. During the COOL period, the LH system is mainly inactivated and does not desynchronize the theta and irregular slow-wave activity in the hippocampus and shows little evidence of the activation pattern. The unopposed tonic activity in the MH system is probably responsible for the mixed theta and irregular slow waves. During the POSTCOOL period, when the temperature at the LH cryoprobe is returned to normal, LH stimulation again produces a strong desynchronizing and activating influence that overrides tonic MH influence.

In other records not shown here, reticular stimulation in certain regions also induces hippocampal theta-rhythm activity and it is blocked by the same lesion, or cooling, in the MH pathway, thus indicating that more caudally initiated stimulation in the lower brain stem uses this same medial pathway in its theta production. Bilateral lesions of the dorsal fornix prevented MH stimulation from producing hippocampal theta rhythm, thereby implicating the septum and fornix in the synchronizing system that generates hippocampal theta rhythm. The fornix lesions did not affect the ability of LH stimulation to produce desynchronization and activation effects on hippocampal electrical activity. This seems to indicate that the LH desynchronizing system is separate from that of the MH synchronizing system. However, their interactions may take place in part at the septum, and at the hippocampus by an extraseptal route. The latter is indicated by the fact that septal and fornix lesions do not block the activation effect (fast activity in hippocampus) when LH is stimulated. Evidence for the former was presented by Wilson and Lindsley (1974) and has since been illustrated (Lindsley & Wilson, 1975) by showing that LH stimulation that desynchronizes hippocampal activity may have either an excitatory or an inhibitory effect upon the firing pattern of certain septal cells. It is as yet uncertain by what extraceptal route the LH system reaches the hippocampus. If the LH system is to be identified with the medial forebrain bundle or a part of it in the diencephalon, it may be somewhat tortuous for the medial forebrain bundle has been shown to become diffuse and ramify extensively in this region (Millhouse, 1969).

Much of the study by Anchel and Lindsley (1972) was conducted on acute cats immobilized with gallamine triethiodide (Flaxedil), protected from pain by thorough and repeated infiltrations of local anesthetic at all cut surfaces and pressure points, and maintained on artificial respiration. In such acute preparations, it was possible to vary our stimulating sites, our lesion and cryogenic blocking sites, and our recording sites until we found the most efficacious locations for permanently implanting electrodes and cryoprobes in awake and behaving chronic preparations. Having determined where our stimulating electrodes could be placed for optimal generation of hippocampal theta rhythm, and for its desynchronization, we proceeded to develop five chronic cat preparations so that we could observe the effects of stimulation not only on the changes in hippocampal electrical activity but also upon behavior. These studies were quite preliminary in scope but nevertheless resulted in our obtaining some cogent and relevant observations.

Stimulation via electrodes in MH caused hippocampal theta rhythm in these awake and behaving animals, as did cryogenic blockade of the LH system, although stimulation effects were more marked and time related to the stimulus. Each procedure separately produced similar behavioral effects consisting of head turning, searching, and orienting. Because both procedures caused hippocampal theta rhythm, it was inferred that theta rhythm in the hippocampus is associated with such behaviors, either as a cause or as a consequence. A quite different pattern of behavior was associated with the desynchronization caused by LH stimulation or by cryogenic blockade of the MH system. It consisted of arrest of on-going behavior and attentive fixation of gaze and posture. These results were so promising that several subsequent studies were planned to test the effects of manipulating hippocampal electrical activity by means of stimulation or blockade of these two brain-stem-hypothalamic-hippocampal systems in order to note the associated changes in behavior under both spontaneous and trained conditions.

Before such studies were undertaken, however, we wished to learn more about the origins of these two-system pathways in the lower brain stem. We also initiated a program of investigation of the rostral course of the pathways and especially on the nature of the theta synchronizing mechanism. It was suggested that this mechanism might reside in the septum, or in its reciprocal connections with the hippocampus (Lindsley & Wilson, 1975; Wilson, Motter, & Lindsley, 1976).

With respect to the caudal origins of these contrasting systems of influence on hippocampal electrical activity, Macadar, Chalupa, & Lindsley (1974) initiated a program of systematic stimulation mapping of the brain stem in the region of the midbrain and pons. The region of study extended from frontal plane A-6 to P-8. Surgery and stereotaxis were accomplished under general halothane anesthesia. Thereafter the cats were maintained under a mixture of nitrous oxide and oxygen, and millimeter by millimeter stimulation was begun. Only a few electrode penetrations were made in each cat in order to avoid a pincushion effect.

Responses to stimulation were classified and plotted on four frontal-plane maps between A-6 and P-8 (A-4.1, P-0.2, P-3.1, P-6.0) and on two parasagittal plane maps 0.3 and 2.5 mm from the midline. Stimulation points that elicited hippocampal theta rhythm were marked by solid circles, desynchronization responses were represented by open circles, mixed responses by open squares, and no-effect stimulations by open triangles. Fig. 15.9 shows the data for one frontal plane, P-0.2, to illustrate the procedure and a portion of the results.

Briefly, the results, including those plotted on other frontal-plane maps and on the parasagittal maps, show that five regions had heavy concentrations of solid circles indicating that stimulation caused hippocampal theta activity. The regions were: *periaqueductal grey substance, nucleus reticularis pontis oralis, nucleus locus coeruleus, midbrain tegmentum,* and *nucleus reticularis gigantocellularis*. The regions where stimulation caused desynchronization of hippocampal electrical activity were: *nucleus reticularis pontis caudalis* and *nuclei of the raphe*.

Fig. 15.10 shows the types of responses recorded in the hippocampus and cortex elicited by stimulation in each of the just-mentioned regions except nucleus reticularis gigantocellularis in the pons. The four pairs of traces in the upper left reveal that stimulation in each of the four regions induced hippocampal theta

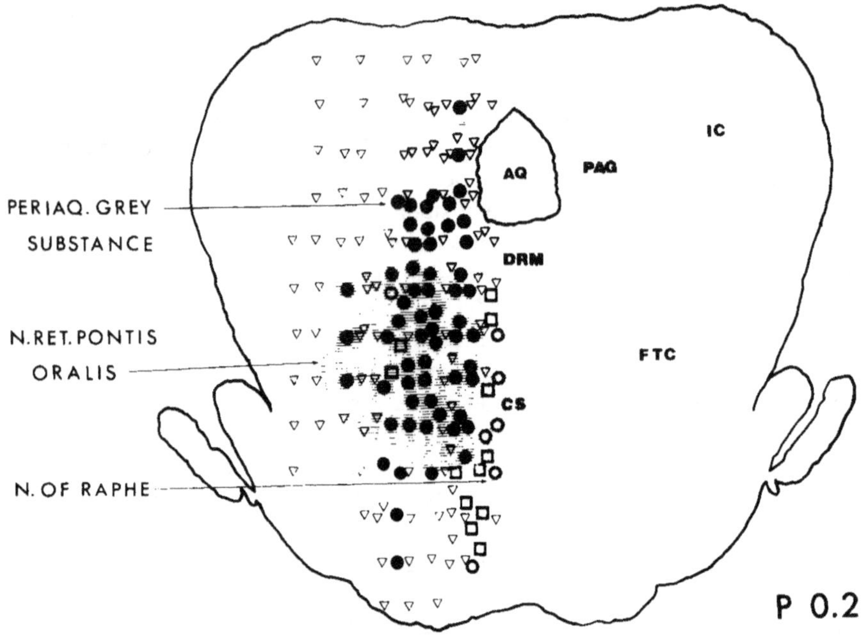

FIG. 15.9. Brain-stem stimulation sites in the cat, which cause hippocampal theta rhythm (solid black circles), other sites mainly in raphe, which desynchronize theta and other slow waves of hippocampus (open circles), sites showing mixed theta and desynchronization patterns (open squares), and sites having no effect (open triangles). See text for details. From Macadar et al., 1974. By permission.

activity although it varied in magnitude and frequency from region to region, indicating that they are not homogeneous with respect to their influences upon the septum and hippocampus. In the case of each of these theta-eliciting sites, the neocortex tends to show desynchronization, thus upholding the general rule of Green and Arduini (1954) that theta activity in hippocampus is usually accompanied by neocortical desynchronization. In two instances there appears to be clearly detectable theta-like activity in a regional area of the cortex only (right anterior cortex for periaqueductal grey, and left posterior cortex for pontis oralis). Although unilateral stimulation of these brain-stem sites usually produces the same bilateral effects in the hippocampus, the anterior and posterior regions of the neocortex on the side contralateral to the site of stimulation may vary in their responses from those on the ipsilateral side, suggesting that neocortex is more differentially controlled and regulated than is the hippocampus.

The bottom two sets of traces on the left show quite clearly that stimulation in nucleus reticularis pontis caudalis and in the superior central nucleus of the raphe elicits a desynchronizing response in the hippocampus. Those traces on the right

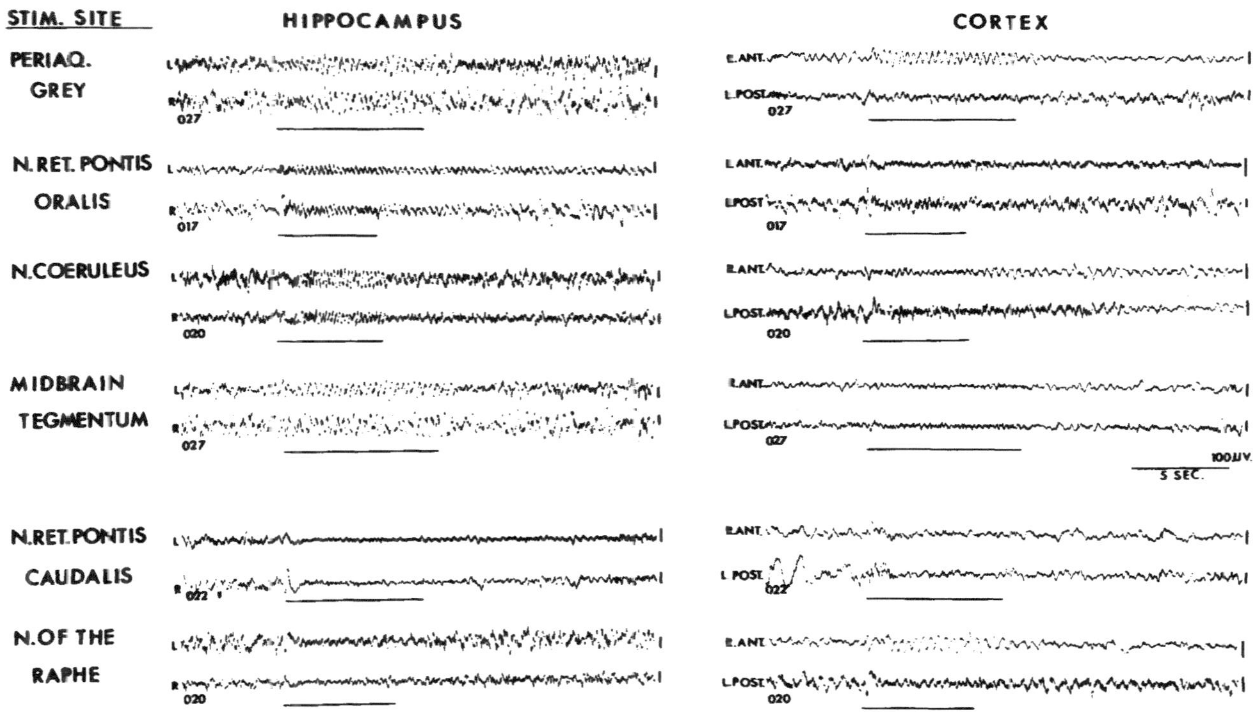

FIG. 15.10. Stimulation sites in midbrain and pons in the cat, which induce hippocampal theta rhythm (upper four pairs of tracings from left and right dorsal hippocampus) but usually an inverse desynchronization effect in cortical records shown on right; see text for exceptions). Also two stimulation sites that induce hippocampal desynchronization (lower left) with tendency to reciprocal effects in neocortical records. Calibrations: 100 uV; 3 sec. From Macadar et al. 1974. By permission.

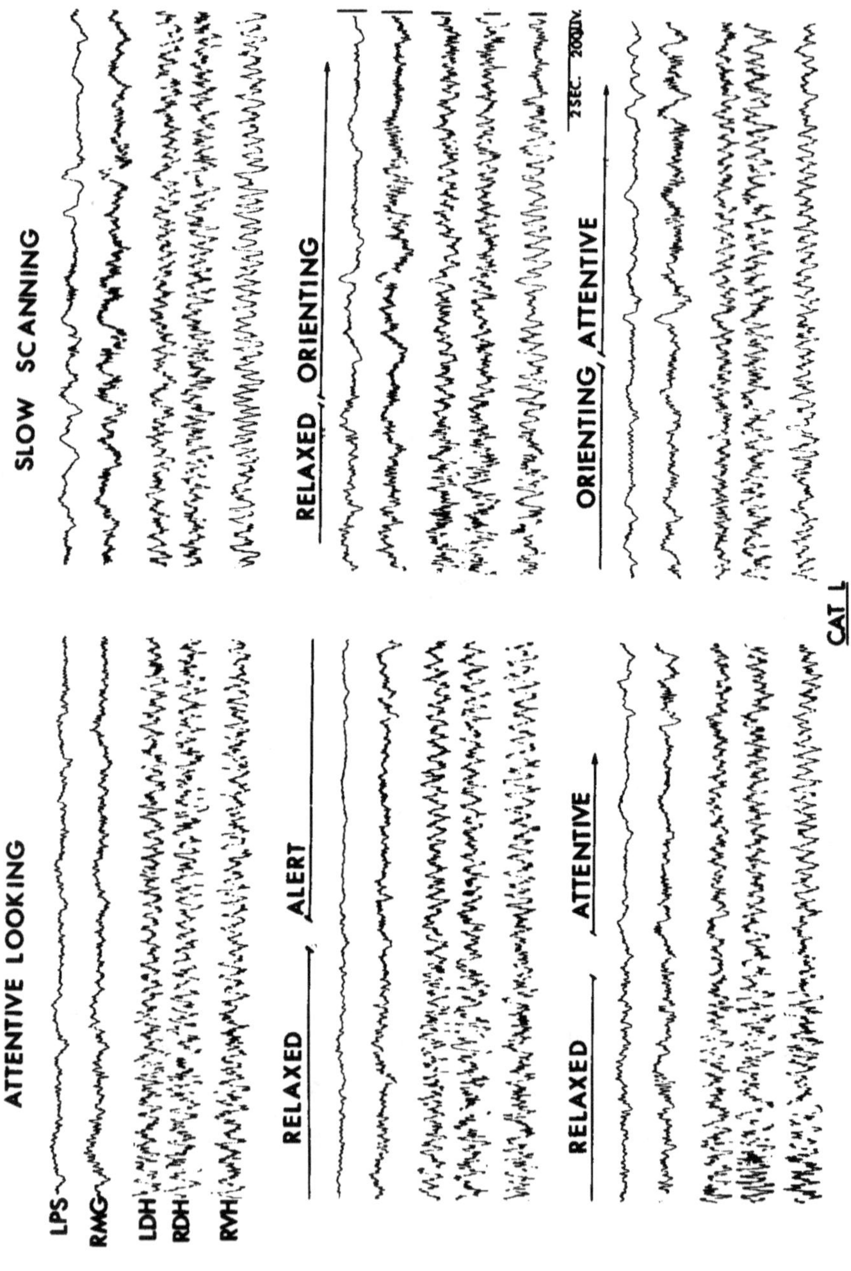
ATTENTIVE LOOKING
SLOW SCANNING
LPS
RMG
LDH
RDH
RVH
RELAXED
ALERT
RELAXED
ORIENTING
RELAXED
ATTENTIVE
ORIENTING
ATTENTIVE
2 SEC.
200µV.
CAT L

show that pontis caudalis stimulation attenuated on-going neocortical activity and left low-amplitude theta-like activity, whereas raphe stimulation induced strong theta-like activity on the right and less strong and less well-organized theta like activity on the left in the posterior region.

During the late 1950's and the 1960's much energy and enthusiasm were manifested by investigators around the world for finding behavioral and psychological correlates of hippocampal electrical activities, both of the tonic, steady-state and of the phasic, sporadic varieties. A few representative studies may be mentioned (Grastyan, 1959; Grastyan, Karmos, Vereczkey, & Kellenyi, 1966; Grastyan, Karmos, Vereczkey, Martin, & Kellenyi, 1965; Grastyan, Lissak, Madarasz, & Donhoffer, 1959; Adey, 1967; Adey, Dunlop, & Hendrix, 1960; Adey, Walters, & Lindsley, 1962; Bennett, 1970, 1971, 1973a, 1973b; Kemp & Kaada, 1975; Paiva, Lopes da Silva, & Mollevanger, 1976; Wishaw & Vanderwolf, 1973). Among the functions associated with the hippocampal theta rhythm are orienting responses, arousal, alerting and attentive states, scanning for information, investigatory behaviors, motivation, discrimination and information registry, learning and memory consolidation, voluntary behaviors, and response inhibition.

In order to advance our studies of the relation of hippocampal theta rhythm to behavior, we studied spontaneous behavior in chronic cat preparations and also the effect of stimulation of medial and lateral hypothalamic systems upon behavior and the electrical activity of dorsal and ventral hippocampus and neocortex (Coleman & Lindsley, 1975). The cats were free to move about in a small soundproof box with one-way visibility for observing spontaneous behavior. After the cats adjusted to the experimental chamber for several days, recordings and observations were made each day during a variety of spontaneous and free behaviors ranging across various states of waking and the different stages of sleep. Fig. 15.11 illustrates some of the variations in electrical activity recorded in hippocampus and neocortex during spontaneous changes in waking behavior. After much observation of the individual cats day after day, it became possible on the continuously running electrical records to classify and record the states and phasic shifts of behavior quite accurately and reliably.

Although there was nothing in the soundproof box to manipulate or attract attention, there were periods of attentive looking as in the upper record on the left, or continuous slow scanning behavior as in the upper record on the right. In

FIG. 15.11. Hippocampal and neocortical electrical activity in the cat during free spontaneous behavior states and specific behavior changes. Throughout free behavior states of attentive looking (A), slow scanning of head and eyes (D), theta rhythm was predominant; bursts of theta rhythm accompany onset of specific behavior changes such as in (B), relaxed to alert (C), relaxed to attentive (E), relaxed to orienting (F), during shifts from orienting to attentive state. Abbreviations in this and next figure: LPS—left posterior sigmoid; RMG—right marginal gyrus; LDH and RDH—left and right dorsal hippocampus; RVH—right ventral hippocampus. Calibrations as shown on Figs. From Coleman and Lindsley, 1975. By permission

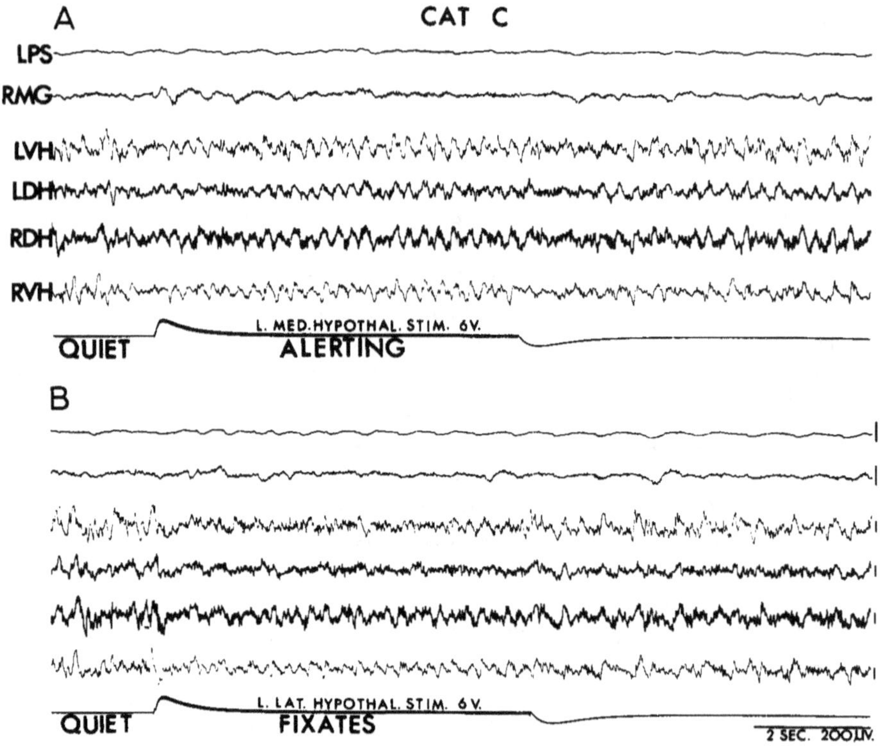

FIG. 15.12. Contrasting behavior and hippocampal electrical effects in the cat from 100 Hz stimulation of medial and lateral posterior hypothalamic sites. Inverse effects in neocortex sites. (A) Stimulation of right medial hypothalamus induces theta rhythm at all hippocampal sites, but not in neocortex. (B) Lateral hypothalamic stimulation causes fixation of gaze and posture and desynchronization of theta and other waves. From Coleman and Lindsley, 1975. By permission.

both instances the hippocampus exhibited continuous theta activity throughout. The middle records on the left and right, and the record on the lower left, began with the cat quiet and relaxed, but midway in each record there was a phasic shift in behavior accompanied by a change in the electrical activity of the hippocampus from an irregular mixed pattern to one of rhythmic theta activity. The behavior change was from quiet relaxation to alerting, orienting, or attentiveness. In the lower right record, the cat was first orienting and then became attentive. Both behaviors were accompanied by a more or less continuous theta activity. Many other observations were made, but arousal, alerting, orienting, scanning, searching, and investigatory behavior were always accompanied by continuous theta activity or shifts from an irregular pattern to a theta pattern.

Fig. 15.12 shows the effects of stimulating either the medial or lateral hypothalamus at 100 Hz and 6 volts for short periods of time, usually about 5 seconds. Record A illustrates the effect of stimulating the MH theta-producing system. At the start of the record there is irregular slow-wave activity while the cat is quiet, but as soon as stimulation starts theta rhythms appear in all four hippocampal traces and low-level, fast activity appears over the right marginal gyrus of the cortex. Record B shows a contrasting effect when the LH desynchronizing and activating system is stimulated. On-going irregular slow waves at the start during quiet behavior are desynchronized for the duration of the stimulus, especially in the left dorsal and ventral hippocampus. Some evidence of theta rhythm appears in the right dorsal and ventral hippocampal traces. This sometimes happens when the LH stimulating electrodes are near the margin of the MH. The important thing is that not only do MH and LH stimulation produce contrasting hippocampal effects, but result in contrasting behaviors as well. Here MH stimulation caused the cat to become alert (at other times, there might be orienting or scanning behavior) whereas LH stimulation caused the cat to assume a posture and gaze of fixation.

In a subsequent study, Coleman and Lindsley (1977) trained cats to bar press for water with continuous reinforcement present. At the start, when the cats were struggling to adjust to the problem and when close attention to the water well and to the bar were necessary, synchronous theta activity was frequently present in the hippocampus and the cortical activity was desynchronized. Later, when the cat was trained to bar press about once per second without having to pay attention to either the water well or the bar, low-voltage, fast activity and irregular slow waves were very much the rule, as during more relaxed periods in spontaneous behavior. During a second phase of the training, 10-second periods of reinforcement were alternated with 10-second periods of nonreinforcement and theta activity increased during nonreinforcement. Initially, the cats had difficulty withholding responses during the nonreinforcement period but, as they learned to withhold, theta diminished and desynchronization increased. Such a change in hippocampal activity suggests that it accompanies learned-response inhibition or differential extinction, as Bennett and Gottfried (1970) have found when a cat is required to withhold responses under differential reinforcement of low rate (DRL) following training under continuous reinforcement (CRF).

Another phase of this study involved stimulus-cued alternating reinforcement with tone presented during the first 10 seconds followed after 2 seconds by a single light-flash cue and then 10 more seconds of nonreinforcement. As the cat learned the significance of the tone on and flash cue as signals for nonreinforcement and reinforcement periods, respectively, greater attention to the task was required and hippocampal theta activity increased.

A final phase of the study was the effect of MH and LH stimulation on these learned behaviors. Only one situation is mentioned here because of its uniqueness. In advanced stages of training, when a cat was pressing the bar at a rate of about one press per second during a reinforcement period, stimulation of the MH or LH systems was introduced. Medial hypothalamic stimulation as usual caused hippocampal theta rhythm and one or more of the following behaviors: alerting, orienting, scanning, and investigatory activity. Bar pressing ceased immediately and strikingly was not renewed for long periods, 1-44 minutes with a mean of 10 minutes. During such a nonresponsive period, the cats showed no interest in or attention to the manipulanda as they had shown before such stimulation. They were not drowsy and did not become inactive; instead, while showing theta rhythm, they continued to orient, scan, or investigate the chamber. Lateral hypothalamic stimulation briefly interrupted bar pressing but in a matter of a few seconds it was reinstated at the usual rate. The puzzling thing is why, after MH stimulation, such prolonged periods of nonpressing occurred. It was not due to satiation or loss of drive strength because when bar pressing resumed, the once-per-second rate continued. Though the cat appeared distracted from the task, it was not inattentive to other things, and alert, orienting, attentive, and scanning behavior occurred. This effect of MH stimulation on bar pressing for reward is not unlike the interruption of bar pressing that followed lesion or cryogenic blockade of the ITP in the study by Skinner and Lindsley (1967). In that experiment, cooling of the peduncle stopped learned bar pressing for reward, the cat turned away from the bar as if no longer interested, and explored the immediate environment, without drowsiness or fearfulness. There was no evidence of pain or fear as a result of MH stimulation. It was as if memory for the learned habit and the consequences of its performance were held in abeyance, or as if some disruption of the mechanism of attention made it impossible to focus upon and integrate the sensory cues provided by the manipulanda with the drive state and the learned motor performance necessary to consummate the act. It may be a combination of temporary memory loss induced by internal distraction and loss of some attentive mechanism focussing on recently learned acts that satisfy a drive state.

Perhaps this is an example of how two systems of arousal, alerting, and attention may work in parallel, one being the brain-stem-reticulo-thalamo-cortical activating system effective in influencing neocortex and specific decision and information-processing channels, the other being a brain-stem-hypothalamic-hippocampal system possibly concerned with processing information into memory and retrieval from memory and perhaps with an emotional or motivational reinforcing effect. Stimulation of the reticular activating system tends to desynchronize neocortical alpha activity and arouse or alert the organism to attend and act; stimulation of the medial hypothalamic (MH) system tends to synchronize hippocampal electrical activity with resulting theta waves and associated behavior involving arousal, alerting, attention, and scanning for information. W. Grey Walter (1953) once proposed that neocortical alpha rhythms scan for pattern in visual signals, whereas theta rhythms may scan for pleasure!

It is of particular interest that in the study by Macadar et al. (1974), five somewhat different groups of cells or fibers of passage trigger theta rhythms in the hippocampus but of slightly different frequency and other characteristics.

Some of these influence hippocampus and neocortex via pathways in the MH and some by pathways forming a part of the MFB. Also, a part of the MFB must be presumed to carry fibers from the raphe nuclei and perhaps nucleus reticularis pontis caudalis, the two regions that, when stimulated, cause desynchronization of hippocampal activity. With the tremendous surge of knowledge in neurochemistry and neuropharmacology, particularly with respect to the monoamine substances of which some nuclear groups such as n. locus coeruleus (norepinephrine) and the raphe nuclei (serotonin) are said to be composed, and whose transmitter substances may be widely disseminated rostrally, it would seem to be important to categorize and analyze the roles and interactions of the five nuclei or cell groups that contribute to the induction of hippocampal theta and the two that desynchronize hippocampal activity. The nature and source of their afferents and their efferent targets, and the neuro-transmitter substances released at efferent terminals, coupled with electrophysiological and behavioral data relative to their functions will help to advance our understanding of these interacting systems.

Role of the Pulvinar in a Secondary Visual System: Eye movements, Attention, and Information Processing

My interest in n. pulvinaris was first generated by publications of the British anatomist-anthropologist, Sir Wilfrid E. Le Gros Clark (Clark, 1932; Clark & Northfield, 1937) and the American neurological surgeon, A. Earl Walker (Walker, 1938). Clark emphasized the progressive phylogenetic differentiation and growth of the pulvinar in infraprimates and primates. Walker studied cortical projections of thalamic nuclei, including the pulvinar, in monkeys by retrograde degeneration using the Nissl technique.

Later, in 1955, as a participant in an international symposium on the thalamus held at Montevideo, my interest in the thalamus was further enhanced, but not because of great enlightenment about the pulvinar. Only two of the extensive presentations dealt briefly with the pulvinar. Hassler (1955) emphasized the integrative role of the pulvinar and mentioned that it receives visual input from the LGB via fibers ascending in lamella lateralis and terminating in the caudal part of the pulvinar and a few connections that end in the inferior pulvinar. He also said that it receives auditory input from the MGB. No mention was made of somatosensory input to this complex and little understood structure, the largest of the nuclei in the thalamus in monkey and man. In his paper entitled, "The Meaning of the Thalamus," Walker (1955) had this to say about the pulvinar: "At the present time the pulvinar is the terra incognita of the thalamus. Although its afferent connections may be assumed to be from its adjacent nuclei, and its efferent projection to the cerebral cortex is fairly well established, its functional role is largely conjecture [p. 940]." He predicted that only after we know more about the dynamic process of temporal integration, as well as spatial organization of the systems of fibers in the thalamus, will we know something about the meaning of the thalamus.

Prior to this (Lindsley, 1953, 1954), I had been recording electrical responses in the central visual pathways of the cat from eye to cortex and occasionally had as many as three electrodes in the LGB. Once, postexperiment histology revealed that one of the electrodes just missed the caudal tip of the LGB and landed in the MGB; another time one of the electrodes was slightly dorsal and medial to the LGB and in the pulvinar. The MGB electrode, although only 1 millimeter from the LGB, showed no response to the photic flash, but the one in the pulvinar did. This led me to believe that it might be worthwhile to explore the pulvinar for responsivity to visual, auditory, and somatosensory stimuli, particularly because others (Buser, Borenstein, & Bruner, 1959; Mountcastle & Henneman, 1949, 1952) had noted casually some response to somatic or visual and auditory stimuli. Unfortunately, I did not follow this up until 1965 when a young physician, Dr. Chuong Huang, from the National Taiwan University came to UCLA seeking a Ph.D. in Physiology and asked to work with me in the Brain Research Institute.

I proposed a systematic mapping of evoked responses to visual, auditory, and somatosensory stimuli in the region encompassing the pulvinar and adjacent nuclei of the posterolateral thalamus in the cat. The millimeter by millimeter mapping, which was spread across cats to avoid a "pincushion" effect, included the nuclei lateralis posterior, posterior, suprageniculatus, lateralis dorsalis, and some overlapping of the specific sensory nuclei, LGB, MGB, and ventralis posterior lateralis and medialis. This was done under pentobarbital, alpha chloralose, and in the unanesthetized brain of animals immobilized with gallamine triethiodide and protected from pain by local anesthesia. Pentobarbital proved to be too suppressive of responses in all areas, but the other procedures revealed the pulvinar to be a polysensory convergence center. The thesis was completed in 1968, the same year that Roumanian investigators (Kreindler, Crighel, & Marinchescu, 1968) reported a study in cats with similar observations. Our study (Huang & Lindsley, 1973), published later, involved more conditions and parameters of evaluation, including latencies of response components in all regions, successive recovery cycles, intermodality interaction to paired stimuli and microelectrode recordings from some pulvinar and adjacent regions (see also Chalupa, Macadar, & Lindsley, 1974).

We found that the pulvinar was responsive to each of the three modalities of stimulation, but not equally in all regions. Visual responses were more prominent and widespread than auditory or somatic responses, although the latter were usually enhanced in those regions of the pulvinar that were closer to their specific thalamic nuclei. Latencies of both early and late responses in the pulvinar and other posterolateral nuclei were longer than those in thalamic relay nuclei, except for nucleus posterior, which was the same as LGB. Microelectrode recordings confirmed the regional differences for the three stimuli and showed rhythmic bursting often time-locked to the field potentials. Of special interest were the recovery-cycle results and thc intermodality interactions of paired stimuli. Briefly, successive recovery cycles were short for primary sensory pathways and for thalamic relay nuclei and showed response amplitude decrement only when the interstimulus intervals (ISIs) were shorter than 1 second. In contrast, the nonspecific or association nuclei of the posterolateral thalamus (pulvinar and lateralis posterior) had longer recovery cycles and showed progressive decrement of the amplitude of the response to the second stimulus starting with full amplitude at an ISI of 2.0 seconds and steadily dropping to near zero at an ISI of 0.1 second. Thus, there was a distinct difference in the speed with which structures of the specific sensory input channels can process information relative to that with which association nuclei or nonspecific systems function.

Another interesting result was that there were marked differences in the way in which intermodality interactions occur. For example, a visual stimulus exhibited dominance over an auditory stimulus, and an auditory stimulus over a somatic stimulus when different stimulus modalities were paired at progressively shorter interstimulus intervals. The more dominant stimulus for a particular region of the pulvinar showed less attenuation of its amplitude and longer resistance to change as ISIs decreased when it was preceded by a stimulus of less dominance for that region. A pairing in the order visual-somatic showed marked reduction of the somatic response when the ISI was 250 msec but the visual response in a somatic-visual pairing showed no attenuation even at a 70 msec ISI.

There were many other important results too numerous to mention here. We concluded our discussion with the following paragraph (Huang & Lindsley, 1973):

> These regional and interaction differences would seem to provide a potential code for attention and discrimination so that the visual region of the pulvinar hierarchy of precedence would be in the order of visual, auditory and somatosensory. In the auditory region the order of dominance would be auditory, visual and somatosensory. Although all three stimuli may have access to a given region, the order of dominance would favor selective attention and discrimination. On the other hand such regional and spatial codes might be superceded by temporal codes imposed by influences from other systems, either specific or nonspecific sensory systems, whose pacemaker or synchronizing influences might shift the action from one region to another and in so doing shift the balance of influence of the pulvinar (and possibly other association nuclei of the lateral nuclear group) upon the cortical area to which it projects. In man this would be the critically important integrative center at the junction of the occipital, parietal and temporal lobes, usually designated as the supramarginal and angular gyri and sometimes identified as part of Wernicke's area [pp. 277-278].

In 1970 Leo M. Chalupa, who had just completed a Ph.D. thesis under Professor William S. Battersby of Queens College in the City University of New York, came to work with me as a postdoctoral visitor. His thesis had been on the effects of stimulation of the reticular formation, pulvinar and superior colliculus upon the responsivity of the visual cortex in the cat. He was eager to continue work along these lines and, like myself, he was interested in the role of the pulvinar. During the next few years, he took a leading part in experiments on the pulvinar and related structures in the cat and monkey.

Two studies carried out in the cat by Chalupa, Anchel, and Lindsley (1972, 1973) were concerned, respectively, with functional sources of visual input to the pulvinar, and the functional influence of the pulvinar upon visually evoked responses in primary visual cortex (marginal gyrus) and visual association cortex (supramarginal gyrus). In the first study, surprisingly, it was found that with a small cryoprobe cooled at 15°C we could partially block the function of the three laminae of the cat geniculate selectively. Cooling the A lamina diminished the response of the visual cortex to contralateral eye stimulation by approximately 50%, whereas the response to ipsilateral eye stimulation, mediated by the A_1 lamina, was relatively unchanged, and vice versa when the ipsilateral eye was stimulated. Cooling the A or A_1 lamina had no effect on the visual response in the pulvinar, but cooling of the B lamina did, thus suggesting that it was one source of input to the pulvinar.

By similar cooling in the midportion of the suprasylvian gyrus, in the dorsal layers of the superior colliculus (SC), and in the optic tract, each was shown to have an effect upon some component or aspect of the pulvinar response to a brief flash of light. The optic tract had an effect upon the initial positive component, the B lamina of the LGB and the midportion of the suprasylvian gyrus when cooled each reduced the negative component but not the positive one, and SC cooling enhanced both the early positive and later negative components. This enhancement effect suggested that the SC might exert a tonic inhibitory effect upon the pulvinar so that when SC was cooled, the effect of other inputs to the pulvinar would increase its response to visual stimulation.

In the second study, using contralateral eye stimulation, cooling of the pulvinar or the B layer of the LGB, shown earlier to be a scurce of input to the pulvinar, markedly diminished both the early and late components of the visually evoked response on the suprasylvian gyrus, but affected only the late components or after discharge on the marginal gyrus, which was shown to be mediated via the suprasylvian gyrus. Cooling the A layer caused a reduction of only the primary response components on the marginal gyrus. The results overall support the concept of two visual systems, one via the geniculostriate pathways and another from the B layer of the LGB via the pulvinar to the suprasylvian gyrus. The former is mainly responsible for the primary response of the marginal gyrus and the latter the late components.

The cryogenic reversible blocking methods used in our laboratories were described initially by Skinner and Lindsley (1968). The procedures, apparatus, and cryoprobes were designed and built by Skinner when he was a graduate student in my laboratories, but have since gone through a series of further refinements by him. He is now professor in the Department of Physiology of Baylor University College of Medicine in Houston.

Electrophysiological and Behavioral Studies in Monkeys. The following three studies on *Macaca nemestrina* monkeys are examples of several we have done that involve visual-discrimination tasks. The visual stimuli are presented in pairs tachistoscopically and simultaneously on two adjacent viewing panels. The brevity of the flash has been important in the various studies we have done, particularly in our studies of the functions of the pulvinar. Our earlier visual-masking studies also required brief test and masking stimuli separated by ISIs of 10 to 100 msec or more.

The apparatus we have used in these studies of pattern or brightness discriminations is somewhat unique. It was developed over a period of years and has been modified and refined from time to time to suit particular purposes. Initially, at my request, James M. Whitehouse, who held a postdoctoral fellowship with me in 1960–1962, started to construct such an apparatus, but it only came to workable fruition later in the hands of Lester G. Fehmi and Joel W. Atkins, who used it in their Ph.D. studies under my direction. Descriptions of it as used at that time are in Adkins, Fehmi, and Lindsley (1969) and Fehmi, Adkins, and Lindsley (1969).

A semisoundproof chamber, actually the shell of an old refrigerator, was arranged to hold a portable plastic restraining chair in which a monkey sits and views two Lucite panels upon which stimuli may be rear-projected. The stimuli are usually presented simultaneously for 10 msec but duration and intensity of a glow modulator tube can be varied. This light-emitting tube replaces the regular light source of a Kodak Carousel Projector. A special arrangement permits randomization of a given stimulus pattern on the right or left viewing panels. After shaping and preliminary training, the apparatus is programmed to accommodate the monkey's performance for 100 to 120 daily trials, the first 20 being practice or warm-up trials. Microswitches on the panels and other circuits connected with a start lever for initiating each trial and for the flashes that follow the lever press permit the temporal recording of each event, including stimulus presentations, reaction times, right and wrong responses, and so forth. These are recorded on polygraph tape, and on digital counters and timers. Electrophysiological recordings are made on an EEG machine and on FM tapes for later analysis of individual and averaged potentials.

Fig. 15.13 shows a monkey in the apparatus pressing the positive stimulus (the square pattern), picking up the banana pellet reward, and eating it. (For

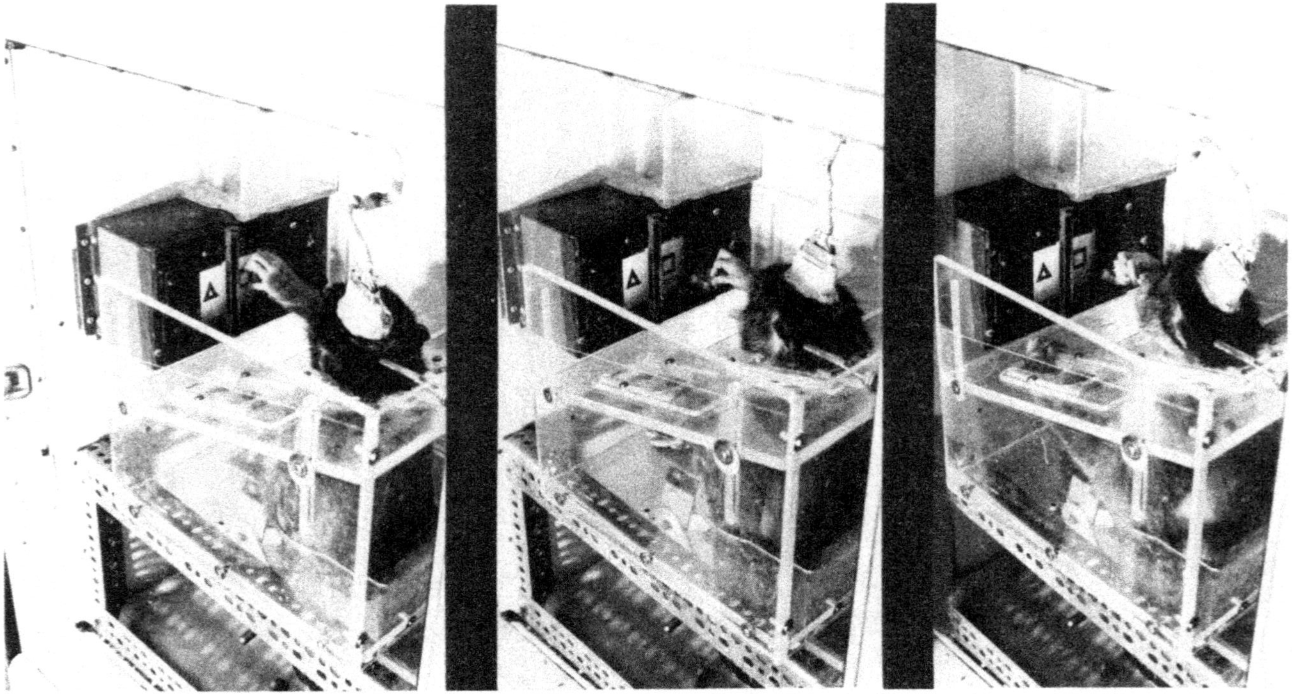

FIG. 15.13. Monkey in special simultaneous, visual pattern discrimination demanding alertness and attention. Details given in text. At left monkey presses panel with positive stimulus and, center, gets banana pellet reward, which is retrieved and eaten at right. The entire sequence is programmed and performance and reaction time recorded. When cortical and/or deep sites are recorded electrically along with behavioral performance, the connections are made at the pedestal of acrylic mounted on skull by screws. Monkeys after training to criterion maintain very stable performance. From Adkins et al., 1969. By permission.

purposes of this illustration, the photos were taken with the panels illuminated; normally the stimulus flash would have disappeared before the monkey's panel press.) Briefly, the monkey learns to press and release the lever to start a trial; 300 or 500 msec later the patterns are flashed on the panels for 10 msec. The monkey has learned that he must fixate the very dimly illuminated panels, separated by a divider strip, in an alert and attentive manner. A banana pellet appears in the little cup above the lever only for a correct response. As soon as a response on one of the panels has been made, a tone or a dim light comes on and continues for the 15-second time out, either to munch the pellet or wait for another trial. When the tone or light goes off, another lever press and release may be made to start a new trial. Over a period of a few weeks with 120 trials per day, monkeys normally attain levels of 90 to 98% correct. Performance tends to remain stable once criterion level has been reached, unless experimental procedures introduce distractions or other difficulties in making discriminations, such as variations in the patterns, the omitting or adding to parts of the basic patterns, changing stimulus parameters, or adding a second masking flash following the test flash as was done in the Adkins et al. (1969) and Fehmi, et al. (1969) studies.

In order to "perceive" the patterns in such briefly presented flashes, a monkey must be *alert* and *attentive* and motivated to perform for the reward. It is assumed that the monkey discovers during early training with longer stimulus durations what to look for in the stimuli—perhaps an "hypothesis" or learning set such as a human might begin with.

The first study in a series of three was by Gould, Chalupa, and Lindsley (1974). The goal was to record electrically from several brain sites while the monkey learned to discriminate between a square and a diamond pattern and to determine whether there were any changes in the electrical responses, averaged over daily trials, that could be correlated with the progress in learning the discrimination to criterion level (90% or better for three successive days). The patterns were identical in shape and size but differed by 90 degrees in orientation. The monkeys were first trained to criterion level on a simpler brightness task. During this phase, they learned procedure and developed a set for solving the simultaneous brightness task—namely, pressing the brighter panel to receive the reward. Electrodes were then implanted in LGB and the *medial striate cortex*, representing the geniculostriate system, in the *pulvinar* (inferior and medial divisions) and the *prestriate cortex*, representing the secondary visual system, and in the *midbrain reticular formation* and *hippocampus*. A 2-week period was allowed for recovery from the operation and then the monkey was tested and retrained on the brightness discrimination task to criterion level. At this point training on the square-diamond pattern discrimination was begun with electrical recordings being made throughout training.

No changes were observed in the averaged evoked potentials of the midbrain reticular formation, the hippocampus, or the medial pulvinar during the course of training. In contrast there were distinctly prominent and consistent changes in LGB and in the striate cortex. Similarly, in the inferior pulvinar and in the prestriate cortex of the secondary visual system, there were striking changes in the component waves of the responses as the performance of the visual pattern discrimination increased from chance level through the acquisition phase to criterion level. These changes in specific components and overall waveform are illustrated for the four responsive brain regions in Fig. 15.14.

Specifically, it may be noted in the LGB records that an early sharp positive wave (downward deflection) with a peak latency of 45 msec increases threefold in amplitude from 71% correct performance in the task to the 92 and 94% levels. The immediately following sharp negative wave peaking at 78 msec is nearly double in amplitude at 92 and 94% over chance and 71% levels. These two early-response components maintain a consistently stable latency throughout all levels of performance. A late negative wave of long duration peaking at about 250 msec at chance level is reduced to less than half its amplitude at the 71% level, and disappears entirely or is displaced by a broad positive-going wave at criterion level and is followed by a low-amplitude, long-duration negative wave. The medial striate cortex records, like the geniculate, show sharp waves but of longer latency followed by a large, long-duration wave of fairly constant latency and amplitude throughout. A particularly striking change in the medial striate record occurs during the acquisition phase of the discrimination at 71% performance level. An early negative sharp wave with a peak latency of 52 msec first appears at 71% and grows about twofold in amplitude at criterion level, while maintaining a constant latency.

The inferior pulvinar and prestriate average evoked potentials of the secondary visual system differ considerably from the wave patterns in the geniculostriate system. They show no sharp positive and negative waves. The first prominent wave (negative) in the inferior pulvinar peaks at about 52 msec, and maintains constant value throughout from chance to criterion level. A similar negative wave in prestriate cortex first appears at the 71% level and peaks at about 60 msec and maintains that latency thereafter. Its amplitude diminishes gradually as performance in the discrimination improves. It is followed by a long-duration positive wave of about 218 msec at 71% and its latency decreases to about 200 msec at 94%. It is notable that none of these waves in the prestriate cortex seem to appear in the chance-level records at 48 and 55%. The most prominent wave (negative) in the inferior pulvinar, peaking at about 200 msec, has its largest amplitude at 71% and diminishes in amplitude to half that value and to a latency of about 175 msec at 94% performance. From 71% on to criterion level it is followed by a long-duration positive wave of increasing voltage, which may account in part for the decreasing amplitude of the preceding negative wave as performance increases to criterion level.

The inferior pulvinar's major negative wave, which peaked at about 210 msec at chance level and about doubled in amplitude by 71% performance level and decreased in latency to 200 msec, decreased further in latency and voltage at

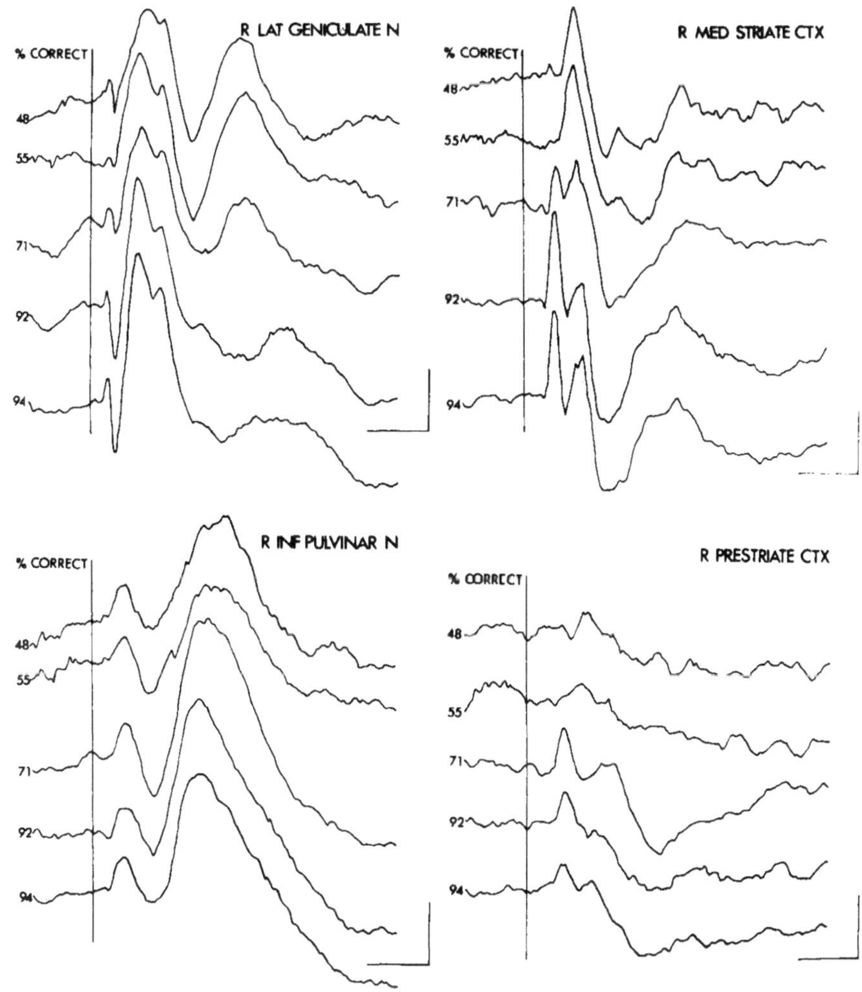

FIG. 15.14. Averaged evoked potentials to discriminative pairs of flashed (10 msec) patterns presented simultaneously (as in Fig. 15.13). These potentials from four brain sites (two in primary visual system—lateral geniculate and striate cortex)—and two in secondary visual system—inferior pulvinar and prestriate) at three stages of acquisition of the discrimination learning, chance level (48 and 55%), midlevel (71%), and above 90% criterion level (92 and 94%). See text for details of changes in evoked potentials as a function of learning the discrimination task. Calibrations: 40 uV and 100 msec. From Gould et al., 1974. By permission.

criterion level; the voltage almost returned to chance level. The prestriate cortex also showed this reduction in amplitude effect from midway in the performance range (71%) to criterion level and beyond. This may signify that arousal and attention are highest during the acquisition of this visual habit and then fall off to lower levels as performance becomes habitual and easier and requires less attention than during the active stages of learning. By the same token, assuming a reduction in the activity in the ascending reticular activating system, its seems likely that the amplitude of early responses in LGB and primary visual cortex should be enhanced for that is what Skinner and Lindsley (1967) found when they blocked the reticular activating influence in the ITP by lesion or cryogenic reversible blockade.

Here are some common examples at the human level that show heightened arousal and attention in learning certain stressful new tasks or even performing familar ones under emotional stress. The increased amplitude of the major potential components of the inferior pulvinar and prestriate cortex in monkeys midway in the acquisition of this rather difficult visual pattern discrimination may signal increased arousal and attention to the task and be comparable to what occurs when an inexperienced person begins to learn to drive a car. Initially, arousal, alertness, and attention are high, and often mental and physical tension are also. As the task is learned and becomes more habitual, tension eases off and attention and performance come under better control. Even an experienced airplane pilot may be anxious and apprehensive on takeoff but once flight altitude is reached in calm weather the pilot may put the plane on "automatic-pilot" conditions. At this point the pilot's arousal, alerting, and attention level may subside somewhat as he or she shifts to a relaxed attentive state perhaps characteristic of vigilance but not arousal, anxiety, apprehensiveness, and rapid phasic attention shifts as during takeoff.

In the preceding study, the prestriate electrodes were stainless steel screws implanted in the skull of the monkey over Brodmann's area 19 in a region over gyrus parietalis inferior and immediately anterior to the lunate sulcus. The inferior pulvinar projects to it, and among others, to the temporal lobe, the posterior parietal lobe, and prestriate and striate cortex (Benevento & Rezak, 1976; Rezak & Benevento, 1979). The prestriate cortex also has reciprocal connections with several of these. The medial striate electrodes were over the dorsomedial region of area 17 of Brodmann. The reference electrodes were four skull screws interconnected along the frontal margin of the frontal lobe. The fact that inferior pulvinar showed electrical response changes during visual-discrimination learning and the medial pulvinar did not is important beca se it is the inferior pulvinar that apparently receives, rostrally, laterally, and caudally, projections from the SC (Benevento & Fallon, 1975; Trojanowski & Jacobson, 1975), and in turn projects to several cortical regions, mainly reciprocally. Recently, using both anterograde (autoradiographic technique) and retrograde (horseradish peroxidase) tracing procedures, Yoshida and Benevento (1981) seem to have found projections from the dorsal LGB to extrastriate or prestriate regions of the cortex that also receive projections from the inferior pulvinar, thus possibly providing additional loci of cross-correlation and integration between primary and secondary visual systems.

In another study, Chalupa, Rohrbaugh, Gould, and Lindsley (1976) found an interesting relationship between reaction times (RTs) in monkeys and the amplitude of certain components of the evoked potentials. Using the data of the preceding experiment on brightness discrimination at criterion level of performance, they did a special computer analysis of the average evoked potentials and the trial-by-trial evoked potentials with respect to amplitude of the various components, and they correlated these with RTs. Two of the brain-recording sites, both in the geniculostriate system, showed statistically significant inverse correlations with RT—that is, higher amplitude with short RTs, and vice versa. Both in the averaged responses and the trial-by-trial responses and early component of the geniculate response and a late component (P3) of the striate cortex showed this result. The responses of inferior pulvinar and prestriate cortex of the second visual system did not, nor did any of the other brain-recording sites except hippocampus, which showed an opposite result—namely, an association between low-amplitude responses and short RTs and high-amplitude responses and long RTs. Such a reversal between hippocampus and neocortex results may reflect the inverse relationship between hippocampal arousal (synchronous theta waves) and neocortical arousal (desynchronization of alpha waves) systems described earlier. Other areas such as the midbrain reticular formation and medial pulvinar showed no significant positive or negative correlations of their responses to Rts.

Ten years earlier, Donchin and Lindsley (1966) found a similar correlation between spontaneous fluctuations in RT and experimentally manipulated RTs in human subjects and the amplitude of evoked responses recorded over the visual cortex. Eason, Harter & White (1969) observed correlations between RTs and evoked potentials during conditions that varied arousal and attention in human subjects. In still earlier studies of attention and vigilance by Haider et al. (1964) and of selective attention by Spong et al. (1965), it was found that the amplitude of average evoked potentials was enhanced not only for specifically detected signals embedded in a prolonged vigilance task, but also for nonsignal stimuli early in the task in contrast to later ones during waning vigilance. Also, when selective attention was manipulated by instructions for attention to visual or auditory modalities, the amplitude of the cortically evoked responses was enhanced by selective attention. These results seem to be consistent with what we have found in monkeys and what other investigators have observed in both animals and humans.

A third study involving the pulvinar is an investigation by Chalupa, Coyle, and Lindsley (1976), which has differentiated by local regional or divisional lesions of the pulvinar the performance of *Macaca nemestrina* monkeys on a pattern discrimination demanding of a high degree of alertness and attention. The apparatus for training and testing the monkeys was essentially as previously described. The procedure was much the same as in the Gould et al. (1974) study with the monkeys first being trained to criterion level on a simultaneous brightness discrimination. The monkeys were then randomly assigned to three groups: three unoperated controls, four monkeys with medial and lateral pulvinar lesions, one of which also had lesions of the inferior pulvinar bilaterally, and four monkeys with inferior pulvinar lesions.

None of the animals, including the controls, had training during a 6-week post-surgical recovery period. Then all were retrained to criterion level on the brightness discrimination and were thoroughly familiar with the apparatus procedure and the two-panel discriminanda and manipulanda (pressing lever to start a trial, then discriminating and pressing the panel containing the positive brightness value). Next came training in the simultaneous visual pattern discrimination (N and Z patterns, identical except for 90-degree rotation of the Z pattern), again with the goal of establishing learning to a 90% criterion level. All monkeys were given a series of neurobehavioral tests prior to surgery and again just prior to sacrifice. All were found to be normal at both testings, including those with pulvinar lesions. The tests included: orientation to visual and auditory stimuli, visual acuity, eye movement, pupillary constriction to light, and visual-motor coordination. Histology revealed that all lesions were located within the divisions of the pulvinar intended, without overlap of other visual structures such as the LGN. Reaction times were automatically recorded on digital counters.

The three control monkeys learned the N-Z pattern discrimination to criterion performance level in 1000, 2300, and 4300 trials (100 trials per day). After the 6-week period without training, each animal relearned the task to criterion level in 4 to 5 days. Each animal was penalized by distraction stimuli or interference overlays but quickly recovered to criterion level. Three monkeys with medial and lateral pulvinar lesions learned the N-Z discrimination in comparable time and trials to that of the control animals: 2100, 2500, and 3200 trials; the fourth monkey with medial and lateral pulvinar lesions, but also bilateral inferior pulvinar lesions, was unable to learn the task in nearly 10000 trials. This was undoubtedly due to the lesions of the inferior pulvinar and not the medial and lateral lesions. Of the four monkeys with only bilateral inferior pulvinar lesions, two were unable to learn the task in over 9000 trials and remained at or very near chance level throughout the training period. Two other monkeys with inferior pulvinar lesions eventually learned the discrimination, but very slowly, requiring 6900 and 7400 trials. Both of these animals were greatly penalized by the distraction patterns (circles surrounding the N and Z patterns); one never regained criterion-level performance under this condition in nearly 5000 trials; the other one required 2300 trials to meet criterion level again under the distraction condition. Of the three control monkeys subjected to the distraction pattern (circle surround), one required 900 trials to regain criterion performance, the others required 1100 and 1300. Of the three monkeys with only medial and lateral pulvinar lesions, the distraction circles required 600, 700, and 800 trials to regain criterion level.

All of the monkeys able to learn the visual pattern discrimination, even though some took much longer than others, showed a pattern of RTs that was comparable. That is, RTs were low during the period of chance-level (around 50%) performance, but as soon as a monkey apparently began to get a clue or developed an "hypothesis" that led to acquisition of the habit either rapidly or slowly, the RTs of individual trials increased markedly (now presumably requiring more time to make a decision before pressing a panel) until the performance level was about 70% or better. Thereafter, RTs decreased, as if the monkey was now confident that it knew how to perform correctly to obtain the reward.

The results seem to implicate the inferior pulvinar in this visual discrimination, but not those medial and lateral regions of the pulvinar that were lesioned, although in extent they were equal to or greater than the inferior pulvinar lesions. Recent neuroanatomical studies have indicated that the inferior pulvinar in various species of monkeys receives input from the SC and projects to various regions of the cortex, including occipital cortex, especially prestriate, the inferotemporal cortex, and posterior parietal cortex; furthermore, it receives projections from most of these cortical regions and more are being discovered gradually. Thus, it seems to be an important part of the so-called secondary visual system.

The functions of the second visual system are far from known as yet. So far, speculations concerning the role of the pulvinar have been made in terms of the regions from which it receives projections. These have been growing steadily in recent years as new anterograde and retrogarde methods of tracing pathways have become available. Some years ago, Mishkin (1972) reviewed some of the literature. He discussed his results in the light of a pulvinar-relay hypothesis and a prestriate-relay hypothesis, and described pathways from SC to the pulvinar and from the pulvinar to the inferotemporal cortex (Chow, 1950; Mishkin, 1972).

Of particular importance were the results obtained by Iwai and Mishkin (1969) and in their subsequent unpublished study. In terms of various learning and relearning tasks before and after lesions combining small regions along the middle and inferior temporal gyri extending caudally to the inferior occipital sulcus, they found that the posterior two-thirds was involved in visual functions. Dividing this region into an anterior and posterior part, they observed that the anterior was more concerned with visual memory and the posterior with visual-pattern discrimination and, significantly, with visual attention. Their retrograde degeneration observations indicated that this posterior part receives a projection from the inferior pulvinar and the anterior portion does not. Such results of lesions in the posterior part of the temporal visual area are consistent with our results of lesions in the inferior pulvinar involving pattern discrimination of briefly presented stimuli demanding attention (Chalupa et al., 1976).

Mishkin (1972) also mentioned a study by Snyder and Mishkin (unpublished) in which complete destruction of the pulvinar in monkeys produced no deficit on visual discrimination. Much earlier, Chow (1954) found no impairment in visual-pattern discrimination in monkeys after pulvinar lesions. Unlike our tachistoscopic studies requiring alertness and attention, their tasks allowed unlimited time to scan the stimulus patterns or objects and did not place a premium upon attention. Furthermore, our results were based upon the acquisition of a visual-pattern discrimination after lesions of the inferior pulvinar, rather than retention measured in terms of relearning as were theirs. In three of our monkeys given retention tests, one an unoperated control, one with medial, and one with inferior pulvinar lesions, none showed significant memory losses and in a few days reached criterion level.

Considering all of the projections of the visual cortical areas to and from the pulvinar, including striate cortex, extrastriate, and inferotemporal cortex, it seems quite likely that special integrative functions are subserved by the pulvinar. It receives ocular spatial orientation, eye movement, and fixation data from the colliculus. From the geniculostriate system, either directly or by various extrastriate relays, it apparently receives information concerning visual-pattern resolution. The mechanism by means of which these data from different sources are somehow integrated temporally and spatially probably depends to a high degree on attention. There may well be temporal gating factors associated with eye-movement saccades and fixations. There may also be internal timing and gating mechanisms as suggested by the rhythmic burst discharges of pulvinar units after visual flash stimuli (Huang & Lindsley, 1973; Perryman & Lindsley, 1977) and by the excitatory and inhibitory intervals observed after eye movements (Perryman, Lindsley, & Lindsley, 1981).

One might even speculate that reciprocal circuits between pulvinar and cortex may have something to do with temporary delay or memory holding mechanisms that circulate partially processed information until a decision is reached to hold and store, or erase and wipe out. The pulvinar as a polysensory convergence center may function in cross-modality association and integration as in bimodality conditioning—for example, visual-auditory or visual-somesthetic, or auditory-proprioceptive. It might also be a control center for cross-modality association and integration taking place elsewhere—for example, frontal cortex with which it has connections, or caudate and hippocampus immediately below it. This may be wild speculation, but with the various reciprocal connections of pulvinar, even involving intralaminar nuclei and frontal cortex, there is a wide span of alternatives and possibilities to be sifted out by future research.

Pulvinar Studies in Squirrel Monkeys. I turn now to recent studies on visually evoked potentials recorded in the geniculostriate system and in the pulvino-extrastriate system in squirrel monkeys using patterned and unpatterned stimuli (Perryman & Lindsley, 1977) and to another study (Lindsley, Perryman, & Lindsley, 1980; Perryman et al., 1980) on pulvinar neuron responses associated with spontaneous and trained eye movements.

The first study was largely a parametric investigation of summated evoked potentials recorded in dorsal LGN, striate cortex (area 17) and extrastriate cortex (area 19), and in the pulvinar using both field-potential recordings and single-cell responses simultaneously recorded there. Our concern was to establish some of the response characteristics in the different structures when diffuse light flashes of standard luminance level were compared to higher or lower levels of fixed amount, and similarly for checkerboard and vertical stripe patterns varying in contrast border and contour density. These stimulus parameters were tested under dark- and light-adapted conditions, first in chronic, unanesthetized monkeys, and terminally under a paralyzed state to eliminate eye movements.

A variety of results too detailed to report here were obtained. In the geniculate there were no differences in responses to patterned and unpatterned stimuli, equated for luminance level. There were changes in each of the other recording sites, especially for those patterned flashes of higher contrast border and contrast density (small checkerboard squares and fine vertical striations in black and white). These differences were not observed in the paralyzed state with all eye movements eliminated. Microelectrode poststimulus time histograms were recorded from the pulvinar in relation to the onset of patterned and unpatterned stimuli. Various excitatory and inhibitory response patterns were found. A fairly wide range of onset latencies and modal peak latencies were observed. The inferior pulvinar tended to have three distinct latencies of modal rate of discharge that corresponded to peak latencies of three components of the visually evoked field potentials recorded in the same area. The responses in the inferior pulvinar showed higher concentrations of unit discharge around modal points in time to patterned stimuli than to the unpatterned stimuli, and those patterns with the higher contrast border had the higher firing rates. The results have proved useful for further experimental planning, and the methods and technical accomplishments contributed very significantly to the planning and execution of the following study of cellular responses in the pulvinar of squirrel monkeys (*Saimiri sciureus*) and their relationship to spontaneous and trained eye movements. My son, Dr. David F. Lindsley of the Department of Physiology of the School of Medicine, University of Southern California, like Dr. Perryman and myself, has an interest in the neurophysiological mechanisms of attention and perception and joined us in this study.

Our publication (Perryman et al., 1980) stresses the importance of eye movements in visual attention and perception, indicates the role of eye movements in visual scanning of the environment for information, and suggests that foveation of visual objects in space is associated with attention and detailed resolution of visual pattern. Our paper also provides references to the very considerable literature (too extensive to be included here) supporting the following assertions. The SC is involved in eye movements, and unit discharges recorded in the intermediate and deep layers usually precede saccadic eye movements in the dark. Electrical stimulation in these regions of the SC elicits eye movements, and lesions there cause oculomotor impairment. In monkeys the cells of the superficial layers of the SC send projections to the medial portion of the inferior pulvinar and cells of the deep layers project to junctional borders of the medial and lateral subdivisions of the pulvinar.

The pulvinar in primates also receives projections from striate and prestriate cortex, and from certain parts of temporal, parietal, and frontal cortex. The projections to area 7 of the posterior parietal cortex are of special interest because the discharges of cells in this region have been shown to be related to shifts of visual attention and direction of gaze (Lynch, Mountcastle, Talbot, & Yin, 1977; Mountcastle, Lynch, Georgopoulos, Sakuta, & Acuna, 1975: Yin & Mountcastle, 1977, 1978). Electrical stimulation of the pulvinar in humans at time of surgery has been reported to elicit eye movements.

The goal of this experiment was to determine the responsiveness of cells in the medial, lateral, and inferior regions of the pulvinar to light flashes, but mainly to spontaneous eye movements in the dark and light (Ganzfeld), and during specially trained horizontal saccades.

Three results may be noted. First, certain pulvinar cells (about 10% of 1200 sampled) were responsive to spontaneous eye movements made under homogeneously lighted field conditions. Approximately one-quarter of these cells were responsive to spontaneous eye movements made in complete darkness. Cells that responded to eye movements in the dark almost uniformly responded to a diffuse light flash of brief duration in the dark, but cells responsive to eye movements in the light responded to light flash in the dark only to the extent of about half. Only about half of the cells responsive to eye movements in the light responded to trained eye movements. The second finding of significance was that cells responding to eye movements, whether in the dark or light, showed only postsaccadic responses. No cells were found that fired before the onset of a saccade, as is the case with superior colliculus cells. Thirdly, it is significant that all cells that responded to eye movements in the dark, in the light, or during trained eye movements were found only in narrow vertical zones extending throughout the rostral-caudal extent of the pulvinar. These are illustrated schematically in Fig. 15.15 on two frontal planes, A 2.5 and A 1.5.

Certain deductions may be made on the basis of specific findings in this study and these deductions lead to certain conclusions about the functioning of the pulvinar. First, all of the cells sampled in the vertical zone of the inferior pulvinar that were responsive to eye movement in the dark, in the absence of light or pattern, accordingly must be driven by eye-movement related input alone. On the other hand, all of these neurons were also responsive to light flash in the dark, the light flash being homogeneous in areal luminance and without pattern. Thus, these neurons are responsive to either eye movement alone or light input alone. Other eye-movement cells in the vertical zone cutting across medial and lateral pulvinar divisions were only responsive to eye movements in the light, indicating that eye movement input alone was insufficient. Only a small proportion (25%)

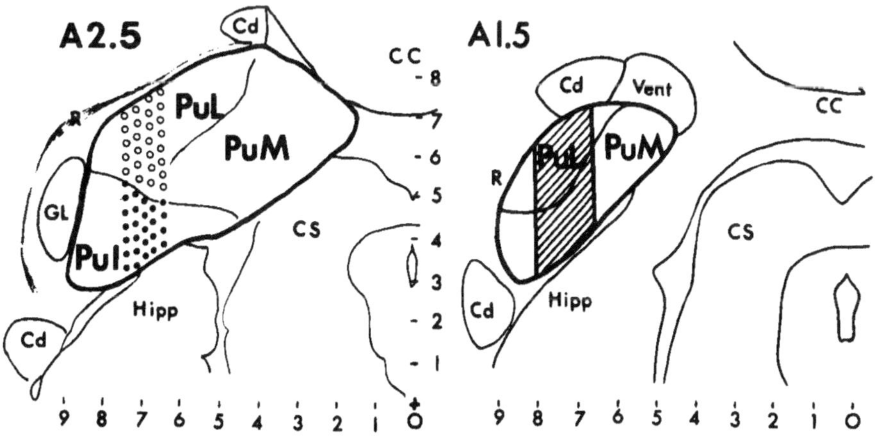

FIG. 15.15. Single neuron responses to eye movements in the light, dark, and during trained eye saccades were recorded in the three divisions of pulvinar: inferior (PuI), lateral (PuL), and medial (PuM), but were found to be only postsaccadic rather than presaccadic as in superior colliculus, and limited to a narrow vertical column, extending from rostral to caudal and mainly cutting across inferior and lateral divisions. Details are given in the text. Points are plotted on two frontal planes; open circles are eye movements in light, solid circles in dark, and in dark at cross-hatching of A 1.5. From Perryman, Lindsley, and Lindsley, 1981. By permission.

of eye-movement cells in the light were responsive to eye movements in the dark, thus suggesting that their responsiveness was potentiated by light input.

These results support the concept that there is convergence and interaction of visual and oculomotor input in the pulvinar. This reinforces the notion that primary and secondary visual systems may be integrated at the level of the pulvinar. Because eye movements are usually associated with shifts of attention during scanning for information and retinal foveation of objects in space, we believe that the convergence of both visual and oculomotor input at the pulvinar implies that it plays a role in visual attention. The results of the other studies we have done on the pulvinar have emphasized the high degree of attention required by the visual task and therefore seem to support the idea that visual attention may be one of the functions subserved by the pulvinar. If the inferior pulvinar receives feature-detecting information from complex and hypercomplex cells of the prestriate visual cortex, it may provide synthesis and integration of visual patterns from these elements appropriately oriented in space and oculomotor information received from the SC.

Cells responsive to eye movements in the light were found throughout the anterior–posterior strip cutting across the inferior, lateral, and medial divisions of the pulvinar. Only eye-movement responsive cells in the light were found in the lateral pulvinar; eye-movement responsive cells in the dark were found only in the inferior pulvinar. Cells responding to trained eye movements were found only in the cross-hatched region illustrated on frontal plane section A 1.5.

None of the 120 cells responding to eye movements showed presaccadic responses, only postsaccadic responses ranging in latency from 25 msec to 250 msec. Responses consisted of suppression or inhibition of firing, excitation, or combinations of inhibition and excitation. In contrast, SC cells sampled showed both pre- and postsaccadic responses associated with eye movements, and the LGN showed no response to eye movements.

The data suggest that eye-movement responsive cells also respond to light flashes (about half of the cells responding in light, and nearly all responding in the dark). Furthermore there is indication that a tonic light discharge may be responsible for more of the eye-movement responsive cells responding in the lighted environment. However, in some cells, especially those dark-responding cells that are found only in the inferior pulvinar, there seems to be no need for light reinforcement by tonic light discharge. Yet, almost all dark cells could be fired by light flash. These observations suggest that there are interactions of oculomotor and visual input and that such convergence and integration of primary and secondary visual-system influences at the pulvinar may be important in information processing where both attention and visual-oculomotor information play a role. But just what the nature of that information input is seems very vague at the moment, and so also does the mechanism of integration. Yet much new information has been brought to bear on the pulvinar and secondary visual system in the very recent years (see Chalupa 1977). It is no longer a terra incognita, completely, as Walker said!

Human-Evoked Potentials and Information Processing

In our human psychophysiology laboratory we were one of the pioneering groups in the use of average evoked potentials (AEPs) to study various psychological and behavioral events. We began such work as soon as facilities for averaging potentials by special-purpose computers became available in the early 1960's. I have already mentioned a few of the studies we carried out dealing with attention, perception, visual masking, and RT. In recent years we have engaged in a series of studies in which we have sought to analyze some of the factors that underlie information processing and related psychological functions. Following are sample results from two kinds of studies.

In the first study with Seales & Wilson reported here for the first time, AEPs were recorded bilaterally over visual association cortex (Brodmann's area 18) and over an intermodality association zone (Brodmann's area 40 and 39) during visual-pattern information-processing tasks involving three levels of complexity. As a nonvisual control we recorded from the vertex (Cz) over motor cortex (Brodmann's area 4). The subjects sat in a sound-attenuated, electrically shielded room before a computer-controlled display scope with the head positioned by a chin rest and a viewing hood. The display area was dimly lit and contained a central, continuously lighted fixation point. We wanted to keep the discrimination aspect of the task as simple as possible and accordingly used three lines of unequal length connected at two points in such a manner as to form various angles and shapes unidentifiable by name. Five patterns are shown at the left in Fig. 15.16 together with their code numbers and a sixth pattern (D). The patterns were presented on the display scope at the fixation point and defined a visual angle of 1.5°, the code numbers 0.5°; all well within foveal range. Serially programmed by the computer, the five patterns were presented in random order every 3–5 sec at a duration of 9 msec. When the code number was used, it appeared 0.5 sec after its stimulus pattern for the duration of 1 msec.

Three levels of complexity of visual-information processing were incorporated in three separate experiments using different subject groups. Although the general outcome of all three are described briefly here, only data from Experiment I are presented and they are illustrated for only one recording site, the left visual-association cortex. It shows the main effect—that is, the difference in the AEPs for the simplest level of processing, merely viewing the patterns as presented—versus the most complex level, identifying the patterns by a code number.

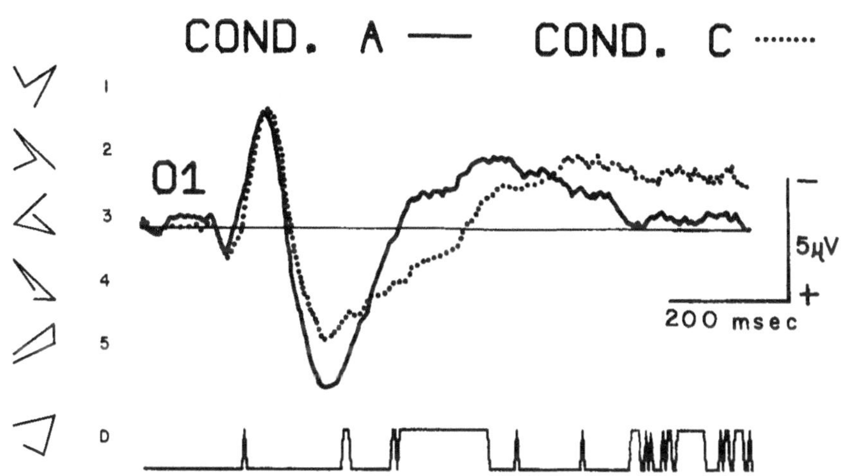

FIG. 15.16. Changes in late component of average evoked potentials after learning a pattern code, visual-visual association, in Condition B. The difference is shown between Condition A (simplest level of information processing—*just looking* at visual patterns presented singly at random for 100 presentations) versus Condition C (giving a readout of code number for each pattern), the most complex level of three used. Details given in text. Reliability of differences in waveforms shown by Wilcoxon signed-ranks statistic on bottom line; p value .05 or less. Unpublished data by D. B. Lindsley, D. M. Scales, and G. F. Wilson.

Experiment I had three conditions, A, B, and C. In Condition A the five unnameable patterns were each presented 20 times randomly mixed for a total of 100 stimulus presentations. The subjects were told to keep their gaze on the fixation point and simply view the patterns as they were presented. There was no task involved other than to look and observe. This was taken to be the *simplest level of visual-information processing,* without any specified or implied goal. During Condition B, the same procedure was followed, but now 0.5 sec after the pattern disappeared the code number was flashed. The subjects were told to learn the code name for each pattern and that in a subsequent test they would be asked to identify the patterns by their code numbers. In terms of the number and kinds of operations involved, this was the *complex level of visual-information processing*. It meant essentially learning to discriminate and distinguish each pattern from the other patterns and at the same time associate each with its code number. Learning the pattern code required visual-visual association between an unknown and unnameable pattern and a known and nameable pattern, the code number.

Condition C was identical to Condition A except that the subject task was to give a ''readout'' of the code number approximately 2 sec after the pattern disappeared from the display scope. The 2-sec delay was to avoid contamination of the 1-sec recording epoch by the verbal response and preparation for it. Subjects usually learned the pattern-code task to 95–100% accuracy by about half-way through Condition B.

AEPs were computer averaged across the 100 identical stimulus presentations of Conditions A, B, and C for each of seven subjects and then averaged again across subjects. This was done for each of the recording sites, but for simplicity and clarity only the AEPs recorded from the left visual association area (01) are illustrated in Fig. 15.16 where the AEPs for Conditions A and C may be contrasted. Because the stimulus patterns and presentations in A and C were identical, the prominent differences in the A and C waveforms cannot be due to physical differences in the stimulus patterns or to differences in their presentation sequences, which followed the same random presentation. The differences would appear to be the result of intervening information processing learned during Condition B, which in Condition C gives each pattern an identity. Each pattern now has significance and meaning and can be identified by a previously learned code name.

Comparison of the AEPs for Conditions A and C shows the waveforms to be identical for the first 150 msec (the first 50 msec of the epoch preceded the stimulus). This period includes a small positive (downward) wave (P1) and a larger following negative (upward) wave (N1). As the next positive wave (P2) starts downward, there is a gradual divergence of the two waveforms that becomes markedly increased thereafter. The P2 wave of Condition C has less amplitude and longer duration than the P2 wave of Condition A. It also ascends more slowly in a negative direction and crosses the baseline to become N2 later than in Condition A. Similarly, the N2 long-duration wave above the baseline persists longer and does not return to baseline by the end of the 1-sec epoch, whereas the N2 of Condition A does. These differences in waveform are shown to be reliably different by a Wilcoxon signed-ranks statistic computed on a point-by-point basis across the epoch where the criterion was a p value of .05 or less. The upward deflections of the bottom line indicate the regions where this criterion is met, and it may be noted that these are at the peak region of P2, the transition region from P2 to N2, and in the N2 towards the end of the epoch.

In a separate experiment with seven different subjects, an effort was made to determine whether the amplitude difference in P2 and the broadening of that wave might be due to habituation. In the three conditions of the preceding experiment, each of the five stimulus patterns had been presented 60 times for a total of 300 stimulus presentations. Conceivably, this might have led to amplitude attenuation of the P2 wave and an increase in its duration, although there was no indication that the early components of the waveform in Condition C were attenuated in amplitude. In this habituation test, three Condition A series were run (A1, A2, A3) for a total of 300 stimulus presentations to match the 300 of the A, B, and C conditions of the preceding information-processing experiment. A comparison of the AEPs for the A1 and A3 conditions showed that they were almost identical throughout and showed no significant modification in the amplitude or duration of the P2 and N2 components. Therefore, we conclude that the results of the information-processing experiment cannot be accounted for in terms of an habituation effect.

Next we made a test of the effect of information processing upon the AEPs using a task more difficult or demanding than merely viewing the five patterns, but less difficult and requiring fewer operations than the pattern-code discrimination learning of Condition C in the preceding experiment. This experiment involved the pattern D shown at the left in Fig. 15.16. The procedure was the same as in Condition A of the first experiment, except that prior to beginning with a new group of subjects, we showed them the pattern D on the display scope and told them to take careful note of it and remember it. They were told that the D pattern would appear among five other patterns that would be presented and they were to keep a count of the number of times that the D pattern appeared. This meant that each pattern that appeared would have to be discriminated from the iconic or memory image they retained from the preexposure of pattern D. The results show that the AEPs following this procedure, which we consider to be an *intermediate complexity level,* showed the same type of change as in the *complex level* but the differences were less marked. Thus we believe that degrees of complexity of visual-information processing have been demonstrated in the AEPs recorded over visual association cortex. Those recorded over bilateral intermodality association areas of the cortex (Brodmann's areas 40 and 39), in a region sometimes referred to as Wernicke's and Dejerine's areas, showed a similar but less marked effect. However, we are dealing here with visual-information processing involving a visual-visual association (pattern-code discrimination learning) and therefore the major effects were to be expected over the visual area of the cortex. In a subsequent study carried out with Diana S. Woodruff and John W. Rohrgaugh, both visual-visual and visual-auditory associations were used. It was confirmed that the major effect for visual-visual associations were over the visual cortex, and for the visual-auditory intermodality associations, the effect was greater over the intermodality association areas (Brodmann's areas 40 and 39).

In the study described above by Lindsley, Seales, and Wilson, there was a recording from a control area of the cortex along with the other sites of recording. This control recording was over the motor cortex at the midline vertex (Cz). The AEPs recorded there had a different waveform than over the sensory association zones and the waveforms for the A and C conditions were essentially identical and showed no changes in amplitude, duration, latency, or overall waveform. This is contrary to what has been observed by other investigators who have found the so-called P300, sometimes associated with information processing, over widespread areas, including motor and frontal cortex. Therefore it does not seem to be modality specific, or even sensory specific in nature. Furthermore, when it has been observed over visual cortex and elsewhere, it has been reported to be of increased amplitude with more complex information processing, which is contrary to what we have found and reported here.

The second kind of average evoked potential study with which we have been concerned involves slow negative potential shifts occurring during an interval between some kind of sensory warning stimulus and a following imperative or command signal requiring a mental or motor response. This phenomenon was first observed by W. Grey Walter and colleagues (Walter, Cooper, Aldridge, McCallum, & Winter, 1964) at the Burden Neurological Institute in Bristol, England, and because it seemed to be contingent upon an exciting or forewarning stimulus (S1) and a second stimulus (S2) triggering a response, they called it a Contingent Negative Variation (CNV). In a variety of experiments, they became convinced that it involved anticipation or expectancy, and in this respect it seemed to have possibilities as a means of investigating higher mental processes of a cognitive variety. Many other studies have since been conducted around the world in an effort to define the phenomenon and to determine more precisely what psychological or behavior events it might reflect (for a recent review, see Haider, Groll-Knapp, & Ganglberger, 1981). Kornhuber and Deecke (1965) soon described another slow negative potential shift associated with preparation for a voluntary motor response, which they called a "Bereitschaftspotential," most pronounced over motor cortex, The CNV was found most prominently over motor, premotor, and frontal cortex. There has, accordingly, been a good deal of discussion about the extent to which these two phenomena overlap or are interrelated in other ways—for example, being components of an overall negative wave pattern such as the CNV or successive sensory and motor potentials leading to a motor response. Deecke, Scheid, and Kornhuber (1969) next described a negative potential shift that they called a readiness potential, then a premotion positivity, followed by a more phasic motor potential preceding or accompanying voluntary finger movements. In our laboratory, Syndulko and Lindsley (1977) reported on a maximal focus of negativity over motor cortex during motor preparatory tasks. This was of larger amplitude over motor cortex of the hemisphere contralateral to the hand used in unimanual tasks.

These and other developments led us to investigate AEPs topographically displayed over the head, but especially over the region extending from parietal to anterior frontal cortex. In an experimental study by Rohrbaugh, Syndulko, and Lindsley (1976), a first effort was made to separate possible components of the CNV. Others before us had used the strategy of separating the S1 warning stimulus from the S2 imperative stimulus by an interval greater than the 1 or 2 sec typically used. Employing a 4-sec interval with long-time constant amplifiers to faithfully reproduce slow potential changes therein, we soon found that the usual CNV phenomenon that seemed to be a continuous process between S1 and S2 clearly revealed a response to S1 that partially subsided, and then renewed negativity started up about midway in the interval between S1 and S2. This led to recording responses to the S1 alone and to uncued motor responses alone without S2, using the motor key-press to time-lock the averaging of potentials.

The results showed that by putting these separately recorded responses together it was possible to duplicate the potential shifts observed when the S1 and S2 were paired but with a 4-sec interval separating them. This was followed up by other confirming and extending experiments (Rohrbaugh, Syndulko, & Lindsley, 1978, 1979; Rohrbaugh, Syndulko, Sanquist, & Lindsley, 1980; Sanquist, Beatty, & Lindsley, 1981) in which a considerable number of factors were tested against the components of the waveforms in even longer intervals of separation of S1 and S2. Among the variables and conditions tested were the effects of different tasks such as passive listening, pitch discrimination, counting of stimuli, relevance, and probability of occurrence of stimuli, and so forth, using stimuli of visual and auditory modes. Also the effects of modality, intensity, and rate of stimulation were investigated. Considering a variety of detailed results brought out by special methods of analysis of waveforms, the general conclusions reached were that there are two major components comprising the CNV, or at least during the interval in which it occurs. One of these is a negative afterwave apparently arising from S1 and it varies with the modality of stimulation used as well as with the rate of stimulation, but not with intensity. Tasks, and the instructions given for them, may influence significantly the extent and degree to which the negative afterwave and its possible components reflect factors residing in the S1 or warning stimulus.

We have tentatively concluded from these various results that the negative afterwave is a consequence of the properties of the S1 or warning stimulus. If S1 is a brief, moderate-intensity auditory stimulus, it may reflect arousal, orienting, and alerting to attention. If, regardless of intensity, it carries meaning or significance (e.g., a low-tone or dim-light S1 means respond with right hand to S2, or a high-tone or bright-light S1 means respond with left hand to S2), it may still have an enhancing effect on the negative afterwave. Thus, the S1 warning stimulus may be endowed with various properties of a psychological nature that are reflected in the rise time, amplitude, and duration of the negative afterwave. In this respect, the negative afterwave may have importance for investigating the various psychological properties that may be attached to the S1 warning stimulus, by previous experience or instructions.

If the waiting interval for S2 is extended, the negative afterwave may persist and fuse with the slow negative shift (readiness potential) that accompanies preparation for the mental (verbal) or motor response indicated by the instructions and triggered by the S2 or imperative stimulus. A somewhat brief and phasic electrical response (especially over motor or premotor regions) may then intervene as the response act is performed and be overlapped or quickly followed by a large positive wave sometimes identified as the P300 response, which has been thought by some investigators to be related to cognitive processes or information processing, such as acquisition and retention in learning and short-term memory situations. But it may be, in part, an aftereffect or afterdischarge associated with the motor act itself because it seems to be maximal at the vertex and spread widely anteriorly and posteriorly. As mentioned earlier, this aspect of the P300 wave suggests that it is a nonspecific, and perhaps nonsensory, influence of the reticular activating system enhancing the excitability of the cortex as in arousal, alerting, and attention. This, of course, does not deny its importance for the processing of information and in cognitive functions, because attention is an important element in perception and learning.

Tasks involving the amount and kind of associative processing and encoding in memory of verbal and conceptual materials at a cognitive level, in contrast to simple sensory and perceptual events, appear to produce a broader late positive wave that peaks later (500 msec) than the P300 wave. This has been observed in a recent study in our laboratory (Sanquist, Rohrbaugh, Syndulko, & Lindsley, 1980b), in situations or tasks where the judging of pairs of stimuli as "same" or "different" were observed with regard to three classes or levels of information processing. The simplest processing level, the *orthographic*, consisted of word pairs in upper- or lower-case type. An intermediate level, the *phonemic*, consisted of pairs of words that were judged as to whether or not they rhymed. The most complex level, the *semantic*, was comprised of word pairs judged as to whether or not they were synonyms.

Some interesting preliminary results were reported. The late positive component (LPC), and its extension in a positive slow wave of negative-going direction. showed a progressive change in amplitude and duration for the S2 word when it was judged "same" as opposed to when it was judged "different." The LPCs for "same" were larger in amplitude than those for "different" as the complexity of information processing increased from the simplest level to the most complex. Also, the increase in complexity of information processing caused marked increases in the rise-time and amplitude of late negative-going slow wave. In the orthographic situation, it rose faster and crossed the baseline to become a late negative wave, but in the phonemic and semantic conditions, it reached, but did not cross, the baseline when S2 was judged "same."

These differences were similar to those reported and illustrated earlier when the changes recorded were principally over the visual cortex. In that study, the information processing ranged from the simple sensory awareness of visual patterns to a complex level of visual discrimination of one pattern from another and the forming of visual-visual associations between each pattern and its code number. In this study the tasks involved verbal materials in which the letters in upper and lower case composing words were different in size and pattern or the same if of the same type case—for example, all capital letters. In the second level of complexity, the words were phonemically the same or different in sound, thus rhyming or not rhyming. At the most complex level, they were semantically and conceptually different or the same in meaning.

After completing the judging of pairs as "same" or "different," the subjects were tested on their recognition memory for the S2 items. Sixty S2 words in the judgment tasks were randomly mixed with 60 new words, and on brief and fairly rapid presentation the subjects were required to say whether each word was "old" or "new." This test was repeated with new word lists. It was found that recognition memory for items was considerably superior for the more complex levels of processing; semantic was highest and orthographic lowest for items that had been judged "same." Test cases in the phonemic and semantic series yielded a higher positivity for the LPC and later negative-going slow wave.

The concluding remarks of the study included the following: (Sanquist, et al., 1980a)

> Thus, it appears that ERP (Event-Related Potential) components reflect not only neural activity associated with short-term memory performance, but also the more elusive processes of differential perceptual processing and long term memory trace formation. The fact that these processes are indexed by brain potentials suggests that ERP analyses of long term memory and its input will provide a useful tool in the *continuing search for the engram* [p. 660; parentheses and underlining added].

The preceding reference to a search for the elusive engram seems an appropriate place to end this discussion, for it was Lashley, who, in the critically incisive *In Search of the Engram* ended with a despairingly humorous sentence. He wrote (Lashley, 1950), "I sometimes feel, in reviewing the evidence on the localization of the memory trace, that the necessary conclusion is that learning just is not possible. [p. 477]."

But despite Lashley's discomfiture at not being able to solve the problem of memory and the nature and localization of the engram, he was able to present and clarify "information about what and where the memory trace is not." Furthermore, he stated a number of his conceptualizations and insightful speculations that had, and still have, great value for anyone motivated and willing to think deeply about the neural structure and functional organization of the brain and nervous system in relation to psychological processes and behavior. Three years after Lashley's famous article, Sir John Eccles (winner of a Nobel award in 1963), in a unique and stimulating book entitled, "*The Neurophysiological Basis of Mind,*" (1953) presented basic background information in neurophysiology and electrophysiology and then brought some of it to bear on the brain-mind problem, including perception, memory, conditioning, and learning. In it he acknowledges, and seems to agree, with some of Lashley's concepts.

Much later, in a brief autobiographical review of his scientific career Eccles (1975) disavows some of his earlier convictions:

> I have come to recognize that I was mistaken in my original belief that an understanding of the synapse would contribute substantially to a solution of the brain-mind problem. . . . But the functional performance of the higher levels requires postulates of a global kind: neuronal systems forming continuously operating and interacting dynamic loops of immense complexity and variability—the "enchanted loom" imagined by Sherrington [p. 477].

Three other distinguished neuroscientists, all Nobel laureates—Adrian and Sherrington in 1932, Granit in 1967—have, from time to time, turned their attention and thought to problems of psychological processes and behavior, based on their knowledge and experience gained in working with the nervous system. Their midcentury books reveal their concern and acknowledge the complexity of neural networks required to accomplish even the simplest of perceptual and cognitive functions. Adrian (1947) wrote on *The Physical Background of Perception,* Granit (1955) on *Receptors and Sensory Perception,* and Sherrington (1951) on the broader topic *Man on His Nature*.

Like Lashley and Eccles, Granit (1975), in an autobiographical sketch, wrote of the need to look at the larger picture of neural organization in the brain. He said (Granit, 1975):

> It must now be common knowledge that the organ of highest control, our brain, cannot be discussed as if it were a question of localization versus general representation. . . . We now realize that there are highly localized functions, even tricks—if I may say so—that only certain aggregates of cells can perform, as well as functions that require coactivation of several cortical areas widely apart. As we penetrate problems of localization, we tend to end up with problems of organization [p. 328].

In this light, it may be that the "systems approach" described here will help to detect and clarify the organizational and reorganizational patterns in neural networks of the cortical matrix believed to be associated with perception, learning, and memory. These studies include the reticular activating system and its upward extension in the nonspecific thalamo-cortical systems that regulate the synchronization and desynchronization of cortical rhythms, two brain-stem-hypothalamic-hippocampal systems having contrasting effects upon behavior and the synchronous theta activity of the hippocampus and inverse effects upon the rhythms of the hippocampus and the neocortex, the role of the polysensory pulvinar in mediating interaction and integration of the primary and secondary visual systems, perhaps also similar arrangements for the auditory and somatosensory modalities, and finally, the use of computer methods in the study of the factors involved in information processing as revealed by AEPs over the different topographical regions of the head.

REFERENCES

Adey, W. R. EEG studies of hippocampal system in the learning process. In P. Passouant (Ed.), *Physiologie de l'hippocampe*. Paris: C.N.R.S., 1962 (No. 107), 203-222.

Adey, W. R. Hippocampal states and functional relations with cortico-subcortical systems in attention and learning. In W. R. Adey & T. Tokizane (Eds.), *Progress in brain research: Structure and function of the limbic system*. Amsterdam: Elsevier, 1967.

Adey, W. R., Dunlop, C. W., & Hendrix, C. E. Hippocampal slow waves: Distribution and phase relationships in the course of approach learning *Archives of Neurology*, 1960, *3*, 74-90.

Adey, W. R., Walter, D. O., & Lindsley, D. F. Subthalamic lesions: Effects on learned and correlated hippocampal and subcortical slow-wave activity. *Archives of Neurology*, 1962, *6*, 194-207.

Adkins, J. W., Fehmi, L. G., & Lindsley, D. B. Perceptual discrimination in monkeys: Retroactive visual masking. *Physiology and Behavior*, 1969, *4*, 255-259.

Adrian, E. D. *The basis of sensation: The action of sense organs*. London: Christophers, 1928.

Adrian, E. D. Potential changes in the isolated nervous system of *Dysticus marginalis*. *Journal of Physiology*, 1931, *72*, 132-151.

Adrian, E. D. *The mechanism of nervous action: Electrical studies of the neurone*. Philadelphia: University of Pennsylvania Press, 1932.

Adrian, E. D. *The physical background of perception*. Oxford: Clarendon Press, 1947.

Adrian, E. D., & Buytendijk, F. J. J. Potential changes in the isolated brain stem of the goldfish. *Journal of Physiology*, 1931, *71*, 121-135.

Adrain, E. D., & Matthews, B. H. C. The Berger rhythm: Potential changes from the occipital lobes of man. *Brain*, 1934, *57*, 355-385.

Anchel, H., & Lindsley, D. B. Differentiation of two reticulo-hypothalamic systems regulating hippocampal activity. *Electroencephalography and Clinical Neurophysiology*, 1972, *32*, 209-226.

Andersen, P., & Andersson, S. A. *Physiological basis of the alpha rhythm*. New York: Appleton-Century-Crofts, 1968.

Bartley, S. H., & Bishop, G. H. The cortical response to stimulation of the optic nerve in the rabbit. *American Journal of Physiology*, 1933, *103*, 159-172. (a)

Bartley, S. H., & Bishop, G. H. Factors determining the form of the electrical response from the optic cortex of the rabbit. *American Journal of Physiology*, 1933, *103*, 173-184. (b)

Beach, F. A. Karl Spencer Lashley, 1890-1958. In *Biographical Memoirs: National Academy of Sciences*. New York: Columbia University Press, 1961, *35*, 161-204.

Benevento, L. A., & Fallon, J. H. The ascending projections of the superior colliculus in the rhesus monkey (*Macaca mulatta*). *Journal of Comparative Neurology*, 1975, *160*, 339-362.

Benevento, L. H., & Rezak, M. The cortical projections of the inferior pulvinar and adjacent lateral pulvinar in the rhesus monkey (*Macaca mulatta*): An autoradiographic study. *Brain Research*, 1976, *108*, 1-24.

Bennett, T. L. Hippocampal EEG correlates of behavior. *Electroencephalography and Clinical Neurophysiology*, 1970, *28*, 17-23.

Bennett, T. L. Hippocampal theta activity and behavior—A review. *Communications in Behavioral Biology*, 1971, *6*, 37-48.

Bennett, T. L. The effects of centrally blocking hippocampal theta activity on learning and retention. *Behavioral Biology*, 1973, *9*, 541-552. (a)

Bennett, T. L. Hippocampal theta activity and the attention component of discrimination learning. *Behavioral Biology*, 1973, *8*, 173-181. (b)

Bennett, T. L., & Gottfried, J. Hippocampal theta activity and response inhibition. *Electroencephalography and Clinical Neurophysiology*, 1970, *29*, 196-200.

Berger, H. Über das Elektrenkephalogramm des Menschen. I. *Archiv fur Psychiatrie und Nervenkrankleiten*, 1929, *87*, 527-570.

Berger, H. Über das Elektrenkephalogramm des Menschen. II. *Journal fur Psychologie und Neurologie, Lpz*, 1930, *40* 160-179.

Berger, H. Über das Elektrenkephalogramm des Menschen. III. *Archiv fur Psychiatrie und Nervenkrankheiten*, 1931, *94*, 16-60.

Berger, H. Das Elektrenkephalogramm des Menschen und seine Bedeutung für die Psychophysiologie. *Zeitschrift fur Psychologie*, 1932, *126*, 1-13.

Berger, H. Über das Elektrenkephalogramm des Menschen. IV. *Archiv fur Psychiatrie und Nervenkrankheiten*, 1932, *97*, 6-26.

Berger, H. Über das Elektrenkephalogramm des Menschen. XIV. *Archiv fur Psychiatrie und Nervenkrankheiten*, 1938 *108*, 407-431.

Bishop, G. H. Cyclic changes in excitability of the optic pathway of the rabbit. *American Journal of Physiology*, 1933, *103*, 213-224.

Bishop, G. H. Electrical responses accompanying activity of the optic pathway. *Archives of Ophthalmology, Chicago*, 1935, *14*, 992-1019.

Bishop, G. H. The interpretation of cortical potentials. *Cold Spring Harbor Symposium Quantitative Biology*, 1936, *4*, 305-319.

Bishop, G. H., & O'Leary, J. Response of the optic cortex of the cat. *Proceedings of the Society of Experimental Biology, N.Y.*, 1935, *38*, 532-535.

Bishop, G. H., & O'Leary, J. Components of the electrical response of the optic cortex of the rabbit. *American Journal of Physiology*, 1936, *117*, 292-308.

Bishop, G. H., & O'Leary, J. Electrical activity of the lateral geniculate of cats following optic nerve stimulation. *Journal of Neurophysiology*, 1940, *3*, 308-322.

Brain Research Institute, UCLA, Directory—From origin to 1972. Los Angeles: University of California, 1972.

Bremer, F. Cerveau "isolé" et physiologie du sommeil. *C. R. Soc. Biol. (Paris)*, 1935, *118*, 1235-1242.

Bremer, F. Nouvelles recherches sur le mécanisme du sommeil. *C. R. Soc. Biol. (Paris)*, 1936, *122*, 460-464.

Bremer, F. L'activité électrique de l'écorce cérébrale et le problème physiologique du sommeil. *Bolletino della Societa Italiana di Biologia Sperimentale*, 1938, *13*, 271-290.

Bremer, F., & Stoupel, N. De la modification des réponses sensorielles corticales dans l'éveil réticulaire. *Acta Neurologica Belgica*, 1958, *58*, 401-403.

Bremer, F., & Stoupel, N. Facilitation et inhibition des potentiels évoqués corticaux dans l'éveil cerebral. *Archives Internationales de Physiologie*, 1959, *67*, 240-275.

Brodal, A. *The reticular formation of the brain stem: Anatomical aspects and functional correlations*. Springfield, Ill.: Thomas, 1958.

Brouwer B. Über die Projektion der Makule auf die Area striata des Menschen. *Jahrbuch fur Psychiatrie und Neurologie Leipzig*, 1930, *40*, 147-159.

Buser, P., Borenstein, P., & Bruner, J. Etude des systemes ''associativs'' visuelles et auditifs chez le chat anesthesie au chloralose. *Electroencephalography and Clinical Neurophysiology*, 1959, *11*, 305-324.

Chalupa, L. M. A review of cat and monkey studies implicating the pulvinar in visual function. *Behavioral Biology*, 1977, *20*, 149-167.

Chalupa, L. M., Anchel, H., & Lindsley, D. B. Visual input to the pulvinar via the lateral geniculate, superior colliculus, and visual cortex in cat. *Experimental Neurology*, 1972, *36*, 449-462.

Chalupa, L. M., Anchel, H., & Lindsley, D. B. Effects of cryogenic blocking of pulvinar upon visually evoked responses in the cortex in cat. *Experimental Neurology*, 1973, *39*, 112-122.

Chalupa, L. M., Coyle, R. S., & Lindsley, D. B. Effect of pulvinar lesions on visual pattern discrimination in monkeys. *Journal of Neurophysiology*, 1976, *39*, 354-369.

Chalupa, L. M., Macadar, A. W., & Lindsley, D. B. Responses of pulvinar and lateralis posterior units to visual and auditory input in the cat: Interactions with cortex, lateral geniculate and superior colliculus. *Electroencephalography and Clinical Neurophysiology*, 1974, *36*, 210.

Chalupa, L. M., Rohrbaugh, J. W., Gould, J. E., & Lindsley, D. B. Cortical and subcortical visual evoked potential correlates of reaction time in monkeys. *Journal of Comparative and Physiological Psychology*, 1976, *90*, 119-126.

Chang, H.-T. The repetitive discharges of cortico-thalamic reverberating circuit. *Journal of Neurophysiology*, 1950, *13*, 235-258.

Chang, H. -T. Changes in excitability of cerebral cortex following single electric shock applied to cortical surface. *Journal of Neurophysiology*, 1951, *14*, 95-112.

Chang, H. -T. Cortical response to stimulation of lateral geniculate body and the potentiation thereof by continuous illumination of retina. *Journal of Neurophysiology*, 1952, *15*, 5-26.

Chang, H. -T., & Kaada, B. R. An analysis of primary response of visual cortex to optic nerve stimulation in cats. *Journal of Neurophysiology*, 1950, *13*, 305-318.

Chow, K. L. A retrograde cell degeneration study of the cortical projection field of the pulvinar in the monkey *Journal of Comparative Neurology*, 1950, *93*, 313-340.

Chow, K. L. Lack of behavioral effects following destruction of some thalamic association nuclei in monkey. *Archives of Neurology and Psychiatry*, (*Chicago*), 1954, *71*, 762-771.

Clark, G., & Ward, J. Responses elicited by combined stimulation of pairs of fixed electrodes in the unanestheized monkey. *American Journal of Physiology*, 1949, *158*, 474-477.

Clark, W. E. Le Gros. The structure and connections of the thalamus. *Brain*, 1932, *55*, 406-470.

Clark, W. E. Le Gros, & Northfield, D. W. C. The cortical projection of the pulvinar in the macaque monkey, *Brain*, 1937, *66*, 263-290.

Coleman, J. R., & Lindsley, D. B. Hippocampal electrical correlates of free behavior and behavior induced by stimulation of two hypothalamic-hippocampal systems in the cat. *Experimental Neurology*, 1975, *49*, 506-528.

Coleman, J. R., & Lindsley, D. B. Behavioral and hippocampal electrical changes during operant learning in cats and effects of stimulating two hypothalamic-hippocampal systems. *Electroencephalography and Clinical Neurophysiology*, 1977, *42*, 309-331.

Dahlström, A., & Fuxe, K. Evidence for the existence of monoamine-containing neurons in the central nervous system. I. Demonstration of monoamines in the cell bodies of brain stem neurons. *Acta Physiologica Scandinavica Supplement* (197), 1965, *232*, 1-55.

Dawson, G. D. Cerebral responses to nerve stimulation in man. *British Medical Bulletin*, 1950, *6*, 326-329.

Dawson, G. D. A summation technique for the detection of small evoked potentials. *Electroencephalography and Clinical Neurophysiology*, 1954, *6*, 65 81.

Deecke, L., Scheid, O., & Kornhuber, H. H. Distribution of readiness potential, pre-motion positivity, and motor potential of the human cerebral cortex preceding voluntary finger movements. *Experimental Brain Research*, 1969, *7*, 158-168.

Dempsey, E. W., & Morison, R. S. The interaction of certain spontaneous and induced cortical potentials. *American Journal of Physiology*, 1942, *135*, 301-308. (a)

Dempsey, E. W., & Morison, R. S. The production of rhythmically recurrent cortical potentials after localized thalamic stimulation. *American Journal of Physiology*, 1942, *135*, 293-300. (b)

Donchin, E., & Lindsley, D. B. Retroactive brightness enhancement with brief paired flashes of light. *Vision Research*, 1965, *5*, 59-70. (a)

Donchin, E., & Lindsley, D. B. Visually evoked response correlates of perceptual masking and enhancement. *Electroencephalography and Clinical Neurophysiology*, 1965, *19*, 325-335. (b)

Donchin, E., & Lindsley, D. B. Average evoked potentials and reaction times to visual stimuli. *Electroencephalography and Clinical Neurophysiology*, 1966, *20*, 217-223.

Donchin, E., & Lindsley, D. B. (Eds.). *Average evoked potentials: Methods, results, and evaluations*. Washington, D.C.: NASA-U.S. Government Printing Office, 1969.

Donchin, E., Wicke, J. D., & Lindsley, D. B. Cortical evoked potentials and the perception of paired flashes. *Science*, 1963, *141*, 1285-1286.

Dumont, S., & Dell, P. Facilitations specifiques et non-specfiques des réponses visuelles corticales. *Journal de Physiologie (Paris)*, 1958, *50*, 261-264.

Dumont, S., & Dell, P. Facilitation reticulare des mecanismes visuels corticaux. *Electroencephalography and Clinical Neurophysiology*, 1960, *12*, 769-796.

Dusser de Barenne, J. G., Garol, H. W., & McCulloch, W. S. Functional organization of sensory and adjacent cortex of the monkey. *Journal of Neurophysiology*, 1941, *4*, 324-330.

Dusser de Barenne, J. G., & McCulloch, W. S. Functional organization of the sensory cortex of the monkey (*Macaca mulatta*). *Journal of Neurophysiology*, 1938, *1*, 69-85.

Dusser de Barenne, J. G., & McCulloch, W. S. Physiological neuronography of the cortico-striatal connections. *Research Publications of the Association for Nervous & Mental Disease*, 1941, *21*, 246-266. (a)

Dusser de Barenne, J. G., McCulloch, W. S. Suppression of motor response obtained from area 4 by stimulation of area 4s. *Journal of Neurophysiology*, 1941, *4*, 311-323. (b)

Eason, R. G., Harter, M. R., & White, C. T. Effects of attention and arousal on visually evoked cortical potentials and reaction time in man. *Physiology and Behavior*, 1969, *4*, 283-289.

Eccles, J. C. *The neurophysiological basis of mind: The principles of neurophysiology*. Oxford: Clarendon Press, 1953.

Eccles, J. C. Under the spell of the synapse. In F. G. Worden, J. P. Swazey, & G. Adelman (Eds.), *The neurosciences: Paths of discovery*. Cambridge, Mass.: MIT Press, 1975.

Fehmi, L. G., Adkins, J. W., & Lindsley, D. B. Electrophysiological correlates of visual perceptual masking in monkeys. *Experimental Brain Research*, 1969, *7*, 299-316.

Flourens, M. J. F. *Recherches experimentales sur les propriétés et les fonctions du systeme nerveux dans les animaux vertebres*. Paris: Crevot, 1824.

Forbes, A., & Thacher, C. Amplification of action currents with the electron tube in recording with the string galvanometer. *American Journal of Physiology*, 1920, *52*, 409-471.

Fox, J. C., Jr., & German, W. J. Macular vision following cerebral resection. *Archives of Neurology and Psychiatry, Chicago*, 1936, *35*, 808-826.

Franz, S. I., & Lashley, K. S. The retention of habits by the rat after destruction of the frontal portion of the cerebrum. *Psychobiology*, 1917, *1*, 3-18.

French, J. D. Brain lesions associated with prolonged unconsciousness. *Archives of Neurology and Psychiatry, Chicago*, 1952, *68*, 727-740.

French, J. D., Hernandez-Peon, R., & Livingston, R. B. Projections from cortex to cephalic brain stem (reticular formation) in monkey, *Journal of Neurophysiology*, 1955, *18*, 44-55.

French, J. D., & Magoun, H. W. Effects of chronic lesions in central cephalic brain stem of monkeys. *Archives of Neurology and Psychiatry, Chicago,* 1952, *68,* 591-604.

Fuster, J. M. Effects of stimulation of brain stem on tachistoscopic perception. *Science,* 1958, *127,* 150.

Fuxe, K., Hökfelt, T. & Ungerstedt, U. Morphological and functional aspects of central monoamine neurones. *International Review of Neurobiology,* 1970, *13,* 93-126.

Gasser, H. S., & Erlanger, J. A study of the action currents of nerve with the cathode ray oscillograph. *American Journal of Physiology,* 1922, *62,* 496-524.

Gerard, R. W., Marshall, W. H., & Saul, L. G. Electrical activity of the cat's brain. *Archives of Neurology and Psychiatry, Chicago,* 1936, *36,* 675-738.

Gibbs, F. A., Davis, H., & Lennox, W. G. The electro-encephalogram in epilepsy and in conditions of impaired consciousness. *Archives of Neurology and Psychiatry, Chicago,* 1935, *34,* 1133-1148.

Gloor, P. (Ed). Hans Berger on the electroencephalogram. *Electroencephalography and Clinical Neurophysiology Supplement, 28.* Amsterdam: Elsevier, 1969. (English translation of 14 of Berger's original publications from 1929 to 1938.)

Gould, J. E., Chalupa, L. M., & Lindsley, D. B. Modifications of pulvinar and geniculo-cortical evoked potentials during visual discrimination learning in monkeys. *Electroencephalography and Clinical Neurophysiology,* 1974, *36,* 639-649.

Granit, R. *Sensory mechanisms of the retina.* London: Oxford University Press, 1947.

Granit, R. *Receptors and sensory perception.* New Haven: Yale University Press, 1955.

Granit, R. Half a century in the neurosciences: Personal comments on choices and decisions. In F. G. Worden, J. P. Swazey, & G. Adelman (Eds.), *The neurosciences: Paths of discovery.* Cambridge, Mass.: MIT Press, 1975.

Grastyan, E. The hippocampus and higher nervous activity. In M. A. B. Brazier (Ed.), *The central nervous system and behavior.* New York: Josiah Macy, Jr. Foundation, 1959.

Grastyan, E., Karmos, G., Vereczkey, L., & Kellenyi, L. The hippocampal electrical correlates of the homeostatic regulation of motivation. *Electroencephalography and Clinical Neurophysiology,* 1966, *21,* 34-53.

Grastyan, E., Karmos, G., Vereczkey, L., Martin, J., & Kellenyi, L. Hypothalamic motivational processes as reflected by their hippocampal electrical correlates. *Science,* 1965, *149,* 91-93.

Grastyan, E., Lissak, K., Madarasz, I., & Donhoffer, H. Hippocampal electrical activity during the development of conditioned reflexes. *Electroencephalography and Clinical Neurophysiology,* 1959, *11,* 409-430.

Green, J. D., & Arduini, A. A. Hippocampal electrical activity in arousal. *Journal of Neurophysiology,* 1954, *17,* 531-557.

Haider, M., Groll-Knapp, E., & Gangelberger, J. A. Event-related slow (DC) potentials in the human brain. *Review of Physiology Biochemistry Pharmacology,* 1981, *88,* 125-197.

Haider, M., Spong, P., & Lindsley, D. B. Attention, vigilance and cortical evoked potentials in humans. *Science,* 1964, *145,* 180-182.

Halstead, W. C., Walker, A. E., & Bucy, P. C. Sparing and nonsparing of "macular" vision associated with occipital lobectomy in man. *Archives of Ophthalmology, Chicago,* 1940, *24,* 948-966.

Hartline, H. K. Intensity and duration in the excitation of single photoreceptor units. *Journal of Cellular & Comparative Physiology,* 1934, *5,* 229-247.

Hartline, H. K., & Graham, C. H. Nerve impulses from single photoreceptor units. *Journal of Cellular & Comparative Physiology,* 1932, *1,* 227-295.

Hartline, H. K., Wagner, H. G., & MacNichol, E. F., Jr. The peripheral origin of nervous activity in the visual system. *Cold Spring Harbor Symposia Quantitative Biology,* 1952, *17,* 125-141.

Hassler, R. Functional anatomy of the thalamus. *Congreso Latinoamericano Neurocir., VI, Montevideo,* 1955, 754-787 (Symposium de Talamo).

Head, H. *Aphasia and kindred disorders of speech* (2 vols.). New York: Macmillan, 1926.

Hebb, D. O. *The organization of behavior.* New York: Wiley, 1949.

Heron, W., & Anchel, H. Synchronous sensory bombardment of young rats: Effects on the electroencephalogram. *Science,* 1964, *145,* 946-947.

Hess, W. R. Hirnreizversuche über den Mechanismus des Schlafes. *Archiv fur Psychiatrie und Nervenkrankheiten,* 1929, *86,* 287-292. (a)

Hess, W. R. Lokalisatorische Ergebnisse der Hirnreizversuche mit Schlafeffekt. *Archiv fur Psychiatrie und Nervenkrankheiten,* 1929, *88,* 813-916. (b)

Hess, W. R. Das Schlafsyndrom als Golge dienzephaler Reizung. *Helvetica physiologica et pharmacologica Acta,* 1944, *2,* 137-147.

Hess, W. R. The diencephalic sleep center. In J. F. Delafresnaye (Ed.) *Brain mechanisms and consciousness.* Springfield, Ill.: Thomas, 1954.

Horsley, V. A., & Clarke, R. H. The structure and functions of the cerebellum examined by a new method. *Brain,* 1908, *31,* 45-124.

Huang, C. C., & Lindsley, D. B. Polysensory responses and sensory interaction in pulvinar and related postero-lateral thalamic nuclei. *Electroencephalography and Clinical Neurophysiology,* 1973, *34,* 265-280.

Iwai, E., & Mishkin, M. Further evidence on the locus of the visual area in the temporal lobe of monkeys. *Experimental Neurology,* 1969, *25,* 585-594.

Jasper, H. H. Cortical excitatory state and synchronism in the control of bioelectric autonomous rhythms. *Cold Spring Harbor Symposia on quantitative Biology,* 1936, *4,* 320-338.

Jasper, H. H. Diffuse projection systems: The integrative action of the thalamic reticular system. *Electroencephalography and Clinical Neurophysiology,* 1949, *1,* 405-420.

Jasper, H. H., & Carmichael, L. Electrical potentials from the intact human brain. *Science,* 1935, *81,* 51-53.

Jasper, H. H., & Ajmone-Marsan, C. Thalamocortical integrating mechanisms. *Research Publication of the Association for Nervous and Mental Diseases,* 1952, *30,* 493-512.

Jeffress, L. A. (Ed.). *Cerebral mechanisms in behavior: The Hixon Symposium.* New York: Wiley, 1951.

Jouvet, M. The role of monoamines and acetylcholine-containing neurons in the regulation of sleep-waking cycle. *Ergebnisse der Physiologie, Biologischen Chemie und Experimentellen Pharmakologie,* 1972, *64,* 166-307. (a)

Jouvet, M. Some monoaminergic mechanisms controlling sleep and waking. In A. G. Karcznar & J. C. Eccles (Eds.), *Brain and human behavior.* New York/Heidelberg/Berlin: Springer-Verlag, 1972. (b)

Kawamura, H., Nakamura, Y., & Tokizane, T. Effect of acute brain stem lesions on the electrical activities of the limbic system and neocortex. *Japanese Journal of Physiology,* 1961, *11,* 564-575.

Kemp, I. R., & Kaada, B. R. The relation of hippocampal theta activity to arousal, attentive behaviour and somato-motor movements in unrestrained cats. *Brain Research,* 1975, *95,* 323-342.

Kennard, M. A., & Ectors, L. Forced circling in monkeys following lesions of the frontal lobes. *Journal of Neurophysiology,* 1938, *1,* 45-54.

Kennard, M. A., & McCulloch W. S. Functional organization of frontal pole in monkey and chimpanzee. *Journal of Neurophysiology,* 1944, *7,* 37-40.

Kennard, M. A., Spencer, S., & Fountain, G., Jr. Hyperactivity in monkeys following lesions of frontal lobes. *Journal of Neurophysiology,* 1941, *4,* 512-524.

Kleitman, N. *Sleep and wakefulness*. Chicago: University of Chicago Press, 1939 (2nd ed. 1963).

Kreindler, A., Crighel, E., & Marinchescu, C. Integrative activity of the thalamus pulvinar-lateralis posterior complex and interrelations with the neocortex. *Experimental Neurology*, 1968, *22*, 423-435.

Kornhuber, H. H., & Deecke, L. Hirnpotentialänderungen bei wilkerbewegungen und passiven bewegungen des menschen: Bereitschaftspotential und reafferente potentials. *Pfluger's Archiv fur die gesamte Physiologie*, 1965, *284*, 1-17.

Lansing, R. W., Schwartz, E., & Lindsley, D. B. Reaction time and EEG activation under alerted and nonalerted conditions. *Journal of Experimental Psychology*, 1959, *58*, 1-7.

Lashley, K. S. *Brain mechanisms and intelligence*. Chicago: University of Chicago Press, 1929.

Lashley, K. S. In search of the engram. In *Symposia of the Society for Experimental Biology, No. 4, Animal Behavior*. Cambridge, Eng.: Cambridge University Press, 1950.

Lashley, K. S. The problem of serial order in behavior. In L. A. Jeffress (Ed.), *Cerebral mechanisms in behavior: The Hixon Symposium*. New York; Wiley, 1951.

Lashley, K. S., & Franz, S. I. The effects of cerebral destruction upon habit formation and retention in the albino rat. *Journal of Comparative Psychology*, 1917, *1*, 71-139.

Leão, A. A. P. Spreading depression of activity in the cerebral cortex. *Journal of Neurophysiology*, 1944, *7*, 359-390.

Leão, A. A. P. Pial circulation and spreading depression of activity in the cerebral cortex. *Journal of Neurophysiology*, 1944, *7*, 391-396.

Leão, A. A. P., & Morison, R. S. Propagation of spreading cortical depression. *Journal of Neurophysiology*, 1945, *8*, 33-45.

Lindsley, D. B. Electroencephalography. In J. McV. Hunt (Ed.), *Personality and the behavior disorders* (Vol. 2). New York: Ronald Press, 1944.

Lindsley, D. B. Emotions and the electroencephalogram. In M. L. Reymert (Ed.), *Feelings and emotions: The Mooseheart Symposium*. New York: McGraw-Hill, 1950.

Lindsley, D. B. Emotion. In S. S. Stevens (Ed.), *Handbook of experimental psychology*. New York, Wiley, 1951.

Lindsley, D. B. Brain stem influences on spinal motor activity. *Research Publication of the Association for Nervous and mental Diseases*, 1952, *30*, 174-195. (a) (Also appears in P. Bard (Ed.), *Patterns of organization in the central nervous system* (Chapter 9). Baltimore: Williams and Wilkins, 1952).

Lindsley, D. B. Psychological phenomena and the electroencephalogram. *Electroencephalography and Clinical Neurophysiology*, 1952, *4*, 443-456.

Lindsley, D. B. Effect of photic stimulation in visual pathways from retina to cortex. *Science*, 1953, *117*, 469.

Lindsley, D. B. Electric response to photic stimulation in visual pathways of the cat. *Electroencephalography and Clinical Neurophysiology*, 1954, *6*, 690-691.

Lindsley, D. B. Basic perceptual processes and the EEG. *Psychiatric Research Reports*, 1956, *6*, 161-170.

Lindsley, D. B. Psychophysiology of motivation. In M. R. Jones (Ed.), *Nebraska symposium on motivation*. Lincoln: University of Nebraska Press, 1957.

Lindsley, D. B. Psychophysiology and perception. In R. Patton (Ed.), *The description and analysis of behavior*. Pittsburgh: University of Pittsburgh Press, 1958. (a)

Lindsley, D. B. The reticular system and perceptual discrimination. In H. H. Jasper, L. D. Proctor, R. S. Knighton, W. C. Noshay & R. T. Costello (Eds.), *Reticular formation of the brain*. Boston: Little, Brown, 1958. (b)

Lindsley, D. B. Attention, consiciousness, sleep and wakefulness (Chap. 64). In J. Field (Ed.), *Handbook of Physiology, Section 1, Neurophysiology* (Vol. 3). Washington, D.C.: American Physiological Society, 1960.

Lindsley, D. B. Common factors in sensory deprivation, sensory distortion and sensory overload. In P. Solomon et al. (Eds.), *Sensory deprivation*. Cambridge, Mass.: Harvard University Press, 1961. (a)

Lindsley, D. B. The reticular activating system and perceptual integration. In D. E. Sheer (Ed.), *Electrical stimulation of the brain*. Austin, Tex.: University of Texas Press, 1961. (b)

Lindsley, D. B. Electrophysiology of the visual system and its relation to perceptual phenomena. In M. A. B. Brazier (Ed.), *Brain and behavior* (Vol. 1). Washington, D.C.: American Institute of Biological Sciences, 1961. (c)

Lindsley, D. B. The ontogeny of pleasure: Neural and behavioral development. In R. G. Heath (Ed.), *The role of pleasure in behavior*. New York: Hoeber, 1964.

Lindsley, D. B. Neurophysiological mechanisms of attention and perception: Their role in information processing in the visual system. In D. P. Kimble (Ed.), *Readiness to remember*. New York: Gordon and Breach, 1969.

Lindsley, D. B. The role of nonspecific reticulo-thalamo-cortical systems in emotion. In P. Black (Ed.), *Physiological correlates of emotion*. New York: Academic Press, 1970.

Lindsley, D. B., Bowden, J. W., & Magoun, H. W. Effect upon the EEG of acute injury to the brain stem activating system. *Electroencephalography and Clinical Neurophysiology*, 1949, *1*, 475-486.

Lindsley, D. B., & Emmons, W. H. Perception time and evoked potentials. *Science*, 1958. *127*, 1061.

Lindsley, D. B., & Hunter, W. S. A note on polarity potentials from the human eye. *Proceedings of the National Academy of Science, Washington*, 1939, *25*, 180-183.

Lindsley, D. B., & Griffiths, R. S. Differential response of eye and optic pathways to intensity and wave-length. *Science*, 1955, *122*, 976.

Lindsley, D. B., Schreiner, L. H., Knowles, W. B., & Magoun, H. W. Behavioral and EEG changes following chronic brain stem lesions in the cat. *Electroencephalography and Clinical Neurophysiology*, 1950, *2*, 483-498.

Lindsley, D. B., Schreiner, L. H., & Magoun, H. W. An electromyographic study of spasticity. *Journal of Neurophysiology*, 1949, *12*, 207-216.

Lindsley, D. B., & Wilson, C. L. Brain stem-hypothalamic systems influencing hippocampal activity and behavior. In R. L. Isaacson & K. H. Pribram (Eds.) *The hippocampus*. Vol. 2, New York: Plenum Press, 1975.

Lindsley, D. B., Wilson, G. F., and Seales, D. M. Evoked potentials and information processing. *Electroencephalography and Clinical Neurophysiology*, 1974, *36*, 213.

Lindsley, D. F., Perryman, K. M., & Lindsley, D. B. Brain mechanisms of attention and perception. In R. F. Thompson, L. H. Hicks, & V. B Shvyrkov (Eds.), *Neural mechanisms of goal-directed behavior and learning*. New York: Academic Press, 1980.

Lynch, J. C., Mountcastle, V. B., Talbot, W. H., & Yin, T. C. T. Parietal lobe mechanism for directed visual attention. *Journal of Neurophysiology*, 1977, *40*, 362-389.

Macadar, A. W., Chalupa, L. M., & Lindsley, D. B. Differentiation of brain stem loci which affect hippocampal and neocortical electrical activity *Experimental Neurology*, 1974, *43*, 499-515.

Magoun, H. W. Caudal and cephalic influences of the brain stem reticular formation. *Physiological Review*, 1950, *30*, 459-474.

Magoun, H. W. An ascending reticular activating system in the brain stem. *Archives of Neurology and Psychiatry*, 1952, *67*, 145-154.

Magoun, H. W. An ascending reticular activating system in the brain stem. *Harvey Lectures*, 1952, *48*, 53-71.

Magoun, H. W. The ascending reticular system and wakefulness. In J. F. Delafresnaye (Ed.), *Brain mechanisms and consciousness*. Springfield, Ill.: Thomas, 1954.

Magoun, H. W. *The waking brain*. Springfield, Ill. Thomas, 1958, (2nd ed. 1963.)

Magoun, H. W., & Fischer, C. Walter R. Ingram at Ranson's Institute of Neurology, 1930-1936. *Perspectives in Biology and Medicine*, 1980, *24*, 31-56.

Magoun, H. W., & Rhines, R. An inhibitory mechanism in the bulbar reticular formation. *Journal of Neurophysiology*, 1946, *9*, 127-132.

Marquis, D. G. Effects of removal of the visual cortex in mammals with observations on the retention of light discrimination in dogs. *Research Publications of the Association for Nervous and Mental Diseases*, 1934, *13*, 558-592.

Marquis, D. G., & Hilgard, E. R. Conditioned responses to light in monkeys after removal of the occipital lobes. *Brain*, 1937, *60*, 1-12.

Marshall, W. H. The relation of dehydration of the brain to the spreading depression of Leão. *Electroencephalography and Clinical Neurophysiology*, 1950, *2*, 177-185.

Marshall, W. H., Essig, C. F., & Dubroff, S. J. Relation of temperature of cerebral cortex to spreading depression of Leão. *Journal of Neurophysiology*, 1951, *14*, 153-166.

Marshall, W. H., & Talbot, S. A. Recent evidence for neural mechanisms in vision leading to a general theory of sensory acuity. *Biological Symposia. VII. Visual mechanisms*. Lancaster, Pa.: Jacques Cattell Press, 1942, 117-164.

McCulloch, W. S. Cortico-cortical connections. In P. C. Bucy (Ed.), *The precentral motor cortex. Illinois Monographs in the Medical Sciences*, 1944, *4* (Nos. 1-4), 212-242. (a)

McCulloch, W. S. The functional organization of the cerebral cortex. *Physiological Review*, 1944, *24*, 390-407. (b)

McCulloch, W. S. Machines that want and think. In W. C. Halstead (Ed.), *Brain and behavior: A symposium*. Berkeley/Los Angeles: University of California Press, 1950.

McCulloch, W. S. Why the mind is in the head. In L. A. Jeffress (Ed.), *Cerebral mechanisms in behavior: The Hixon Symposium*. New York: Wiley, 1951.

McCulloch, W. S., & Pitts, W. A logical calculus of the ideas immanent in nervous activity. *Bulletin of Mathematical Biophysics*, 1943, *5*, 115-133.

McCulloch, W. S., & Pitts, W. The statistical organization of nervous activity. *Biometrics*, 1948, *4*, 91-99.

Millhouse, O. E. A Golgi study of the descending medial forebrain bundle. *Brain Research*, 1969, *15*, 341-363.

Mishkin, M. Cortical visual areas and their interaction. In A. G. Karczmar & J. C. Eccles (Eds.), *Brain and human behavior*. New York/Heidelberg/Berlin: Springer-Verlag, 1972.

Moore, R. Y. Monoamine neurons innervating the hippocampal formation and septum: Organization and response to injury. In R. L. Isaacson & K. H. Pribram (Eds.), *The hippocampus* (Vol. 1). New York: Plenum Press, 1975.

Morison, R. S., & Dempsey, E. W. A study of thalamocortical relations. *American Journal of Physiology*, 1942, *135*, 280-292.

Moruzzi, G. The sleep-waking cycle. *Ergebnisse der Physiologie, Biologischen Chemic und Experimentellen Pharmakologie*, 1972, *64*, 1-65. (Also published as separate monograph: Reviews of Physiology, Ergebnisse der Physiologie. Berlin/Heidelberg/New York: Springer-Verlag, 1972.)

Moruzzi, G., & Magoun, H. W. Brain stem reticular formation and activation of the EEG. *Electroencephalography and Clinical Neurophysiology*, 1949, *1*, 455-473.

Mountcastle, V. B., & Henneman, E. Pattern of tactile representation in thalamus of cat. *Journal of Neurophysiology*, 1949, *12*, 85-100.

Mountcastle, V. B., & Henneman, E. The representation of tactile sensibility in the thalamus of the monkey. *Journal of Comparative Neurology*, 1952, *97*, 409-440.

Mountcastle, V. B., Lynch, J. C., Georgopoulos, A., Sakata, H., & Acuna, C. Posterior parietal association cortex of the monkey: Command functions for operations within extrapersonal space. *Journal of Neurophysiology*, 1975, *38*, 871-908.

Mowrer, O. H., Ruch, T. C., & Miller, N. E. The cornea-retinal potential difference as a basis of the galvanometric method of recording eye movements. *American Journal of Physiology*, 1936, *114*, 423-428.

O'Leary, J., & Cohen, L. A. The reticular core 1957. *Physiological Review*, 1958, *38*, 243-276.

Paiva, T., Lopes da Silva, F. H., & Mollevanger, W. Modulating systems of hippocampal EEG. *Electroencephalography and Clinical Neurophysiology*, 1976, *40*, 470-480.

Perryman, K. M., & Lindsley, D. B. Visual responses in geniculo-striate and pulvino-extrastriate systems to patterned and unpatterned stimuli in squirrel monkeys. *Electroencephalography and Clinical Neurophysiology*, 1977, *42*, 157-177.

Perryman, K. M., Lindsley, D. F., & Lindsley, D. B. Pulvinar neuron responses to spontaneous and trained eye movements and to light flashes in squirrel monkeys. *Electroencephalography and Clinical Neurophysiology*, 1981, *49*, 152-161.

Peterson, E. W., Magoun, H. W., McCulloch, W. S., & Lindsley, D. B. Production of postural tremor. *Journal of Neurophysiology*, 1949, *12*, 371-384.

Petsche, W., Stumpf, C., & Gogolak, G. The significance of the rabbit's septum as a relay station between the midbrain and hippocampus. I. The control of hippocampal arousal activity by the septum cells. *Electroencephalography and clinical Neurophysiology*, 1962, *14*, 202-211.

Pitts, W., & McCulloch, W. S. How we know universals; the perception of auditory and visual forms. *Bulletin of Mathematical Biophysics*, 1947, *9*, 127-147.

Ranson, S. W., & Magoun, H. W. The hypothalamus. *Ergebnisse der Physiologie, Biologischen Chemie und Experimentellen Pharmakologie*, 1939, *41*, 56-163.

Ratliff, F. (Ed.). *Studies on excitation and inhibition in the retina. A collection of papers from the laboratories of H. Keffer Hartline*. New York: Rockefeller University Press, 1974.

Renshaw, B., Forbes, A., & Morison, B. R. Activity of isocortex and hippocampus; electrical studies with microelectrodes. *Journal of Neurophysiology*, 1940, *3*, 74-105.

Rheinberger M. B. & Jasper, H. H. Electrical activity of the cerebral cortex in the unanesthetized cat. *American Journal of Physiology*, 1937, *119*, 186-196.

Rezak, M., & Benevento, L. A. A comparison of the organization of the projections of the dorsal lateral geniculate nucleus, the inferior pulvinar and adjacent lateral pulvinar to primary visual cortex (area 17) in the macaque monkey. *Brain Research*, 1979, *167*, 19-41.

Rhines, R., & Magoun, H. W. Brain stem facilitation of cortical motor response. *Journal of Neurophysiology*, 1946, *9*, 219-229.

Rohrbaugh, J. W., Chalupa, L. M., & Lindsley, D. B. Evoked potentials related to decision confidence in a visual discrimination task. In E. Donchin, G. Galbraith, & M. Kietzman (Eds.), *Neurophysiology and psychology: Basic mechanisms and clinical applications*. New York: Academic Press, in press.

Rohrbaugh, J. W., Syndulko, K., & Lindsley, D. B. Brain wave components of the contingent negative variation in humans. *Science*, 1976, *191*, 1055-1057.

Rohrbaugh, J. W., Syndulko, K., & Lindsley, D. B. Cortical slow negative waves following non-paired stimuli: Effects of task factors. *Electroencephalography and Clinical Neurophysiology*, 1978, *45*, 551-567.

Rohrbaugh, J. W., Syndulko, K., & Lindsley, D. B. Cortical slow negative waves following non-paired stimuli: Effects of modality, intensity and rate of stimulation. *Electroencephalography and Clinical Neurophysiology*, 1979, *46*, 416-427.

Rohrbaugh, J. W., Syndulko, K., Sanquist, T. F., & Lindsley, D. B. Synthesis of the contingent negative variation brain potential from noncontingent stimulus and motor elements. *Science*, 1980, *208*, 1165-1168.

Rossi, G. F., & Zanchetti, A. Brain stem reticular formation. Anatomy and physiology. *Archives Italiennes de Biologie*, 1957, *95*, 199-435.

Sanquist, T. F., Beatty, J. T., & Lindsley, D. B. Slow potential shifts of human brain during forewarned reaction. *Electroencephalography and Clinical Neurophysiology*, 1981, *51*, 639-649.

Sanquist, T. G., Rohrbaugh, J. W., Syndulko, K., & Lindsley, D. B. An event-related potential analysis of coding processes in human memory. In H. H. Kornhuber & L. Deecke (Eds.), *Motivation, motor and sensory processes in the brain. Progress in Brain Research* (*Vol. 54*). Amsterdam: Elsevier/North Holland Biomedical Press, 1980. (a)

Sanquist, T. F., Rohrbaugh, J. W., Syndulko, K., & Lindsley, D. B. Electrocortical signs of levels of processing: Perceptual analysis and recognition memory. *Psychophysiology*, 1980, *17*, 568-576. (b)

Saul, L. J. & Davis, H. Action currents in the central nervous system. I. Action currents of the auditory tracts. *Archives of Neurology and Psychiatry*, 1932, *28*, 1104-1116.

Saul, L. J. & Davis, H. Action currents in the central nervous system. Archives of Neurology and Psychiatry, 1933, *29*, 255-259.

Schreiner, L. H., Lindsley, D. B., & Magoun, H. W. Role of brain stem facilitatory systems in maintenance of spasticity. *Journal of Neurophysiology*, 1949, *12*, 207-216.

Schwartz, A. S., & Lindsley, D. B. Critical flicker frequency and photic following in the cat. *Boletin del Instituto de Estudios Medicos y Biologicos* (*Mexico*), 1964, *22*, 249-262.

Seales, D., & Lindsley, D. B. Modification of human visually evoked potentials by complexity and cerebral lateralization of information processing. *Electroencephalography and Clinical Neurophysiology*, 1975, *38*, 101.

Segundo, J. P. The reticular formation, a survey. *Acta Neurologica Latinoamericana*, 1956, *3*, 245-281.

Sherrington, C. S. *The integrative action of the nervous system*. New York: Charles Scribner's Sons, 1906. (Reprinted in 1911, 1914, 1916, 1918, 1920; 2nd ed. New Haven; Yale University Press, 1947, 1948.)

Sherrington, C. S. *Man on his nature*. Garden City, N.Y.: Doubleday, 1951.

Schreiner, L. H., Lindsley, D. B., & Magoun, H. W. Role of brain stem facilitatory systems in maintenance of spasticity. *Journal of Neurophysiology*, 1949, *12*, 207-216.

Skinner, J. E., & Lindsley, D. B. Electrophysiological and behavioral effects of blockade of the nonspecific thalamo-cortical system. *Brain Research*, 1967, *6*, 95-118.

Skinner, J. E., & Lindsley, D. B. Reversible cryogenic blockade of neural function in the brain of unrestrained animals. *Science*, 1968, *161*, 595-597.

Skinner, J. E., & Lindsley, D. B. Effect of cryogenic blockade of a nonspecific thalamo-orbito-cortical synchronizing system upon sensory evoked responses. *Electroencephalography and Clinical Neurophysiology*, 1969, *26*, 333-334.

Skinner, J. E., & Lindsley, D. B. Enhancement of visual and auditory evoked potentials during blockade of the non-specific thalamo-cortical system. *Electroencephalography and Clinical Neurophysiology*, 1971, *31*, 1-6.

Skinner, J. E., & Lindsley, D. B. A nonspecific mediothalamic-frontocortical system: Its influence on electrocortical activity and behavior. In K. H. Pribram & A. R. Luria (Eds.), *Psychophysiology of the frontal lobes*. New York: Academic Press, 1973.

Skinner, J. E., & Yingling, C. D. Regulation of slow potential shifts in nucleus reticularis thalami by the mesencephalic reticular formation and the frontal granular cortex. *Electroencephalography and Clinical Neurophysiology*, 1976, *40*, 288-296.

Skinner, J. E., & Yingling, C. D. Central gating mechanisms that regulate event-related potentials and behavior. In J. E. Desmedt (Ed.), *Attention, voluntary contraction and slow potential shifts*. Basel: Karger, 1977.

Sloan, N., & Jasper, H. The identity of spreading depression and "suppression." *Electroencephalography and Clinical Neurophysiology*, 1950, *2*, 59-78.

Spong, P., Haider, M., & Lindsley, D. B. Selective attentiveness and cortical evoked potentials to visual and auditory stimuli. *Science*, 1965, *148*, 395-397.

Starzl, T. E., & Magoun, H. W. Organization of the diffuse thalamic projection system. *Journal of Neurophysiology*, 1951, *14*, 133-146.

Starzl, T. E., & Whitlock, D. G. Diffuse thalamic projection system in monkey. *Journal of Neurophysiology*, 1952, *15*, 449–468.

Stumpf, C., Petsche, H., & Gogolak, G. The significance of the rabbit's septum as a relay station between the midbrain and the hippocampus. II. The differential influence of drugs upon both the septal cell firing pattern and the hippocampus theta activity. *Electroencephalography and Clinical Neurophysiology*, 1962, *14*, 212–219.

Syndulko, K., & Lindsley, D. B. Motor and sensory determinants of cortical slow potential shifts in man. In J. E. Desmedt (Ed.) *Progress in clinical neurophysiology*. Vol 1. Attention, voluntary movement and event-related potentials. Basel: Karger, 1977.

Talbot, S. A., & Marshall, W. H. Physiological studies on neural mechanisms of visual localization and discrimination. *American Journal of Ophthalmology*, 1941, *24*, 1255–1265.

Thomas, L. B. Spontaneous and evoked patterns of activity of single cortical cells in auditory and visual cortex. *Electroencephalography and Clinical Neurophysiology*, 1952, *4*, 376.

Tokizane, T., Kawamura, H., & Imamura, G. Hypothalamic activation upon electrical activities of paleo- and archicortex. *Neurol. medicochir.*, 1960, *2*, 63–76.

Trojanowski, J. Q., & Jacobson, S. A combined horseradish peroxidase-autoradiographic investigation of reciprocal connections between superior temporal gyrus and the pulvinar in squirrel monkey. *Brain Research*, 1975, *85*, 347–353.

Velasco, M., & Lindsley, D. B. Role of orbital cortex in regulation of thalamo-cortical electrical activity. *Science*, 1965 *149*, 1375–1377.

Velasco, M., & Lindsley, D. B. Effect of thalamocortical activation on recruiting responses. II. Peripheral and central neural stimulation. *Acta Neurologica Latinoamericana*, 1968, *14*, 188–199. (a)

Velasco, M., & Lindsley, D. B. Effect of thalamocortical activation on recruiting responses. III. Reticular lesions. *Acta Neurologica Latinoamericana*, 1968, *14*, 271–282. (b)

Velasco, M., Skinner, J. E., Asaro, K. D., & Lindsley, D. B. Thalamo-cortical systems regulating spindle bursts and recruiting response. I. Effect of cortical ablations. *Electroencephalography and Clinical Neurophysiology*, 1968, *25*, 463–470.

Velasco, M., Skinner, J. E., Asaro, K. D., & Lindsley, D. B. Thalamo-cortical systems regulating spindle bursts and recruiting responses. II. Effect of thalamic lesions. *Acta Neurologica Latinoamericana*, 1975, *21*, 31–39.

Velasco, M., Skinner, J. E., & Lindsley, D. B. Thalamo-cortical systems regulating spindle bursts and recruiting responses. III. Effects of lesions in the forebrain and rostral diencephalon. *Acta Neurologica Latinoamericana*, 1976, *22*, 1–9.

Velasco, M., Weinberger, N. M., & Lindsley, D. B. Effect of thalamocortical activation on recruiting responses. I. Reticular stimulation. *Acta Neurologica Latinoamericana*, 1968, *14*, 99–115.

Verzeano, M., Lindsley, D. B., & Magoun H. W. Nature of recruiting response. *Journal of Neurophysiology*, 1953, *16*, 183–195.

Walker, A. E. *The primate thalamus*. Chicago: Chicago University Press, 1938.

Walker, A. E. The meaning of the thalamus. *Congreso Latinoamericana de Neurocir., VI*. 1955, 926–946 (Symposium de Talamo).

Walter, W. G. Normal rhythms—their development, distribution and significance. In J. D. N. Hill & G. Parr (Eds.), *Electroencephalography*. New York: Macmillan, 1950.

Walter, W. G. *The living brain*. New York: Norton, 1953.

Walter, W. G., Cooper, R., Aldridge E. J., McCallum, W. C., and Winter, A. L. Contingent Negative Variation-an electrical sign of sensorimotor association and expectancy in the human brain. *Nature*, 1964, *203*, 380–384.

Weinberger, N. M. & Lindsley, D. B. Behavioral and electroencephalographic arousal to contrasting novel stimulation. *Science*, 1964, *144*, 1355–1357.

Weinberger, N. M., Velasco, M., & Lindsley, D. B. Differential effects of reinforced and non-reinforced stimuli upon electrocortical recruiting responses. *Psychonomic Science*, 1965, *2*, 129–130. (a)

Weinberger, N. M., Velasco, M., & Lindsley, D. B. Effects of lesions upon thalamically induced electrocortical desynchronization and recruiting. *Electroencephalography and Clinical Neurophysiology*, 1965, *18*, 369-377. (b)

Weinberger, N. M., Nakayama, K., & Lindsley, D. B. Electrocortical recruiting responses during classical conditioning. *Electroencephalography and Clinical Neurophysiology*, 1968, *24*, 16-24.

Weinberger, N. M., Velasco, M., & Lindsley, D. B. The relationship between cortical synchrony and behavioral inhibition. *Electroencephalography and Clinical Neurophysiology*, 1967, *23*, 297-305.

Weinberger, N. M., Yeudall, L., & Lindsley, D. B. EEG correlates of reinforced behavioral inhibition. *Psychonomic Science*, 1968, *10*, 11-12.

Weiss, P. Selectivity controlling the central-peripheral relations in the nervous system. *Biological Review*, 1936, *11*, 494-531.

Weiss, P. *Principles of development*. New York: Holt, 1939.

Weiss, P. A. The deplantation of fragment of nervous system in amphibians. I. Central reorganization and the formation of nerves. *Journal of Experimental Zoology*, 1950, *113*, 397-461.

Wicke, J. D., Donchin, E., & Lindsley, D. B. Visual evoked potentials as a function of flash luminance and duration. *Science*, 1964, *145*, 83-85.

Wilson, C. L., & Lindsley, D. B. Effects of hypothalamic stimulation upon septal pacemaker mechanisms influencing hippocampal theta rhythm. *Society for Neurosciences Abstracts*, 1974, 479.

Wilson, C. L., Motter, B. C., & Lindsley, D. B. Influences of hypothalamic stimulation upon septal and hippocampal electrical activity in the cat. *Brain Research*, 1976, *107*, 55-68.

Wishaw, I. Q., & Vanderwolf, C. H. Hippocampal EEG and behavior: Changes in amplitude and frequency of RSA (theta rhythm) associated with spontaneous and learned movement patterns in rats and cats. *Behavioral Biology*, 1973, *8*, 461-484.

Worden, F. G., & Livingston, R. B. Brain-stem reticular formation. In D. E. Sheer, (Ed.), *Electrical stimulation of the brain*. Austin, Tex.: University of Texas Press, 1961.

Yin, T. C. T., & Mountcastle, V. B. Visual input to the visuomotor mechanisms of the monkey's parietal lobe. *Science*, 1977, *197*, 1381-1383.

Yin, T. C. T., & Mountcastle, V. B. Mechanisms of neural integration in the parietal lobe for visual attention. *Federation Proceedings*, 1978, *37*, 2251-2257.

Yingling, C. D., & Skinner, J. E. Regulation of unit activity in nucleus reticularis thalami by the mesencephalic reticular formation and the frontal granular cortex. *Electroencephalography and Clinical Neurophysiology*, 1975, *39*, 635-642.

Yingling, C. D., & Skinner, J. E. Selective regulation of thalamic sensory relay nuclei by nucleus reticularis thalami. *Electroencephalography and Clinical Neurophysiology*, 1976, *41*, 476-482.

Yoshida, K., & Benevento, L. A. The projection from the dorsal lateral geniculate nucleus of the thalamus to extrastriate visual association cortex in the macaque monkey. *Neuroscience Letters*, 1981, *22*, 103-108.

16 Cortico-Cortical and Thalamo-Cortical Inputs to Precentral Motor Cortex in the Monkey

Edward V. Evarts
Laboratory of Neurophysiology
National Institute of Mental Health
Bethesda, Maryland

When I arrived at the Yerkes Laboratories of Primate Biology in 1949, Lashley suggested that I investigate the functional role of visual association areas 18 and 19, and I embarked upon a study of the effects of prestriate lesions on auditory-visual association in the monkey (Evarts, 1952). Lashley had asked me to do this study because of his interest in the more general question of the function of cortico-cortical connections: during the decade between 1940 and 1950 the technique of strychnine neuronography had provided maps of these connections, and there had been a series of papers on their role in the functional organization of the cerebral cortex. Always the iconoclast, Lashley had challenged the widely accepted formulations of the neuronographers—pointing out that the surprisingly slight effects of lesions interrupting cortico-cortical fibers made it unlikely that cortico-cortical connections via association areas provided essential links between different primary sensory receiving areas (e.g., visual and auditory areas) or between sensory and motor areas (e.g., postcentral and precentral gyri). Other work on cortico-cortical connections had been carried out in Orange Park prior to my arrival, and the results of these earlier experiments had been largely negative (as were the results of my own studies). For example, Sperry (1947) carried out some technically elegant (but negative) experiments on effects of subpial cuts eliminating cortico-cortical connections within motor cortex of monkey; it was only later that he combined chiasm and callosum sections and made his great discoveries on the role of the cortico-cortical connections linking the two hemispheres.

Lashley seemed pleased with the negative results we were coming up with—because he felt that the map makers of the forties had drawn an overly simplistic picture of the role of cortico-cortical connections in brain organization. But in spite of our negative results and his negative attitude toward neuronographic maps, Lashley knew perfectly well that cortico-cortical connections had to be of great significance—and he motivated those of us who worked with him to come up with positive experimental results that could withstand his keen, critical analysis. Lashley also recognized the importance of understanding the relative functional roles of cortico-cortical and cortico-subcortical connections, and this problem—as it was singled out by Lashley in the forties—remains at the forefront of brain research in the eighties. And so for my contribution to this book, *Neuropsychology after Lashley,* I thought it might be appropriate to discuss some current ideas on the relative roles of cortico-cortical and thalamo-cortical connections.

CORTICO-CORTICAL AND THALAMO-CORTICAL INPUTS TO MOTOR CORTEX

My interest in the relative roles of cortico-cortical and thalamo-cortical connections was recently reawakened by observations on motor cortex pyramidal tract (PT) cell responses to afferent feedback occurring in the course of voluntary movements in monkeys. Sensory responses in motor cortex had been observed by Malis, Pribram, and Kruger (1953) and by a number of subsequent investigators, but it was not until Phillips (1969) proposed that the changes in cortico-motoneuronal (CM) activity with changed loads might in part depend on feedback that the role of these sensory inputs began to be understood. Phillips (1969) stated:

> One may hazard the speculation that the increased discharge of the PT cell . . . was in response to a signal of mismatch between "intended" and actual displacement. Whether this signal is a crude one from the muscle spindles, or whether the mismatch has been computed by the cerebellum is still unknown; nor . . . can the contributions of joints, skin and vision be assessed. But however "instructed", the CM projection would transfer the "instruction" for increased force to the alpha-motoneurons with maximum directness [p. 168].

Phillips' statement made it clear that when we view the PT neuron (PTN) as a summing point in a transcortical servo loop, we can interpret the increased PTN discharge with increased loads not simply as a "force command" (Evarts, 1968) but rather as an error signal corresponding to a mismatch between intended and actual displacement.

In retrospect, it probably should have been clear (even prior to Phillips' insightful paper) that motor cortex outputs would reflect both central motor programs and afferent feedback from the periphery. Perhaps the delay in accepting the idea that motor cortex outputs are reflexly controlled by feedback during volitional movements stemmed from the view that reflex and volitional movements were opposites, and that if a given motor cortex neuron was exhibiting reflex discharge, it could not at the same time be exhibiting volitionally determined discharge. Furthermore, since it was known that outputs from motor cortex were under volitional control, it seemed to follow that motor cortex outputs could not at the same time be under reflex control. And after it was demonstrated (Evarts, 1966) that motor cortex PTNs discharged 100 msec in advance of muscular contraction in learned volitional limb movements (before the influx of any afferent feedback), it seemed reasonable to assume that feedback to motor cortex was relatively unimportant in the behaving animal. But support for the broad features of Phillips' "transcortical servo" hypothesis has now been obtained in a number of studies (Conrad, Matsunami, Meyer-Lohmann, Wiesendanger, & Brooks, 1974; Conrad, Meyer-Lohmann, Matsunami, & Brooks, 1975; Evarts, 1973; Evarts — Tanji, 1976; Porter, 1976), and the results of these studies make it clear that there are strong feedback loops to motor cortex. Given the powerful actions of the afferent information reaching motor cortex, it becomes of interest to consider the routes whereby this afferent information is transmitted; and it is in this connection that we return to the matter of cortico-cortical and thalamo-cortical inputs to motor cortex.

As to the inputs reaching motor cortex from the thalamus, studies by Lemon and Burg (1979) and by Horne and Tracey (1979) have shown that neurons in thalamic nucleus VPL_0 receive short-latency (6- to 10-msec) inputs from nerves of the arm and transmit these signals to the arm area of the motor cortex. In these studies, motor cortex was electrically stimulated to allow antidromic activation of the VPL_0 neurons projecting to motor cortex, and it was found that many of the neurons projecting to motor cortex were activated at short latency by peripheral inputs. Injections of HRP into motor cortex confirmed the location of antidromically activated neurons within the region of VPL_0 projecting to motor cortex.

The short latency of the sensory responses in VPL_0 ruled out a transcerebellar pathway for the sensory inputs to VPL_0, and Lemon and Burg (1979) concluded that the "neurones in VPL_0 both receive a clear peripheral input and project to the motor cortex, and that these neurones may be partly responsible for the short-latency transmission of information from the moving limb to the motor cortex [p. 460]." In essence, then, the latencies of signals to MI from SI and VPL_0 are about the same, and it follows that latency cannot be used to exclude either zone as a source of the MI discharges in response to feedback.

Another dimension (in addition to somatosensory response *latency*) according to which somatosensory inputs to SI and VPL_0 may be contrasted is their origin. For SI the evidence is abundant: SI receives its signals via the ventrobasal complex, which in turn receives several somatosensory submodalities via the medial lemniscus. But what is the origin of somatosensory inputs to VPL_0? This question has been addressed in a recent study by Tracey, Asanuma, Jones, and Porter (1980) on afferent pathways from brain stem, cerebellum, and spinal cord to VPL_0 in monkeys. Using HRP and tritiated amino acid injections, it was demonstrated that lemniscal inputs fail to reach VPL_0. In spite of being "negative," the evidence supporting this conclusion was compelling. The results obtained by anterograde transport of tritiated protein and retrograde transport of HRP were in agreement, for the part of VPL_0 that projected to MI (as shown by anterograde transport) failed to receive inputs from the dorsal column nuclei (as indicated by failure of HRP to be retrogradely transported from VPL_0 to cell bodies in these nuclei). Instead of labeling the dorsal column nuclei, HRP injections localized in VPL_0 caused intense retrograde labeling of cell bodies in the dentate nucleus of the cerebellum.

Given the fact that signals relayed by the dorsal column nuclei can reach MI by cortico-cortical connections (via the ventrobasal complex projections to SI and SII) but not by direct thalamo-cortical connections, it becomes critical to determine the extent to which dorsal column signals are necessary for transmission of sensory feedback to MI. This question was addressed in a recent study by Brinkman, Bush, and Porter (1978), who recorded MI neuron responses to peripheral stimuli in monkeys with dorsal column lesions, and found that short-latency feedback to motor cortex was virtually eliminated by section of the cuneate fasciculi. Such a lesion should not have deafferented VPL_0 (which does not receive inputs from the cuneate nucleus), and it follows that the afferent signals from VPL_0 to MI (even though of short latency) are *not sufficient* to generate short-latency discharges in motor cortex. Furthermore, by showing that dorsal column signals *are necessary* for short-latency MI discharges, the study of Brinkman et al. (1978) indicates that the brain areas generating short-latency MI discharges must receive lemniscal inputs. The most obvious zones having these attributes are SI areas 3a, 3b, 1, and 2 and the second somatic area, SII.

Further evidence in support of the hypothesis that postcentral inputs to motor cortex mediate the feedback underlying "reflex" discharges of motor cortex neurons in response to kinesthetic inputs has been provided by studies on long-loop reflexes in patients with a variety of lesions of the central nervous system. Marsden, Merton, Morton, and Adam (1978) found that lesions of the posterior columns in the cervical cord eliminated the long-latency stretch reflexes in the human thumb. In addition, these investigators found that lesions affecting sensorimotor cortex or capsular cortico-motoneuron pathways also eliminated the long-latency stretch reflex. In conclusion, Marsden et al. stated (1978) that the investigations

> established that lesions of the posterior columns, medial lemniscus, sensori-motor cortex, and capsular corticomotoneurone pathways abolish or depress the long-latency automatic servo responses in the long thumb flexor produced by perturbations applied to the top joint of the thumb during voluntary movement. All this

> evidence is compatible with the notion that the responses are the result of operation of a long loop transcortical stretch reflex pathway. None of this proves that servo action is based on such a pathway (the stretch reflex might still use a spinal arc facilitated from the cortex), but the theory would have fallen to the ground had the results been the opposite [p. 341].

Thus, current evidence is consistent with the hypothesis that cortico-cortical pathways have a significant role in transmitting short-latency kinesthetic inputs to motor cortex. As proposed by Rosén and Asanuma (1972), the peripheral afferent inputs to the monkey motor cortex must play a role in the feedback of information for continuous modulation of output from the motor cortex. Indeed, as Desmedt and Godaux point out (1978): "The motor cortex of man appears to have developed into a highly specialized area for the integration of movement-related kinesthetic and skin inputs. Thus independent finger movements that require detailed regulation by somatosensory input are extensively represented in area 4 [p. 24]."

PATHWAYS TRANSMITTING CENTRAL PROGRAMS TO MOTOR CORTEX

The pathways from postcentral gyrus to motor cortex provide inputs that can continuously control motor cortex output in the closed-loop mode. But what are the pathways giving rise to motor cortex discharges that underlie centrally programmed movements in the open-loop mode? In considering this general problem, Brooks (1979) has proposed that the lateral cerebellum is important in events occurring just before and after movement onset, but that the prior formation of goals is probably subserved by other parts of sensorimotor cortex (e.g., area 6) or by basal ganglia. It is of note that whereas cerebellar projections to thalamus are directly relayed to motor cortex via VPL_0, those regions of thalamus receiving inputs from globus pallidus project in large part to premotor cortex (supplementary motor area and lateral area 6), areas that in turn project to motor cortex via cortico-cortical connections. Thus, in line with formulations of Brooks (1979) and of Arbib (1981), it would appear that *initiation* of movement would in many cases involve prefrontal, temporal, and parietal association cortex projections via striatum and globus pallidus to VL-VA and thence to premotor cortex. Such a sequence would imply that discharges of the premotor cortex would be earlier (for centrally programmed movement) than discharges of motor cortex or dentate nucleus. According to these notions, at the time of initiation of a centrally programmed movement, motor cortex would be receiving inputs both from the premotor area (via cortico-cortical inputs) and from the cerebellum (via the cerebello-thalamo-cortical pathway). It is of note that there are strong projections from premotor cortex (via pontine nuclei) both to the dentate nucleus of the cerebellum and to the lateral parts of the cerebellar hemispheres. Thus, in initiation of centrally programmed movement, there are pathways that could generate discharge of neurons in the dentate nucleus of the cerebellum prior to discharge of neurons in motor cortex. Such a temporal relationship has been observed by Thach (1975) in the case of a ballistic arm movement in the monkey.

Direct evidence showing that the cerebello-thalamo-cortical pathway is involved in centrally programmed open-loop control has been provided by the work of Strick (1978), who recorded activity of single nerve cells in dentate and interposed nuclei of the monkey in the paradigm in which preprogrammed arm movements were triggered by displacements of the arm that was to move. Such a displacement evokes a reflex motor cortex response whose properties are consistent with transmission via the pathway utilized during the continuous control of the closed-loop feedback mode. This feedback-generated activity is followed by a second component of motor cortex discharge, which is dependent upon the motor set of the monkey (i.e., the movement that the monkey is prepared to make) rather than on the specific properties of the triggering afferent feedback; this second component of motor cortex discharge must be driven by an open-loop control system. Strick found that motor set had profound effects upon the responses of 67% of dentate neurons. In examining the effect of prior instruction on dentate activity, it was critical to determine whether or not these "instruction-dependent" changes of dentate activity occurred at a sufficiently short latency to play a role in the intended component of motor cortex discharge. Earlier studies (Evarts & Tanji, 1976) had shown that limb displacement could trigger preprogrammed open-loop discharges of motor cortex at a minimum latency of 40 msec. Strick (1978) found that for many dentate neurons, the instruction-dependent activity began as early as 30 msec. Such dentate activity, dependent upon prior instruction and occurring at 30 msec, presumably has a role in the centrally programmed activity beginning at 40 msec in the motor cortex.

Further evidence for separate pathways underlying the reflex and intended components of motor cortex discharge have come from the experiments of Vilis, Hore, Meyer-Lohmann, and Brooks (1976) on the effects of cerebellar cooling on precentral responses to limb displacements. These motor cortex neuron responses to limb displacements involved an early phase of discharge (20 to 50 msec) and a second phase of response (50 to 100 msec). This second phase corresponds to what we referred to earlier as the intended or centrally programmed component of motor cortex output. Cerebellar nuclear cooling produced no change in the early component of motor cortex response, demonstrating that a transcerebellar route was not necessary for the early feedback-dependent phase. Cerebellar nuclear cooling did, however, decrease the second phase (peak 50 to 100 msec). The authors concluded that this decrease in the second component of the cortical response pointed to a role of the cerebellum in the central programming of movement. Additional evidence for the cerebellar participation in motor programming has been provided by the work of Meyer-Lohmann, Hore, and Brooks (1977). In this study, motor cortex unit discharge was recorded in a simple visual reaction-time (RT) paradigm, and individual neurons were observed before, during, and after cooling of the dentate nucleus. Such cooling increased RTs for both EMG and movement onset by up to 100 msec without any slowing of the initial velocity of the movement. More marked cerebellar cooling resulted in further increases in RT and in a slowing of the velocity of movement. Increases in RT were associated with increases in response latency of motor cortex neurons. Involvement of the cerebellum in the initiation of fast ballistic movements was also demonstrated by Lamarre and Jacks (1978) in a study in which "monkeys were trained to perform a fast ballistic flexion or extension of the elbow in response to a sound cue. The reaction time was about 250 ms in the normal monkey and remained so after deafferentation of the operant arm. In a cerebellectomized animal, the reaction time was consistently longer, being on the average 400 ms. This was associated with an equal retardation in the onset of neural changes in the motor cortex [p. 446]." These results indicated that the cerebellum participated in the generation of programs underlying ballistic limb movement. Additional studies on the effects of dentate cooling on percentral unit activity have been carried out by Meyer-Lohmann, Conrad, Matsunami, and Brooks (1975). In agreement with the findings of Vilis et al. (1976), dentate cooling had no effects on "early" precentral responses to limb displacement.

CONCLUSIONS

But let's return to Lashley now and try to guess how he might have reacted to my proposals that cortico-cortical projections from SI to motor cortex relay somatosensory feedback, whereas projections from area 6 to motor cortex, as well as thalamic projections to motor cortex, are relatively more important in relaying central programs. I think we can be quite sure that Lashley would have had many criticisms. For example, he could have pointed out (1) that postcentral SI lesions have only slight effects on afferent-evoked responses in motor cortex (Malis et al., 1953), and (2) that thalamic lesions have only slight effects on centrally programmed movements, actually being used as a *treatment* for the disturbance of movement in patients with Parkinson's disease.

In answering these criticisms I could respond as follows: (1) As to the fact that SI lesions fail to eliminate afferent-evoked responses in MI, it should be noted that SII and/or area 3a remained intact in these studies. Lashley's own results showed that even a small residue of cortex could provide remarkable capacities (e.g., in vision). Thus, negative effects of lesions totally sparing SII and partially sparing area 3a do not force me to abandon the view that cortico-cortical projections from SI and/or SII to MI are important pathways for afferent feedback to motor cortex. (2) As to the use of VL lesions to improve motor performance in Parkinson's disease, I could point out that such lesions may lead to amelioration of tremor and rigidity but at the same time lead to exacerbation of akinesia. It has actually been shown that akinesia may be *produced* by VL lesions that relieve other parkinsonian symptoms. Of course, Lashley's criticisms would not have stopped here, for the points I have raised are but two of the many facts that he would have called to my attention. Indeed, Lashley's ability to inspire and then to criticize provided some of his greatest contributions to his students: He excited their interest and enthusiasm to understand how the brain works while giving them to understand that he would always be there to smile at their oversimplified wiring diagrams. And though Lashley would probably disagree with the ideas that I have expressed in this chapter, I can at least hope that he would smile at them.

REFERENCES

Arbib, M.E. Perceptual structures and distributed motor control. In *Handbook of physiology: Motor control* Section 1, Volume 2, Part 2, Chapter 33 (American Physiological Society). Baltimore: Williams & Wilkins, in preparation, 1981.

Brinkman, J., Bush, B. M., & Porter, R. Deficient influences of peripheral stimuli on precentral neurones in monkeys with dorsal column lesions. *Journal of Physiology (London)*, 1978, *276*, 27–48.

Brooks, V. B. Motor programs revisited. In R. E. Talbott & D. R. Humphrey (Eds.), *Posture and movement: Perspective for integrating sensory and motor research on the mammalian nervous system*. New York: Raven Press, 1979.

Conrad, B., Matsunami, K., Meyer-Lohmann, J., Wiesendanger, M., & Brooks, V. B. Cortical load compensation during voluntary elbow movements. *Brain Research*, 1974, *71*, 507–514.

Conrad, B., Meyer-Lohmann, J., Matsunami, K., & Brooks, V. B. Precentral unit activity following torque pulse injections into elbow movements. *Brain Research*, 1975, *94*, 219–236.

Desmedt, J.E., & Godaux, E. Ballistic skilled movements: Load compensation and patterning of the motor commands. In J. E. Desmedt (Ed.), *Cerebral motor control in man: Long-loop mechanisms, progress in clinical neurophysiology* (Vol. 4). Basel: Karger, 1978.

Evarts, E. V. Effect of ablation of prestriate cortex on auditory-visual association in monkey. *Journal of Neurophysiology*, 1952, *15*, 191–200.

Evarts, E. V. Pyramidal tract activity associated with a conditioned hand movement in the monkey. *Journal of Neurophysiology*, 1966, *29*, 1011–1027.

Evarts, E. V. Relation of pyramidal tract activity to force exerted during voluntary movement. *Journal of Neurophysiology*, 1968, *31*, 14–27.

Evarts, E. V. Motor cortex reflexes associated with learned movement. *Science*, 1973, *179*, 501–503.

Evarts, E. V., & Tanji, J. Reflex and intended responses in motor cortex pyramidal tract neurons of monkey. *Journal of Neurophysiology*, 1976, *39*, 1069–1080.

Horne, M. K., & Tracey, D. J. The afferents and projections of the ventroposterolateral thalamus in the monkey. *Experimental Brain Research*, 1979, *36*, 129–141.

Lamarre, Y., & Jacks, B. Involvement of the cerebellum in the initiation of fast ballistic movement in the monkey. In W. A. Cobb & H. Van Duijn (Eds.), *Contemporary clinical neurophysiology* (EEG Suppl. 34). Amsterdam: Elsevier, 1978.

Lemon, R. N., & Burg, J. van der. Short-latency peripheral inputs to thalamic neurones projecting to the motor cortex in the monkey. *Experimental Brain Research*, 1979, *36*, 445–462.

Malis, L. I., Pribram, K. H., & Kruger, L. Action potentials in "motor" cortex evoked by peripheral nerve stimulation. *Journal of Neurophysiology*, 1953, *15*, 161–167.

Marsden, C. D., Merton, P. A., Morton, H. B., & Adam, J. The effect of lesions of the central nervous system on long-latency stretch reflexes in the human thumb. In J. E. Desmedt (Ed.), *Cerebral motor control in man: Long-loop mechanisms, progress in clinical neurophysiology* (Vol. 4). Basel: Karger, 1978.

Meyer-Lohmann, J., Conrad, B., Matsunami, K., & Brooks, V. B. Effects of dentate cooling on precentral unit activity following torque pulse injections into elbow movements. *Brain Research*, 1975, *94*, 237–251.

Meyer-Lohmann, J., Hore, J., & Brooks, V. B. Cerebellar participation in generation of prompt arm movements. *Journal of Neurophysiology*, 1977, *40*, 1038–1050.

Phillips, C. G. Motor apparatus of the baboon's hand. *Proceedings of the Royal Society of London Series B*, 1969, *173*, 141–174.

Porter, R. Influences of movement detectors on pyramidal tract neurons in primates. *Annual Review of Physiology*, 1976, *38*, 121–137.

Rosén, I., & Asanuma, H. Peripheral afferent inputs to the forelimb area of the monkey motor cortex: Input-output relations. *Experimental Brain Research*, 1972, *14*, 257–273.

Sperry, R. W. Cerebral regulation of motor coordination in monkeys following multiple transection of sensorimotor cortex. *Journal of Neurophysiology*, 1947, *10*, 275–294.

Strick, P. L. Cerebellar involvement in "volitional" muscle responses to load changes. In J. E. Desmedt (Ed.), *Cerebral motor control in man: Long-loop mechanisms, progress in clinical neurophysiology* (Vol. 4). Basel: Karger, 1978.

Thach, W. T. Timing of activity in cerebellar dentate nucleus and cerebral motor cortex during prompt volitional movement. *Brain Research*, 1975, *88*, 233–241.

Tracey, D. J., Asanuma, C., Jones, E. G., & Porter, R. Thalamic relay to motor cortex: Afferent pathways from brain stem, cerebellum and spinal cord in monkeys. *Journal of Neurophysiology*, 1980, *44*, 532–554.

Vilis, T., Hore, J., Meyer-Lohmann, J., & Brooks, V. B. Dual nature of the precentral responses to limb perturbations revealed by cerebellar cooling. *Brain Research*, 1976, *117*, 336–340.

17 On Sensory Interactions with Motor Programs

A. J. Berman, M.D.
Neurosurgical Research Laboratory
Veterans Administration Medical Center
Bronx, New York

The year was 1917, a time when simple principles of input–output relationships influenced the perspective of most students of behavior. Neurophysiology was dominated by Sherrington's (1906) reflex arc explanation of movement; psychology, by Watson's (1913) behaviorism; ethology, by Loeb's (1913) "tropisms." It all made so much intuitive sense that few people challenged these mechanistic notions, particularly when dealing with the issue of movement control. Into the realm of this dogma entered the perennial iconoclast, Karl S. Lashley. In a landmark article (1917) on sensorimotor integration, he presented the problem thusly:

> For psychology the problem of motor activity has been largely one of the perception of movement. Discussion has centered about the questions of the receptors which are excited differentially by changes in extent and force of movement, about the psycho-physics of the constant error, the influence of the emotions upon the perception of movement, the relation of the "will impulse" to the perception of movement; with the result that the equally important questions of the nervous mechanism of initiation, continuation and cessation of adaptive movements have been dealt with only incidentally as throwing light upon this perception. Whether such an attitude on the part of investigators is the result of the general concept of psychology which would restrict its scope to the study of sensation, or is a consequence of the relative ease with which the problems of sensory and motor physiology may be attacked, the result has been an almost total neglect of the neurological problems presented by skilled movements.
>
> In many cases the perception and control of movement may be one and the same phenomenon, but certain experimental data and facts of everyday experience indi-

> cate a certain degree of independence of the accuracy of movement from any stimulation resulting from the movement itself. Such is the accuracy of automatic movements as seen in the production of steps of uniform length, or, more strikingly, the swift movements of the musicians, many of which are made more quickly than the briefest cortical reaction time. These movements are frequently regulated in extent and force with the utmost nicety, under conditions where any reflex control from excitations arising in the moving hand seems excluded. Again, the evidence obtained by Bowditch and Southard, Loeb, Woodworth and others, while by no means conclusive, indicates a partial independence of the motor control from afferent processes originating in the moving organ. The re-establishment of walking movements in the dog after section of the dorsal roots gives further evidence for the same view [pp. 169–170].

The thrust of Lashley's argument is obvious: Movements are not dependent on continuous sensory input for their execution, as the peripheralists would have it, but can be controlled by central processes alone. As one of his critics (Hunter, 1930) phrased it, the central engram for a movement sequence "unwinds like some Victrola record [p. 459]."

The data upon which Lashley based this view have been severely criticized. He entered the fray as a result of his studies of a spinal-cord-injured patient, on the questionable assumption that all peripheral input to the involved limb was abolished. Subsequently, in his animal studies, his surgically lesioned rats could barely walk, let alone run a maze (Hunter, 1929); the surgical procedures may not have been complete (Pavlov, 1932); there may have been extraneous cues available to his operated animals (Honzik, 1936). Nevertheless, despite these misgivings, most of us would join with Adams (1976) in calling Lashley the "founder of motor programming [p. 92]." His clarity of thought exposed many a psychological dogma to reevaluation and experimental test, and in his 1917 paper, Lashley fueled a controversy over the nature of movement control that has hardly abated over the years.

In summing up a symposium held in 1970 to answer the question, "How and to what extent is motor output controlled by sensory input?" Evarts (1972) commented:

> In almost any symposium on motor control, feedback is inevitably a conspicuous topic and there are often lengthy arguments as to its importance in this or that type of motor performance. . . . It often seems to be the case that such discussions generate more heat than light. This symposium was no exception in respect to the extent to which feedback was discussed [p. 86].

Today, pure centralists or peripheralists are hard to find. Most researchers would agree that movements result from a constant interaction between "feedback" and "feedforward" control, for as Evarts pointed out: "Present evidence suggests that the same segmental mechanisms that subserve classically-defined reflex functions may also be utilized in some measure in movements specified by central patterning [p. 9]." Nevertheless, a bias toward one view or the other tends to flavor the writings of most authors. Thus, Granit (1977) states that "most voluntary acts are merely triggered in the sense that the act is voluntarily demanded but accomplished automatically [p. 134]"; whereas Easton (1972) argues that "normal motor coordination is based to a large extent on reflexes. They may very probably underlie all or most voluntary movements in man and the lower animals, and their involvement is certainly great enough to justify the fruitful hypothesis that the muscles engaged in associated movements are functionally connected by reflexes [p. 591[." When one recalls that Lashley found himself in battle with the "reflexologist" school of thought, which argued that reflex chains underlie serially patterned movements, one cannot help but feel that the issue has moved from the qualitative to the quantitative level but still has not fully been resolved.

When first drawn into this controversy, Lashley was anything but a centralist. As he later (1931) recalled:

> I began life as an ardent advocate of muscle twitch psychology. I became glib in formulating all problems of psychology in terms of stimulus and response and in explaining all things as conditioned reflexes. . . . I embarked enthusiastically upon a program of experiments to prove the adequacy of the motor chain theory of integration [p. 14].

But for Lashley, the interest quickly moved from whether a movement could be performed in the absence of sensory control to whether a series of movements could be learned and then repeated in the absence of sensory control. The issue became not so much a matter of defining what could be done as of explaining how it was done. In fact, throughout the 1920s Lashley conducted an experimental odyssey in search of the motor engram. He never discovered it, perhaps because of the technical limitations of the time. Nevertheless, in the face of a *zeitgeist* of peripheralism, fostered by Sherrington's teachings, he remained convinced of the possibility of coordinated movement sequences generated by higher centers alone.

LASHLEY, SHERRINGTON, AND REFLEXOLOGY

It will be recalled that Sherrington (1906) had restated the Jacksonian concept of hierarchical organization of motor control as tiers of reflex arcs, impinging from "higher" upon "lower." Between the afferent (sensory) and efferent (motor) arms of these reflex arcs are intercalated internuncial neurons. But Sherrington did not distinguish "higher" from "lower" reflexes by the number and complexity of internuncial connections. Rather, the higher reflexes were so categorized because of the more varied inputs that impinge upon their internuncials. Thus, whereas the motoneurons constitute the "final common path" upon which all these hierarchical reflexes terminate, "the internuncial path is itself a common path [p. 328]" for increasingly large numbers of afferent inputs as one ascends through each level toward the cortex. For example, Sherrington defined the pyramidal tract as "another instance of an internuncial path . . . characteristic of the mammalian nervous system [p. 329]." Receiving cortico-cortical inputs at the level of the motor cortex from all over the cerebrum, "it furnishes a path of internuncial character common to certain arcs that have arisen indirectly from various receptors of various species and are knitted together in the cerebral hemisphere [p. 329]." What makes the pyramidal and other corticofugal internuncials "higher" is that they receive exteroceptive as well as proprioceptive inputs and integrate them into complex movements (Sherrington, 1906):

> By the distance receptors are initiated and guided long series of reactions of the animal as a whole. Other receptive reactions integrate individual segments; the reactions of the distance-receptors integrate the whole series of segments. It is in the sphere of reactions of those "distance-receptors" that the most subtle and complex adjustments of the animal therefore arise. In their neural machinery not only short arcs but long arcs, involving extensive internuncial tracts, figure largely. Chains of reactions conducive to a final reaction relatively remote are more evident with them than with other arcs. If appeal to psychical evidence be ventured on, it is to the field of operation of the arcs of these distance receptors that higher feats of associative memory accrue, and though the phrase is hardly permissible here except with curtailed scope conation becomes more intelligent [p. 349].

The purpose of this quote is to indicate that for Sherrington, "lower" reflexes are hard-wired, each bound to its "local sign"; whereas "higher" reflexes are more adaptive, allowing the operation of "mind" upon input from "distance receptors."

Lashley had no quarrel with Sherrington. His attack was leveled at the "reflexology" school, which—using Sherrington's concept of CNS structure as a physiological substrate—sought to explain learning in terms of reflexes. Prominent amongst these reflexologists was Pavlov (1927), who bluntly stated: "It is obvious that the different kinds of habits based on training, education and discipline of any sort are nothing but a long chain of conditioned reflexes [p. 395]." There is little doubt that Pavlov considered Sherrington's model of spinal reflex activity as the substrate for his own theory:

> It is obvious that in its intrinsic nature our work is closely allied to the work of Sherrington and his co-worker upon the spinal cord, and it is impossible not to notice in how many points the different aspects of the nervous activity of the cortex correspond with those described in the physiology of the spinal cord; a fact which seems strong evidence of a similarity of the fundamental laws governing the nervous activity in the two cases [p. 378].

However, unlike Sherrington, who viewed the internuncial path at higher levels as a simple one upon which complex inputs impinge, Pavlov thought of the cortex as a complex network into which all sensory input projects and from which motor output emanates.

Since reflexology was Lashley's prime target, it was an obvious strategy for him to attempt to demonstrate that behavior could be carried out after deafferentation. Deafferentation, according to the Sherringtonian model, would leave intact the cognitive processes that activate the motor side of higher reflexes, so that learned behaviors should persist. According to the Pavlovian view, however, deafferentation would preclude movement, which is dependent on sensory input (Pavlov, 1932). Lashley was, in effect, challenging a view stated by William James in 1890: "In action grown habitual, what instigates each new muscular contraction to take place in its appointed order is not a thought or a perception, but the sensation occasioned by the muscular contraction just finished [p. 115]." Watson (1907) had argued that the ability of blinded rats to continue to run a maze indicates that maze running is dependent on proprioceptive input only. Lashley downgraded the importance of proprioception, arguing instead that "the engram of the maze habit consists of some central organization in which the general direction and succession of turns are so recorded that, once the series is initiated, the essential sequence of movements may be performed in the absence of sensory control" (Lashley& Ball, 1929, p. 97).

It is ironic that Sherrington, who was considered by the reflexologists to have suggested a physiological substrate for their theoy, in fact provided Lashley with the basis for his notion of motor independence from sensory control. Leyton and Sherrington (1917) observed that upon electrical stimulation of the motor cortex in chimpanzee and orangutan, they obtained "combinational sequences" or movements that were "so to say, eloquent of purpose in most instances [p. 177]." From this, they concluded that the motor cortex serves an executive function, as the "synthetic organ for motor acts," composing the "local items" of lower levels or breaking up "compounds already constructed by lower centers" to produce "longer combinations varied in character and serviceable for purposes of different and varied kind [p. 178]." They further concluded that voluntary movements produced by the motor cortex made possible the bypassing of hard-wired segmental and midbrain reflexes. Motor acts would thus result from activation of the efferent arm of segmental reflexes and *not* from activation of the afferent arm: "It would seem that in order to preserve the possibility of being interchangeably compounded in a variety of ways, successive or simultaneously, these movements must lie, as more or less discrete and separable elements, within the grasp of the organ which has the varied compounding of them [p. 178]."

Lashley (1951), who had sought data on motor control "requiring the postulation of some central nervous mechanism which fires with predetermined intensity and duration or activates different muscles in predetermined order [p. 123]," and Sherrington (1953), who argued that "there is good evidence that some of our old motor acts are being uplifted so to say from old more primitive places in the brain into this newer 'thinking' part [p. 249]," are generally considered on opposite sides of the issue of motor control. Perhaps this is because Lashley himself did not seem to grasp fully the importance of Sherrington's view of "encephalization" to his attack on reflexology. Rather than recognizing that Sherrington's model was consistent with the postulation of some form of central programming, Lashley concluded that his notion of motor engrams lacked a physiological substrate (Lashley, 1931) and conceded that "as an explanatory process it is empty, but it may perhaps be filled by continued research [p. 18]."

DORSAL RHIZOTOMY AND PURPOSIVE MOVEMENTS

It was the initial goal of our research to contribute to a resolution of the centralist versus peripheralist controvery regarding movement. Toward this end, we utilized the same experimental strategy as Lashley, studying behavior in animals after interrupting the afferent side of the reflex arc. Lashley, however, had tried to remove sensory input by lesions at secondary levels of the somesthetic system and had been criticized on the ground that relevant avenues for somatic input might have remained intact. We thought, in common with others (e.g., Jankowska, 1959; Lassek, 1953; Mott & Sherrington, 1895; Twitchell, 1954), that we could avoid this problem by making lesions at the dorsal root level. We showed that animals prepared in this fashion could, in the absence of vision, execute movements that had been learned preoperatively and could learn new movements after surgery (Taub & Berman, 1968). Not long after this, however, evidence that sensory fibers traversed ventral, as well as dorsal roots began to appear (e.g., Coggeshall, Coulter, & Willis, 1974). This was not the first time, by any means, that such a possibility had been suggested (e.g., Windle, 1931), but it was the first time that results of studies from several laboratories, using different techniques, converged on the same conclusion. For a while it appeared that the dorsal rhizotomy approach was subject to the same criticism as the deafferentation studies of Lashley; the animals were not completely deprived of sensation from their limbs. It now appears, though, that this concern is unfounded. Most ventral root fibers originate from cell bodies in the dorsal root ganglia (Maynard, Leonard, Coulter, & Coggeshall, 1977). Furthermore, Goldberger (1977) has shown that whether deafferentation is produced by dorsal root ganglionectomy or by dorsal rhizotomy, there is no difference in the behavior of the animals; recovery is identical, and the spinal cord histology is the same. Furthermore, a recent study by Wylie, Barro, and Taub (1979) indicates that brachial plexus stimulation does not evoke electrical activity in the spinal cord of dorsal rhizotomized monkeys.

Willis and Coggeshall (1978) stated:

> If only the myelinated sensory fibers are considered then the numbers are so few that they probably do not require a revision of the law of separation of function of the spinal roots and they are probably not very significant in terms of the sensory mechanisms of the spinal cord [p. 45].

There is recognition, then, among the investigators whose work was the basis for the resurgence of interest in the possibility of ventral root pathways for somesthesis that dorsal rhizotomy is, in all probability, the equivalent of deafferentation; and until there is more compelling evidence to the contrary, we share this view.

On the other hand, Adams (1976) argues that the motor performance of dorsal rhizotomized animals may not be independent of sensory control, basing this argument on two points. He persists in the belief that meaningful sensory input is carried via ventral roots and contends that in any case, there is always some source of sensory input available to control movement—if not through proprioception, then through some other sensory modality; and if not correlated with the movement, then associated with the results of the movement. With regard to the first point, even if some somatic sensation does survive dorsal rhizotomy, Adams does not distinguish between the dual roles of sensory input—as a stimulus and as a component of information. This distinction is discussed later. With regard to the second point, it is undoubtedly true that total deafferentation of all senses cannot be accomplished. It is a valid question, therefore, susceptible to experimentation, as to what precise role different aspects of sensory experience play in the execution of movements when somesthesis is not present. However, we have evidence—and this also is discussed later—indicating that the role of sensory input is not necessarily facilitative to movement.

SENSORY INPUT AS STIMULUS OR INFORMATION

Sensory input that produces specific excitatory or inhibitory effects or that triggers movement can be classified as a stimulus. When sensory input, rather than provoking an output, undergoes processing to extract its meaningfulness in order to compose or adjust movements, it can be categorized as information. The output initiated by trigger stimuli is fixed and of short latency; that initiated by information is delayed, because of the processing time needed to extract meaning. The effect of information input on movement is much more complex and less predictable than that of trigger stimuli.

Proprioceptive input reaching the motor cortex within 10 msec (Devanandan & Heath, 1975) may be classified as a stimulus producing a given effect, but for this input to become meaningful, it must undergo a good deal of processing, and such processing takes time. Stimuli are individually quite potent as input, affecting output at the segmental level, but no matter how rapidly they reach motor cortex, they lose their impact at these higher levels. Fast sensory afferents to the cortex were once thought to control cortical reflexes such as contact placing and grasping (Asanuma, 1975). Asanuma, Larsen, and Yumiya (1979) concluded, however, that this fast cortical loop is too weak and too rigid to shape movements. Rather, it is one of several facilitatory loops that help to "set" the motor cortex for subsequent input. In fact, single-cell recordings taken from the motor cortex of monkeys performing conditioned movements, before and after dorsal rhizotomy, show that movement-related activity patterns are unaltered despite the loss of sensory input (Lamarre, Bioulac, & Jacks, 1978). Denny-Brown (1966) showed that cortical reflexes depend upon input via slower cortical loops. It is when input to the motor cortex through slow nonsensory loops is eliminated, rather than when fast sensory input is removed, that motor cortex is severely affected (Lamarre & Jacks, 1978).

Sensory stimuli must be processed to extract their information-carrying qualities, and this information can then be used to compose movement commands. It is these commands that constitute the input reaching motor cortex via the slow nonsensory loops. "Voluntary" movement must await the participation of these mechanisms, for as pointed out by Davson and Segal (1978): "The pyramidal tract neurons are the executors of a willed task, not the elaborators of it [p. 338]." We should not underestimate the possible importance of rapid somatosensory input to the motor cortex in such functions as the fine tuning and coordination of movement and in the presetting of motor cortex. It is clear, nevertheless, that whatever role cortical reflexes may play in the execution of voluntary movements, they do not initiate them.

VISION AND THE CONTROL OF MOVEMENT AFTER DORSAL RHIZOTOMY

Feedback associated with movement can take one of three forms and occurs at all stages—before, during, and after movement. Reefference, or feedback from the effector system, is returned via collateral fibers to the effector systems themselves or can function to "preset" affectors. It occurs before movement. Reafference results from activation of proprioceptors during movement. Knowledge of results is any change, recorded by exteroceptors, providing feedback about the consequences of a movement and occurs, of course, after the movement. Of these three types of feedback, it must be emphasized, only reafference is eliminated by dorsal rhizotomy.

The possibility was suggested by Konorski (1962) that after dorsal rhizotomy, animals function on the basis of reefference. He proposed that the relevant substrate consisted of a loop from pyramidal collaterals to the dorsal column nuclei and back to sensorimotor cortex. This particular pathway seems unlikely, however, based on some recent findings from our laboratory. We showed

(Berman, Teodoru, Tran & Blau, 1979) that lesion of the dorsal column nuclei enhances, rather than retards, recovery after dorsal rhizotomy. If it is true that the major recfferent route involves the dorsal column nuclei, this would suggest that reefferents may actually impede motor function when afferent input is absent. This question is now receiving further investigation in our own laboratory.

The possibility that the third source of feedback, knowledge of results, is useful in recovery of motor function after dorsal rhizotomy cannot be denied. Adams' suggestion to this effect is, actually, nothing more than a restatement of our own position (Taub, Schlossberg, Teodoru, & Berman, 1967). The difference seems to be that we recognized that feedback associated with the results of movement occurs after the movement, whereas Adams appears to regard it as similar in effect to proprioceptive afferents to motor cortex, for he would have it control ongoing movements. Considering the rapidity with which rhizotomized monkeys make movements, most being ballistic in character, knowledge of results can only prove useful in execution of *subsequent* movements.

Failure to recognize the significance of the delay imposed on exteroceptive feedback runs like a thread through much of the criticism of deafferentation research. For example, Adams (1976) criticized our demonstration that dorsal rhizotomized monkeys could flex their arms in response to a click in a trace-avoidance conditioning paradigm because, though not allowed to see the responding dorsal rhizotomized limb, they could see the inside of the test chamber above the neck collar. Thus, "Correlative movements of the head or eyes could have given visual feedback that would come to be informative about movement progress over learning trials [p. 94]." If one considers that limb flexion is completed within 150 msec, it is hard to imagine how visual inputs, delayed even at the periphery by retinal processig (Mortimer, 1975), could undergo higher-level analysis and still be useful to ongoing movements. The delay inherent in visual processing means that the use of this modality for feedback control of limb movement is useless even when it provides a direct report of limb position. In this regard, Eidelberg and Davis (1976) trained monkeys to track a moving spot on an oscilloscope screen by moving a manipulandum horizontally. The trained forelimb was then deafferented, and the animals were retested. Not one was able to track the moving spot, even when provided with a visual cue reporting manipulandum position relative to the target; the response continuously lagged behind the target.

We do not argue that vision is useless to a dorsal rhizotomized animal. It seems, though, that the effects of vision can be either beneficial or detrimental, depending on the circumstances. Allen (1978) showed that monkeys could make accurate reaching movements to a brief light flash with dorsal rhizotomized limbs in darkness, but that after training in darkness, if the testing chamber was lit, the same movements became ataxic. Similarly, Gilman, Carr, and Hollenberg (1976) reported severe ataxia in monkeys reaching for a target with a seen dorsal rhizotomized limb, whereas Taub, Goldberg, and Taub (1975) reported no such ataxia in reaching in a paradigm in which the dorsal rhizotomized limb was unseen.

We interpret these results as follows: In the dark, when reaching for a light flash, monkeys use visual spatial cues to program a reaching movement that brings the hand on target. However, in the presence of light, they attempt to guide the movement visually. The distinction lies in the fact that all processing is done *before* the movement begins in the former case and *during* execution of the movement in the latter. Since delay in a feedback loop may be the cause of instability in the output (Houk, 1980), visual feedback delay may produce ataxia whenever it is the sole guide to movement. When the movement is visually triggered, however, feedback plays little, if any, role in movement control, and loop delay is then irrelevant; ataxia under such a condition abates (Teodoru, Tran, Herskovic, & Berman, 1979). Though the time required for somatosensory input to influence motor output is only one-fourth that of visual input (Evarts, 1974), feedback loop delay is also a consideration for that modality. Fromm and Evarts (1978) recently showed that whereas the pyramidal cells whose firing frequency is associated with a slow guided movement were very sensitive to proprioceptive input provided by mechanical jerking of the responding hand, the cells associated with a ballistic movement were unaffected. They concluded that in the latter case, where the movement is preprogrammed, sensory input is blocked so that it does not interfere with the movement. In the former case, where the movement is slow and under sensory control, there is enough time for processed sensory input to affect the movement, and it is given access to motor centers. Movements made under sensory guidance are, in contrast to ballistic movements, ''discontinuous'' (Kozlovskaya, Uno, Atkin, & Brooks, 1970). This characteristic probably reflects the delay inherent in the somatosensory feedback loop.

Rather than assist the execution of programs, somatosensory input may in fact inhibit their operation. Extralemniscal somatosensory pathways, mainly the spinocervical tract, are under inhibitory suppression by dorsal column medial lemniscal system (DCMLS) in the intact animal. These extralemniscal systems project to the posterior parietal cortex via dorsolateral thalamus (Graybiel, 1974), and there is reason to suspect that these projections participate in sensory guidance of movements, possibly by denying movement programs access to motor centers (Teodoru, Tran, & Berman, unpublished data, 1980). We have observed that after DCMLS interruption, when extralemniscal systems are released from inhibition (Angel, 1977), monkeys are incapable of executing a ''precision grip,'' consisting of thumb-index apposition (Teodoru, Tran, & Berman, 1978). Such a movement appears to be hard-wired, in that sensory input from the index facilitates execution of this movement by the thumb, and vice versa (McCloskey & Gandevia, 1978). Despite this, a central program for the precision grip also appears to exist, for the precision grip is one of the earliest movements to reappear after complete deafferentation (Teodoru & Berman, 1980). Furthermore, if dorsal rhizotomy is superimposed on DCMLS interruption, the precision grip returns more rapidly than with DCMLS lesion alone (Berman, Teodoru, Tran, & Blau, 1979).

ATTEMPTED MOVEMENT AND RECOVERY AFTER DORSAL RHIZOTOMY

Although the movements of dorsal rhizotomized monkeys can be identified as to purpose and general form, they clearly differ from the same movements made by intact monkeys in such aspects as force buildup (Hepp-Reymond, Trouche, & Wiesendanger, 1973), agonist-antagonist interaction (Terzuolo, Soechting, & Ranish, 1974), stereotyping (Taub, Williams, Barro, & Steiner, 1978), and interjoint coordination (Liu & Chambers, 1971). It has become increasingly clear that these differences are not the result of decreased sensory feedback but are due to physiological (Porter, 1976) and morphological (Chambers, Liu, & McCouch, 1973) alterations at lower levels of the CNS, resulting from the rhizotomy. Ruch and Patton (1979), noting these aberrations in movement after dorsal rhizotomy, have argued that "too much has been made of the fact of movement, too little of the gross ataxia [p. 103]."

Since Sherrington, it has been recognized that sensory stimuli maintain the excitability levels of CNS neurons, each neuron constantly summating the many varied facilitatory (EPSP) and inhibitory (IPSP) stimuli impinging upon it. Assuming that commands from higher centers further contribute to the activity of the cell, there is, at all times, an unpredictable state of neuronal excitability and an unpredictable response to any given input. In the case of the motor neuron, the influence of sensory, propriospinal, recurrent, supraspinal, and other stimuli makes its responsiveness to corticospinal input somewhat uncertain. Even at the level of the muscle, there is still room for variability. Muscle output, in the absence of a functioning "gamma loop," is not linearly related to motoneuron input (Stein, 1974). In fact, Houk (1976) has proposed that one of the functions of the "gamma loop" is to adjust the excitability of motoneurons to the stiffness of muscles—a property that is, according to Nichols and Houk (1976), primarily a mechanical attribute of muscle, independent of neural factors. Motor output is in this way rendered linear to neural input.

We would like to suggest that in the intact animal, fast sensory pathways to motor centers may play a role in modulating motor command output after an initial "test signal"—such as suggested by Allum (1975)—informs the CNS of the state of the muscle, thus permitting the CNS to select an appropriate preprogrammed response. After dorsal rhizotomy, however, these fast feedback loops have been eliminated. In addition, the excitability of spinal cord and brain stem neurons has been so altered (Young & Rowley, 1968) that postsynaptic translation of presynaptic commands becomes truly unpredictable, How, then, does a dorsal rhizotomized monkey regain control over the deafferented limbs?

It cannot be stated at this time whether the rhizotomized monkey compensates for the interruption of the gamma loop, permanently depriving it of reflex control of, and direct feedback from, the muscles. (Hepp-Reymond et al, 1973). That motor control in such a preparation operates exclusively via an "alpha route" may explain the persistent abnormalities we observe in animals 1 year after surgery (Tran, Teodoru, & Berman, 1980). However, though deprived of reafferent feedback, the rhizotomized monkey is not deprived of reefferent feedback, which may—as Konorski (1962) suggested—play a role in motor recovery.

Oscarsson (1973) pointed out that of some 20 spinocerebellar tracts, only 2 carry information about peripheral events. The remainder provide the anterior and intermediate cerebellum with reefferent input from lower levels of the CNS. These same regions of the cerebellum also receive input from the motor cortex, enabling a comparison to be made between the command output from the motor cortex and the translation of that output at different levels of the CNS. The cerebellum projects back to the motor cortex from the interpositus nucleus via the ventrolateral thalamic nucleus and to the spinal cord via the red nucleus and the rubrospinal tract. It is conceivable that after comparing the command signal with its translation at every lower level, the cerebellum functions to update command at the cortical level or to alter the responsiveness of motor units at the spinal level, to compensate for whatever discrepancy may exist.

It may very well be that this cerebellar comparator is in large part responsible for recovery of postrhizotomy motor control. Being able to compare presynaptic input with postsynaptic output, it can compute the excitability at every level of the CNS. It can then either alter the excitability of lower levels via the rubrospinal pathway or adjust command output to the excitability of lower levels via the cerebello-cerebral pathway.

It would follow from the foregoing explanation that in recovery after dorsal rhizotomy, the more synapses intervening between the motor cortex and the motoneurons, the more difficult the recovery. Since pyramidal tract input to the motoneurons controlling hand muscles is strong and monosynaptic (Phillips & Porter, 1964) whereas that to the shoulder is weak and polysynaptic (Bernhard & Bohm, 1954), one would expect that digital movements would recover before whole arm movements. This is indeed the case (Teodoru & Berman, 1980).

It would further follow that for this process of recovery to operate, commands must be issued and movements attempted. Without such attempted movements, data are not available to the comparator, and it cannot "learn" how to control movements. This would explain why, when unilaterally rhizotomized monkeys that exhibit total disuse of the operated limb 3½ months after surgery are induced to use the rhizotomized limb, they follow the same pattern and rate of recovery as do unilaterally rhizotomized monkeys induced to use the limb the 1st day after surgery (Teodoru & Berman, 1980).

CONCLUSION

Despite the great advances made in neurophysiology over the half century since Lashley first proposed that sensory input does not control movements, we have yet to delineate the limits of its role in motor function. The problem remains much as it appeared to Weiss (1941): "Nobody in his senses would think of questioning the importance of sensory control of movement. But just what is the precise scope of that control? Is the sensory influx a constructive agent, instrumental in building up the motor patterns, or is it a regulative agent merely controlling the expression of autonomous patterns without contributing to their differentiation [p. 407]?" This question is very hard to answer because sensory input impinges on motor mechanisms at all levels and motor output in turn impinges on sensory mechanisms at all levels. Part of the answer was given at the conference on feedback control. Evarts (1972) summarized it concisely: "Many participants felt that it might be misleading to speak of sensory input as being translated into motor output. Instead, it seemed more fruitful to look upon the sensory input as serving to select one or another stored pattern (or program) of motor behavior [p. 8]." Our own work leads us to a similar conclusion.

T. D. M. Roberts (1978) pointed out:

> While it is reasonable to suppose that our experiences and our conclusions about external objects are in some way related to the activity of our nervous systems, we must not forget that this activity consists entirely of successions of activity-cycles in individual neurons. Physicists' variables, such as force and length are not directly represented. Our conclusions about such abstract parameters are based upon recognition processes as elaborate as those involved in distinguishing the faces of our friends or the validity of a signature on a cheque . . . and we can continue to perform such recognition acts even in the face of considerable modifications of our sensory equipment [p. 159].

This places the burden of rendering sensory input informative upon the receiving areas rather than upon the receptors. The perceptual capabilities of the human brain, even in the presence of severe sensory lesions, suggest that almost any contingent cue can become informative.

Stimulus-processing delays precede movement, so that elaborate sensory perceptions come to serve as triggers for behavioral programs that are played out with only modest adjustment and updating via rapid reflex loops (responding in fixed, graded fashion to fixed and graded stimuli). The rapidity of the movement is only limited by the motor capacity of the system. In such a scheme, all elements of a rapid series of movements are encoded in the program rather than being triggered by reafferents from the preceding element. Such triggering only occurs at the onset of a movement sequence.

We challenge the peripheralist viewpoint, not on grounds that sensory input plays no role in motor function, but on the grounds that sensory input has attributes that make it difficult for it to control ongoing voluntary movements. Sensory input contains a great deal of "noise" as well as irrelevant information that must be filtered before meaningful information can be extracted. Although this undoubtedly occurs, it takes time—too much time to allow the processed sensory input (i.e., information) to control ongoing movement. When subjects attempt to use sensory guidance for a motor task, they find themselves moving slowly and clumsily. However, when they use sensory stimuli to "trigger" whole movement programs, well rehearsed, they can move very rapidly and effortlessly. The brain must have available a storage bank of movement programs upon which it draws in order to respond to sensory information, much as Lashley proposed so long ago. The "association" cortical areas along with the primary projection and primary motor areas must play a role in sensory analysis and in motor program elaboration and selection. In motor learning, these association areas exhibit an expectancy character upon which their operations are based. Each movement thus serves the dual role of attempting to reach a goal as well as generating information upon which the "set" of higher centers is updated. Because of the processing time involved, the set of the association areas may not affect an ongoing movement, but it certainly dominates the next movement. Thus in motor learning, the evolution of a movement may reflect the evolving set of the association areas more than the fine tuning of sensorimotor mechanisms executing the movement. As Levitt (1978) phrased it:

> Pyramidal tract neuron discharges, EMG responses, sensorimotor reaction times and systematic errors of voluntary movement are all determined by the subject's mental set. Contemporary neurophysiology, striving to comprehend the elemental neural mechanisms of proprioception and motor control in the analytic terms of input and output, must acknowledge and contend with the pervasive dynamic central process that underlies mental sets.

As an interphase between sensory and motor mechanisms, higher cortical centers play a critical role both in transforming sensory input into sensory information and in preparing, selecting, and adjusting motor programs based on the information locked in sensory input.

REFERENCES

Adams, J. A. Issues for closed-loop theory of motor learning. In G. E. Stelmach (Ed.), *Motor control: Issues and trends*. New York: Academic Press, 1976.

Allen, G. C. *Dorsal rhizotomy in rhesus monkeys: Reaching without visual guidance*. Unpublished doctoral dissertation, City University of New York, 1978.

Allum, J. H. J. Responses to load distrubances in human shoulder muscles: The hypothesis that one component is a pulse test information signal. *Experimental Brain Research*, 1975, *22*, 307–326.

Angel, A. Processing of sensory information. *Progress in Neurobiology*, 1977, *9*, 1–122.

Asanuma, H. Recent developments in the study of the columnar arrangement of neurons within the motor cortex. *Physiological Reviews*, 1975, *55*, 143–156.

Asanuma, H., Larsen, K. D., & Yumiya, H. Direct sensory pathways to the motor cortex in the monkey: A basis of cortical reflexes. In H. Asanuma & V. J. Wilson (Eds.), *Integration in the nervous system*. Tokyo: Igaku-Shoin, 1979.

Berman, A. J., Teodoru, D. E., Tran, T. A. & Blau, A. Dorsal column nuclei lesions eliminate disuse of dorsal rhizotomized forelimb. *Neuroscience Abstracts*, 1979, *5*, 362.

Bernhard, C. G., & Bohm, E. Cortical representation and functional significance of the corticomotoneuronal system. *Archives of Neurology and Psychiatry* (Chicago), 1954, *72*, 473–502.

Chambers, W. W., Liu, C. N., & McCouch, G. P. Anatomical and physiological correlates of plasticity in the central nervous system. *Brain, Behavior and Evolution*, 1973, *8*, 5–26.

Coggeshall, R. E., Coulter, J. D., & Willis, W. D. Unmyelinated axons in the ventral roots of the cat lumbosacral enlargement. *Journal of Comparative Neurology*, 1974, *153*, 39–58.

Davson, H., & Segal, M. D. *Introduction to physiology* (Vol. 4). London: Academic Press, 1978.

Denny-Brown, D. *The cerebral control of movement*. Springfield, Ill.: Charles C Thomas, 1966.

Devanandan, M. S., & Heath, C. D. A short latency pathway from forearm nerves to area 4 of the baboon's cerebral cortex. *Journal of Physiology* (London), 1975, *248*, 43P–44P.

Easton, T. A. On the normal use of reflexes. *American Scientist*, 1972, *50*, 591–599.

Eidelberg, E., & Davis, F. Role of proprioceptive data in performance of a complex visuomotor tracking task. *Brain Research*, 1976, *105*, 588–590.

Evarts, E. V. Central control of movement. *Neurosciences Research Program Bulletin*, 1972, *9*, 1–170.

Evarts, E. V. Sensorimotor cortex activity associated with movements triggered by visual as compared to somesthetic inputs. In F. O. Schmitt (Ed.), *The neurosciences: Third study program*. Cambridge, Mass.: MIT Press, 1974.

Fromm, C., & Evarts, E. V. Motor cortex responses to kinesthetic input during postural stability, precise fine movement and ballistic movement in the conscious monkey. In G. Gordon (Ed.), *Active touch*. Oxford: Pergamon, 1978.

Gilman, S., Carr, D., & Hollenberg, J. Kinematic effect of deafferentation and cerebellar ablation. *Brain*, 1976, *99*, 311–330.

Goldberger, M. E. Locomotor recovery after unilateral hindlimb deafferentation in cats. *Brain Research*, 1977, *123*, 59–74.

Granit, R. *The purposive brain*. Cambridge, Mass.: MIT Press, 1977.

Graybiel, A. Studies on the anatomical organization of posterior association cortex. In F. S. Schmitt (Ed.), *The neurosciences: Third study program*. Cambridge, Mass.: MIT Press, 1974.

Hepp-Reymond, M. C., Trouche, E., & Wiesendanger, M. Effects of deafferentation and vibration on precision grip in monkey and man. *Brain Research*, 1973, *49*, 492–493.

Honzik, C. H. The sensory basis of maze learning in rat. *Comparative Psychological Monographs*, 1936, (Whole No. 64).

Houk, J. C. An assessment of stretch reflex function. *Progress in Brain Research*, 1976, *44*, 303–314.

Houk, J. C. Homeostasis and control principles. In V. B. Mountcastle (Ed.), *Medical physiology* (13th ed., Vol. 1). St. Louis, Mo.: Mosby, 1980.

Hunter, W. S. The sensory control of the maze habit in the white rat. *Journal of Genetic Psychology*, 1929, *36*, 505–527.

Hunter, W. S. A consideration of Lashley's theory of the equipotentiality of cerebral action. *Journal of General Psychology*, 1930, *3*, 455–468.

James, W. *Principles of psychology* (Vol. 1). New York: Holt, 1890.

Jankowska, E. Instrumental scratch reflex of the deafferented limb in cats and rats. *Acta Biological Experimentalis* (Warsaw), 1959, *19*, 233–242.

Konorski, J. Changing concepts concerning physiological mechanisms of animal motor behavior. *Brain,* 1962, *85,* 277-294.

Kozlovskaya, I., Uno, M., Atkin, A., & Brooks, V. B. Performance of a step-tracking task by monkeys. *Communications in Behavioral Biology,* 1970, *5,* 153-156.

Lamarre, Y., Bioulac, B., & Jacks, B. Activity of precentral neurons in conscious monkeys: Effects of deafferentation and cerebellar ablation. *Journal de Physiologie* (Paris), 1978, *74,* 253-264.

Lamarre, Y., & Jacks, B. Involvement of the cerebellum in the initiation of fast ballistic movement in the monkey. *Electroencephalography and Clinical Neurophysiology,* 1978 (Supplement No. 34), 441-447.

Lashley, K. S. The accuracy of movement in the absence of excitation from the moving organ. *American Journal of Physiology,* 1917, *43,* 169-194.

Lashley, K. S. Cerebral control versus reflexology. *Journal of General Psychology,* 1931, *5,* 3-19.

Lashley, K. S. The problem of serial order in behavior. In L. A. Jeffres (Ed.), *Cerebral mechanisms in behavior.* New York: Wiley, 1951.

Lashley, K. S., & Ball, J. Spinal conduction and kinaesthetic sensitivity in the maze habit. *Journal of Comparative Psychology,* 1929, *9,* 71-106.

Lassek, A. M. Inactivation of voluntary motor function following rhizotomy. *Journal of Neuropathology and Experimental Neurology,* 1953, *3,* 83-87.

Levitt, M. On the role of mental set involuntary movements. *Behavioral and Brain Sciences,* 1978, *1,* 154-155.

Leyton, A. S. F., & Sherrington, C. S. Observations on the excitable cortex of the chimpanzee, orangutan and gorilla. *Quarterly Journal of Experimental Physiology,* 1917, *11,* 135-222.

Liu, C. N., & Chambers, W. W. A study of cerebellar dyskinesia in the bilaterally deafferented forelimbs of the monkey (Macaca mulatta and Macaca Speciosa). *Acta Neurobiologea Experimentalis,* 1971, *31,* 263-289.

Loeb, J. *Die Tropismen* (Vol. 4). Berlin: Handb-Vergleich, Physiology, 1913.

Maynard, C. S., Leonard, R. B., Coulter, J. D.,& Coggeshall, R. E. Central connections of ventral root afferents as demonstrated by the HRP method. *Journal of Comparative Neurology,* 1977, *172,* 601-608.

McCloskey, D. I., & Gandevia, S. C. Role of inputs from skin, joints and muscles and of corollary discharges in human discriminatory tasks. In G. Gordon (Ed.), *Active touch.* Oxford: Pergamon Press, 1978.

Mortimer, J. A. Cerebellar responses to teleceptive stimuli in alert monkeys. *Brain Research,* 1975, *83,* 369-390.

Mott, F. W., & Sherrington, C. S. Experiments upon the influence of sensory nerves upon movement and nutrition of the limbs. Proceedings of the Royal Society (London), 1895, *57,* 481-488.

Nichols, T. R., & Houk, J. C. The improvement in linearity and the regulation of stiffness that results from the action of the stretch reflex. *Journal of Neurophysiology,* 1976, *39,* 119-142.

Oscarsson, O. Functional organization of spinocerebellar paths. In A. Iggo (Ed.), *Handbook of sensory physiology* (Vol. II). Berlin: Springer-Verlag, 1973.

Pavlov, I. P. *Conditioned reflexes.* Oxford: Oxford University Press, 1927.

Pavlov, I. P. The reply of a physiologist to psychologists. *Psychological Review,* 1932, *39,* 91-127.

Phillips, C. G., & Porter, R. The pyramidal projection to motoneurons of some muscle groups of the baboon's forelimb. *Progress in Brain Research,* 1964, *12,* 222-242.

Porter, R. Influences of movement detectors on pyramidal tract neurons in primates. *Annual Review of Physiology,* 1976, *38,* 121-137.

Roberts, T. D. M. The transmission of parameters by neural messages. *Behavioral and Brain Sciences,* 1978, *1,* 159-160.

Ruch, T., & Patton, H. D. *Physiology and biophysics* (20th ed., Vol. 1). Philadelphia: Saunders, 1979.

Sherrington, C. S. *Integrative action of the nervous system.* New York: Scribner, 1906.

Sherrington, C. S. *Man on his nature.* Garden City, N.Y.: Doubleday, 1953.

Stein, R. B. Peripheral control of movement. *Physiological Review,* 1974, *54,* 215-243.

Taub, E., & Berman, A. J. Movement and learning in the absence of sensory feedback. In S. J. Freedman (Ed.), *The neuropsychology of spatially oriented behavior.* Homewood, Ill.: Dorsey, 1968.

Taub, E., Goldberg, I. A., & Taub, P. Deafferentation in monkeys: Pointing at a target without visual feedback. *Experimental Neurology,* 1975, *46,* 178-186.

Taub, E., Schlossberg, S., Teodoru, D. E., & Berman, A. J. *Deafferentation in monkeys and sensory prosthesis.* Paper presented at the Meeting of the Psychonomic Society, St. Louis, Missouri, 1967.

Taub, E., Williams, M., Barro, G., & Steiner, S. Comparison of the performance of deafferented and intact monkeys in continuous and fixed ratio schedules of reinforcement. *Experimental Neurology,* 1978, *58,* 1-13.

Teodoru, D. E., & Berman, A. J. The role of attempted movements in recovery from unilateral dorsal rhizotomy. *Neuroscience Abstracts,* 1980, *6,* 25.

Teodoru, D. E., Tran, T. A., & Berman, A. J. Forelimb function after dorsal column nuclei lesion or dorsal rhizotomy. *Neuroscience Abstracts,* 1978, *4,* 307.

Teodoru, D. E., Tran, T. A., Herskovic, J., & Berman, A. J. Visual aspects of post-deafferentation ataxia and dysmetria. *Neuroscience Abstracts,* 1979, *5,* 388.

Teodoru, D. E., Tran, T. A. & Berman, A. J. Unpublished data, 1980.

Terzuolo, C. A., Soechting, J. F., & Ranish, N. A. Studies on the control of some simple motor tasks. V. Changes in motor output following dorsal root section in squirrel monkey. *Brain Research,* 1974, *70,* 521-527.

Tran, T. A., Teodoru, D. E., & Berman, A. J. Effects of dorsal rhizotomy and dorsal column medial lemniscal system interruption on performance of a bimanual task. *Neuroscience Abstracts,* 1980, *6,* 25.

Twitchell, T. E. Sensory factors in purposive movement. *Journal of Neurophysiology,* 1954, *17,* 239-254.

Watson, J. B. Kinaesthetic and organic sensation: Their role in the reactions of the white rat to the maze. *Psychological Review Monographs* (Supplement), 1907, *8* (Whole No. 33).

Watson, J. B. Psychology as a behaviorist views it. *Psychological Reviews,* 1913, *20,* 158-177.

Weiss, P. Does sensory control play a constructive role in development of motor coordination? *Schweizerische Medizinische Wochenschrift,* 1941, *71,* 406-407.

Willis, W. D., & Coggeshall, R. E. *Sensory mechanisms of the spinal cord.* New York: Plenum Press, 1978.

Windle, W. D. Neurones of the sensory type in the ventral roots of man and other mammals. *Archives of Neurology and Psychiatry,* (Chicago), 1931, *26,* 791-800.

Wylie, R. M., Barro, G., & Taub, E. Electrophysiological evidence that deafferentation by dorsal rhizotomy abolishes afferent inputs to segmental levels of the spinal cord in the monkey. *Experimental Neurology,* 1979, *66,* 423-443.

Young, J., & Rowley, W. F. Structural and histochemical change in ventral-horn cells resulting from sensory deprivation. *Recent Advances in Biological Psychiatry,* 1968, *10,* 53-73.

18 Cultivating Abstraction in an Ape's Mind: Conceptual versus Sensory*

Dr. David Premack
University of Pennsylvania

It would seem extremely risky for a species to live at the limit of its capacity. Any change in the environment increasing the demands on individual members of the species could lead to extinction. Suppose each leap of a brachiating species required its maximum strength. A slight increase in the average distance between branches, a decrease in the density of food, or an increase in the density of predators could be disastrous. Considerations of this kind suggest that surviving species possess unused reserves, the nature of the reserve being determined by the specialization of the species. In our own case, for example, we may suppose that we have an unused reserve of intelligence.

Suppose that a superior species took us under its wing, either to cultivate our limited competence—so that we might serve them better—or because—having theories of intelligence—they wished to use us as subjects in testing their theories. In this way, too, we (actually, they) could obtain evidence for unused reserve.

It is some version of this experiment that, rather than having performed on us by a superior species, we have been performing on the chimpanzee. In order to understand intelligence, its nature, and evolution, we have made the ape our drawing board, having instructed it in a number of ways for well over 10 years. This is not the first time that an animal has been exposed to a lengthy training; animals used commercially are sometimes trained for years. But neither the species nor the form of training has been propitious for examining the potential for unused intelligence. On one hand, dogs and elephants, for example, are not specialized in intelligence as are the primates; and on the other, teaching apes to

*Research supported by Grant BNS 77-16853 from the National Science Foundation and Grant 1-P01-HD-10965 from the National Institutes of Health.

ride bikes, smoke cigars, and the like is not the optimal way to examine the present hypothesis.

I have two major objectives in this chapter. One is to describe the surprising advances in cognition that appear to have been brought about in the ape, and the other is to speculate about the nature of the change. There are implications here for the teaching of pathological human populations. The ape has been trained for a decade; perhaps we must be prepared to train impaired humans for an appreciably longer period than is customary. Also, we have not yet stopped the training. When we do, will the ape revert to an earlier level or retain her present one? Certainly if regression ensued when training ended, that would have serious implications for how we deal with impaired human populations—in particular with how we incorporate the gains of training into daily life, something we have not yet done with the ape (in a real sense, she has no daily life except for the training).

BIOGRAPHICAL DATA

The ape, Sarah, was born in Africa, having been captured in an unknown way that is likely to have destroyed her mother, since apparently that was the common manner of capturing infant chimpanzees. She was less than a year old when she entered the laboratory and was therefore maintained largely as a human infant. For the 1st year, she was bottlefed, diapered, and attended through the day by a human caretaker. She had ape companionship as well as human. Gussie, an African-born female of comparable age, shared the nursery with her for the 1st year—and went on to share a jaillike cell for the next 4 years. The transition was less harsh than it sounds, for the cage was sizable and the move did not interrupt either the bottle-feeding or the daily trips outdoors for play and exercise. A half dozen surrogate mothers (and fathers) came and went in this 4-year period, one always on hand to assure an object for their affection. When they were about 5½ years old, the two animals were separated. Sarah was moved to new quarters, a two-compartment cage with an outdoor run, a space appreciably larger than that enjoyed by most university students. Her language training began with her move into the new quarters.

The language training continued intensively, four lessons a day for about 16 months, and was then discontinued. After the intensive training stopped, she was still tested occasionally on language, though perhaps no more than 100 times in the past 10 years. Shortly before her 7th birthday, a few months after the language training was discontinued, she took the fifth of her major plane trips: (1) Africa–New York, (2) New York–Louisiana, (3) Louisiana–Missouri, (4) Missouri-California, and (5) arriving in rural Pennsylvania to find herself in a cage identical to the one she had left in California.

The cage is as barren as all the others in which she has lived, containing only a wooden bench and an occasional piece of human furniture that is replaced as needed. The easy chairs, couches, and wooden swings that she has dismantled over the years have all been used in their time as a bed. Each night she settles herself into whatever is at hand, covering herself from head to toe with a blanket. Should you drop in for a night check, you would find that she lowers the blanket to check on you and then draws it back up over her head.

We have often discussed giving her an assortment of furniture, along with an assortment of objects that she could store in the furniture and take out as she chooses. The point would be to learn whether or not, in time, she would organize her life around such things as picture books, lesson materials, and cooking and cleaning materials, as people have organized their days and even weeks around the objects they possess. She could be depended upon to dismantle the first set of objects given her. But how many would she dismantle before allowing the first set to remain? Unfortunately, we have not been in a position to pursue this question on a large scale and have done only one thing along these lines, quite a modest one. We gave her a notebook whose pages were devoted to the paper-pencil form of the same/different test she had been taught (Premack, Woodruff and Kennel, 1978) and gradually sought to increase the number of pages given her at one time. It was our hope that she would take out the notebook kept in her cage and work on it at her own pace. Had the notebook been part of a larger assortment of material, I think there is a chance she would have done this. But it was not and instead contained the only paper available to her. She did a few tests and then chewed up the rest. I still believe we may induce her to dedicate her daily life to our tests, as people build their lives around office routines and the like. For the present, however, she does our tests as we introduce them, in a schoollike way and not as the activity around which she has organized her life.

Her cage offers three large windows, two permanently uncovered, affording a broad view of the woods, sky, and the humans and animals passing nearby. In the late afternoon, when testing is done, she climbs the mesh, finds a good view, and hangs there for hours, staring out the window. On other occasions, when the third window is open, she looks through it, sitting on her wood bench below the window, her faced pressed to the pane. Often she hoots and pounds on this window, for it overlooks the adjacent cage where a group of four juvenile chimpanzees are housed. All these animals visit Sarah daily, interacting with her through the mesh, as we do.

No one has joined Sarah in her cage for over 10 years; all interactions with her are through the mesh. The young animals scramble about on the outside of her cage even as Sarah scrambles about on the inside. The mesh is wide, and through it they interact easily, engaging in mutual grooming and play. Trainers on good terms with Sarah also groom her, scratching her back and shoulders even as she grooms them in turn. The restrictions on entering her cage are not based on her viciousness. She is, of course, a dangerous animal—as are all adult chimpanzees—vastly stronger than we are and by no means faithfully acquiescent as are pet dogs and cats. When working in direct contact with her, we keep a close eye on her. Nevertheless, it is not this degree of danger that prevents us from entering her cage. With sufficient ingenuity, a cage could be devised that would enable visitors to enter, interact directly with her, and leave without being accompanied by her. It is because the present cage offers no assurance that one could leave without her that we do not go inside in the first place.

TRAINING VERSUS ASSESSMENT

Since discontinuing serious language training about 10 years ago, we have tested her on a large variety of cognitive tasks. In abandoning language for these more general cognitive topics, the whole approach has been changed. The former emphasis on training has been replaced by one on assessment. We had approached language by a series of operational definitions, each of which generated a behavioral target and a training program to realize the target. Basically, she was given short strings of plastic words such as *red? apple,* where the new term *color of* was taught her by arranging that she replace the question mark with the word, forming the string *red color of apple*. The strings given her were of varying degrees of complexity, but in all of them there was exactly one new word that was to be taught, every other word in the string being known to her from previous training. All of her strings or sentences were *n* term—generally two-term—relations. In teaching her one unknown at a time, new two-term predicates were introduced only after she knew both the arguments of the predicate; a new argument was introduced only after she knew both the predicate and one of the arguments. In this general way we assessed the complexity of the predicates and arguments that she could be taught. When we abandoned the language training, we abandoned both the fixed format and the whole emphasis on training.

In the cognitive phase, we have asked, What can she do—not what can we train her to do? This distinction is nicely shown by one of the earliest cognitive tasks we gave her. We were concerned with the chimpanzee's evident inability to draw, to produce representational forms, wondering whether the inability was mainly cognitive or motor. To find out, we reduced the motor demands, giving her the pieces of a well-known object, requiring only that she reassemble them. Her ability to reassemble the object would prove both that she recognized the object in its disassembled state and also that she knew the betweenness relations among the pieces. We gave her a disassembled photograph of a chimpanzee face, choosing a face because in all human cultures, it is one of the first representational forms that children draw (Kellogg, 1955). We did not intervene even to the extent that a normal parent would; we did not model the face for her. Nor did we praise her for putting the pieces together one way rather than another. We simply gave her the photograph of the chimpanzee head (with the face whited out), along with the four facial elements, and recorded what she did.

As it turned out, she did not play with the pieces—as did the three younger chimpanzees who were tested in the same way—but reassembled the pieces into faces; though crude, her constructions could be defended statistically as facelike configurations (Premack, 1975). This case is a particularly strong example of the difference between the assessment characteristic of the recent cognitive period and the training characteristic of the earlier language period. In training, one drills the individual on the exemplars of some target and then tests the accomplishment by transfer procedures. In assessment, one presents the individual with a representation that is incomplete in one of many possible senses and then invites the individual to demonstrate his or her comprehension by completing the representation.

KNOWLEDGE VERSUS SCHEMATA

Sarah has been in school for nearly 10 years, 5 days a week, 3 to 4 hours a day, with no time off for summer vacations. The differences between her school and a human one are not confined to temporal schedule, however. Human schools emphasize knowledge, or facts. Years of training in geography, history, civics, literature, biology, chemistry, and physics prepare the child to answer such questions as: What is the capital of Ethiopia? Where was Napoleon finally defeated? How many chambers does the frog's heart have? Who wrote the *Ancient Mariner?* Can a naturalized citizen be President of the United States? (The exceptions to this emphasis on knowledge are grammar and math, both being formal systems. However, the teaching of grammar appears to be relatively unsuccessful, and even perhaps gratuitous, since in the end, children's mastery of the sentence owes little to the grammar taught them in school. Arithmetic is a bit reminiscent of grammar, for some of the basic principles of counting are known by children before entering the school; Gelman & Gallistel, 198.) Children's instruction concerns parts of the world they have not seen—some of which they will never see, for it is invisible, and some of which they may yet see. Foreign countries are discussed but also amoebae, gravity, and historical events.

In contrast, Sarah's curriculum has not emphasized knowledge but abstract structures—some of which underlie basic human concepts. In the rest of the chapter, I describe Sarah's cognitive assessment in some detail, concentrating on action or causality, analogies, proportions, and conservation. This will enable us to evaluate the extent to which Sarah's curriculum has exposed her to representations of abstract concepts.

ACTION OR CAUSALITY

Can the ape be said to have a concept of action or causality akin to our own? The basic idea of action can be represented by three elements: an object in both its initial and terminal states, along with an instrument that can be used to produce the transition from initial to terminal state. Sarah was shown sequences in which one of the three elements was missing. Examples of such sequences are an intact apple, a blank space, and a cut apple; a piece of paper, a blank space, and a marked piece of paper. With each such sequence she was given three alternatives: a writing instrument, a cutting instrument, and a container of water. Her task was to fill in the blank by selecting the item that could produce the transformation in question. The blank space was not confined to the instrument but was sometimes located in the third position, thus requiring her to select the terminal or transformed state of the object. For example, given apple, knife, and blank space, her alternatives were sometimes: cut apple, cut orange, and apple pierced as by a nail; or a dry sponge, container of water, blank space, with alternatives: wet sponge, sponge changed in color, wet cloth, etc.

Sarah—and two other younger animals—succeeded on these kinds of tests from the beginning. The very first tests were transfer tests since in one form, the object-implement pairs were unique from one trial to the next and in the other form, the initial and terminal object pairs were unique from one trial to the next. Thus the animal could not memorize the correct answer on one trial and use it on successive trials, for every trial was different (Premack, 1976).

More advanced forms of the test, given only to Sarah, showed that she comprehended two other aspects of the human notion of action (or causality in the physical domain). The first of these is that action has a temporal order—cause precedes effect—even as the initial state of the object precedes the terminal state. In the first series Sarah had been tested on cutting, wetting, and marking, actions with which she had abundant experience. For the new tests, she was given experience on the reverse of these actions—namely, joining, drying, and erasing. Then she was taught to read the sequences from left to right by being given cases identical except for their order. For instance, she was given both the sequences—blank paper? marked paper; and the reverse—marked paper? blank paper; along with the alternatives—container of water, pencil, and eraser. Whereas container of water is irrelevant, the pencil and eraser are not, and to determine which is correct, one must take into account the order of the change. A pencil is needed to change blank paper into marked paper, whereas an eraser is needed to do the reverse. After learning to read the sequences in the prescribed order, she was given a transfer test based on 60 novel cases. She was correct on 40 of the 60 cases, which, with three alternatives, is highly significant ($p < .001$, binomial test).

An additional test emphasized her ability to appreciate the transformational nature of action. She was given trials on which the same terminal state was reached from different initial ones, as well as the reverse—identical initial states paired with different terminal ones. In an example of the first kind, the terminal state was a piece of paper that was severed, wet, and marked. This terminal state was paired with initial states in which the paper was marked and cut but not wet; marked but neither wet nor cut; cut and wet but not marked, etc. Given her usual three alternatives, she was now required to divide them into two groups—those that participated in the transformation and those that did not. On the 60 trials of this kind, she was correct about 69% of the time—highly significant since chance is 1 out of 8. She was also correct on 8 of the first 13 unique trials ($p < .01$). Her success on tests of this kind showed that she could compute the difference between two states of an object and identify the instrument or instruments needed to produce the transiton.

PROPORTIONS

In another series, Sarah and four juvenile chimpanzees were tested on their ability to judge proportions in a match-to-sample format (Woodruff & Premack, 1981). Two quite different types of objects were used. In one case, vertical cuts were made in spherical fruit—apple, grapefruit, potato—producing ¼, ½, ¾, and the intact fruit. In a second case, glass cylinders were filled with tinted water, producing ¼, ½, ¾, and a completely filled cylinder. Each proportion was used as the sample and as both the correct and incorrect alternatives equally often. For example, trials were given on which the sample was ¼ apple and the alternatives consisted of ¼ and ¾ apple. In a second series, comparable tests were given on the glass cylinders; for example, ¼ cylinder of water was used as a sample, and the alternatives consisted of ¼ and ¾ cylinders of water. Here too every proportion served equally as the sample and as both the correct and incorrect alternatives.

Not only Sarah passed these tests but also the four juveniles. Of course, both series—the one based on fruit and the one based on glass cylinders—could be solved on a sensory basis. The shape of the sample had only to be matched with that of the correct alternative. The matching could not be done physically, in the sense of superimposing an alternative on the sample, but had to be done mentally, by picturing one proportion set against another. Yet we already know that apes are quite capable of that. For example, Sarah made same/different judgments in a paper/pencil format requiring that she read a question on one line and answer by choosing among alternatives presented on another line (Premack, Woodruff, & Kennel, 1978). Monkeys faced with stimulus-response separation of this kind fail (Meyer, Treichler, & Meyer, 1965).

In the next series, the sensory factor was eliminated; now the subject was required to match a proportion instanced by a filled glass cylinder to a proportion instanced by some part of the fruit. For example, the animal was given a ½-filled cylinder as the sample and ½ apple and ¾ apple as alternatives. Moreover, all the fruit alternatives were now equated for size (by using large fruit to instance ¼ small fruit to instance ¾, etc.). Once again, each of the four proportions was used equally often as the sample and as correct and incorrect alternatives.

On this series, Sarah and the four juveniles parted company. All of the young animals failed the test, whereas Sarah passed and did so from the beginning. The first eight trials were unique, and she was correct on all of them ($p < .01$).

(Actually the test was a bit more complicated than indicated, involving not only fruit as alternatives but also abstract wooden disks; the latter were used to determine whether proportions might not be more difficult to judge with abstract objects than with natural ones. The hypothesis was weakly confirmed with the juveniles but not with Sarah.)

Given that the third test could only be solved on a conceptual basis, we must now ask for specifics: What conceptual factors could be used to solve this test? To judge the equivalence of proportions of fruit and cylinders—and other items of comparable physical disparity—one must first recognize that both items are some part of a whole. For example, one must see the apple as whole or part of a whole; the cylinder as either a completely filled one or as part of one that is filled. Then, one can go in either of two directions. A common label or description can be assigned to both—for example, half an apple and half a cylinder—provided, of course, that one has such labels, which Sarah presumably does not (or at least none that we had taught her). Alternatively, one could use a form of reasoning akin to analogies. One could observe that the given part of the apple (x) is to the whole apple (X) as the filled part of the cylinder (y) is to the completely filled cylinder (Y)—that is, x/X: y/Y. This would seem more than usually difficult, for one of the terms, the whole apple, is not present and must be inferred. The alternative might also be thought difficult, for it requires observing in the first place that analogies are applicable to the proportions problem. This is not self-evident, especially as the proportions task was not given to Sarah in the explicit format of an analogy—that is, x/X same $?/Y$. If Sarah solved the problem on an analogical basis, it is all the more impressive. Yet on what other basis could she have solved the problem?

ANALOGIES

Fortunately, we now have independent evidence that Sarah can do analogies (Gillan, Premack, & Woodruff, 1981). She was given a format of this kind: A/A' same $B/?$ and was required to select B' from two to four alternatives. For instance, A and A' may consist of a large and small circle, respectively; B, of a large square; and her alternatives, of a small square, a small circle, a large triangle, and a small triangle. In this case, she should choose the small square, producing the analogy: large circle/small circle: large square/small square. In other examples, the relation between A and A' was one of color change, shape change, or change in a specific mark such as an x or a dot superimposed on one of the two items. These are all sensory or figural analogies: The relation between A and A' can be computed simply by looking at the two items; one does not have to know or remember anything about either of them.

In a conceptual analogy one cannot compute the relation between the relevant items simply by looking at them. Suppose that A is a can opener, A' is a can, B is a key, and the alternatives are: lock, key chain, fork, beer bottle. To choose lock and thus produce can opener/can: key/lock, one must know something about the functional relation between the items in question. Merely looking at the items is not sufficient to compute the relation between A and A'.

In a model for analogies proposed by Rumelhart and Abrahamsom (1973), one computes the difference between A and A' and then chooses a B' such that the difference between B and B' equals that between A and A'. (Whether the subject looks exclusively at the relation between A and A' or also takes into account that between A and B, or even A' and B, does not seem a serious matter. At issue is whether the subject simplifies things for the modeler by parsimoniously considering only one of the three relations that he or she might use. The human at least is almost certain to consider all of them (on some occasions), yet the modeler may still get away with the simplifying assumption because for most problems, the subject will not need to consider more than the A/A' relation.)

Notice that the Rumelhart and Abrahamson model, whatever its success with certain cases, cannot be a general model. It will work nicely for Sarah's sensory problems but not for her conceptual ones. Take the case where A and A' are a can opener and a can, respectively, B is a key, and Sarah is required to choose a lock to complete the analogy. A can opener and a can differ in many ways; the same is true for a key and a lock; and the difference(s) important in one comparison may be irrelevant in the other. The conceptual problems cannot be solved by computing differences between the items; one must consider the functional relation between the relevant items, not their physical difference.

Sarah's performance is interesting because she not only passed the conceptual problems but passed them from the beginning. She was correct on all of the first six conceptual problems given her ($p < .05$). Thus, after being shifted from the sensory problems, with which her exposure to analogies began, she did not fail the first few conceptual problems and then gradually master them; she succeeded from the start. Either she did the sensory problems more or less as the Rumelhart and Abrahamson model requires, confronted the conceptual problems, and immediately recognized that they could not be done this way and then devised a different approach; or she did not solve the sensory problems by computing differences in the first place. Instead, she used one and the same approach for both types of problems—in neither case an approach based on computing physical differences. What kind of an approach would work on both kinds of problems?

Both the sensory and conceptual problems can be seen as an example of a transformation. We are already familiar with this idea from the causality or action problem. A transformation can be represented by a three-element sequence in which an item in an initial state is changed, by some instrument or process, into a different or terminal state. The applicability of this paradigm to the conceptual analogy is straightforward. For instance, can opener is to can as key is to lock exactly because in both cases, the first item makes the same kind of change in the second one; keys do to locks what openers do to cans. But transformation is a general notion and can also be applied to the sensory analogy. For instance, to view the change from small to large circle in this light, you need only imagine a process that will have the desired effect. A small circle can become a large one by growing older, being inflated with air, being filled with water, becoming pregnant, being heated, fermenting; the actual process that the individual imagines depends, of course, on his or her knowledge and experience. Whether Sarah actually used this paradigm in solving either or both forms of the analogies is not something we can presently answer. The paradigm can be used in principle, and whether she actually uses it is readily subject to test.

ORDER

For years there has been the impression that chimpanzees and nonhuman animals, generally, have special difficulty with temporal order (e.g., Hebb & Thompson, 1954). The claim has been that they may be able to discriminate spatial patterns but not temporal ones. Interestingly, similar claims can be found for human children. However, recent work has discounted both claims. Altom and Weil (1977) have shown that children acquire information both for the spatial location of words and for the temporal order in which they appeared, and neither form of information had an advantage over the other. We have recently obtained similar results with Sarah (Premack, 1981).

Since words were inappropriate for Sarah, we used nonsense figures—forms cut out of colored paper. We made 24 such items and arranged them in sequences of 3 items each. Sarah was given pairs of such sequences, always consisting of the same elements but either in the same or different order, and she was required to make same/different judgments about them. The sequences were presented spatially (simultaneously) or temporally (successively), or one temporal and the other spatial, so that she had to translate between tham. She was successful on all three forms, though better on the simple cases than on the mixed one. For example, on a recent series in which all three forms were presented in a counterbalanced order, she was 20/24 spatial, 21/24 temporal, and 17/24 mixed ($p < .05$) (with no difference between spatial-temporal and temporal-spatial).*

Despite these positive results, Sarah's overall performance was compatible with the long-standing supposition that order is difficult for nonhuman animals. Sarah's success on these tests was by no means immediate. Almost 2 years of testing went into her final success. In contrast to factors like quantity and proportion, order is evidently not salient for the chimpanzee.

The fact that Sarah can make same/different judgments on order opens the possibility that she may be able to make such judgments on both a sensory and a conceptual basis. The problems given her so far concern sensory order—that is, sequences whose elements are physically identical. To raise the problem of order

*Data collected with G. Woodruff.

from a sensory to a conceptual level, we must use elements that are conceptually the same though physically different. For instance, since Sarah is capable of analogies, we might build the sequences out of elements used in the analogies. A sequence might consist of *A/A′*, *B/B′*, *C/C′*, the first relation involving a change in size; the second, a change in color; and the third, a change in the marking. A second sequence would consist of the same three relations but exemplified by quite different elements. For example, the first sequence could consist of small circle/large circle, red square/green square, and unmarked triangle/triangle with a dot in it; and the second sequence, of small rectangle/large rectangle, red pyramid/green pyramid, and an unmarked sawtooth/sawtooth with a dot in it. The two sequences do not consist of the same physical features; yet at the level of relations—size, color, marking—they are identical.

Of course, we need not use specifically analogical elements to represent conceptual sequence but could use any of a number of elements. We might use sequences consisting of items that Sarah knew belonged to one individual or another. A sequence could consist of, say, Tom's hat, Keith's shirt, and Dave's shoe; another, of Tom's glove, Keith's jacket, and Dave's glasses. Though composed of different items, these sequences, too, are identical on the conceptual level—both being sequences of Tom, Keith, Dave, in that order.

We have not yet tested Sarah on conceptual order, though we have tested her on other problems where the need to use the conceptual level is no less explicit. Indeed, the preceding problem, based on ownership, is related to a kind of problem that she has already solved. This problem is represented in Fig. 18.1. As you may see, it is a match-to-sample problem but one that cannot be done on a physical basis; for there is no more similarity between one of the alternatives and the sample than between the other alternatives and the sample. In the upper panel, the items in each circle consist of pieces of clothing—hat, shoe, dress. In the lower panel, of parts of fruit—stem, seed, peel. Both problems can be solved provided you have additional information and can operate upon that information appropriately.

In the sample shown in Fig. 18.1, the hat, shoe, and dress all belong to Mary; in the left alternative, the hat, dress, and shoe all belong to Jane; whereas in the right alternative, each piece of clothing has a different owner. Hence, both the sample and left alternative instance *all*—all Mary's and all Jane's—whereas the right alternative does not. A similar state of affairs holds for the problem in the lower panel. In the sample, the seed, stem, and peel all come from apples; those on the left alternative all come from oranges; whereas those on the right alternative each come from a different fruit. Hence, in this case, too, both the sample and left alternative instance *all*—all apple, all orange—whereas the right alternative does not. We have not used the clothing problem with Sarah—not yet having established what she knew about the association of clothing and people—but we have used the fruit problem successfully (Premack, 1976). Extensive testing showed that she knew a great deal about the association among the several pieces of a fruit. Indeed, these tests showed that she could use any of the

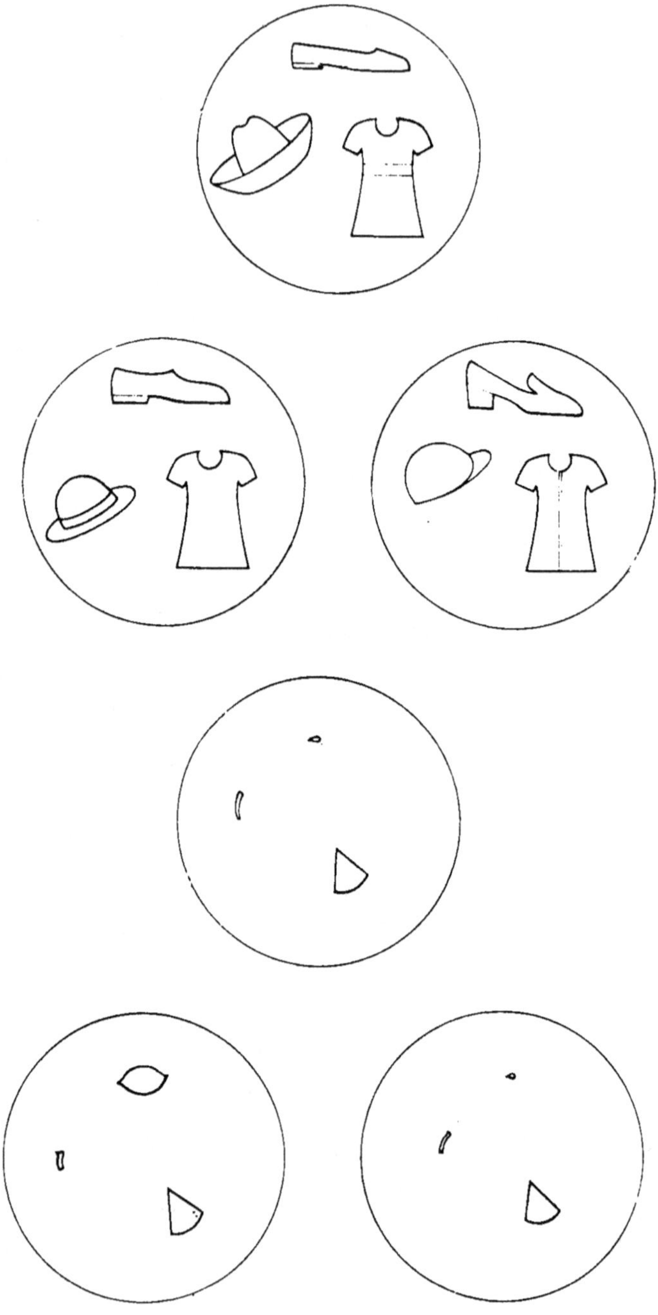

FIG. 18.1. Conceptual match to sample (from Premack, 1976).

seven components—taste, peel, seed, stem, wedge, color, shape—into which we divided a set of eight fruits to identify any other component of the same fruit.

In addition, other tests showed that Sarah could learn the quantifiers. She was taught *all, none, one,* and *some* with the use of sets of crackers varying in the proportion of round and square crackers that each contained. In one set, *all* four crackers were round; in a second set *none* was round; in a third *one* was round; and in the fourth more than one but less than all (i.e., *some*) were round. Not only did Sarah pass the standard transfer tests; she also applied the quantifiers to dimensions different from the training one. Trained on sets that varied exclusively in shape, she spontaneously applied the quantifiers correctly to sets that varied in size in one case and color in another.

Her performance on the foregoing series showed that she could code the stems, peels, seeds, and the like in terms of the fruit from which the pieces came and then quantify over the coded items. Since independent tests showed that she was capable of both the operations involved in the present test—coding the fruit pieces and quantification—it may not seem much of a surprise that she could combine the operations. The fact remains, however, that it is one thing to carry out single operations in particular contexts and another to be able to combine them in yet another context. Moreover, the quantification in the present tests was of a special kind. Whereas in previous tests, the sets of items over which Sarah quantified were physically present or perceptually apprehensible, the items in the present sets were not of this kind. It was not possible to solve the present tests by quantifying over the pieces of fruit as such. Rather, it was only after the pieces had been coded—as apple, orange, etc.—that the test could be solved by quantifying over them.

To clarify this constrast further, compare Sarah's problem with a lesser one in which everything remains the same except for the requirement that the quantification be made on conceptual elements. Picture three circles, as in Fig. 18.1, filled now with dots of different colors. The sample consists of red dots, the left alternative of blue dots, and the right alternative of green, yellow, and pink dots. Once again both sample and left alternative instance *all*—all red and all blue—whereas the right alternative does not. But now the items in the sequence do not have to be coded; the quantification can take place over the features red, blue, etc. Incidentally, it seems reasonable to speculate that monkeys could pass this test but that they would fail the earlier one, being able to quantify over sensory items but not over conceptual ones.

CONSERVATION

The classical Piagetian conservation test represents yet another way to look at the sensory-conceptual distinction. Young children's failure to conserve—for example, their failure to call equal amounts of fluid in different containers the "same"—is said to be the result of their undue reliance on sensory or perceptual factors. They are misled by appearance; whereas older children, having progressed to a more advanced level of intelligence, escape the influence of perception and rely on knowledge or inference. This is the classical view of the conservation data, and though it is not the only possible one—conservation tests are notoriously complex and thus may involve many factors—it is a reasonable interpretation.

We tested Sarah on three forms of conservation—number, liquid, and solid quantity—abandoning number when she failed to pass even the precursor to the conservation test—namely, accurate same/different judgments on numerosity. For the chimpanzee, number is clearly not the salient dimension that it is for the child (cf. Gelman & Gallistel, 1978). Sarah is peculiarly inconsistent in her discrimination of number: Periods in which she makes accurate judgments on numerosity alternate with other periods in which she performs at chance. Although Sarah shows some inconsistency for virtually every distinction, in no other case is the magnitude of her inconsistency comparable to that for number.

Although Sarah failed even the precursor sessions on number, when tested on liquid and solid quantity, she passed not only the precursor sessions but all the conservation tests as well. These complex tests are described in detail elsewhere (Woodruff, Premack, & Kennel, 1978), and I do not repeat the description here except to note that she passed them from the outset. Notice that we did *not* address the question, Can an individual who does not conserve be trained to do so?—which is familiar from the child literature. We did not train Sarah to conserve; we tested her and found that she did.

Sarah's successful conservation of liquid and solid quantity is puzzling because normal children do not pass such tests until they are 5 or 6 years old, and generally Sarah does not pass tests that are failed by normal children of 5 or 6 years of age. The rule of thumb I have come to use is this: If a 3½-year-old child can pass the test, then in all likelihood, so can Sarah (of course I exclude tests of language). But she rarely goes beyond this level. How then does she conserve liquid and solid quantity when even the 5-year-old child often fails to do so?

Before speculating excessively, it was desirable to eliminate a simple alternative. Sarah was not tested in the same way as children are. The child is interrogated, asked to say whether one container has more than the other, etc.; whereas Sarah was restricted to same/different judgments with her plastic words. To obtain comparable tests, we taught children the use of Sarah's same/different plastic words, since the reverse—teaching Sarah the equivalent of a child's language—was not possible. Julie Rosenberger carried out the work as an undergraduate research project. Using six retarded children, ranging in age from about 9 to 12, she first taught the children to make same/different judgments with the plastic words on pairs of objects—toys, fruit, and the like. Then she tested them just as Sarah had been tested, with one difference: The children passed the precursor sessions on numerosity, so she was able to include numerosity in the conservation tests. Briefly, the application of Sarah's test procedures to the children did not alter the child data in the least. Instead, Rosenberger's data essentially verified the child data based on standard verbal tests. The youngest children conserved number but neither liquid nor solid quantity; only the two oldest children conserved both liquid and solid quantity. We are left with the fact that Sarah passed tests that normal children do not pass until about 5 or 6.

Of course, the comparison between children and Sarah is troubled by the fact that we do not know the underlying process in either case. Conservation is hardly a simple procedure, and it may be no more simple at the level of underlying process. We can claim this much, in any case. The tests Sarah passed cannot be done on the basis of sensory information alone. When shown two equal containers of liquid *after* one of them had been transformed, without having been shown them before the transformation, she responded at chance; when given the same comparisons but allowed to see them before the transformation, she succeeded. Thus she could not simply look at the two different containers and observe that they held equal amounts; she had to have seen the two liquids before one was poured into the other container in order to judge them same.

Perhaps the classical interpretation is correct (Piaget, 1974): Conservation requires subjugating sensory or perceptual information—and Sarah is uniquely good at this. Two friends have proposed a clever way to test this interpretation. Both Anne Premack and my colleague Henry Gleitman have made the same suggestion: If Sarah is predisposed to respond on a conceptual level, then when given tests that require responding on the sensory level, she would fail; whereas juvenile apes and perhaps children who fail conservation should succeed when given the same tests. The full design, of course, is to give problems based on sensory criteria in one case, conceptual in another, to both groups. Sarah and older children should do better on the conceptual problem, juvenile apes and young children better on the sensory ones. Gleitman has even proposed a sensory problem that he has used demonstrationally in introductory psychology classes. The student is given a never-ending list of words and is required to identify those that are correct; he or she is given feedback on each trial. The criterion is along these lines: Those words are correct that begin with an *l* and end with a *g*. I am told that college students sometimes require 45 minutes worth of words to solve the problem and that many do not solve it at all. The interests of the demonstration would be substantially enhanced, of course, if it were also the case that fourth graders solved the problem in short order.

We cannot specify the elements in Sarah's experience that may have been responsible for her performance. After all, she was not only given incomplete representations and the like but was also trained on language. Because the language training did not instill much language—by which I mean grammar—does not mean that it may not have contributed in other ways. That it probably did contribute in some fashion is suggested by a comparison involving not Sarah, but two other groups of apes—one group trained on language and one not so trained.

The present juveniles have not been trained on language, in contrast to two animals who were previously in the laboratory, Peony and Elizabeth. Both groups were given the causality tests, the simplest version of them, at about the same age—5 to 6 years. Peony and Elizabeth both passed the tests (Premack, 1976); all four of the present juveniles failed (unpublished data). Although not language trained as were Peony and Elizabeth, the four juveniles have otherwise received no less, and probably more, general training. Exactly what portion of the language training may have contributed to the causality performance is not easily said; language training is a heterogeneous procedure. There is, however, one exact parallel between the two procedures: The task in both cases was akin to sentence completion.

The animal encountered an incomplete string of elements—incompleteness marked either by an interrogative particle or blank space—and was required to select the completing element(s). That the alternatives were plastic words in one case and objects in another seems unimportant. What does seem important is that in neither case could the animal base its choice on either of two forms of responding. The strings could not be completed by choosing items that either physically matched those in the string or that had the more frequent association with those in the string. Both of these peripheral mechanisms may have been weakened by the language training, preparing the animal for a conceptual level of processing.

Data of yet another kind suggest that the language training may have contributed. Children are reported not to sort items at a superordinate level until perhaps 5½ years of age (e.g., Rosch, Mervis, Gray, Johnson, & Boyes-Braem, 1976). Yet we found Sarah to sort items spontaneously at what appeared to be a superordinate level at about 7 years of age. We were interested in whether we could find evidence for something akin to semantic clustering in the chimpanzee, and for this purpose we gave what amounted to delayed match-to-sample problems with a multiple sample. The sample consisted of, say, 12 objects—4 items of food, 4 pieces of doll's clothing, and 4 miscellaneous toys. These were thrown out before the animal in a random order, removed, and then replaced by another set of, say, 16 items. The old set was included in the new set, and the animal's task was to pick out the old set. Actually we were less interested in the animal's ability to choose correctly than in the order of its choice; would it choose in runs—foods followed by toys, etc.? If so, we would have evidence for semantic clustering.

That Sarah spontaneously sorted items at what would appear to be the superordinate level was demonstrated before we reached the matching part of the test. Simply to assure ourselves that she had attended to the many items in the complex sample, we required her to pick the items up one at a time and hand them over to us. As it turned out, even at this stage of the experiment, she did not pick the items up in a random order but showed definite runs. Often semantic clustering is attributed to mnemonic factors; it is considered a good strategy for dealing with a limited memory. Although Sarah also showed runs in the matching part of the experiment, when memory was a factor, she showed runs earlier in the experiment when memory was not a factor; the latter displays were if anything stronger than the former (Premack, 1976).

CONCLUSIONS

Our major speculation is that exposing the chimpanzee to a particular kind of material produced change in the animal not unlike the change that is produced in people by school or formal pedagogy. Unfortunately, we cannot at this time unravel the chimpanzee's experience and isolate the critical elements, nor be certain that the effect really depends upon a "long" experience, nor even be confident about the exact nature of the change. The change appears to be a predilection to respond on the conceptual rather than the sensory level—that is, a disposition to choose items that *complete* partial representations as opposed to items that merely physically match or were associated with some part of the representation.

We are not in an ideal position to prove these claims, for to prove that experience and not simply maturation transformed Sarah, we need chimpanzees of Sarah's age who were not given her experience; it may be years before we have them, if we ever do. Moreover, the consistent contrast between Sarah's performance and that of the four juveniles is not helpful, for this difference could come either from age or from experience (ultimately, these animals should equal Sarah's performance, for they are receiving experience comparable to hers). Zoo animals might be tested on at least some of Sarah's tasks, provided we could find zoo animals tame enough to be tested at all. Yet another possible comparison is that between Sarah and a comparable animal given different experience—experience emphasizing the sensory level (matching and paired associates). Even if the transition from sensory to conceptual were largely maturational, the transition might be either accelerated or delayed by specific experience. But we have none of these controls.

Not having the needed experimental controls, we must fall back on other kinds of arguments. As substitutes for experimental controls, these arguments must seem dubious, for the celebrated status of the experiment or controlled comparison is not based on illusion. To some extent, neotony can be used to support the claim that Sarah's competence is not maturational but is based upon special experience. Neotony is the view that related species mature at a rate proportional to the evolutionary age of the species. The oldest primate—the prosimians—mature most quickly, monkeys next most quickly, followed by the apes, and finally by man, the most recent primate and the slowest to mature. Regrettably, for our purposes, the data on neotony scarcely touch on cognition but concern anatomical and motor development. The suitability of anatomy and motor skills is obvious: Grasping, locomotion, self-feeding, and the like ultimately appear in all members of the group, making direct comparison of maturational rates straightforward. In cognition, however, some milestones may not even appear in some members of the group—for example, the ability to make computations on conceptual rather than sensory items, conservation, and the like—making comparison of maturational rates impossible. These problems notwithstanding, let us assume for the sake of discussion that neotony applies not only to anatomy and motor skills but also to cognitive development.

If we make this assumption, then we see that Sarah's performance—and, to a lesser extent, those of the juvenile apes—do not accord with neotony, for by the time Sarah passed the most impressive of her tests, she was appreciably older than are children when they pass. This point suffers from the fact that we cannot claim to have tested Sarah at the earliest age at which she may have been able to pass the tests. (Had she failed when first tested and then succeeded later, we would, of course, have a good sense of the age at which she could first pass; unfortunately, she passed from the beginning.) Fortunately, the juvenile animals provide a way around this dilemma, for they have been given the same experience as Sarah except for the language training, and they fail all the tests at an age far older than that at which children pass the tests. For example, (1) children pass the causality tests when 3½ years old and may do so when younger; they have not yet been tested at an earlier age (Bullock & Gelman, 1979); none of the juveniles passed the causality tests. (2) None of the juveniles give any evidence of attributing intention to the other one (in the videotape tests) (Premack & Woodruff, 1978), whereas about 50% of 3½-year-old and virtually all 4-year-old children do. (3) Indeed, videotape cannot even be used in testing chimpanzees until they are perhaps 5 or more, whereas it can be used with children when they are 3 and probably much earlier. (4) The conceptual proportions afford yet another comparison: They were failed decisively by the juvenile apes and passed by nearly all 3½-year-old children. If we equate Sarah and the (brightest of the) juveniles with regard to native ability, we can say that chimpanzees passed the tests in question somewhere between the 6th and 15th year—the juveniles failed at 6, whereas Sarah passed at 15—in comparison to children who pass the same tests when about 3½ years old. If neotony applies to cognitive development, we have the paradoxical fact that the ape achieves cognitive milestones after (rather than before) the child. I take this to suggest that the ape would not achieve these milestones at all were it not for special experience.

Of course, in its general form there is nothing novel about this argument; we know that in our own species, maturation alone does not guarantee all forms of cognition. School, introduced into a technologically primitive human group, changes the cognitive and mnemonic skills of children and even adults in the group (Cole, Gay, Glick, & Sharp, 1971). Interestingly, the intervention in this case occurs on a within-, rather than between-, species basis; teacher and student differ technologically, not biologically. The intervention appears to have been successful in both cases. Yet the parallel must be qualified by two factors: First, the advance in the ape did not carry it to the level of the child. Pedagogy can serve only to bring the individual closer to the limits of its species; it cannot change the genetic envelope of one species into that of another. Second, the pedagogy came exclusively from human beings—human teaching human in one case, human teaching ape in another. In the human species, pedagogy—manipulation of the behavior of the other one—is an *intrinsically* maintained disposition. This is not to deny that apes intentionally modify each other's behavior. Apes can be observed to manipulate one another, in both a degree and manner that is often startling (e.g., Premack & Woodruff, 1978), but in all cases with immediate benefit to the manipulator—therefore an *extrinsically* maintained disposition. Moreover, nothing I have every observed suggests that apes possess behavioral ideals, concepts of the form that behavior should take, and intervene to modify behavior that falls short of the ideal. In the development of culture, tradition has given language great emphasis; I suspect that the human pedagogic impulse deserves equal emphasis.

If the contrast described here is sustained by further data and is backed up by more direct controls, we can confirm our opening thesis. Successful species do not dwell at the peak of their capacity; they have a reserve—for species specialized in intelligence, a reserve in intelligence. If such species fall into the hands of "superior" species and are properly treated, they will attain a level of competence beyond their usual one. This change may take specifically the form of concentrating on the conceptual as opposed to the sensory level of processing. This appears to be the case with Sarah, an African-born female ape who has been in a kind of school for well over 10 years. We hope to carry her still further in the next decade—indeed, to extract from her meager brain (and hairy body) an answer to the question, What is intelligence?

REFERENCES

Altom, M. W., & Weil, J. Young children's use of temporal and spatial order information in short-term memory. *Journal of Experimental Child Psychology*, 1977, *24*, 1-17.

Bullock, M, & Gelman, R. Preschool children's assumptions about cause and effect: Temporal ordering. *Child Development*, 1979, *50*, 89-96.

Cole, M., Gay, J., Glick, J. A., & Sharp, D. W. *The cultural context of learning and thinking*. New York: Basic Books, 1971.

Gelman, R., & Gallistel, R. *The child's understanding of number*. Cambridge: Harvard University Press, 1978.

Gillan, D., Premack, D., & Woodruff, G. *Reasoning: I. Analogical reasoning in chimpanzee. J. Exp. Psych.. Animal Beh. Proc.*, 1981, *1*, 1-17.

Hebb, D. O., & Thompson, W. R. The social significance of animal studies. In G. Lindzey (Ed.), *Handbook of social psychology* (Vol. I) *Theory and Method*. Reading, Mass.: Addison-Wesley, 1954.

Kellogg, R., *What children scribble and why*. San Francisco: Author, 1955.

Meyer, D. R., Treichler, F. R., & Meyer, M. Discrete-trial training techniques and stimulus variables. In A. M. Schrier, H. F. Harlow, & F. Stollnitz (Eds.), *Behavior of nonhuman primates*, New York: Academic Press, 1965.

Piaget, J. *Understanding causality*. New York: Norton, 1974.

Premack, D. Putting a face together. *Science*, 1975, *188*, 228-236.

Premack, D. *Intelligence in ape and man*. Hillsdale, N.J.: Lawrence Erlbaum Associates, 1976.

Premack, D. Characteristics of an upgraded mind. In W. Michaelis (Ed.), *Bericht über den 32 Kongress der Deutschen Gesellschaft für Psychologie in Zürich 1980*, Zürich: Verlag für Psychologie, 1981.

Premack, D., & Woodruff, G., Does the chimpanzee have a theory of mind? *The Behavioral and Brain Sciences*, 1978, *4*, 515-526.

Premack, D., Woodruff, G. & Kennel, K. Paper-marking test for chimpanzee: simple control for social cues. *Science*, 1978, *202*, 903-905.

Rosch, E., Mervis, C. B., Gray, W. D., Johnson, D. M., & Boyes-Braem, P., Basic objects in natural categories. *Cognitive Psychology*, 1976, *8*, 382-439.

Rumelhart, D. E., & Abrahamson A. A. A model for analogical reasoning. *Cognitive Psychology*, 1973, *5*, 1-28.

Woodruff, G., Premack, D., & Kennel, K., Conservation of liquid and solid quantity by the chimpanzee. *Science*, 1978, *202*, 991-994.

Woodruff, G. & Premack, D. Primitive mathematical concepts in the chimpanzee: proportionality and numerosity. *Nature*, 1981, *293*, 568-569.

19 Prenatal Protein Deprivation and Early Behavioral Development

A. J. Riopelle
Louisiana State University

INTRODUCTION: LASHLEY AND ANIMAL MODELS

It is remarkable that 50 years after the publication of Karl Lashley's *Brain Mechanisms and Intelligence* (1929) and 21 years after his death in 1958, he still remains one of the anchor points in the development of our thinking about how the brain affects behavior; this volume organized by Dr. Orbach is adequate testimony to the fact. We are prone to think of neuropsychology when we think of Lashley, but we should not forget that Lashley was more than a neuropsychologist: He was an animal behaviorist, a biologist, a comparative psychologist, a philosopher of science, and a methodologist. It is no wonder that with the breadth of his background and the range of his interest, he saw patterns and interrelationships of data missed by others of his time.

Knowledge of interspecies differences was essential for using animal models to study human problems. As Henry Nissen, his colleague at Yerkes Laboratories, has remarked (1951): "Whether we are impressed more by the similarities or by the differences of behavior within the animal kingdom depends on the scale of observation used. The broader the category the more do the similarities stand out and vice versa [p. 352]." The breadth of Lashley's comparisons has enabled us to recognize the origin of his emphasis on the organizational unity of animals. The mind and brain, for Lashley, was one—not two.

But the title of this volume is *Neuropsychology After Lashley,* and the advances that have occurred in psychology and biology, as well as in other neurosciences, cause us to recognize the fact that physiological organization lies principally within individuals of a given mammalian species, not between them. The similarities we observe among species are human abstractions from samples that are themselves quite diverse. Accordingly, not just any species can be used as a model for humans in any project we choose. Yet we need not despair of their use as models, for despite their diversity, all species of any complexity pass through a period of development—if only from a single cell to a multitude of cells and a multiplicity of organs. Each organ, including the brain or, more precisely, the organs of the brain, is subject to the environment's opportunities and constraints, and each is at the mercy of the available nutrients and victim of the toxins to which it is exposed.

THE NUTRITION-BRAIN PROBLEM

Extent and Severity

In recent years we have seen growing concern about widespread malnutrition and its role in development. If inadequate early nutrition resulted merely in a small body, little attention would be paid to it, despite the fact that upwards of one-quarter of the world's population, by some estimates (F.A.O., 1963; McGovern, 1979), experience malnutrition at some time in their lives. However, the structural and functional integrity of the individual, his or her intellectual functioning and personality development, might be compromised by the early malnutrition; this suggests that those with limited educational and economic opportunities, who need to muster all the intellectual resources with which they are genetically endowed, are the very ones who might be the victims of malnutrition. This possibility has led to worldwide awareness of the problem. The conclusion that these victims are twice afflicted seems plausible in light of the well-known fact that children born into families where the plane of nutrition is low are small at birth, have neurological and developmental anomalies, and have a high incidence of perinatal mortality, especially among those infants of low birth weight whose gestational period was longer than would be expected from their weight (Gruenwald, 1964). Difficulty in language development is frequently seen, and deviant behavior such as autism, hyperkinesis, and involvement in childhood accidents is more common than in the normal population. Academic achievement, physical growth, and motor behavior are also adversely affected (Caputo & Mandell, 1970; Drillien, 1968). It was a study by Stoch and Smythe in South Africa (1963) that directly connected low intellectual achievement to early malnutrition. Although Stoch and Smythe could not prove their point with finality because of inadequate controls for social factors, other corroborating studies soon followed. Subsequent publications showed that monovular twins of widely disparate birth weights, denoting differences in prenatal nutrition, had intelligence quotients that accorded with their birth weights: The lower the birth weight, the lower the IQ

(Willerman & Churchill, 1967). It was also known that the identical twin with the lower birth weight tends to have lower verbal and performance IQs in later life (Kaelber & Pugh, 1969). "Small-for-date" babies may be more seriously impaired mentally than are chronologically immature babies of the same birth weight, for they are thought to suffer intrauterine growth retardation (Baird, 1945).

Theoretical Background

These findings have been rationalized in terms of two dominant theories, both of which emphasize the consequences of malnutrition during early development (Davison & Dobbing, 1968). Davison and Dobbing have observed that morphologic development occurs in stages. The first stage terminates when multiplication of neuroblasts ceases. Stage 2 lasts from then until the end of the period of rapid myelination and other growth. Stage 3 occurs through maturity, and Stage 4 is the stage of senile regression. Dobbing has proposed that vulnerability to adversity is greatest during the period of fastest growth, Stage 2. Teratological studies show that viruses, drugs, and ionizing radiation produce gross anatomical deformity if the insult occurs during this stage. Restricting the rate of growth during the growth spurt, when fetal demands are proposed to be most critical, may retard development and possibly reduce its ultimate extent, resulting in a small adult having a small brain and few constituents, particularly myelin, and possibly some distortion of the normal structural pattern.

Winick's alternative hypothesis (1968) is based directly on Enesco and Leblond's principle (1962) that except for a few organs that exhibit continuous cell division, growth begins with hyperplasia (increasing cell number) and follows with hypertrophy (increasing cell size), the two stages overlapping. If, because of the unavailability of essential nutrients, cell proliferation cannot be completed within the restricted time allotment, permanently reduced cell number results, despite later rehabilitation. The brain, in this respect, is like the other organs. Although it is true that glial cells outnumber neurons 9 to 1 in the brain, the effects should be the same on both components.

The dominant dogma before the research and the hypotheses just cited came to the fore was that the fetus is not significantly influenced by the dietary intake of the mother during pregnancy. The fetus was thought to be a perfect parasite, and only severe and prolonged malnutrition could impair obstetrical performance. The newer hypotheses implied the opposite—that the mother is only an imperfect filter, passing to the fetus what remains after extracting, more or less adequately, her own requirements. The two animals, then, are competitors for the nutrients, and the fetus might occasionally be the loser.

The two hypotheses assume that the mother has no adequate reserves of the essential nutrients on which the fetus can draw—the labile stores, with the exception of fat, being limited to only a few days' supply. Both hypotheses also assert that rehabilitation cannot be totally effective or complete if it begins after the deadline.

Human studies confirmed that the greatest detriment to growth and function occurs when malnutrition is early. The autopsy studies of Winick, Rosso, and Waterlow (1970), conducted on Chilean and Jamaican babies who died of malnutrition before 2 years of age, showed that the children had a deficiency in brain cells. Parekh, Pherwani, Udani, and Mukherjee (1970) studied the brains of malnourished Indian children and found them severely underweight. These authors concluded that nutritional deficiency had its severest impact during the last 3 months of gestation or the first 3 months after birth. The clear implication of these studies is that brain development parallels development in other organs; therefore, studies of these organs will reveal secrets of the brain.

NUTRITIONAL MECHANISMS AND INFANT GROWTH

Feto-placental Relations

Intervening between mother and fetus is the placenta, the proximate source of fetal nutrition. It is obvious that if the placenta is limited in its capacity through infection or inadequate nutrition for its own complete growth, the nutrients available to the infant will be inadequate. Placental insufficiency has long been a hypothesized cause of intrauterine growth retardation (IUGR). This notion arose in part from the long-known fact that large infants have large placentas and small infants, small placentas. Infants who survived the neonatal period, for example, had, in one study, a mean placental weight of 446 g; infants who died during the neonatal period had a mean placental weight of 321 g; and those who were stillborn had placentas that weighed 316 g (Sedlers, Berends, Kim, Stone, Weiss, Deutschberger, & Jackson, 1967).

Both normal and IUGR infants weigh approximately eight times the placenta upon delivery. The exact value of the ratios have little meaning, because different investigators discard different amounts in preparing the placentas for weighing; but the similarity in feto-placental ratios between the growth retarded and the normal is to be expected, regardless of whether the fetus controls the placenta or vice versa. What is surprising in the study of these data is that a wide range of ratios exists in both groups. The ratios for the IUGR group were between 5.5 and 11.6 to 1.0 and, for the normal-term infants, between 4.6 and 11.7 to 1.0. The great overlap and the wide range of ratios suggest that the materno-fetal coupling is very loose, and accordingly, we may not be able to attribute birth deficiencies directly to placental defects in size or cellularity.

To evaluate directly the importance of placental integrity, Wigglesworth (1964) ligated the artery of one uterine horn of a rat during the latter part of its pregnancy. When born, the infants were stunted, and they showed organ changes characteristic of small, malnourished babies: large, well-developed brains; small livers; and histological maturity of the organs in accordance with gestational age.

A parallel study was conducted on rhesus monkeys by Myers, Hill, Holt, Scott, Mellits, and Cheek (1971), who at the 100th gestational day ligated the fetal umbilical vessels attached to the secondary placental disc, isolating it from the fetus. Postoperative interruption of pregnancy was high, but 7 of the 13 animals reached 150 to 160 days of gestation, when they were delivered by cesarean section. The smallest animals weighed, on the average, about two-thirds as much as the control animals. The brain, adrenals, kidneys, and pituitary gland were affected less than the lungs, pancreas, liver, and spleen. Hill, Myers, Holt, Scott, and Cheek (1971) found cerebellar DNA of the IUGR group to be low.

The experiment was repeated by Portman, Alexander, Neuringer, Novy, Illingworth, and Uno (1977). They, too, ligated the vessels bridging the two discs of the bidiscoid rhesus placenta, but at Day 90. All infants survived to Day 155, when they were delivered by cesarean section, but three of them died within 2 weeks. The survivors were fed a low-protein formula (3.6% of energy as protein) for 40 days, after which they were sacrificed for analysis. Significant reductions in brain weights and in the weights of brain stems and cerebella were found, but no significant reduction was observed in total content of DNA, protein, or any of the lipid constituents of the cerebellum or cerebrum. How much of the glycolipid deficiency that was found in the brain stem can be ascribed to the period of pregnancy and how much to the postnatal period cannot be determined. The study does point to the possible reserve capacity of the monkey placenta and to the resistance of brain DNA to undernutrition.

PRENATAL DEPRIVATION

Species Comparisons and Deficiency Definition

Placental ligation studies, if conclusive, would point directly to the mechanism involved in intrauterine growth retardation. They are less useful for determining whether or not the starvation and malnutrition experienced by millions of mothers are causative factors in low birth weight and in the hypothesized physiological and behavioral incompetence. Because of the circumstances of ignorance, lack of intellectual and social stimulation, and social disorganization that accompany severe malnutrition in humans, epidemiologic studies can only suggest factors that might be involved in the relation of low protein to low birth weight. Obviously, experiments involving deprivation cannot be conducted with human subjects, so animals are required as models.

We are likely to run some risk of illegitimate comparisons of prenatally or early postnatally deprived animals of different species because the act of birth occurs for them at different stages of fetal development. We, of course, are interested in humans, so the usefulness of other animals must be judged in terms of the likelihood of their contributing to an understandning of the human situation. A number of deprivation studies have been conducted with laboratory animals and with farm animals, and they have determined that food deprivation of the mother, inflicted at different stages of her pregnancy, will differentially affect the various organs of the fetus because at any one instant, the organs are in different stages of development and, hence, of vulnerability. But we are interested in knowing whether limitation of food intake of the pregnant human has adverse consequences for the birth status and development of the infant.

It would be ideal to study the effects of single-nutrient deficiencies, for prevention or repletion programs could then be most precisely targeted, but such pure deficiencies are uncommon in human experience. For that reason, the term *protein-calorie malnutrition* is very useful for describing the situation in the world at large. Although the term is intentionally vague, in order to describe a complex situation, the nutritional problem may nevertheless be somewhat more precise than that indicated by the term. There is reason to believe that whether protein alone is deficient or both protein and calories are lacking, the basic deficit is in protein. Indeed, protein deficiency alone is as adverse in effect as is calorie deficiency.

Rodent Studies

Churchill and his colleagues (1961; 1967; Churchill, Neff, & Caldwell, 1966) found that the young of rats fed a protein-deficient diet during pregnancy had difficulty in learning. Studies by Barnes, Moore, Reid, and Pond (1968), by Dobbin (1968), and by Stewart and Platt (1968) suggest that protein deficiency produces different and usually more serious effects on the central nervous system than does mere food restriction. Protein is also one of the more expensive components of diets, so with families and cultures in which economic factors are of considerable importance in determining the composition of the diet, protein is one of the first items to be foregone. Miller, in particular, has adduced evidence to support the idea that protein, not calories, is the most limiting nutrient in such studies (1970). He noted a net accumulation of fat amounting to 240% during the suckling period of rats, a fact that implies an excess of calories in a neonatal diet. Moreover, when animals were placed on a diet low in protein, weight gain was restricted. Replacing the protein calories with carbohydrates did not restore the weight gain to its original rate. Accordingly, it has been proposed that the undernourished infant suffers a protein deficit because the protein consumed is diverted to energy expenditure rather than to tissue formation.

Brains of the offspring of rats maintained, in another study, on an 8% diet contained less DNA and protein than did the progeny of well-fed females. Because the rat brain at birth contains mostly neurons, the reduction in DNA denotes that the dietary restriction resulted in a permanent brain-neuron deficiency (Zamenhof, Van Marthens, & Margolis, 1968). A number of other investigators have corroborated the finding that the offspring of rats prenatally deprived of protein are undersized at birth (Hawrylewicz, Kissane, Blair, & Hepner, 1973; Rosso, 1977; Zeman, Shrader, & Allen, 1973; Zeman & Stanbrough, 1969). Mice may respond slightly differently. The protein content, but not the DNA content, of the cerebra of newborn mice was reduced, as was the total brain weight of the offspring of dams fed low-protein diets (Nehrich & Stuart, 1978).

Similar adverse effects on the offspring of rats occur if the mothers are deprived of calories during pregnancy (Chow & Lee, 1964; Smart, Adlard, & Dobbing, 1972; Zamenhof, Van Marthens, & Grauel, 1971). As indicated earlier, protein deficiency may result when caloric intake is insufficient, because the protein ingested is probably consumed as energy rather than distributed for tissue accretion. A 20% drop in birth weight and persistent stunting was noted for male offspring of mothers fed a diet containing 50% of the calories but no reduction in protein (Rider & Simonson, 1973).

Cortical thickness at several positions was significantly reduced in the young of rats that were maintained on a calorie-deficient diet. The reduction in cortical thickness is approximately double that expected from the reduction in cerebral weight, a finding that suggests that cerebral cortex itself is more affected by such malnutrition than the cerebrum as a whole. The deficiencies were most evident at birth (Clark, Zamenhof, Van Marthens, Grauel, & Kruger, 1973).

The data are not entirely confirmatory. For example, Naismith (1969) noted that the birth weight of rats was not substantially lower when the mother consumed a low-protein diet during pregnancy. Suggesting that the fetus lives as a parasite, having a prior claim on the nutrients circulating in the maternal bloodstream, he observed that a 54% reduction in the dietary protein intake reduced fetal weight by no more than 11%. Yet most reviewers of the literature dealing with rodents agree that on many measures of physical integrity or behavioral capacity, the young of rats fed diets during pregnancy that are deficient in proteins, calories, or both are themselves deficient in a number of respects. Moreover, diets containing as much as 10% to 15% protein have sometimes produced deficits in infant rats. Despite the few negative reports, the literature is preponderately in favor of the view that there is a deleterious effect of maternal protein or calorie deficiency on the offspring. The brain can be seriously affected in infant rodents if the mother is deprived of protein or calories during pregnancy.

Studies in Primates

Some of the data from studies on pregnant primates have come from our laboratory. Preliminary to conducting studies of protein deprivation in pregnant monkeys, we needed some idea of the requirements for nonpregnant animals, and our first studies were directed to this end. A literature search uncovered widely different estimates of the requirements for rhesus monkeys. A good deal of this variation is probably attributable to different ages of the animals (often unspecified or unknown). Nothing was found of the requirements for pregnant animals, so parallels were drawn with human data. It is accepted and, indeed, recommended that women consume more calories and protein when pregnant than they do when they are not pregnant. Since the differential may be in the neighborhood of 20% and since we guessed from the published data that the nonpregnant young-adult animal would need approximately 100 Cal. per kilogram of body weight per day, we devised a diet that we thought would be optimal for the pregnant animals, assuming they consumed 120 Cal. per kilogram of body weight per day. This diet was arranged to afford 4 g protein per kilogram of body weight each day and contained 13.4% protein as casein. (Some commercial monkey diets contain 25% protein; most contain 10% to 15% protein.) Additional isocaloric diets were confected having one-half, one-fourth, or one-eighth the amount of protein of the control diet; that is, they contained 6.7%, 3.35%, or 1.68% protein. Since it turned out that even the nonpregnant animals consumed about 115 cal per kilogram of body weight per day for the first three groups, actual consumption was close to 4 g, 2 g, or 1 g of protein per kilogram

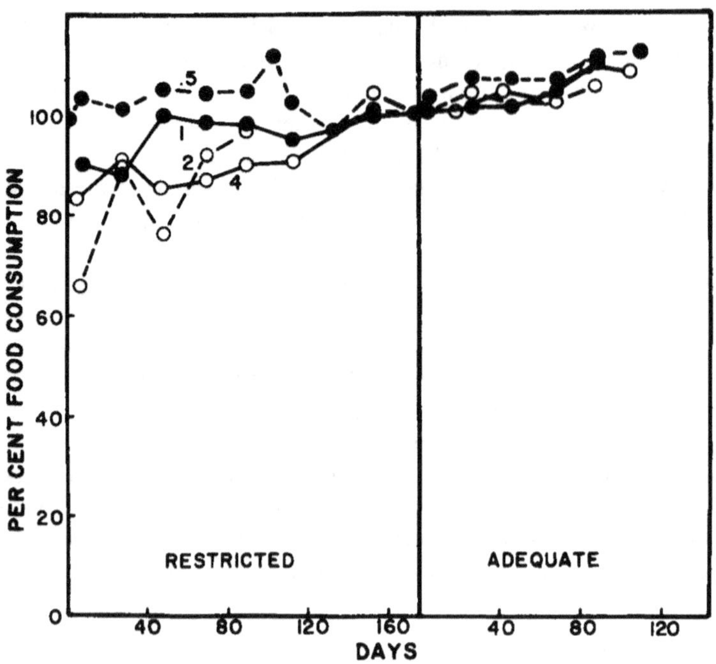

FIG. 19.1. Daily food consumption of four groups of nonpregnant monkeys expressed as a percentage of consumption at the end of the restriction. (From the *American Journal of Clinical Nutrition.*)

of body weight per day. The last group—nominally, the ½-g group—lost considerable weight but continued to eat the amount it ate at the beginning of the experiment; so its protein intake per kilogram of body weight actually was higher than ½ g.

The exact relations between food consumption and body weight are shown in the first few figures. Figure 19.1 shows the amount of food eaten by the nonpregnant animals during the 6 months they were fed the experimental diets and during the subsequent 4 months, when they were returned to the control diet. Daily consumption is expressed in terms of the percentage of food consumed at the end of the restricted period. The initial effect of the transfer to the restricted diet was a temporary disruption of appetite. A general upward trend exists in the data, indicating that the animals, young adults, were still growing. Another point to be noted is that the ½-g-diet animals consumed more food right from the beginning than did the animals on the other diet. Their curve is at the top of the group. Finally, note that the consumption curves during repletion are identical for all animals, deprived or not. This fact indicates that none of the animals, even those fed low-protein diets, ate excessively when returned to the high-protein diet.

Figure 19.2 shows the body-weight curves for the same period. The animals

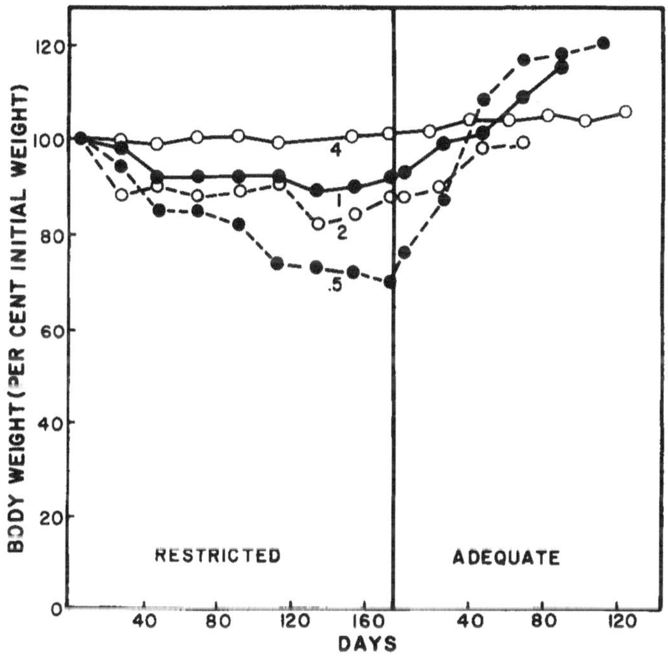

FIG. 19.2. Weights of four groups of nonpregnant monkeys fed isocaloric diets varying in protein concentration over a 6-month period. (From the *American Journal of Clinical Nutrition*.)

on the 4-g diet gained weight slowly throughout the experiment, whereas the animals fed the 2-g, the 1-g, or the ½-g diet lost weight. Upon returning to the 4-g diet, they recovered their weight loss; indeed, some even overshot the weight of the 4-g animals. Only later did they fall to their "normal" weight. The decline in weight during the low-protein period and the rapid weight recovery during rehabilitation indicate plainly that the animals were deprived during the restricted-protein period. Evidence from other sources corroborates this. An analysis of the ratio of the nonessential to the essential amino acids in the circulating plasma revealed exactly what we would expect: The animals on the low-protein diet depleted their stores of amino acids, so that instead of one-third of the amino acids being essential (normal), only one-ninth were essential amino acids. Return to normal values was prompt upon resuming the diet containing 13.4% protein (Riopelle, Hill, Li, Wolf, Seibold, & Smith, 1974). Clearly, our experimental diets are deficient for rhesus monkeys.

The food intake during this experiment, when it was repeated in pregnant animals beginning on the 30th day of pregnancy and continuing until delivery—with diets containing 13.4%, 6.7%, and 3.35% protein—is shown in Fig. 19.3. All animals ate about the same amount of diet before and during the first 30 days of pregnancy, while they were still on the 4-g diet. By the end of pregnancy, however, the 4-g animals were eating more than the 2-g animals,

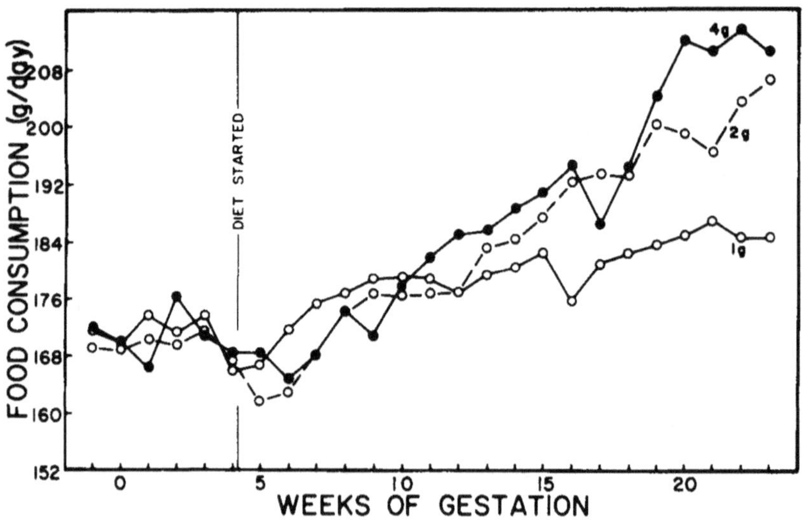

FIG. 19.3. Daily food consumption of three groups of pregnant animals fed isocaloric diets varying in protein concentration, beginning at 30 days of pregnancy and continuing until delivery. (From the *American Journal of Clinical Nutrition.*)

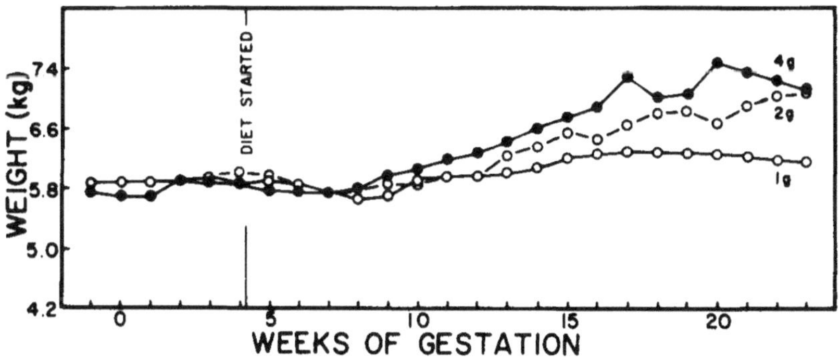

FIG. 19.4. Weights of three groups of pregnant animals fed different concentrations of protein from the 30th day of pregnancy until term. (From the *American Journal of Clinical Nutrition*.)

which in turn ate more than the 1-g animals. Figure 19.4 shows that there is a precisely parallel increase in the body weight of the pregnant animals; the 4-g animals gained more than did the 2-g animals, which in turn gained more than the 1-g animals did. Note that even the low-protein animals gained weight during pregnancy; yet they were eating diets that caused nonpregnant animals to lose weight (Riopelle, Hill, Li, Wolf, Seibold, & Smith, 1975). The daily food consumption per kilogram of body weight of the three groups followed relatively similar courses. The most important conclusion to be drawn from this finding is that in terms of unit body weight, the 1-g animals ate as much as the 2-g or the 4-g animals did. In other words, it is unlikely that these animals were deficient in minerals, proteins, or calories per unit of body weight.

We might note further, as Fig. 19.5 shows, that after delivery, when all animals were returned to the high-protein diet, those who were fed the 1-g diet during pregnancy did not gain weight as the nonpregnant, low-protein animals did when they were refed the high-protein diet (Riopelle & Shell, 1978).

It appears, then, that the mother holds her own status rather than losing tissue during pregnancy, even though she may be fed a diet containing as little as 3.35% protein, roughly equivalent to a daily intake of 1 g of protein per kilogram of body weight. Accordingly, the mother does not deplete her reserves in order to provide adequate support for her infant. As early as 1919, Slemons asserted, on the basis of balance studies, that the mother gains rather than loses during pregnancy. It would seem that her needs have considerable priority, so that if she is engaged in competition for nutrients with the fetus, she competes quite effectively with it. It does not necessarily follow, however, that if the mother proceeds through pregnancy with little or no deficit to herself, the fetus must necessarily suffer as a consequence.

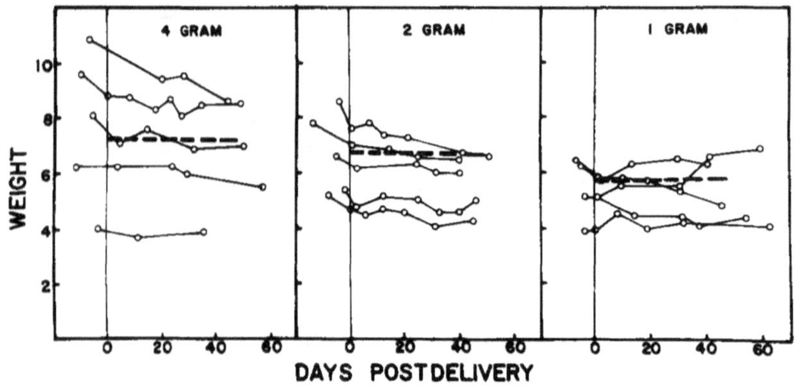

FIG. 19.5. Postdelivery weights representative of individual protein-deprived and nondeprived pregnant animals. Note that deprived animals gained no weight when they were returned to the protein-rich diets. (From the *American Journal of Clinical Nutrition*.)

To evaluate this alternative, we need to examine the birth status of the infants of these mothers and follow their growth and behavioral development. But before we do, we should note that fetal wastage increased slightly but not significantly in the low-protein group; that is, slightly more prenatal deaths occurred in the low-protein groups than in the control group (Riopelle, Hill & Li 1975). The infants of the three groups weighed the same when delivered normally at term. It appears that if the fetus does not develop properly, it is aborted or stillborn.

INFANT BEHAVIOR

Let us now turn our attention to the behavior of the infants born of these three groups of mothers. The standard infant regime was as follows: When a baby was born, it was taken from its mother, brought to the nursery, cleaned, weighed, offered food, and installed in its own cubicle. The front and one wall of the cubicle were transparent, allowing sight of the nursery activities and of the animals in the adjacent cubicle. Infants were not deprived nutritionally; they were fed a commercial formula designed for humans. Animals were held in the hand while feeding for the first 30 days of life. Later, they frequently were fed on mechanical bottle holders. In the beginning we gave seven feedings daily, but the number was reduced to three by the 50th day.

Forty-nine infants participated in our first study—19 from mothers fed the 3.35% protein, 15 from mothers fed the 6.7% protein, and 15 from mothers fed the 13.4% protein.

Early Behavior Battery

The intent of the first experiment was to assess the behavior of the animals as soon as feasible after birth, and tests were selected that might identify animals having obvious behavioral deficits. The tests consisted mostly of reflex and muscular coordination tests. The animals were tested at two stages, depending on the age of onset and of disappearance of the behavior we examined. The tests were taken or adapted from those described by Mowbray and Cadell (1962). The first block of testing was conducted within the first 20 days; and the second block, more variable, began at the 8th and continued to Day 50 for some tests. The tests were: (1) *rooting,* mouthing an object that touches the nose or cheek; (2) *visual orientation,* following with the head and eyes a small, bright object moving across the visual field; (3) *extending,* reflexly extending the arms and legs upon loss of support; (4) *body orientation,* righting oneself when placed on a 60-cm circular disc, tilted 30° off the horizontal and rotated about its pivot; (5) *clasping,* placing the arms and legs around an object that touched the ventral body surface; (6) *righting,* righting after being lowered, back downward, onto a table while hanging from a cylinder; (7) *placing,* appropriate positioning of arms while being held and moved forward until the suspended arms touched the near edge of the table; (8) *rod walking,* crawling suspended along a rod to an end platform; (9) *rope crawling,* crawling suspended along a moderately taut rope line; (10) *tunnel,* moving through a transparent plastic tunnel, at one end of which was a wig incentive; (11) *platforms,* stepping down off three platforms of varying heights, each approximately 250 mm square; (12) *startle,* flinching in response to the sound of two short, wooden boards being clapped together behind the monkey's back; (13) *visual cliff,* differential response to depth when placed on a narrow board, 50 cm long, centered on a piece of transparent glass. (A solid surface was located immediately below the glass on one side of the board, but on the other side, the solid surface was some distance below the glass. This test measures innate response to depth.)

The scores for the two age blocks, one shown in solid lines and the other in dashed lines, are portrayed for the 13 tests in Fig. 19.6. Each panel of the figure shows an individual test. We are not especially concerned here with individual test results. Rather we observe two things: (1) The dashed line representing the performance of the second age block is generally higher than that of the solid line of the first age block; and (2) the lines for all tests are essentially horizontal. That is, no significant differences occurred on any of the tests as a result of the diet of the mother. Indeed, not even the slightest suggestion of a trend is apparent.

These data, when published, evoked a number of comments and suggestions. One was that the tests were too insensitive or the scoring too coarse to detect any changes. In reply, we can note that in the first place, the differences between age

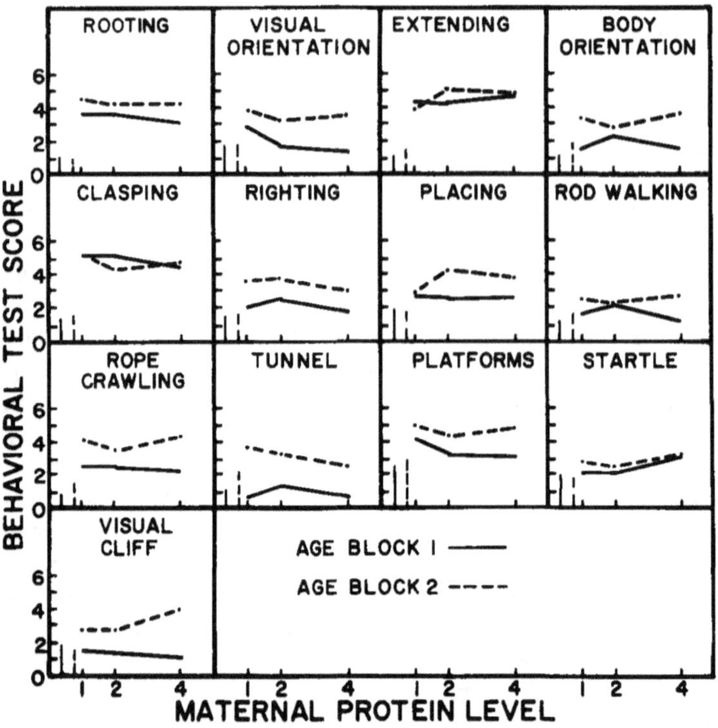

FIG. 19.6. Performance of infants of protein-deprived mothers on a series of early behavior tests. (From the *American Journal of Clinical Nutrition.*)

blocks achieved significance levels adequate to please even the most fastidious researcher, so the present scoring system was adequate for detecting changes. Secondly, unreliability that would arise from coarse measurement would not alter any trend that might exist, and as can be seen, no trend existed among the groups. Another person suggested that differences will become evident when the animals are older or that the differences will appear when we study emotional and social behaviors. We had no quarrel with these suggestions, but we were reluctant to issue promissory notes when the data that might bear on these points would eventually arrive and be able to speak for themselves.

In a subsequent study, the social behavior of 15 animals was investigated. They were observed eight times in each of two age blocks: 30 to 70 days and 130 to 170 days. First one animal was put alone for 10 minutes into a play cage that served as the experimental arena; then a second animal was added, and each animal was observed for two 15-minute periods. Then the first animal was removed, and the second was observed alone for 10 minutes. Each animal was tested with the next oldest and the next youngest peer. In general, a number of behavioral categories were defined that involved social or nonsocial activities. The categories were subdivided into four classes: emotional responsiveness, exploratory behavior, activity level, and social behavior. In the nonsocial conditions, it was obvious that all the animals were distressed when they were placed in the play cage. While cooing and screeching, they ran about the play cage, clawing at the entry door and the corners. If they were not moving, they stared at the clear observation screen, sucked a finger or toe, or wrapped their arms about themselves, clutching vigorously. The infants were rarely silent. In view of their attachment to the blankets in the home cages, it was surprising to note that very little time was spent in contact with the blanket that was located in the play cage. When the animals were older, they became more active, jumped more, and climbed the different toys more often.

When the second infant was introduced into the playpen, both animals became highly emotional. A few changes in behavior were seen between the first and second 15 minutes of each session; the animals mouthed and manipulated the environmental objects significantly more in the latter part of each session. They screeched frequently, and they explored the environment by biting and manipu-lating objects in the cages. One pair of males clung to each other ventrally every time they were together, but most of the infant–infant contact merely involved one animal briefly brushing against another. No significant diet differences were found among any of the behavioral categories.

Although the infants always showed a high level of emotionality in the open field while alone during the presocial condition, they were even more distressed after peer separation. They cooed, screeched, and sucked and clung to themselves more vigorously than before, and they explored the environment less than when initially placed in the playroom.

The picture that emerged from these data is that the adequately fed infants of protein-deprived mothers are as responsive to environmental stimulation as are those of adequately fed mothers. They were all highly emotional, alert to changes in the environment, and not at all apathetic, listless, or irritable, as is reported for children with kwashiorkor or marasmus. Behavior of the maternally deprived infants was indistinguishable in any persistent way from that of the infants whose mothers received adequate protein (Hale, Hillman, & Hendricks, 1975).

BEHAVIOR OF JUVENILES ON PERCEPTUAL-LEARNING TASKS

After the animals were 1 year old, they were made familiar with the standard discrimination testing apparatus. In this apparatus, the caged monkey faced a table on which was placed a retractable tray bearing two food wells, over one of which was a small, distinct object. Monkeys were trained in the general testing procedure until they were capable of displacing a single test-object promptly from a food well for reward. When adapted, they began a series of four perceptual-learning tests using the simultaneous discrimination procedure and the noncorrection method.

Twenty-trial Problems

The task on each trial of the first group of problems was merely to displace that one of two dissimilar stimulus objects that covered a baited food well on a stimulus tray. Each trial began when an opaque screen was raised, exposing the problem to the animal; it ended immediately after the animal displaced a single object and either got the reward or viewed an empty food well. The pairs of discriminanda constituting the consecutive problems differed in multiple characteristics including size, color, shape, and texture. For example, one problem might have consisted of a rubber heel versus an oilcan; another, a wooden block versus a plastic doll head; and so on. No two objects were alike, and no problem was presented more than once to any animal. Thirty-seven animals participated in this experiment and were given 36 simple discrimination learning problems each for 20 trials. Each daily testing session consisted of a single pair of discriminanda presented for 20 trials, adequate for nearly complete learning. Figure 19.7 shows the scores for each block of six problems. All the animals improved in performance when we recorded the percentage of correct responses in the 20 trials. Group differences were variable and did not reflect dietary deficiency.

Multiple Discrimination Learning

In this test, often called *learning set,* the animals were tested on 6 problems each day, 5 days a week, for 10 weeks—for a total of 300 problems. Each problem consisted of only six trials, regardless of the animal's proficiency. Progressive improvement in learning occurred over the problems, but we saw no differences among the groups.

The results were essentially the same for a spatial delayed-response task administered over a period of 10 days. In this task the monkey is shown under which of two identical stimuli the food reward is hidden. It need merely remember which location is correct after a delay of 0, 5, or 10 sec. Performance improved from the first to the second block of 5 days, but differences between groups were not significant. Overall proficiency scores were 76%, 72%, and 81% correct for the 1-g, 2-g, and 4-g infants, respectively.

Concurrent Discrimination Learning

The final learning task was designed to test retention and learning in the presence of interference from other problems. In the 1st week, the monkeys got three 10-trial problems per day, all problems being presented concurrently; that is, Trial 1 was given for all three problems; then Trial 2 was given for all problems;

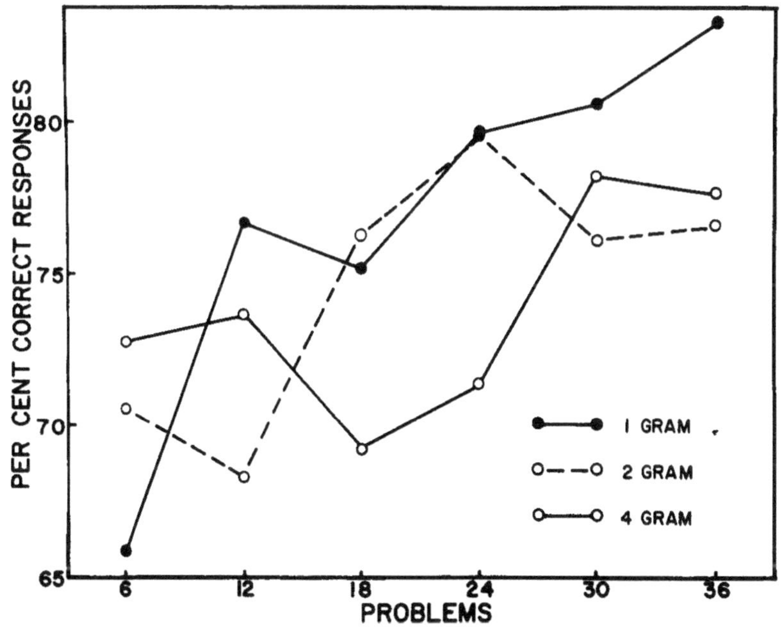

FIG. 19.7. Performance of 1-year-old infants born of mothers fed diets containing different concentrations of protein on 36 object-quality, discrimination learning tasks. (From the *American Journal of Clinical Nutrition.*)

and so on until completion. In the 2nd week, they learned five and, on the final week, seven similar problems, all presented concurrently. On this task the animals demonstrated that they could learn concurrently as many as seven separate problems. Their overall accuracy was 84%, and about 70% of their second-trial responses were correct. As the tasks became harder due to the increased interproblem interference, response accuracy decreased but not greatly. Dietary differences were both practically and statistically insignificant (Fig. 19.8) (Hillman, Khalid, Riopelle, 1978).

Birth Weight and Test Performance

The view is widely held that infants who are "poorly born" suffer numerous maladies including reduced intelligence and adaptive capacity (Churchill et al., 1966; Drillien, 1969; Stoch & Smythe, 1963). In view of the potential importance of perinatal attributes in intellectual competence, we reanalyzed our data to determine whether or not their neonatal status irrespective of prenatal nutrition would have a bearing on their test performance. A thorough examination of the data using powerful regression techniques showed that neither birth weight nor skeletal maturity at birth had any bearing whatsoever on test performance.

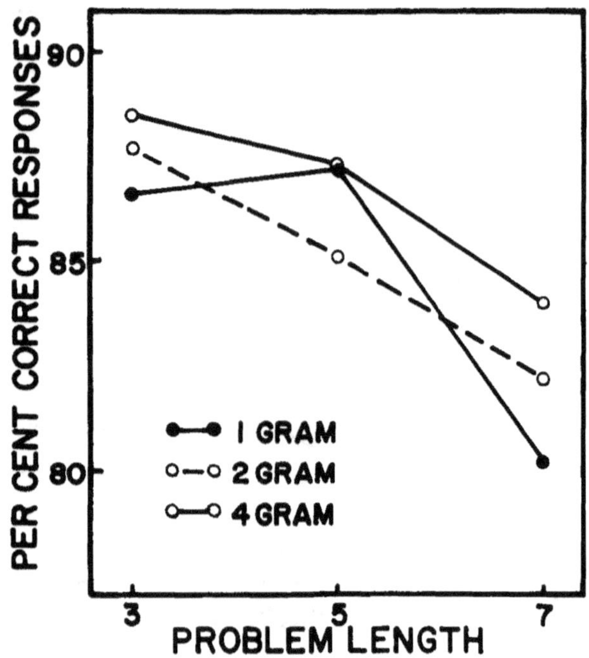

FIG. 19.8. Performance of juvenile rhesus monkeys on concurrently learned discrimination problems. (From the *American Journal of Clinical Nutrition.*)

We may summarize the behavioral data by saying that we have yet to find a significant difference in behavior attributable to dietary deficiency of the mother.

PRENATAL NUTRITION, NEONATAL HEALTH STATUS, AND SUBSEQUENT GROWTH

Absence of Intrauterine Growth Retardation in Infants of Deprived Mothers

The crucial question before us, then, is: How do we account for the failure to obtain a behavioral difference despite substantial reduction in prenatal protein intake? To answer this question, we need to ask whether the babies of the low-protein mothers were physically smaller than the infants of the high-protein mothers. Does any evidence exist to show that the infants suffered intrauterine growth retardation? The answer to all these questions is abundantly clear. No significant differences occurred in birth weights, in body length as measured by the length of the radius shaft, or in body conformation as measured by the ratio of the weight to radius length at birth. Skeletal maturity at birth varied among the infants but not among the groups (Riopelle, Hale, & Watts, 1976). Growth of these infants in terms of weight, of radius length, of the weight-radius index, of food intake, relative food intake, and food utilization efficiency was equal for all groups (Riopelle & Favret, 1977). In short, we have no evidence—behavioral, anatomical, or nutritional—to indicate that the infants of the low-protein mothers were any different from those of the high-protein mothers. Plainly, they were not deprived.

Data similar to ours have been reported from other laboratories. Cheek, Holt, London, Ellenberg, Hill, and Sever (1976) noted that infants of mothers fed diets that provided 1.2 g of protein per kilogram daily weighed only 4% less than the infants of the control mothers when they were delivered by cesarean section at the 157th day of gestation. A number of brain parameters, including DNA, RNA, phospholipids, cholesterol, and protein, were statistically analyzed, and no differences were found between the two groups. In a similar study, Portman et al. (1977) fed a diet that supplied 3.6% of the calories as protein. After delivery by cesarean section at 160 days gestational age, the control infants weighed 485 g, whereas the infants of the protein-deficient mothers weighed 408 g. The animals were kept on the low-protein diet for 7 weeks and were then sacrificed. The protein-deprived were smaller in body weight, brain weight, cerebrum, cerebellum, and brain stem weights. The greatest reduction was in the weight of the brain stems of the protein-deficient animals. Since the infant diet supplied only 3.6% of the calories as protein for the deprived animals, we cannot be certain whether the brain deficiencies at necropsy were primarily due to prenatal or to postnatal undernutrition.

Some lower limit obviously must exist, below which the protein concentration causes substantial harm to the infant. Kohrs, Harper, and Kerr (1976) noted disastrous consequences in pregnant monkeys fed a diet that afforded only .5 g protein per kilogram of body weight per day. In addition to the protein deprivation, the experimental animals reduced their food intake about 20% during the latter part of pregnancy. The infants of the deprived mothers weighed about 15% less than the infants of normally fed mothers, and maternal and fetal mortality were high in the low-protein group. It would appear, then, that maternal protein intakes of .5 g or less per kilogram of body weight per day, or about 5% of the calories, exceed the adaptive capacity of the mother, especially if this low-protein diet is accompanied by a reduction in caloric intake. It should be noted that diets containing less than 5% of the calories as protein are not characteristic of even the populations normally considered to be underfed (Hegsted, 1977).

The conclusion from the primate research on prenatal undernutrition conducted so far is that behavioral differences were not obtained; and they should not have been obtained, because despite the maternal dietary differences, the infants themselves were adequately fed during gestation.

Comparison of Animal Models and the Human Condition

We have seen that rodents are highly susceptible to prenatal undernutrition whereas primates are not. Diets low in protein and probably in calories can be withstood by the pregnant primate but not by the rodent. Cheek (1973) first called attention to the differences in rodents and primates on theoretical grounds. He doubted that prenatal protein-calorie restriction would produce in the offspring of primates the deleterious effects that are seen in rodents. He proposed, in other words, that the deficiency syndrome may be peculiar to small animals. For one thing, the metabolic stress of pregnancy, as represented by the ratio of the total birth weight to the gestation time, is significantly lower in primates than it is in lower orders of animals (Payne & Wheeler, 1968). Pregnant rats accumulate protein and water stores for the rat fetus at a rate that is 25 times higher than that of the monkey and 60 times higher than that of the human. But that fact alone is not a sufficient explanation. Probably one critical factor is the long gestation time of primates. The rat must produce within 21 days a litter of perhaps 10 pups that collectively, with the other products of conception, weigh 25% of the mother's weight at time of conception. The rhesus monkey takes 5.5 months to produce a single infant and the other conceptional products, which collectively weigh 5% to 10% of the mother. Some 200 species of primates are recognized, and variation would be expected in these parameters. For example, New World monkeys have higher fetal-maternal weight ratios than do rhesus monkeys. The difference, however, is probably a reflection of their evolutionary specialization to a habitat with little seasonal variation.

Another factor is involved: Because the rodent produces a large litter, the mother cannot adjust her blood nutrient supplies to fit the requirements of each of the individual fetuses. Hence, one or more may be underfed. The rhesus mother, on the other hand, who has only a single infant to nourish, can adjust the conditions of the pregnancy on the basis of feedback from the fetus in order to keep its development within acceptable bounds. An exquisitely sensitive technique available to the rhesus is to modify the gestation length. Studies of our own animals (Riopelle & Hale, 1975) show that gestation length is modified by the protein intake of the mother, her conception weight, the season of the year in which she becomes pregnant, and the sex and size of her infant.

The evolutionary adaptation of the primate with respect to pregnancy is quite different from that of the rodent in another respect. Consider the single versus the multiple birth. In general, monotocus animals produce infants that are physiologically competent at time of delivery to withstand most of the environmental insults they will encounter. If they do not, the infants will die and the species will terminate. Both the mother and the infant must be able to withstand the rigors of the environment. Because no excess infants are born, the strategy, then, is to maximize the competence of the mother and the infant to enable survival of the single infant. The situation with litter-bearing animals is quite different. Such species can perpetuate themselves, with a lower percentage of infants surviving, by producing many infants. Not all of the infants in a litter need survive to allow the species to continue. Accordingly, a higher percentage of rodents will be adversely affected by prenatal environmental insults than will be the case for primates. Accordingly, we are not surprised that rats born of protein-deprived mothers are more affected than their monkey counterparts. It is precisely this principle that makes rodents the species of choice for the assessment of environmental pollutants, carcinogens, and other toxic agents.

Rodents can survive despite susceptibility to nutritional deficiency during pregnancy by deferring mating until optimal nutrients are available. Since gestation is brief, mating and delivery are likely to occur in the same season, so the nutritional conditions that apply at the time of conception will hold through delivery and probably through lactation. The length of the gestation period of the primate, lasting 5.5 months for rhesus monkeys, spans at least two seasons, during one of which the food supply to the mother is likely to be reduced either in quality or in quantity. Indeed, many monkeys deliver their babies just before or just after the beginning of the rainy season in spring. This implies that pregnancy occurs and transpires through a dry season. Thus, the species has opted for a rigorous pregnancy. The champion spartan primates seems to be the Japanese Macaque, which conceives in September or October and delivers in the springtime. Gestation, then, is carried through the snowy winter months when food supply is reduced to absolute minimums. To have evolved such long gestation periods, primates must also have evolved adequate means to accommodate the intervening periods of suboptimal nutrition.

The goal of any model is to understand the human problem. If our conclusions about the robustness of primates are correct, they ought to hold for human populations as well. Comparisons are never perfect between feral animals and industrialized populations, who have canned goods and frozen foods to eliminate the seasonal variations in diet. Nevertheless, some human data are at hand that are not entirely contrary to what we have reported. Protein seems not to be the limiting factor for birth weight in the diets of pregnant Guatemalan women (Habicht, Yarborough, & Klein, 1974). Supplementation with protein during pregnancy has only a minor effect on birth weight. The resistance of survivors who were exposed to prenatal maternal deprivation during wartime is documented by Stein, Susser, Saenger, and Marolla (1975). They could find no evidence that prenatal malnutrition caused by the siege of Holland impaired mental competence in young adults.

We have not made a survey of seasonal distributions of birth in relation to dietary intakes, but Wilmsen (1978) examined the seasonal dietary intakes of the Kalahari San. They, like rhesus monkeys in their natural habitat, experience periodic feast and famine conditions. They are not, by any measure, malnourished. Conception is timed so that the model numbers of birth occur during the months of March and April. The peak months of meat consumption are, in contrast, April, May, and June, which are during or after the peak birth season. During the latter part of pregnancy, cucumbers and berries, foods that are low in protein, are most often eaten. It is not inconceivable that the human reproductive adaptation to seasonal fluctuations in food supply is to time mating so that pregnancy takes place during a period when the mother is physiologically most capable, through increased metabolic efficiency, to withstand the lowered plane of nutrition. The failure of the rhesus monkey to show the spurt in weight upon the return to the high-protein diet, after bearing an infant and prolonged low-protein intake, testifies to her improved metabolic efficiency during pregnancy. A remarkable human case that has some similarity was reported by Montgomery and Pincus (1955). Their young patient was made metabolically inefficient by the surgical loss of much of her small intestine. Her state of health was precarious at best. When she became pregnant, she gained weight, felt good, and delivered a healthy, normal baby, after which she promptly returned to her unfortunate state of health.

CAVEATS AND CONCLUSIONS

A wise person has said that a model is a device we use that allows us to believe we know more about something than we actually do. This counsel gives cause for caution. It would be erroneously hasty for us to overgeneralize our findings. Some limits on exegesis are required. The studies reviewed were directed toward an understanding of mechanisms that might operate to affect brain growth and behavioral capacity adversely if nutritional insult might occur during the period of cell proliferation and rapid growth. That problem is not exactly the same as the one faced by the millions of persons who are the malnourished subjects of the report of the World Food Council (summarized in McGovern, 1979). The typical problem for these unfortunates began generations before they were born and continued throughout their entire lives—not, as in our study, beginning during gestation and ending at delivery. Moreover, our infants were well nourished from delivery forward. Our experiments do not simulate the human problem; rather, they parallel only unusual circumstances, those of war, or sudden (moderately long, but not permanent) famine caused by a natural disaster among a normally adequately nourished people. As the Stein et al. (1975) studies show, however, they are not beyond human experience.

The finding that rhesus monkeys (and, by extension, those species that must experience a period of suboptimal nutrition during pregnancy) are—with their long gestations and single-offspring births—more resistant to malnutrition during pregnancy than are the litter-bearing species most common in research laboratories has implications for our selection of animal models in laboratory studies of nutrition during development. Rats are not miniature monkeys with white hair and pink eyes, and monkeys are not little humans with fur coats. Each species has its special characteristics and its appropriate usefulness and limitations in research. The value of the data they produce to the understanding of physiological processes and to the solution of human problems will depend to a great extent on the wise recognition and utilization of their differences in research.

ACKNOWLEDGMENT

The author's research reported herein was supported by grant HD 0749 from the National Institute of Child Health and Human Development of the National Institutes of Health, U.S. Public Health Service.

REFERENCES

Baird, E. The influence of social and economic factors on stillbirths and neonatal deaths. *Journal of Obstetrics and Gynaecology of the British Empire*, 1945, *5*, 36–42.

Bandera, E., & Churchill, J. Prematurity and neurological disorders. *Henry Ford Hospital*, 1961, *9*, 414–418.

Barnes, R. H., Moore, A. U., Reid, I. M., & Pond, W. G. Effects of food deprivation on behavioral patterns. In N. S. Scrimshaw & J. E. Gordon (Eds.), *Malnutrition learning & behavior*. Cambridge, Mass.: MIT Press, 1968.

Caldwell, D. F., & Churchill, J. A. Learning ability in the progeny of rats administered a protein deficient diet during the second half of gestation. *Neurology*, 1967, *17*, 95–99.

Caputo, D. V., & Mandell, W. Consequences of low birthweight. *Developmental Psychology*, 1970, *3*, 363–383.

Cheek, D. B. Brain growth and nucleic acids: The affect of nutritional deprivation. In F. Richardson (Ed.), *Brain and intelligence: The ecology of child development*. Hyattsville, Md.: National Educational Press, 1973.

Cheek, D. B., Holt, A. B., London, W. T., Ellenberg, J. A., Hill, D. E., & Sever, J. L. Nutritional studies in the pregnant rhesus monkey—the effect of protein-calorie or protein-deprivation on growth of the fetal brain. *American Journal of Clinical Nutrition* 1976, *29*, 1149–1157.

Chow, B. F., & Lee, C. J. Effect of dietary restriction of pregnant rats on body weight gain of the offspring. *Journal of Nutrition*, 1964, *82*, 10–18.

Churchill, J. A., Neff, J. W., & Caldwell, D. F. Birth weight and intelligence. *Obstetrics and Gynecology*, 1966, *28*, 425–429.

Clark, G. M., Zamenhof, S., Van Marthens, E., Grauel, L., & Kruger, L. The effect of prenatal malnutrition on dimensions of cerebral cortex. *Brain Research*, 1973, *54*, 397–402.

Davison, A. N., & Dobbing, J. The developing brain. In A. N. Davison & J. Dobbing (Eds.), *Applied neurochemistry*. Oxford: Blackwell, 1968.

Dobbing, J. Effects of experimental malnutrition on development of the nervous system. In N. S. Scrimshaw & J. E. Gordon (Eds.), *Malnutrition, learning and behavior*. Cambridge, Mass.. MIT Press, 1968.

Drillien, C. M. Studies in mental handicap. II: Some obstetric factors of possible aetiological significance. *Archives of Diseases of Childhood*, 1968, *43*, 283–294.

Drillien, C. M. School disposal and performance for children of different birth weight, born 1953–1960. *Archives of Diseases of Childhood*, 1969, *44*, 562–570.

Enesco, M., & Leblond, C. P. Increase in cell number as a factor in the growth of the organs of the young male rat. *Journal of Embryology and Experimental Morphology,* 1962, *10,* 530-561.

F.A.O. *Third World Food Survey* (Freedom from Hunger Campaign Basic Study II). Rome: F.A.O., 1963.

Gruenwald, T. Infants of low birth weight among 5,000 delivered. *Pediatrics,* 1964, *34,* 157-162.

Habicht, J. P., Yarborough, C., & Klein, R. E. Assessing nutritional status in a field study of malnutrition and mental development: Specifically, sensitivity and congruity of indices of nutritional status. In J. Cravioto, L. Hambraeus, & B. Vahlquist (Eds.), *Symposium of the Swedish Nutrition Foundation* (Vol. 12), *Early malnutrition and mental development.* Uppsala: Almqvist and Wiksell, 1974.

Hale, P. A., Hillman, N. M., & Hendricks, D. *Protein deprivation in primates. IX. Individual and social behaviors of infants born of deprived mothers.* Unpublished, 1975.

Hawrylewicz, E. J., Kissane, J., Blair, W. H., & Hepner, C. A. Effect of maternal protein nutrition on neonatal lung development and mitochondrial function. *Nutrition Reports International,* 1973, *7,* 253-270.

Hegsted, D. M. Safe allowance of protein (letter). *American Journal of Clinical Nutrition,* 1977, *30,* 465-466.

Hill, D. E., Myers, R. E., Holt, E. B., Scott, R. E., & Cheek, D. B. Fetal growth retardation produced by experimental placental insufficiency in the rhesus monkey. II. Chemical composition of the brain, liver, muscle, and carcass. *Biology of the Neonate,* 1971, *19,* 68-82.

Hillman, N. M., Khalid, S. R., & Riopelle, A. J. Protein deprivation in primates: X. Test performance of juveniles born of deprived mothers. *American Journal of Clinical Nutrition,* 1978, *31,* 388-393.

Kaelber, C. T., & Pugh, T. F. Influence of intrauterine relations on intelligence of twins. *New England Journal of Medicine,* 1969, *280,* 1030-1034.

Kohrs, M. B., Harper, A. E., & Kerr, G. R. Effects of a low-protein diet during pregnancy of the rhesus monkey: I. Reproductive efficiency. *American Journal of Clinical Nutrition,* 1976, *29,* 136-145.

Lashley, K. S. *Brain mechanisms and intelligence.* Chicago: University Chicago Press, 1929.

McGovern, G. Human rights and world hunger. *National Forum, The Phi Kappa Phi Journal,* 1979, *49,* 7-10.

Miller, S. A. Nutrition in the neonatal development of protein metabolism. *Federation Proceedings,* 1970, *29,* 1497-1502.

Montgomery, T. L., & Pincus, I. J. A nutritional problem in pregnancy resulting from extensive resection of the small bowel. *American Journal of Obstetrics and Gynecology,* 1955, *69,* 865-868.

Mowbray, J. B., & Cadell, T. E. Early behavior patterns in rhesus monkeys. *Journal of Comparative and Physiological Psychology* 1962, *55,* 350-357.

Myers, R. E., Hill, D. E., Holt, A. B., Scott, R. E., Mellits, E. D., & Cheek, D. B. Fetal growth retardation produced by experimental placental insufficiency in the rhesus monkey. I. Body weight organ size. *Biology of the Neonate,* 1971, *18,* 379-394.

Naismith, D. J. The fetus as a parasite. *Proc. Nutr. Soc.,* 1969, *28,* 25-31.

Nehrich, H., & Stuart, J. A. The effect of prenatal protein restriction on the developing mouse cerebrum. Journal of Nutrition, 1978, *108,* 368-372.

Nissen, H. W. Phylogenetic comparisons. In S. S. Stevens (Ed.), *Handbook of experimental psychology.* New York: Wiley, 1951.

Parekh, U. C., Pherwani, A., Udani, P. M., & Mukherjee, S. Brain weight and head circumference in fetus, infant, and children of different nutritional and socioeconomic groups. *Indian Pediatrics,* 1970, *7,* 347-358.

Payne, P. R., & Wheeler, E. F. Comparative nutrition in pregnancy and lactation. *Proceedings of the Nutrition Society*, 1968, *27*, 129-138.

Portman, O. W., Alexander, M., Neuringer, M., Novy, M., Illingworth, R., & Uno, H. The effects of perinatal malnutrition on lipid composition of neural tissues from rhesus monkeys. *Journal of Nutrition*, 1977, *107*, 2228-2235.

Rider, A. A., & Simonson, M. Effect on rat offspring of maternal diet deficient in calories but not in protein. *Nutrition Reports International*, 1973, *7*, 361-370.

Riopelle, A. J., & Favret, R. Protein deprivation in primates: XIII. Growth of infants born of deprived mothers. *Human Biology*, 1977, *43*, 221-233.

Riopelle, A. J., & Hale, P. A. Nutritional and environmental factors affecting gestation length in rhesus monkeys. *American Journal of Clinical Nutrition*, 1975, *28*, 1170-1176.

Riopelle, A. J., Hale, P. A., & Watts, E. S. Protein deprivation in primates: VII. Determinants of size and skeletal maturity at birth in rhesus monkeys. *Human Biology*, 1976, *48*, 203-222.

Riopelle, A. J., Hill, C. W., & Li, S-C. Protein deprivation in primates. V. Fetal wastage and neonatal status of infants born of deprived mothers. *American Journal of Clinical Nutrition*, 1975, *28*, 983-993.

Riopelle, A. J., Hill, C. W., Li, S-C., Wolf, R. H., Seibold, H. R., & Smith, J. L. Protein deprivation in primates. I. Nonpregnant adult rhesus monkeys. *American Journal of Clinical Nutrition*, 1974, *27*, 13-21.

Riopelle, A. J., Hill, C. W., Li, S-C., Wolf, R. H., Seibold, H. R., & Smith, J. L. Protein deficiency in primates. IV. Pregnant rhesus monkeys. *American Journal of Clinical Nutrition*, 1975, *28*, 20-28.

Riopelle, A. J., & Shell, W. F. Protein deprivation in primates. XI. Determinants of weight change during and after pregnancy. *American Journal of Clinical Nutrition*, 1978, *31*, 394-400.

Rosso, P. Maternal-fetal exchange during protein malnutrition in the rat. Placental transfer of glucose and a non-metabolizable glucose analog. *Journal of Nutrition*, 1977, *107*, 2006-2010.

Sedlers, A., Berends, H., Kim, H.-S., Stone, D. F., Weiss, W., Deutschberger, J., & Jackson, E. The placental weight-birth weight relationship. *Developmental Medicine and Child Neurology*, 1967, *9*, 160-171.

Slemons, J. M. The nutrition of the fetus. *American Journal of Obstetrical Diseases of Women*, 1919, *80*, 194-210.

Smart, J. L., Adlard, P. F., & Dobbing, J. Effect of maternal undernutrition and other factors in the birth weight in the rat. *Biology of the Neonate.*, 1972, *20*, 236-244.

Stein, Z., Susser, M., Saenger, G., & Marolla, F. *Famine & human development*. New York: Oxford University Press, 1975.

Stewart, R. J. C., & Platt, B. S. Nervous system damage in experimental protein-calorie deficiency. In N. S. Scrimshaw & J. E. Gordon (Eds.), *Malnutrition, learning and behavior*. Cambridge, Mass.: MIT Press, 1968.

Stoch, M. B., & Smythe, P. M. Does undernutrition during infancy inhibit brain growth and subsequent intellectual development? *Archives of Diseases of Childhood*, 1963, *38*, 546-552.

Wigglesworth, J. S. Experimental growth retardation in the fetal rat. *Journal of Pathology and Bacteriology*, 1964, *88*, 1-13.

Willerman, L., & Churchill, J. A. Intelligence and birth weight in identical twins. *Child Development*, 1967, *38*, 623-629.

Wilmsen, E. N. Seasonal effects of dietary intake on Kalahari San. *Federation Proceedings*, 1978, *37*, 65-72.

Winick, N. Nutrition and cell growth. *Nutrition Reviews*, 1968, *26*, 195-197.

Winick, N., Rosso, P., & Waterlow, J. Cellular growth of cerebrum, cerebellum, and brain stem in normal and marasmic children. *Experimental Neurology*, 1970, *26*, 393-400.

Zamenhof, S., Van Marthens, E., & Grauel, L. DNA (cell number) in neonatal brain: Alteration by maternal dietary caloric restriction. *Nutrition Reports International*, 1971, *4*, 269–274.

Zamenhof, S., Van Marthens, E., & Margolis, F. L. DNA, cell number, and protein in neonatal brain: Alteration by maternal dietary restriction. *Science*, 1968, *160*, 322-323.

Zeman, F. J., Shrader, R. E., & Allen, L. N. Persistent defects of maternal deficiency in postnatal rats. *Nutrition Reports International*, 1973, *7*, 421-436.

Zeman, F. J., & Stanbrough, E. C. Effect of maternal deficiency on cellular development in the fetal rat. *Journal of Nutrition*, 1969, *99*, 372-382.

20 Elaborations of Hebb's Cell Assembly Theory

D. O. Hebb

A. RECRUITING AND INHIBITING CEREBRAL PROCESSES AS CONTROL MECHANISMS IN PERCEPTUAL LEARNING, ATTENTION AND THOUGHT[1]

Psychology–or physiology–may have given you a picture of learning like this. You may think of a pathway through the brain with a stimulus at this end, a response at that end, and some synapses in between. Each time the stimulus is applied the response follows, getting a little quicker or stronger each time because the connections at the synapses are getting a little closer. But that picture has no relation at all to what actually happens in the home and in the classroom. At most it applies to the case where the child must learn to make some specific response to a specific stimulus. How often does that occur? How big a part is that of the educational process? And even when learning is of that kind, the theory forgets that there are wrong responses to be got rid of, as well as the right one to be strengthened. But the most important kinds of learning are often ones where no specific response is to be made, and where the child must generalize and become prepared to respond in the future in different ways, in various future situations. This learning is not a stimulus-response conditioning, but consists of a modified relation between internal ideational systems. There is no particular response at the time the learning occurs, and whether it has occurred or not becomes evident only when one sees, later, whether the child's behavior has

[1]Excerpted from "Physiological learning theory" by D. O. Hebb, *J. abn. child Psychology*, 1976, *4*, 309–314.

changed the next time he is exposed to that kind of situation–or even a different situation, but one in which the information acquired earlier is relevant.

In real life, if not in the laboratory, learning is less a matter of conditioned responses than of seeing what goes with what, so that later one can act appropriately. This observational learning, as Estes calls it, brings us to the problem of perception, and there are strong suggestions that it is here that the brain-injured child has his difficulties. Relations that are not perceived cannot be learned, and if they are not generalized in perception, beyond the specific features of the learning situation, they can have little value. It is common to blame learning difficulties on a failure of attention, on inability to concentrate or to avoid being distracted, and of course there are such defects of attention. The hyperactive child, certainly, is inattentive. But which is the cause: a primary disorder of attention, or an earlier failure of perceptual learning? I would propose to you that *attention, as such, is not a power of which the child has much or little,* but instead is an aspect of consequence of perception and the concurrent cognitive activity.

What does attention mean, in the sense of keeping one's attention on a particular task, or sticking to a particular line of thought–in short, attention in the sense of ability to concentrate? Clearly, it means that one cortical-cognitive set of activities is able to maintain itself in spite of "noise" from irrelevant sensory stimulation and from the spontaneous activity of neurons, in the brain, that are not part of that cortical-cognitive process.

It may be overlooked that having a big brain is not entirely helpful when it comes to learning one particular thing, or carrying out a particular task. The value of a big brain is in the capacity to learn many things, but the trouble is that there must be many more pathways, or many more neurons, than are needed for any one task. The neural cell is a living thing; it must be active or die. If it is not stimulated, not given its normal job of transmitting excitations, it eventually fires anyway unless it is inhibited. Activity of the "extra" neurons–those unnecessary for the present cognitive activity–will tend to be disruptive, unless they are either inhibited or are somehow incorporated into that present cognitive activity. This clearly points to the importance of inhibition, which is already emphasized in the literature, and I will be returning to that topic. But it does not strike me as plausible to suppose that all of those excess neurons, which must be a great majority, can be inhibited by a very much smaller number, and for a period of minutes or longer; I do not believe that this can be the real function of inhibition (what I think it is I will say later).

Instead, I make the guess that "concentration," and the ability to attend, means that the perceptual process and the ongoing cognitive activity between them have, so to speak, enlisted wide support throughout the brain–much more massive activity, as a total, than necessary, perhaps, but constituting also a large safety factor to ensure the continuance of that line of thought and consequently the maintenance of attention on the relevant aspects of the sensory environment.

In other words, instead of the small minority of neurons–the ones necessary to the thing being learned–being able to inhibit the much greater majority of the rest of the neurons in the brain, the minority may draw in most of the majority and control them by making them part of itself, as an organized total activity. Here it is implied that the brain-injured child's problem of attention is more likely to result from internal than from external noise. In fact, it is even possible that exposure to a familiar interesting environment may help the child to attend rather than distracting him, if this complexity is incorporated into the *Aufgabe,* the controlling idea of the task, and makes it more interesting too.

That can only be possible if there is a past history of complex associative connections of the various mental activities involved, and also a complex perceptual learning, so that the percept is not merely a simple sensory input. I don't mean to embark here on a discussion of thought, nor any detailed discussion of perception, but I must remind you of the complications. Estes (1970) points out that there are hierarchies of perception, and in my own theorizing I have also proposed that perception consists in the arousal of cell-assemblies of lower and higher order, whose activity constitutes representative processes–that is, ideas–that range from the very concrete and specific to the highly abstract. Such proposals gain physiological support, at least in principle, from the parallel with Hubel and Wiesel's (1968) simple, complex, and hypercomplex cells, which are also hierarchically organized. The simple cell is directly excited by a very specific local stimulation. The complex cell is excited by any of a number of simple cells of the same kind but varying somewhat in locus. The activity of a complex cell is a generalization, on a minute scale, since the same response is made to different stimuli; on a minute scale, it is also an abstraction, since it is a response to only a selected part of the information in the stimulus event. And so with the activity of the hypercomplex cell, in being fired only by complex cells. The parallel with first-, second-, third-, and perhaps higher-order cell-assemblies, on a more molar scale, is very close. Activity of a first-order assembly theoretically is a very specific perception, of a horizontal line in the visual field, for example, or a vowel sound, or a sensation of roughness; activity of a second-order assembly is more generalized, as perception of the line anywhere in the field, or the phoneme at a higher or lower pitch, or roughnesses at different loci. Perception of an object or a word would be a still higher level, an assembly of the third or fourth order.

You see how complicated this is getting. I don't intend to go on with it, but I will put it in a more familiar context to give it more meaning. Suppose your eye falls on a cat. What do you perceive? Depending on the situation and on what you are concerned with at the moment, you may perceive a bit of fur, a particular pet, or just *a cat* (more general, more abstract), or even *an animal* (still more so). Or you hear the word *run,* and your perception is of a reference to a particular action, or it may be also of the word as an action word, a verb (Hebb, Lambert, & Tucker 1971). The point is that from all we know about the structure of the brain and its handling of input information, this is the kind of complexity that is demanded of the brain of the growing child, and it is easy to see how minimal brain damage might retard such a perceptual and cognitive development. If these activities are not well established, it is easy to see how the ongoing process might be susceptible to interference from the "noise" of irrelevant sensory inputs and the spontaneous firing of the "unnecessary" neurons of the cortex. Development of normal ability to concentrate and keep attention fixed on an assigned task, I propose, is a matter of first developing those higher-order cell-assembly activities, and secondly enriching them with associative connections interwoven like a tapestry so that the core processes of a given mental activity may reduce conflict, not by inhibiting other activity, but by co-opting and imposing its own order widely throughout the brain. When this can happen we speak of the learning task as "interesting," which clearly means it is one that engages the thought process fully. The necessary richness of associative connections must be a function of the early environment, and from this point of view we can perhaps understand the disastrous and lasting effect, reported by Goldfarb (1943), of 3 early years spent in an orphanage (also see Hunt, 1961). The orphanage must lack the variety of experience to be found in the ordinary home and so fail to develop that complex of associations to the same degree.

Now let me return to the topic of inhibition and what I believe is its true significance. I have two theoretical propositions for your consideration: one, that the secret of the extraordinary efficiency of the normal human brain is to be found in the number of inhibitory neurons it contains, much higher, apparently, than in other species (Rakic, 1975); and two, that the inhibitory neuron may be more fragile, more easily destroyed by anoxia, for example, at birth, than the excitatory neuron. The suggestion is that the child with minimal brain damage may have suffered a selective loss of inhibitory neurons.

The reason for thinking that inhibition has special importance intellectually is this: Thinking is a serial activity, a sequence of events, and when one of the events in the sequence has done its job and excited the following event it should cease; if its activity continues it must be disruptive, and a main function of the inhibitory neurons in the brain, I propose, is to shut off that activity once it has fired the next stage. If thought depends on a series of cell-assembly activities, what I once called a phase sequence, such that assembly A fires assembly B, and B fires C, and so on, When A has fired B it can only be disruptive if A continues to be active itself-like an actor in a play who keeps on repeating his speech and keeps on giving a second actor the cue for his speech.

In *The Organization of Behavior* I proposed that the function of the recurrent circuits of the brain was to maintain firing: The available evidence when I wrote made it appear that a neuron fired once would not fire again for some period of time, lacking specific stimulation, because of the period of subnormality. For repetitive firing I thought that it would have to be restimulated, and that this was the function of the closed circuits. But it seems instead that a neuron fired once tends to fire several times at least, and I am now inclined to think that those circuits may be predominantly inhibitory and serve the purpose of promptly shutting off a cell-assembly once it has performed its function of firing, or taking part in firing, another. A maintained activity I think must be a function of a closed network of assemblies, not of single cells. The system must be less efficient when a component continues active after its function has been performed; without inhibitory neurons thought must be woolly, less precise, less capable of a given train of ideas that are discrete and uncontaminated by associated but irrelevant ideas.

And this must apply to learning too, when learning involves perception and thought-as all cognitive (nonreflexive) learning must. Perception like thought is intrinsically serial, a succession of part-perceptions. If it should be true that minimal brain damage is apt to have a special effect on inhibitory neurons, perception and thought and cognitive learning would not be eliminated but they would be less effective, less capable of the maintained selectivity that we know as concentration on one topic. Thought, learning, and attention—attention in the wider sense—must all suffer on the assumption (1) that the source of the normal high efficiency of the human brain, pound for pound or gram for gram in comparison with that of other species, lies in the known higher frequency of short-axon cells, assumed to be inhibitory in function, and the assumption (2) that these unmyelinated small-diameter neurons are more vulnerable to toxins and nutritive lack-especially anoxia. With such loss no gross signs of brain damage need appear, no specific incapacity at a stimulus-response level need be evident, and yet there would be serious impairment of higher-order cognitive processes.

B. DIVERGENT CONDUCTION IN ASSOCIATION CORTEX[2]

For Lashley, mind or consciousness was an organized activity of the cerebrum. How then could he (1958) say as he did to this Association that "no activity of mind is ever conscious"? He went on to explain what he meant by this-namely, that mind is not conscious of its own processes but did not explain what he himself called the paradox of saying what he did. The explanation lies in recognizing two meanings of the term conscious. The first meaning is a reference to a state of the brain, one phase of the diurnal cycle: the state of the normal, waking, alert, adult human being or higher animal, as contrasted with one that is comatose. The other meaning refers not to the whole organized activity of the cerebrum, nor to the whole activity of mind, but to those parts of the activity of which

[2]Excerpted from "Cerebral organization and consciousness" by D. O. Hebb. In "Sleep and altered states of consciousness," *Proc. Assoc. Res. Nerv. Ment. Dis.*, 1967, *45*, 1-7.

the mind itself is conscious. It is one thing to say that I am conscious-of the world about me. It is another to say that some of my ideas are conscious and mean by this that I am conscious of them. One must question this latter usage. There is reason to believe that there are no ideas of which we are conscious, that introspection does not exist (as a direct awareness, that is, rather than complex inference (Boring, 1953; Humphrey, 1951). In that case the second meaning of conscious is illusory and might be avoided; however, if it is to be used, along with its corollary of an unconscious mind, I would urge that the user should always make clear that he means it in this second and now somewhat doubtful sense.

Modern thought has come a long way from the time, in the 1920's, when it was possible to debate whether consciousness was the result of impulses crossing synapses with high resistance, or low resistance-consciousness being like a kind of juice squeezed out of the neuron. The modern period is mainly marked by emphasis on the brain-stem control of level of consciousness and might be dated from a suggestion of Penfield's in 1938–a suggestion that, I regret to say, I failed to appreciate at the time. He concluded that consciousness must be more closely correlated with some discrete subcortical region than with any specific cortical activity and that "the indispensable substratum of consciousness lies outside the cerebral cortex." With hindsight, one can see this pointing directly to the epochal paper of Moruzzi and Magoun (1949) on the brain-stem activating system, one of the focal points of our present discussion.

Lashley and Penfield are the two outstanding names when one discusses the problem of cerebral organization and consciousness, and I want to take a moment to put their contributions in perspective before going on. Lashley's weakness was an over-reaction from his own early simpleminded Watsonian connectionism, which in effect ended up as an opposition to any form of theory. His theoretical contribution was thus negative and destructive only, but it was at the same time enormously clarifying, and it is to him more than to any other man, I believe, that our understanding of theoretical issues in this field is due. As for Penfield, his great contributions are empirical, in the demonstration of fundamentally important phenomena of brain function. His theory of memory is unsatisfactory, I think, because of not having a behavioristic foundation, of not being an outgrowth of that simpleminded S-R formulation that we all disavow in its cruder forms but that nonetheless is the starting point, the germ from which the theory of learning springs, even for those whose purpose seems to be to destroy S-R theory but to destroy only by modifying and elaborating and making it grow into something more flexible and powerful. But whatever difficulties there may be for the theory, Penfield has made discoveries that are truly fundamental for psychology and the theory of cerebral organization: the astonishing lack of apparent importance of prefrontal lobe in that organization (compared, e.g., to temporal lobe), the major significance of dysfunction for psychological processes, and the special relation, at least, of temporal lobe to memory. These discoveries must have lasting significance. Finally, Penfield's (1959) delineation of the speech areas in conscious patients, of first importance in itself, has a special significance for our understanding of cerebral organization.

The significance lies in the fact that electrical stimulation of speech-area cortex does not produce speech but impairs or prevents it. This is in contrast to stimulation of primary sensory or motor cortex, which mimics the normal function of the tissue instead of being directly opposed. It draws attention to a property of neural transmission in higher centers, and an aspect of cerebral function, that has been little regarded by the neurophysiologist although it appears to be related to the much regarded function of ARAS, the "ascending reticular activating system" or arousal system.

Fundamentally the role of the cerebrum like that of the rest of the central nervous system must be to act as a communications system, a transmitter of excitations. If so, how or why should so much of the cortex consist of the so-called silent areas where electrical stimulation is not transmitted or has only a negative effect? As I see it, the answer has much to tell us about cerebral organization and consciousness–why the activating system is needed for consciousness, as well as the nature of the conscious activities themselves.

The answer (as I see it) is that transmission in the cerebrum is largely via divergent pathways with no automatic provision of summation at the synapse, such as is provided by the overlapping axon collaterals at each synaptic junction in the great afferent and efferent tracts, which are organized in parallel. In divergent pathways, the summation necessary for reliable excitation of the postsynaptic neuron, therefore, must be provided elsewhere; hence, the necessity of bombardment from ARAS, to provide that summation. With it, synaptic transmission in the "silent" regions–which I think would be better known as regions of divergent conduction becomes possible. It is clear that organized activity in these regions must depend on a concordance of neurons at a distance from each other; firing all the neurons in one small region, by electrical stimulation, must negate their normal function, whereas a similar stimulation in a region of parallel conduction would reproduce normal function: for here the neurons that lie side by side are normally excited together.

It seems also that transmission in these divergent-pathway regions of the cerebrum needs the further summation coming from activities that are already going on in the cerebrum, so that only those messages that are related to the concurrent activity tend to be transmitted and have their effect on behavior. These regions have an essential screening function. This is strictly an inference from the behavioral evidence of the selectivity of attention, and of thought generally, so I will not expand on it here. But I cannot speak on the topic of cerebral organization and consciousness without saying at least that I believe consciousness to consist in the activity of the closed or re-entrant circuits of Lorente de Nó, and transmission of excitations from circuit to circuit, with a constant motor outflow as well as constantly varying sensory input to the system.

The importance of divergent conduction in the higher centers of the central nervous system is that it does that screening that I have referred to, in addition to permitting a semiautonomous activity in the system. Without it, man would be an automaton-like stimulus-response animal, programmed by his environment–whereas, in fact, he programs himself to a very large extent in what we call voluntary behavior (Hebb, 1966).

C. TO KNOW YOUR OWN MIND[3]

All available information points to the conclusion that introspection does not exist; knowledge of mind is inferential, not phenomenal. The implications of this state of affairs however seems not to be recognized; psychologists and philosphers, many of them, still talk as if they had first-hand information about mental processes that gives them a sure basis for evaluating theory. Any such discussion today is incompetent. Mind and its activity are as theoretical as the atom, and ideas about their nature must be justified as theoretical ideas are in other fields.

I use the term introspection here in its proper sense of direct self-knowledge by the mind, the immediate awareness of its own content or activity. There is also a looser use with which I am not concerned, which refers simply to the fact that we do have a certain amount of information about what is going on in our minds at any given moment. The point made here is that the knowledge, such as it is (very limited, mostly), is the result of one or more steps of inference.

The authoritative modern critique of introspective data is by Humphrey (1951). His close analysis of the reported introspections of Titchener's group at Cornell shows that they described not sensory content, as they supposed, but the external objects and events that they perceived or imaged. No one has shown error in this analysis or refuted Humphrey's conclusion that

> we perceive objects directly, not through the intermediary of 'presentations', 'ideas', or 'sensations'. Similarly, we imagine objects directly, not through the intermediary of images, though images are present as an important part of the whole activity. (p. 129)

What one is aware of in perception is not a percept but the object that is perceived; what is given in imagination is an illusory external object, not an internal mental representation called an image. This latter, and the percept, are inferred. They undoubtedly exist, as atoms do likewise.

---

[3]By D. O. Hebb. In Nicholas, John M. (ed.), *Images, Perception and Knowledge*. Dordrecht-Holland: D. Reidel Publishing Co., 1977, 213–219.

C. S. Peirce came to the same conclusion over a century ago (Buchler, 1940, pp. 230, 308; Goudge, 1950, p. 232; Gallie, 1952, p. 80). It is hardly necessary to say that Peirce, on this point, has not been refuted either. He has been disregarded instead. It is commonly said that Peirce was ahead of his time, with the apparent implication that we have caught up with him now, but this is a point on which he still is ahead. The point is one of fundamental philosophic significance, affecting any discussion of the nature of mind. If it is not accepted, perhaps because of its connection with other views of Peirce such as his theory of signs, there is still Humphrey's independent analysis as confirmation. It seems therefore that it is not technically competent to go on taking introspective awareness for granted, without first showing how Peirce and Humphrey, both of them, were wrong in denying its existence.

1. HOW THE INFERENCE IS MADE

Having concluded that such self-knowledge is inferential, one has some obligation to ask what the basis of inference is. This was for me a difficult task and I was concerned with it for more than a year – and then discovered that Peirce had found the answer and stated it simply: "all knowledge of the internal world is derived by hypothetical reasoning from our knowledge of external facts" (Buchler, 1940, p. 230). After I had come to this conclusion myself I realized what he was saying, but not before. I report this personal observation for its significance in showing how Peirce's idea could be for so long disregarded. If one in full agreement with the implications of the idea could fail to see what Peirce was saying, in plain English, it is not surprising that others who are less in sympathy with those implications might pass the conclusion by.

Also, Peirce did not deal with the question at length but sounds rather like a man who, having pointed out the obvious, sees no need to elaborate. Goudge (1950, p. 232–3) has summarized the argument as applied to sensation, emotion, and volition – all events that have been regarded as inescapably private. A sensation of redness is known only in the perception of red objects, clearly external to the observer; anger is something known secondarily, the primary perception being that of undesirable behavior on the part of another; and volition – this I find harder to follow – is known in the concentration of attention or abstraction, the two latter being evident in the changing and selective awareness one has of the external world.

The argument needs elaboration, and I must approach it from another direction. Let us start by recognizing that the inference to mind and mental activity concerns something happening inside oneself. The idea of the physical self, objectively known, is therefore fundamental. That idea, and the idea of the other, have been shown to have a common element (Hebb, 1960). The evidence is from adult behavior but it becomes understandable when one realizes that, for the child especially, others are perceived as integral wholes but the self can only be perceived piecemeal; even before a mirror, perspective on oneself is difficult. Inevitably then the baby must form his ideas of a *person* on the basis of other persons, objectively known, and then presumably with difficulty form an idea of himself on this model. The result is an objectively known physical self, a combination of fragmentary perceptions of his own body and the perception of others as wholes. Some perceptions of one's body are of course private – one's aches and pains and muscle tensions are not experienced by others – but they are still objective and of sensory origin: perceptions of things happening in parts of that objectively known body.

A further step comes with the idea of a *mind* as something inside the body that perceives and knows, of which the primary evidence is the peculiar relation that is evident between the posture of the body and events elsewhere. The simplest and most direct example is the relation between the position of the eye-lids and a large part of one's surroundings; at the moment when the eyes close, a segment of existence ceases, in color and shape and size. The eyes, evidently, are a sort of channel from the outside world to something within. Similarly, the ears are a channel for a different kind of information, and so with skin (for hardness, roughness, warmth), lining of the mouth (taste) and the nose (smell). The existence of that something within, mind or soul or demon, is thus inferred from the relation between certain objective phenomena.

The idea of *sensation* is the implied idea of the reception by the mind of that incoming information: an event known by inference, a highly theoretical idea and not an observable.

Of special interest, and closely related to the idea of sensation, is the image; and the first thing to note is a confusion in current discussion that derives from the fact that the term, image, is applied to two quite different entities. One is the imagined object or event that is (apparently) seen or heard or felt; the other is the theoretical activity of mind that is the basis of the experience. When I have a visual after-image, the result of staring at a bright light for a few seconds, I see before me a spot on the wall. Again there is a correlation with a phenomenon of the body, for the spot moves exactly as my eyes move, unlike other spots; the observed relation, also, between the prior exposure of the eye to the bright light and the occurrence of the spot, as well as its transience, permits the inference that what I am really dealing with is something going on inside me, an aberration of a (theoretically known) sensory process. I may refer to this internal event as a mental image, but I do not see it. In that sense of the term I *have* an image; what I *see* is the illusory spot on the wall.

My present deafness provides another example. The deaf man, especially at first, is tempted to conclude that everybody mumbles these days instead of speaking clearly (as they used to do) but it is likely to appear more parsimonious, on further consideration, to suppose instead that he himself has changed; and when he finds that he cannot hear other things that he used to hear, things that others can still hear, the latter conclusion becomes inescapable: changed properties of the objective world, as perceived, require the inference that it is his own sensory processes that have changed.

I could go on: with illusions, which are detected from conflicts of evidence from the external world, and emotions, which are recognized in oneself in the first place as they are in others, namely, by a temporary deviation from an established baseline of behavior (including changes of heart rate etc.). Secondarily, one may learn from associated signs to make the same diagnosis (Hebb, 1946; the onset of stage-fright I now recognize from a disturbed appetite and a peculiar restlessness some time before having to appear on the platform). But the examples given should be sufficient.

2. WIDER IMPLICATIONS

It is not possible logically to prove that there is no introspection – the null hypothesis cannot be proved – but Peirce and Humphrey (and Gilbert Ryle and E. G. Boring) have given us strong reason to doubt its existence, and that view is reinforced when it can be shown how inference may provide what knowledge we do have of our own thought processes. At the very least, an immediate awareness by the mind of its own activity becomes improbable and cannot be taken for granted as a basis of psychological and philosophic investigation. Let us consider some of the implications of this situation.

One concerns current discussions of what philosophers know as the identity hypothesis, the idea that mind is a part or property of the activity of the brain or part of the brain (i.e., the cerebrum). Argument against the hypothesis characteristically assumes an empirical knowledge – empirical as distinct from theoretical knowledge – of mental states and processes and proceeds by asserting that they are unlike what the identity hypothesis would require. A psychologist for example may say that a visual percept, the consciousness of some object in the visual field, cannot consist of a volley of impulses for the consciousness is not the aggregation that would imply but something forming a more smoothly integrated whole; or it may be argued by a philosopher that mind cannot be an activity of brain because mind is not localized and a brain activity obviously is. I do not speak here of the soundness or unsoundness of such theoretical ideas but only make the point that they *are* theoretical, and that the identity hypothesis is not refuted by showing that another theory is not in agreement with it.

An obvious implication, if immediate self-awareness does not exist, is an undermining of the basis of philosophic idealism. The argument here is that all we can know surely is in our own minds, so that other (external) existence becomes uncertain or known only with difficulty. In this case *knowing* becomes a relation between some part of the mind and its sense-data and not, as common sense would have it, between an organism and its environment. Idealism can certainly be maintained as a theoretical view (provided it is carried out consistently, which as far as I can make out is not done, the solipsist for example forgetting that his own body and sense-organs must be counted among the nonexistent objects of the physical world), but cannot be regarded as an inescapable consequence of the 'fact' that what we really know is our sensations. Distinctions such as that of appearance versus reality, or of the phenomenal versus the physical, as usually made, seem to be diluted forms of the same thing. It is true that the physicist's reality is theoretical and inferential and so different from the phenomenal, but the theory is based solidly on direct observation of a physical world whose reality is not brought in question – that is, on galvanometer readings, photographs of cloud chambers, and the like. The sophisticated theory that results cannot raise doubts about the reliability of these phenomena, for in doing so it would invalidate itself.

On another point, the long-standing doubts about the legitimacy of Helmholtz's 'unconscious inference' go up in smoke. There is no other kind of inference, for in this terminology 'conscious inferences' are in the class of mental processes that are open to self-inspection – of which there are none. The dichotomy of conscious and unconscious in this sense is a misconception that goes back to Herbart. It is misconception for two reasons. In the first place it assumes that one part of the mind, the conscious part, is observable, and we have seen what reason there is to deny that possibility. In these terms, there is an unconscious but not a conscious mind. This language however incorporates a fundamental confusion. It is one thing to say that I am conscious, and mean that my mind is active and responsive to my environment; it is very different to say that an idea is conscious, and mean by that that *I* am conscious of *it*. The true meaning of the term conscious is a reference to a state of the organism, as distinct from the state of a man in coma, under anesthesia, or in deep slow-wave sleep. If we accepted Herbart's (and Freud's and Jung's) terminology, we would now find ourselves in the position of having to say that man's consciousness is the result of an activity of his unconscious mind.

So what Helmholtz's 'unconscious inference' means is simply that the subject cannot report how the inference was made. This is the normal state of affairs. We have seen that one may know something of what goes on in one's mind, but the complexity of brain function is such that far more must be going on than one can know about. *All* inference is unconscious in the Herbartian sense, and there is strong independent support for that conclusion in the Würzburg studies of the imageless thought where, for example, it was shown that even elementary arithmetical operations involve an unreportable mental activity.

I have already referred to the topic of imagery, and the fallacy of mistaking the properties of the imagined object for the properties of the imaginal process itself. The nature of the process is a matter of theory, and the only evident basis for theory in this case is in the physiology of perception. In a physiological context it is possible to see the problem of imagery, and of representative processes generally, in a perhaps clearer light. It becomes evident that there may be degrees and degrees of abstraction, suggesting that we should abandon the crude categorization of representative processes as either concrete or abstract, the concrete usually being treated as some kind of image, the abstract usually as verbalization. Hubel and Wiesel (1968) provide direct physiological evidence of three degrees of abstraction in visual sensory processes (the activity of 'simple', 'complex' and 'hypercomplex' cells in visual cortex), and there are indications of a still higher level of abstraction. The cell-assemblies that I have proposed as the basis of representational activity must have a similar hierarchical order. A first-order assembly is representative of a narrow range of sensory stimulations: representative not because it resembles the stimuli but because it has the same physiological effect in the absence of the stimulation. A second-order assembly is one that represents the first-order assemblies that organized it, because it has more or less the same excitatory effect as they have on other thought processes and motor response; and so on. Now this suggests in turn that the importance of imagery is not that it carries the burden of thought – after all, Binet (1903) reported an antagonism between image and thought – but that it is a *reportable* part or accompaniment of thought, consisting of first and second-order assemblies that can function as the actual process of perception does and initiate speech. And, from the point of view of this paper, it has the very important property of providing one with a clue to what is going on within one's own head: its effect is to make one see something or hear or feel something whose existence other evidence does not confirm; the conflict of evidence informs one that the something is illusory, but also provides information about what one's present thought is concerned with.

REFERENCES

Binet, A. *L'Etude Experimentale de l'Intelligence*. Paris: Schleicher, 1903.

Boring, E. G. A history of introspection. *Psychological Bulletin,* 1953, *50,* 169.

Buchler, J. *The Philosophy of Pierce: Selected Papers*. 1940.

Dorland's Illustrated Medical Dictionary, Ed. 24. Philadelphia, W. B. Saunders Co., 1965.

English, H. B., & English, A. C. *A Comprehensive Dictionary of Psychological and Psychoanalytical Terms.,* New York, Longmans, Green and Co., Inc., 1958.

Estes, W. K. *Learning theory and mental development,* New York: Academic Press, 1970.

Gallie, W. B. *Pierce and Pragmatism*. 1952

Goldfarb, W. Effects of early institutional care on adolescent personality. *Journal of Experimental Education,* 1943, *12,* 106–129.

Goudge, T. A. The Thought of C. S. Pierce. 1950.

Hebb, D. O. Emotion in man and animal: An analysis of the intuitive processes of recognition. *Psychological Review,* 1946, *53,* 88–106.

Hebb, D. O. *The organization of behavior*. New York: Wiley, 1949.

Hebb, D. O. The American Revolution. *American Psychologist*. 1960, *15,* 735–745.

Hebb, D. O. *A Textbook of Psychology,* Ed. 2. Philadelphia: W. B. Saunders Co., 1966.

Hebb, D. O., Lambert, W. E., & Tucker, G. R. Language, thought and experience. *Modern Language Journal,* 1971, *55,* 212–222.

Hubel, D. M., & Wiesel, T. N. Receptive Fields and functional architecture of monkey striate cortex. *Journal of Physiology,* 1968, *195,* 215–243.

Humphrey, G. *Thinking*. London: Methuen & Co., Ltd., 1951.

Hunt, J. McV. *Intelligence and experience*. Ronald Press, 1961.

Kleitman, N. *Sleep and Wakefulness*. Chicago: University of Chicago Press, 1939.

Lashley, K. S. Cerebral organization and behavior. *Research Publication of the Association of Nervous and Mental Diseases*. 1958, *36,* 1–18.

Legendy, C. R. On the scheme by which the human brain stores information. *Mathematical Biosciences,* 1967, *1,* 555–597 (Cited by Scott, 1975).

Moruzzi, G., & Magoun, H. W. Brain stem reticular formation and activation of the EEG. *Electroencephalography & Clinical Neurophysiology,* 1949, *1,* 455–473.

Penfield, W. The cerebral cortex in man. I. The cerebral cortex and consciousness. *Archives of Neurology and Psychiatry,* 1938, *40,* 417–442.

Penfield, W., & Roberts, L. *Speech and Brain-Mechanisms*. Princeton: Princeton University Press, 1959.

Rakic, P. Local circuit neurons. *Neurosciences Research Program Bulletin,* 1975, *13,* no. 3.

Scott, A. C. Neurodynamics (a critical survey). *MRC Technical Summary Report No. 1548* (Mathematics Research Center, University of Wisconsin-Madison), October 1975.

21 Forebrain Commissurotomy and Conscious Awareness

R. W. Sperry
California Institute of Technology

The left and right cerebral lobes of the mammalian brain in the natural state are largely separate anatomically except for cables of cross-connecting fibers, the cerebral commissures, most prominent of which is the enormous corpus callosum, the largest fiber system of the brain, estimated to contain in man over 200 million fibers. Experimental investigation of the functional role of the cerebral commissures was stimulated during the early 1940s by a series of clinical reports in which complete surgical section as well as congenital absence of the corpus callosum had seemingly failed to produce any consistent or distinct behavioral symptoms detectable in extensive neurological and psychological testing (Akelaitis 1943; Bremer 1958; Bremer, Brihaye, and André-Balisaux 1956). Animal studies started in the early 1950s, mostly on cats and primates (Myers and Sperry 1953; Sperry, Stamm, and Miner 1956; Sperry 1961; Downer 1962; Myers 1962), showed consistently, however, that each hemisphere after surgical separation functions independently to a very large extent in most higher activities, including perception, learn-

Portions of this article draw substantially on prior presentations for the 9th International Symposium on Brain Research, Netherlands Central Institute for Brain Research, Amsterdam, July 1975, and a symposium on The Psychology of Consciousness, The Institute for the Study of Human Knowledge, San Francisco, May 8, 1976. Work of the author is supported by grant no. MH 03372 of the National Institute of Mental Health and the F. P. Hixon Fund of the California Institute of Technology.

ing, and memory. In objective behavioral tests involving sensory discrimination learning, each surgically disconnected hemisphere was found to sense, perceive, learn, and remember independently of the other.

Although deep surgical bisections are possible experimentally that include the roof of the mid-brain, the supramammillary commissure, and even the cerebellum (Sperry 1964), it was sufficient merely to cut the forebrain commissures that mediate cross communication between the hemispheres proper to prevent interhemispheric transfer of perceptual learning and memory. The collected animal evidence (Sperry 1961) supported the conclusion that each of the disconnected hemispheres develops its own private chain of learning and memory experiences that are cut off from, and inaccessible to, recall through the opposite hemisphere.

Not only did learning remain lateralized to the one hemisphere receiving the critical sensory input but also the two hemispheres could be trained concurrently to perform mutually contradictory tasks (Myers 1962). It was shown further by Trevarthen (1962) that with an optical system of light-polarizing filters the separated hemispheres could be made to perceive two different things occupying the same position in space at the same time. Under these conditions (see Fig. 21.1), in which one or the other of two stimulus panels is selectively activated in a series of trial-and-error responses, one hemisphere perceives itself to be receiving rewards for selecting, for example, circles and avoiding crosses, while at the same time with the same responses the other hemisphere sees itself being rewarded conversely for avoiding circles and selecting crosses. The animals tend to work with one hand in this situation, and the hemisphere controlling the working hand tends to learn more rapidly than does the more passive hemisphere. By forcing use of the inactive hand after learning is established, and by restricting vision to the more passive hemisphere, the cerebral dominance can be shifted, and the animal can be shown to have been learning with the second hemisphere the reverse of what was being learned with the first hemisphere.

Thus the objective animal evidence suggests that in each disconnected hemisphere conscious experience (assuming cats and subhuman primates have consciousness) is cut off from conscious experience in the other. Lack of cross communication of awareness between the two hemispheres is further evident in the inability of the split-brain animal to cross compare or integrate sensory information projected simultaneously partly to one and partly to the other hemisphere (Sperry and Green 1964). However, the same kinds of perceptual cross integration that fail with complete surgical deconnection are readily achieved if the anterior commissure or a small one-centimeter strand of the posterior corpus callosum is left intact (Tieman and Hamilton 1974; Doty 1975). The interhemispheric mediation of higher activities can thus be forcibly narrowed down by surgical and other experimental procedures to a small band of roughly

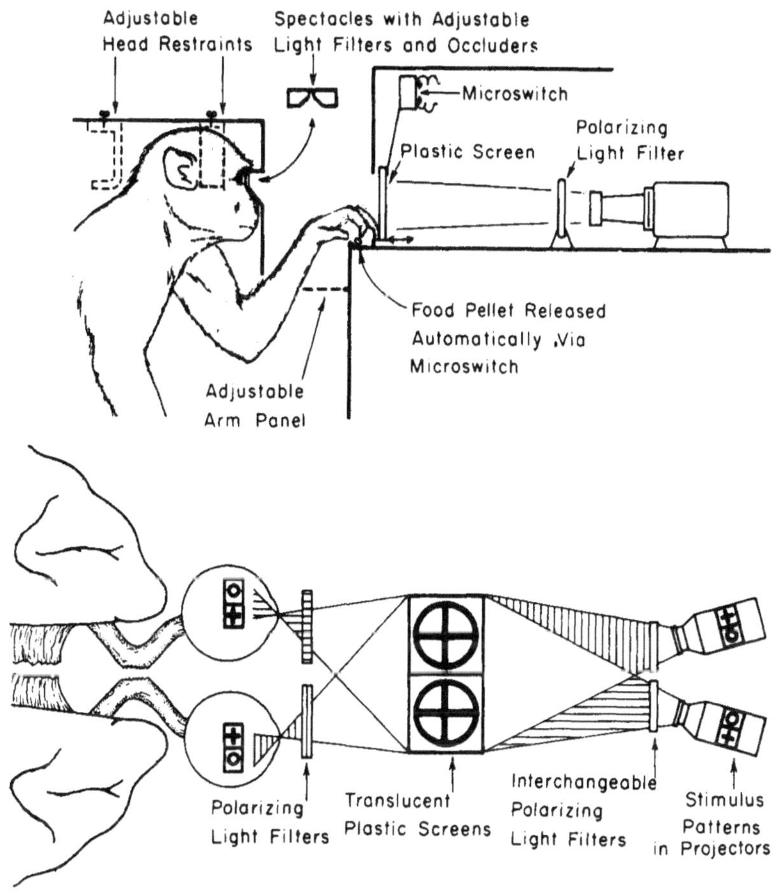

FIG. 21.1. Technique of Trevarthen (1962) for showing split-brain monkey can perceive two different things occupying the same position in space at the same time. Left and right hemispheres trained under these conditions learn mutually contradictory discrimination habits from the same set of trial-and-error responses (from Sperry 1961).

several hundred thousand fibers. Such studies hold promising possibilities for the further dissection and analysis of the anatomical substrate of awareness. Whether the impulse traffic crossing such a minimal remnant of the cross communication system should be regarded as an intrinsic part of the conscious process per se will be considered below in more detail.

Although there is no way to prove firmly that the surgically disconnected hemispheres in the bisected brain of subhuman mammals are separately conscious, this conclusion would seem to follow if one is willing to accept a starting assumption that cats, monkeys, and other mammals normally possess consciousness. The position taken here is that consciousness may be inferred to be present in animals by much the same logic that we infer it to be present in other persons (compare aphasics who have been rendered temporarily mute by brain damage, drugs, or hypnosis, and who may then after recovery be able to recount their conscious experience during the mute period).

SPLIT-BRAIN MAN

In human patients who have undergone cerebral commissurotomy (see Fig. 21.2), carried out for control of intractable epilepsy (Akelaitis 1943; Bogen and Vogel 1976), there similarly is no direct empirical data that can be advanced as firm proof that the surgically separated hemispheres are independently conscious. Human subjects, however, furnish more

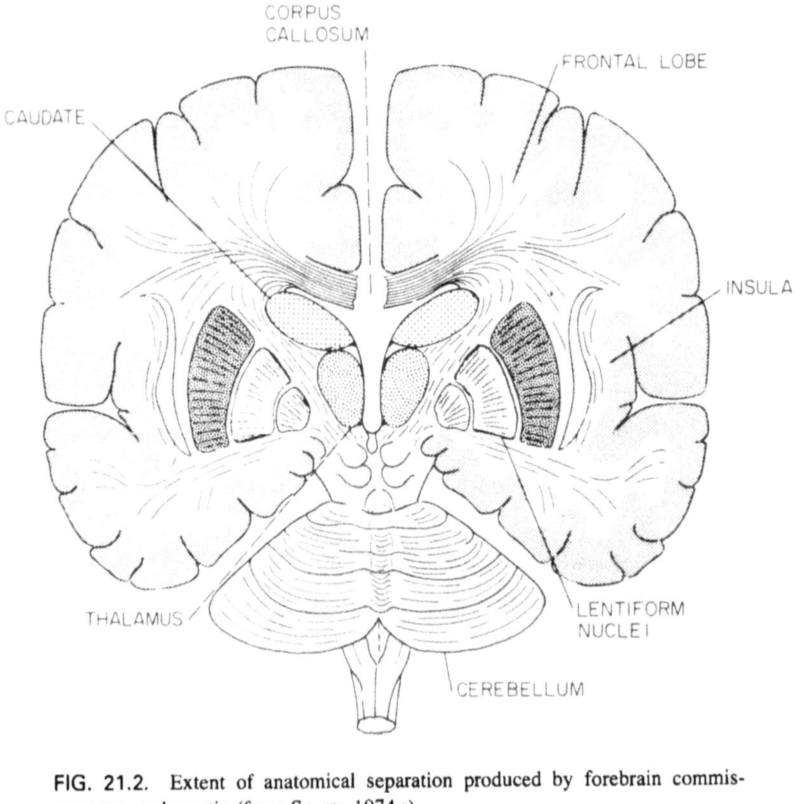

FIG. 21.2. Extent of anatomical separation produced by forebrain commissurotomy, schematic (from Sperry 1974*a*).

direct evidence for this conclusion, since the vocal hemisphere of the human brain readily transmits a verbal report of what it introspectively does or does not experience. As a rule, the surgically disconnected speaking hemisphere disclaims any awareness. Further, the mute hemisphere displays a corresponding lack of ability to respond to stimulus sensory input to its own hemisphere and the subsequent subjective effects. At the same time it conversely disclaims any direct awareness of stimulus input that has been restricted to the opposite hemisphere. Meantime, the nonvocal, mute or "minor" right hemisphere can show by the use of manual signs, nonverbal pointing, or tactual retrieval that it perceives and comprehends correctly the same stimulus input for which the speaking hemisphere disclaims any awareness. Further, the mute hemisphere displays a corresponding lack of ability to respond to stimulus input restricted to the vocal hemisphere. The foregoing applies in general to all sensory modalities thus far tested that can be lateralized, including visual, somaesthetic, olfactory, and auditory. In the case of auditory stimulation the natural bilateralized projection to the cerebral cortex from each ear necessitates the use of competitive dichotic stimulus input in order to obtain lateralization of conscious effects. This apparently works through suppression of conscious perception of the weaker input from the ipsilateral side (Milner, Taylor, and Sperry 1968).

Studies along the above line have repeatedly confirmed over many years of testing the oblivious unawareness of one hemisphere for conscious experience in the other. This applies not only to perception of the sensory input itself but also to more central phases of cognitive processing. It is standard procedure in our human testing to ask the vocal hemisphere, following completion of a task performance by the mute hemisphere, to describe what was in the test performed by its silent partner, the contents of the test material, or what had been done or selected by the silent hemisphere. Where the sensory input has been properly controlled and lateralized, the responses of the speaking hemisphere show that it has no direct awareness of the cerebral processing of the partner hemisphere.

Although commissurotomy subjects show a definite tendency to direct attention selectively either to left or right input at the expense of the other, conscious attention to a task confined to one hemisphere does not necessarily switch off conscious awareness in the other. As described above for the split-brain monkey, it is possible to show also that both hemispheres can commonly be coconscious concurrently in split-brain humans and can perform, in parallel, different and even mutually antagonistic, cognitive tasks. For example, in tests involving right hemisphere performance, the vocal hemisphere often tends to offer throughout a running commentary based on those aspects of the situation not restricted to the mute hemisphere. Because this parallel activity of the second hemisphere may often interfere with the performance of the test hemisphere, the subject is usually instructed to remain silent. Occasionally the commissurotomy subject may become so absorbed in a right hemisphere task that speech and other left hemisphere functions are temporarily depressed to the extent that one questions whether consciousness may not have been shifted entirely to the one working hemisphere. This state of affairs occurs more frequently in the reverse direction, that is, where the vocal hemisphere is dominantly active. Parallel cognitive processing is greatly facilitated when left and right tasks involve a common central background of postural and mental sets and is correspondingly disrupted when the background of cerebral and postural sets are in conflict.

Like the split-brain monkey, the human commissurotomy subject also can be made to perceive two quite different things occupying the same position in space at the same time, something rejected, of course, by the normal brain. The method (Levy, Trevarthen, and Sperry 1972) involves the use of compound left-right stimuli composed of the left and right halves of different pairs of stimulus items joined at the vertical midline (see Fig. 21.3) and projected half to one hemisphere and half to the other. By the laws of perceptual completion and closure each hemisphere automatically tends to fill in its half stimulus across the midline to form a whole bisymmetric percept on each side (Trevarthen 1976).

Other kinds of evidence further confirm that, while one hemisphere is performing, the nondominant less-active hemisphere, though overtly passive in not exerting control over the motor system, may nevertheless be alert and consciously cognizant of what is going on externally. This is indicated, for example, in disgusted shaking of the head or irked facial expressions triggered from the minor hemisphere after it has heard its speaking partner making what it knows to be an incorrect answer. Also, it is not uncommon, while the informed right hemisphere is performing, for the vocal hemisphere to make remarks like, "Now, why did I do that?" "What's the matter with me anyway?"

In sum, cerebral commissurotomy appears to divide not only the brain but also the mind. Two separate realms of subjective awareness are apparent: one in each disconnected hemisphere, and each in itself seems to be remarkably whole, unified, and capable of supporting behavior comparable in many respects to that of the combined intact system. This latter is most impressive with respect to the dominant left vocal hemisphere, the high-level linguistic and related logistic capacities of which seem largely responsible for earlier impressions that cerebral commissurotomy fails to produce any definite behavioral symptoms. It may be remembered in this connection that brain bisymmetry provides each hemisphere with a full complement of basic cerebral mechanisms.

Emotional tone appears to be an exception to the rule that each disconnected hemisphere during lateralized testing remains oblivious of

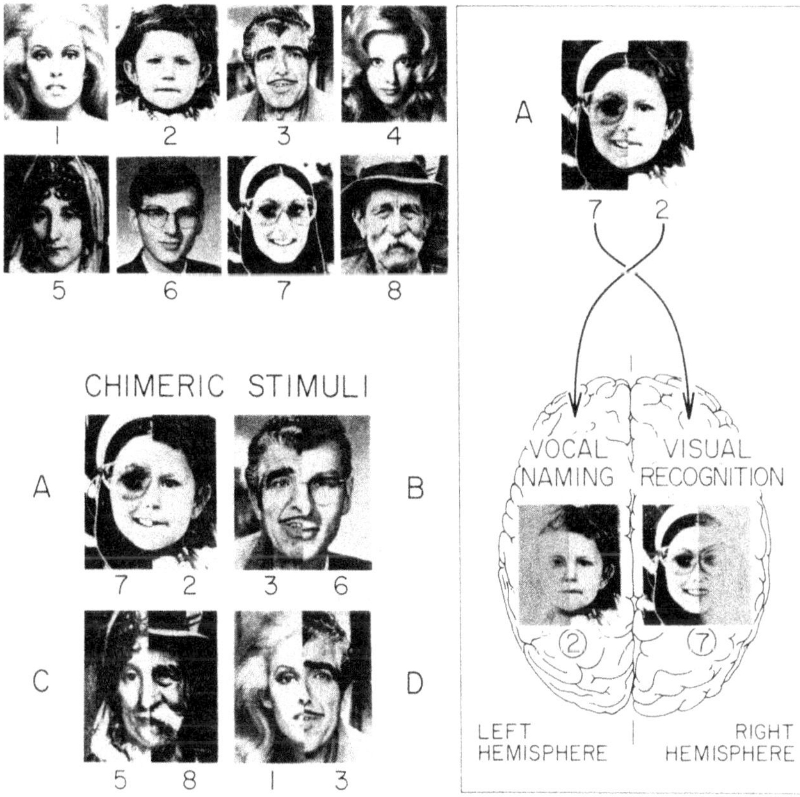

FIG. 21.3. Method by which two hemispheres of split-brain human subjects may be shown to perceive two different and mutually exclusive things at same point in space at same time. With gaze centered on nose of composite stimulus figure, each hemisphere sees a different half stimulus, the missing half of which is automatically completed in each hemisphere to form a bisymmetric whole (from Levy et al. 1972).

the conscious experience of the partner hemisphere. Emotions are rather promptly transferred from one hemisphere to the other, presumably through intact brain-stem mechanisms. Similarly some sensory, attentional, and alertness aspects of awareness are also projected bilaterally via the intact brain stem to both hemispheres, as discussed more fully below. For the present it is important to note that each hemisphere thus contains in functional terms much more than the half mind one might predict at first thought without taking into account the extensive bilateral redundancy in brain organization. With the foregoing in mind, and with some further qualifications to be mentioned below, we can accept the general conclusion that brain bisection yields two conscious minds or selves within the one cranium.

FUNCTIONAL ASYMMETRY

The two disconnected hemispheres of man not only function as if each is independently conscious but also as if each possesses distinctive qualitative properties not equally shared with the other. Linguistic, perceptual, cognitive, motor, attentional, and mnemonic asymmetries have been found (Bogen 1969; Gazzaniga 1970; Levy 1972; Levy et al. 1972; Milner and Taylor 1972; Zaidel 1973; Zaidel and Sperry 1973; Milner 1974; Nebes 1974; Sperry 1974*a*; Dimond 1976; Franco & Sperry 1977), most of which presumably reflect corresponding differences in the content and quality of subjective experience. Most conspicuous among these functional asymmetries is the presence of speech, writing, reading, and calculation in the left hemisphere and the relative absence of these same functions in the right hemisphere.

Prior controversy and uncertainties of the early 1960s as to whether the nonvocal hemisphere has simply lagged behind in human evolution or alternatively has evolved advanced nonverbal specialties of its own (Denny-Brown 1962; Hecaen 1962) seem now to be effectively settled in numerous studies involving direct left-right comparisons within individuals where many otherwise complicating variables cancel out, and in which the so-called subordinate and relatively passive hemisphere has proven to be the superior and dominant hemisphere. It has been possible further to extend the concept of hemispheric specialization to basic modes in cerebral information processing.

Led by Levy (Levy-Agresti and Sperry 1968; Levy 1972), one may interpret hemispheric specialization in man to be a result of the evolutionary differentiation of two mutually conflicting modes of cerebral processing, holistic-spatial and analytic-sequential in nature. In ordinary mental testing of any series of brain-damaged patients, one tends to take for granted that they will show individual differences in cognitive style and in the kinds of mental strategies employed in approaching test tasks. However, when one sees the same individual consistently approaching and solving a set of problems in two distinct ways, like two different persons, depending on whether the left or the right hemisphere is in use, even subtle left-right cognitive differences become meaningful. Prior doubts and uncertainties resolve and the way is clear to further delineate the nature, extent, and functional role of the left-right differences in cerebral processing.

The demonstrated specialties of the minor hemisphere are, first, nonverbal and nonmathematical and mostly involve spatial and visualizing abilities in which a single mental image is more effective than a long series of words. Geometrical discriminations of topological forms, for example, are performed at a high level by the right hemisphere but seem to be extremely difficult or impossible for the left hemisphere

(Franco and Sperry 1977). The prevailing neurological doctrine of the early 1960s, based mainly on symptoms of unilateral brain lesions, had depicted the minor hemisphere as being typically mute, agraphic, word blind and word deaf, and correspondingly agnostic in language-related faculties (Geschwind and Kaplan 1962; Geschwind 1976). This older view has now receded before mounting evidence of positive language performance of the minor hemisphere after commissurotomy. The capacity of the disconnected minor hemisphere to comprehend spoken instructions and even read words flashed to the left field of vision (Gazzaniga and Sperry 1967; Sperry and Gazzaniga 1967; Sperry, Gazzaniga, and Bogen 1969) was found from the start to be much more developed after commissurotomy than anticipated in view of the severe receptive aphasias that have been reported to follow unilateral lesions of the language centers in the dominant hemisphere. Initial inclinations to interpret these right hemisphere language abilities in our commissurotomy cases as an exception to the rule, caused perhaps by diffusing effects of long-term epilepsy or just by individual differences, have now given way to a revised view in which the minor hemisphere of the typical right hander is credited with substantial, though limited and selective, language functions.

The linguistic faculties of the minor hemisphere have been measured more thoroughly and precisely in recent years by Zaidel (1973) using our two best commissurotomy cases and also three hemispherectomy patients, one of the dominant hemisphere. Zaidel (1975) uses a "stabilized image" technique in which a half field occluder is mounted on the eye on a scleral contact lens. The system allows prolonged exposure of visual material with ocular scanning up to one half hour. A high-level vocabulary for the comprehension of single spoken words is confirmed showing in two patients a mental age for the minor hemisphere of eleven and sixteen years, respectively, only two years below that for the vocal hemisphere in these same subjects on the same Peabody Picture Vocabulary Test. In contrast to our earlier results, no specialization was found for nouns as opposed to verbs. The minor hemisphere lexicon appears to follow instead the frequency of word usage. Zaidel finds the right hemisphere to be capable of syntactic and phonetic as well as semantic discriminations.

With respect to reading, writing, and speaking, the results have not much changed our earlier impressions based on tachistoscopic tests. We anticipated that the long exposure and examination of whole sentences instead of single words might reveal a higher level of reading ability, but this is not the case. In general, the ability of the minor hemisphere to process single words stands in marked contrast to its inability to deal with words in series, at least in prose. These limitations do not apply in the same way when words are strung together in singing a familiar melody or in emotional exclamations. In any case, with regard to issues concerning the presence and quality of consciousness in the minor hemisphere, one should keep in mind that the cerebral processing of this hemisphere, though it does not support much speech, is in the current view not at all devoid of linguistic dimensions.

MINOR HEMISPHERE CONSCIOUSNESS

The conclusion that cerebral commissurotomy results in the presence of two largely independent conscious entities, one based in each hemisphere, has not gone unchallenged. Some authorities have preferred to think that the unity of the conscious self is preserved in these subjects with its center in the vocal left hemisphere or in a metasystem in the intact brain stem (MacKay 1966; Penfield 1966; Eccles 1973). These and other theoretically possible ways of interpreting the commissurotomy and related findings have been reviewed in a comprehensive philosophical perspective by Nagel (1971).

Our own impression that both hemispheres, the minor as well as the major, are separately conscious after commissurotomy and that the two disconnected hemispheres may commonly be coconscious in parallel, even in mutually conflicting experiences, is based mainly on the kinds of things that the minor hemisphere has been shown to be capable of doing in the course of a long series of tests over many years. The subjective experience of the minor hemisphere has to be inferred almost entirely, of course, from nonverbal manual performance, although facial, linguistic, and emotional expression generated in the minor hemisphere are also involved. Mute test performances of the minor hemisphere show that it can sense, perceive, learn, and remember all at a characteristically human level. The disconnected mute hemisphere can center and hold a focus of attention, perform high-level spatial reasoning and spatial transformation, generate concepts, make cognitive decisions, and carry out volitional actions. It displays goal preferences and can act on value priorities, and it shows typical human emotional responses in reactions to affect-laden stimuli and situations. It further comprehends spoken single words at a moderately high level and to a lesser extent can also read and comprehend single printed words.

In the face of accumulating evidence along the above lines, earlier claims that the speechless hemisphere is not conscious are now giving way to intermediate positions contending that we must remain agnostic about consciousness in the minor hemisphere or that the minor hemisphere possesses only an elemental form of consciousness not sufficiently advanced to be the basis of a conscious human person or self. Specifically, the nonvocal hemisphere has been interpreted to be lacking in self-awareness (DeWitt 1975). Self-awareness rates as a comparatively advanced and characteristically human form of consciousness appearing relatively late phylogenetically in primate evolution and also late ontogenetically in childhood.

In recent efforts to explore further the upper levels of conscious awareness in the disconnected mute hemisphere (Sperry and Zaidel 1973), we have used the stabilized occluder technique developed by Zaidel to test for a sense of self-consciousness and for general social awareness. If these higher peculiarly human levels of conscious awareness can be shown to be present, one may infer that the lower levels of awareness must be there as well. The subject in these tests wears a scleral contact lens on which is mounted a small optical system with an opaque screen that moves with the eye and blocks out the selected half field of vision wherever the gaze is directed. The procedure is to present to the subject for examination a choice array of pictures or photographs, usually four (see Fig. 21.4), including items for which the subject might have some familiarity, preference, or an emotional response, such as pictures of the subject, of family, relatives, pets and

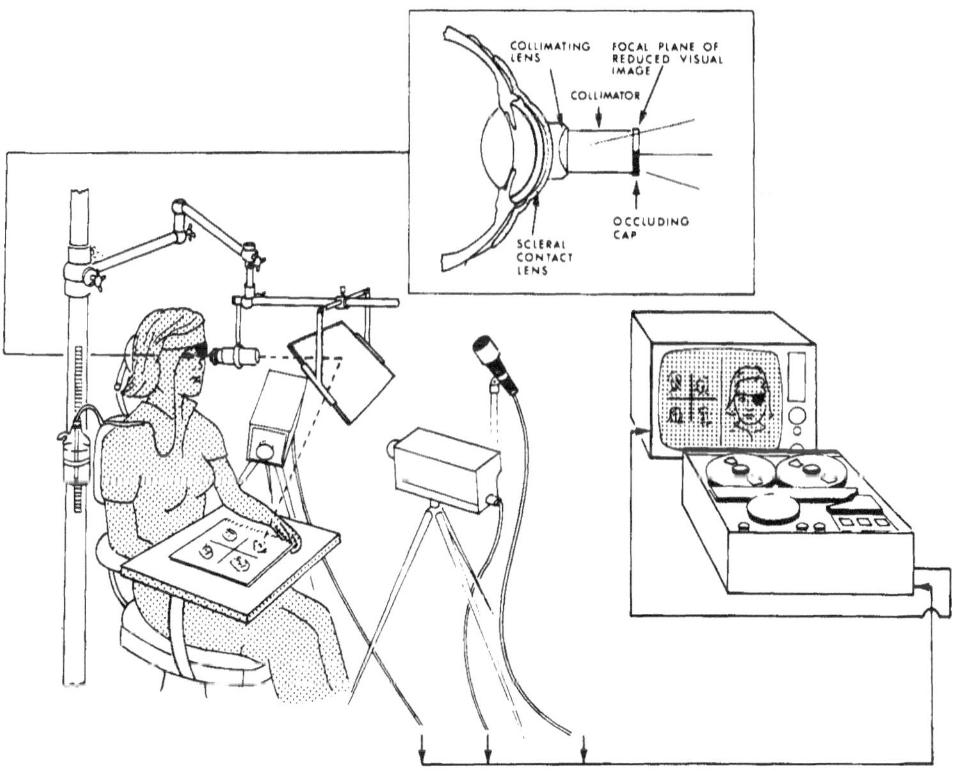

FIG. 21.4. Setup employing contact lens technique of Zaidel which continuously blanks out visual input to one hemisphere, used here to test for upper levels of awareness in minor hemisphere. (This Fig. replaces Fig. 4 in the original paper.)

belongings, political, historical and religious figures, and well-known figures from the entertainment world. After leading questions and remarks by the examiner to establish desired mental sets and associations, the subject is asked to point to the item in the choice array he or she would select for a given situation or reason, the one that he or she most likes or dislikes, might recognize, and to differentiate by "thumbs-up" or "thumbs-down" his or her feelings about selected individuals, etc.

The kinds of reactions obtained from the mute hemisphere in the two patients thus far fitted with the required corneal contact lens (L. B. and N. G.) strongly indicate a characteristic self and social awareness that is generally normal and roughly comparable to that of the language-dominant hemisphere. If anything, the emotional responses generated in the right hemisphere in these two subjects were more intense and less inhibited than those from the left. Minor hemisphere reactions included appropriate emotional outbursts when pictures of the subject's self were introduced by surprise among the test items in an unexpected or unseemly context. The emotional tone of these responses promptly crossed to the other hemisphere, presumably by brain-stem mechanisms, and affected the vocalization of the blinded hemisphere changing the tone of voice, evoking exclamations, etc. From the content of the speech, however, which included comments like "what are they?" "something nice," "whatever it was," it was clear that the speaking hemisphere remained unaware of the particular visual material that had triggered (via the mute hemisphere) its emotional reaction. When the speaking hemisphere was allowed a series of follow-up guesses, however, and eventually came to ask, "Was it me?" "Myself?" the minor hemisphere recognition of the audible stimulus as correct had some kind of a central effect that was registered across and recognized in the speaking hemisphere which thereon settled with satisfaction on this as the answer.

When the subjects were asked directly if they could find a portrait photo of themselves inserted among similar photos in the choice array, they had no trouble doing so, working with either hemisphere. Pictures of pets, other belongings, and of scenes in and outside the home were readily recognized by either hemisphere and evoked appropriate responses. Pictures of well-known public or historical figures, relatives, and acquaintances also were readily pointed out by the minor as well as the major hemisphere. Evaluative judgments from the right hemisphere expressed by preferential pointing and by "thumbs-up" "thumbs-down" gestures were consistent with those obtained verbally from the other hemisphere of the same subject and also in free vision. For example, in a series of trials with L. B., a twenty-one-year-old male subject, the response from the right hemisphere was "thumbs-up" for Churchill, pretty girls, Johnny Carson, and a ballet scene, and "thumbs-down" for Hitler, Castro, and a war scene. A photo of Nixon (the date of testing was pre-Watergate) evoked some indecision, ending in an intentional and definite horizontal neutral. A photo of the subject himself inserted at the end of this same series evoked a definite "thumbs-down" response, but in this case unlike the others, the response was accompanied by a distinct wide, sheepish, and (we think) self-conscious grin generated in the mute hemisphere.

Again, follow-up verbal questioning by the examiner, as well as spontaneous remarks of the subject during testing, indicated that the vocal hemisphere had remained quite unaware of the contents of the test material presented to the minor hemisphere. However, if such verbal questioning were pursued, the subject's left hemisphere was commonly able, with the combined cues from himself and the examiner, to narrow in, after a few exchanges, on the correct category and sometimes on the specific test item. It was concluded that the mute disconnected minor hemisphere does indeed possess self- and social awareness at levels quite comparable to those of the left hemisphere and of the intact brain as a whole.

INCOMPLETENESS OF PSYCHOLOGICAL DIVISION

Although the foregoing and many similar lateralized tests indicate that each surgically disconnected hemisphere has a conscious domain of its own and that the bulk of the content of mental experience in each hemisphere remains cut off from any direct awareness through the other hemisphere, there are important qualifications to be kept in mind in thinking about the degree and nature of this mental separation. This applies especially to behavior under natural nonlateralized conditions. Many unifying factors can be enumerated (Sperry 1968, 1974*a*) that tend to make at least components of the inner experience of the two disconnected hemispheres similar or identical in orientation and content especially during ordinary unrestricted behavior. The bilateral sensory projection systems of the brain, like those for cutaneous sensibility of the face, ensure a bilateral reduplication of symmetric sensations in both hemispheres. Thus, with conscious attention focused on facial, auditory, or other stimuli that get bilateral representation, both hemispheres presumably develop a full bilateral percept with no vertical split between right and left aspects. Scanning movements of the eyes yield a similar duplication with respect to vision (Sperry 1970*a*, 1974*a*). The overall effect in some respects is thus more like a twinning or doubling of the conscious domain of the self rather than midline division. This bisymmetric reduplication of sensory input from proprioception and from some external sources provides a considerable background of left-right unification in the functional organization in both hemispheres and has been an important factor in the concept of two separate minds or selves in the bisected brain. Insofar as mental activities are identical in the two hemispheres, there is no way to prove behaviorally that the two are separate; this can only be extrapolated from analogous conditions where the functions differ.

Unity in conscious experience after hemisphere deconnection tends to be preserved also by cross-integration systems of the intact brain stem like those referred to above that mediate a prompt bilateralization of emotion generated unilaterally. This brain-stem cross-integration we presume involves also mood, alertness, and perhaps subtle shades of these as in the more elemental dimensions of mental sets and attention. This latter is inferred from the ability of the vocal hemisphere in tests for social awareness to sense orientational, categorical, or attitudinal cues generated in the mute hemisphere which then enable the vocal member to center in on the correct general category of a mute hemisphere experience. Cross transmission of some components of auditory verbal images at brain-stem levels remains a possibility. At any rate, some affective, cognitive, and attentional aspects of consciousness seem to be effectively transmitted from one side to the other to further help the two disconnected hemispheres to function together in harmony and in some respects as a unit.

Whether the neural cross integration involved in the foregoing as, for example, that mediating emotional tone, constitutes an extension of a single conscious process or is better interpreted as just a transmission of neural activity which triggers a second and separate bisymmetric conscious effect in the opposite hemisphere remains open at this stage. In any case, it is pertinent to remember that the bilateralizing and unifying mechanisms are largely of the nonfocal, general background category, whereas conscious awareness tends on the other hand to be correlated predominantly with attentional and focal aspects of cerebral function.

When all unifying factors like the above are taken into account in combination with the evidence for functional deconnection, one is led to conclude with respect to ordinary behavior that the bulk of conscious experience after cerebral commissurotomy is separated into two distinct hemispheric domains but that these are usually similar in their attentional focus and have a large common overlap in general content. Differences contributed by the lateral specialization of the hemispheres will, of course, be accentuated whenever the cerebral processing becomes centered exclusively around specialties of either hemisphere like speech, calculation, or topological reasoning.

During lateralized testing, prolonged use of a single hemisphere with deprivation of focal input to the other not uncommonly leads to a state in which there is a suppression of functional alertness in the nonworking hemisphere to the point where several trials may be required with input to this hemisphere to restore a state of proper function. In ordinary unrestricted behavior, on the other hand, it is rare that conditions would thus selectively restrict sensory input or central processing to one hemisphere for an extended period. Thus typically the two disconnected hemispheres appear to be actively, but separately, conscious in parallel, each working and contributing in its own way to the performance on which attention is focused.

The inference that the disconnected hemispheres are commonly in a state of simultaneous separate coconscious awareness receives additional support from many bilateral tests that involve concurrent but different sensory input and different motor response from each hemisphere. The conclusion is reinforced as well by numerous incidental observations like those involving cross-cueing which variously require that the second hemisphere be actively alert while the other is performing. Coconscious involvement is indicated also in Zaidel's (personal communication, 1976) recent evidence that scores for commissurotomy subjects with free vision are superior to those of either hemisphere working alone on the visual reception subtest of the Illinois Test of Psycholinguistic Abilities. Coconsciousness is further inferred from tests involving competitive double performances, like reading aloud or whistling while counting or sorting blocks with left and right hand. When the two tasks involve the same hemisphere there is severe interference, while tasks performed in separate hemispheres can be carried through in parallel (Franco, in press).

IMPLICATIONS FOR CONSCIOUSNESS IN THE NORMAL INTACT BRAIN

It has been argued by Anderson (1974) that, if one can have two coconscious entities occupying the same cranium concurrently, as in commissurotomy subjects, and if two or more different persons can occupy the same body successively, as in multiple personality or fugue states, it follows logically that it is no longer correct to identify a "person" or "self" as being correlated one-to-one with a body. The concepts and definitions of "person," "self," and related terms need accordingly to be more precisely refined in terms of the critical brain states involved. Such definitions become important for medicolegal issues concerning, for example, comatose, anencephalic, or severely deranged mental conditions, in evaluating donors for vital organ transplants, in dealing with different stages in fetal development, etc.

An interesting position in regard to the concept of "personal identity" has been taken by Puccetti (1973, 1976) and Bogen (1969) who infer that each hemisphere must have a mind of its own—not only after brain bisection but in the normal intact state as well; a conclusion apparently accepted also by DeWitt (1975) with the qualification that only the left cerebral member has self-awareness and is therefore qualified as a person. The argument goes like this: if cutting the cross connections between the hemispheres leaves two coconscious minds, and if surgical removal of a whole hemisphere, that is, hemispherectomy, leaves one conscious person or self, regardless of which hemisphere is removed, then there must have been two present to start with. Puccetti contends that we are, therefore, all of us, really a compound of two conscious persons that coexist in the normal brain, one based in each hemisphere, and that this goes undetected when the commissures are intact and the normally conjoined hemispheres work in perfect synchrony. Because a similar proposal regarding the inherent duality of mind was made back in 1844 by Wigan (see Zangwill 1974), modern dual-mind proponents are known as "latter-day Wiganites." Again one is impressed with the need for sharpening definitions of mind, person, self, and related concepts. Regardless of terminology, however, the question of whether the normal intact brain contains only one unified realm of conscious awareness or alternatively maintains two separate conscious systems, or minds, one centered in each hemisphere, poses a rather clear dichotomy that should be subject eventually to a definite empirical answer.

My own position on this question has been a relatively conventional one. I see consciousness and the conscious self as being normally single and unified, mediated by brain processes that typically involve and span both hemispheres through the commissures. This interpretation implies: first, that the fiber systems of the brain mediate the stuff of conscious awareness as well as the switching mechanisms, synaptic interfaces, or other interaction sites of the gray matter; and second, that the fiber cross connections between the hemispheres are not different in this respect from fiber systems within each hemisphere. Third, this interpretation is based on a theory of consciousness that goes back to the early 1950s (Sperry 1952) in which the subjective unity in conscious experience, along with other subjective effects, is ascribed not so much to corresponding spatiotemporal unity in neural activity or to other isomorphic or topological correspondence but rather to the operational or functional effects in brain dynamics. What counts in determining subjective meaning on these terms is the way a given brain process works in the context of cerebral organization. Subjective unity is accordingly conceived in terms of organizational and functional relations which in turn leads to the idea of a functional (thus causal) impact.

When I tried to put some of these threads together back in the mid-1960s, I found to my initial consternation (as well as that of immediate colleagues) that what seemed to be emerging was a conceptual formula for the way that conscious mind could move matter in the brain and exert causal influence in the direction and control of behavior—in direct contradiction, of course, to the central founding precepts of behaviorism and of twentieth-century scientific materialism generally, and contrary to everything that we had always been taught and believed. When this "unthinkable thought" nevertheless continued to hold up under repeated reexamination, I decided to risk a trial-run publication in a humanist lecture (Sperry 1965, 1966) that might allow me to save face should it promptly be shot down. When, instead, it held up in the marketplace with favorable feedback, it was presented more seriously four years later to the National Academy of Sciences (Sperry 1969*a*), since when it has had a fairly wide exposure in the literature (Sperry 1969*b*, 1970*a*, 1970*b*, 1972, 1974*b*; 1976*a*, 1976*b*, 1976*c*, 1976*d*, 1977). The longer it survives, of course, the less casually it is taken.

Since the main concepts have been presented recently in some detail elsewhere, they are reviewed below in rather brief outline to permit added regard for some of the broader implications and humanistic impact. In essence, consciousness was conceived to be a dynamic emergent of brain activity, neither identical with, nor reducible to, the neural events of which it is mainly composed. Further, consciousness was not conceived as an epiphenonmenon, inner aspect, or other passive correlate of brain processing but rather to be an active integral part of the cerebral process itself, exerting potent causal effects in the interplay of cerebral operations. In a position of top command at the highest levels in the hierarchy of brain organization, the subjective properties were seen to exert control over the biophysical and chemical activities at subordinate levels. It was described initially as a brain model that puts "conscious mind back into the brain of objective science in a position of top command . . . a brain model in which conscious, mental, psychic forces are recognized to be the crowning achievement . . . of evolution" (Sperry 1965, 1966). It must be emphasized at the outset that no direct empirical proof is available, any more than proof is available for the opposing behaviorist position. At this stage, we have only a balance in credibility, all things considered, and the most that can be said is that many of us have now come to regard these psychophysical-interaction concepts as being a little more credible in several respects than the older behaviorist-materialist stance.

Broadly speaking, one of the more important revisions brought by the current concepts is a shift in the scientific status of consciousness. In the past, consciousness has been variously dispensed within science as some kind of parallelistic epiphenomenon, aspect, or correlate of brain processing, and has been considered to be entirely passive in cerebral operations without influence on the stream of physical causation in brain activity, and therefore something that objective science could safely ignore. On our new terms, consciousness, as a holistic systemic property and an active dynamic part of high-order brain processing, is now put within the province of science and is something that cannot be ignored where science wants an explanation of higher brain activities. In effect, this change means that the whole value-rich qualitative world of inner-conscious, subjective experience, the world of the humanities, that has long been explicitly excluded from the domain of science on materialist principles, is now reinstated. In the revised scheme, subjective phenomena have a place and a use in brain function and a reason for having been evolved in a physical system.

An overall consequence of this change is that many of the more objectionable materialistic, mechanistic, deterministic, and reductionistic aspects of science that the humanities have always found difficult to accept and relate to, and which have consistently drawn the fire of antiscience, no longer apply in the new framework. Science, behavioral science in particular, acquires a new look in this perspective to become much more mentalistic, subjectivistic, and humanistic. The swing we have witnessed in recent years toward an increased recognition of conscious subjective experience and referred to variously as the "humanist" or "third resolution" in psychology, the "cognitive revolution" or just the "new psychology," can be seen to be more than just a matter of changing attitudes in science or a reflection of general trends of the time. The new subjectivism in psychology has authentic support and grounding in basic theoretical changes in fundamental mind-brain concepts.

The past strength of the materialist-behaviorist movement has rested in no small measure on the seeming inconceivability that the causal march of neuromechanisms could be influenced by the contents of subjective experience. The present undermining of prior convictions in this area has resulted in a floodgate release of all the pent-up subjectivist pressures held back for decades by behaviorist doctrine. All those disciplines in behavioral science which by preference or by necessity work with subjective experience directly, such as the clinical, cognitive, and humanist schools, also acquire in the new framework a corresponding shift in scientific status. Parallel changes have occurred also in philosophy dealing with mind/brain relations. Today one finds mentalists, dualists, and psychophysical interactionists surfacing again in numbers after having been essentially silent and invisible for decades.

It is important to caution that there is nothing in the current theoretical change that makes subjective experience any easier to work with by scientific methodology and that therefore many of the old arguments against the use of introspection in experimentation still apply. One must caution further that the above legitimate changes toward an increased recognition of subjective mental experience supported by theory have been accompanied in recent years by a series of corollary developments not similarly supported by theory but which have opportunistically ridden along on the same upsurge of new interest in mental phenomena. Things like mysticism, occultism, astrology, faith healing, and parapsychology also have enjoyed a new vigor and popular acceptance in the past eight or nine years. The current view of consciousness as an emergent property of the living brain in action with all its anatomical and physiological constraints hardly increases the likelihood of things like mental telepathy, precognition, psychokinesis, or the existence of mental domains of experience separate from brain activity.

FORMULA FOR PSYCHOPHYSICAL INTERACTION

Perhaps the simplest and quickest way to approach and explain our current mind-brain concept is to compare it with better-known preexistent theories and thus, largely by elimination, to state what the present view is by describing what it is not. First, consciousness in the current view is not an acausal epiphenomenon as widely held in materialist theory. Second, consciousness is not just an "internal aspect" of brain activity as in "dual-aspect theory." An internal aspect is conceivable for all neural processing, but consciousness is special. Third, conscious experience is not conceived to be identical to neural events as in "psychophysical-identity theory." In the present view, conscious phenomena are different from, more than, and not reducible to, neural events, though it is correct to say that conscious phenomena are built of neural events as elements and perhaps also of glial and other cerebral events. Fourth, consciousness is not a pseudoproblem conjured into our thinking by semantic gymnastics, or something that will disappear with a proper linguistic approach. In brief, we can thus bypass previous interpretations of the epiphenomenal, parallelistic, passive correlate, dual aspect, psychophysical identity, and semantic pseudoproblem types in order to focus on consciousness as an emergent property of brain activity, as upheld especially by the Gestalt school of psychology in ideas that peaked during the 1930s and early 1940s under Kohler (1929), Koffka (1935), Kohler and Held (1949), and others (see Boring 1942).

It then remains to distinguish our present model from these earlier emergent Gestalt concepts. First, the emergent properties of the present view are not conceived to be correlated with, nor derived from, electrical field or volume current conduction effects in the cortex. They are conceived rather in terms of traditional nerve circuit and nerve integration theory. Second, the brain processes of consciousness are not conceived to depend on isomorphic or topological correspondence with the mental event. Conscious meaning is a functional derivative conceived in terms of functional impact and potential. Third, while the current view agrees with Gestalt theory that the conscious phenomena are not reducible to the neural elements, it does not take the extreme Gestalt position that categorically rejects analysis and explanation in terms of the parts. Fourth, and most important, the emergent properties in the present view are not interpreted to be mere passive, parallel correlates, or passive aspects or byproducts of cortical events, but as active causal determinants essential to the normal cerebral control.

A conceptual explanatory model for psychoneural interaction is provided, stated in terms acceptable to neuroscience without violating the monistic principles of scientific explanation. The main focus is on the feature of causality. By all prior theories of consciousness, at all recognized by science, consciousness was interpreted to be acausal in brain function, and brain research could accordingly confine itself to the neurophysiology, chemistry, and biophysics of brain processing, totally ignoring consciousness, and expect this approach to lead, in principle, to a complete explanation of brain function. This of course is not the case with the present view in which consciousness (to repeat) plays a causal role and is neither identical to, nor reducible to, the neural events.

Given our present perspectives, it is not difficult now to stretch the meaning of terms such as "neural events," "brain events," "brain processes," etc., to include their emergent (i.e., holistic, configurational, organizational, gestalt, pattern) conscious properties and to thus bring psychophysical identity theory into line with the current emergent interpretation. On these terms identity theory tends to fuse with emergentism and is then forced to espouse reductionist philosophy to retain identity. Either way we come around to much the same concept. It has been pointed out (Sperry 1970*b*, 1976*c*) that the theoretical and semantic distinctions that prevailed in philosophy prior to 1965 no longer hold in the same way in the context of current perspectives.

Even after the meaning of neural events is stretched to include the holistic conscious properties, our current model still differs from identity theory in that it identifies consciousness only with the holistic properties of *select* brain processes and then not with their neurophysiological, biophysical, and chemical infrastructure. The holistic conscious properties are recognized to be distinctive "real" phenomena in their own right with their own distinctive causal properties. Though mainly composed of neural events, conscious phenomena are not conceived to be "nothing but" neural events.

The causal power attributed to the subjective properties is nothing mystical. It is seen to reside in the hierarchical organization of the nervous system combined with the universal power of any whole over its parts. Any system that coheres as a whole, acting, reacting, and interacting as a unit, has systemic organizational properties of the system as a whole that determine its behavior as an entity, and control thereby at the same time the course and fate of its components. The whole has properties as a system that are not reducible to the properties of the parts, and the properties at higher levels exert causal control over those at lower levels. In the case of brain function, the conscious properties of high-order brain activity determine the course of the neural events at lower levels (Sperry 1966). The term "interaction" for the psychophysical relation is perhaps not the best descriptively but is used for its historical connotations which still apply in the sense that mental phenomena are conceived to exert causal control influence on neural events.

Emergent properties are generally assumed to have causal potency elsewhere at all levels, and one need merely insist that no exception should be made in the case of the yet-to-be-described aspects of cerebral processing responsible for consciousness. On the foregoing terms, psychology and psychiatry are best interpreted as distinct disciplines in their own right, not reducible or identical to neuroscience or behavioral biology. In other words, "The meaning of the message will not be found in the chemistry of the ink." This exaggeration, however, should not be taken to the extreme of depreciating the tremendous explanatory value of analysis and of subdisciplines in science generally, at least those close to the level of the causal unknowns under investigation. Our concepts of the emergent subjective properties and their causality are still, of course, at a general, abstract level. It remains by this and by any other theory thus far available to explain those critical organizational differences that distinguish brain processes with subjective properties from those without, and to define in exact operational and neural terms the essential functional role played by subjective awareness.

From the standpoint of functional control, one may ask what benefits precisely are conferred by the introduction in evolution of subjective conscious effects? Thinking concerning this question is still preliminary and speculative along lines like the following: consider the tactical difference between responding to the world directly and responding to inner conscious representations of the outside world. Wherever displacements in time or in space are advantageous, as, for example, in mental recall, in thinking, and in the formation of anticipatory sets, the use of inner representations has indispensable organizational advantages. The real world can hardly be manipulated as can inner images. Responses involving perceptual constancies in shape, size, position, etc., would seem also to be more effectively managed through the use of inner representations. Further, the employment of implicit trial-and-error responses to inner mental models, and the avoidance thereby of overt response commitments, with possible errors in the real world, is a central rationale in the evolution of thinking.

The development of an inner subjective world may thus be viewed broadly as part of the evolutionary process of freeing behavior from its initial primitive stimulus-bound condition, providing increasing degrees of freedom of choice and of originative central processing. The subjective effects have additional advantages in the driving and directing of behavior as motivational elements and as positive and negative reinforcers. It is difficult to conceive an efficacious motivational system without subjective properties like pain, pleasure, hunger, etc. These subjective effects evolve into controlling ends in themselves in much of human behavior.

Conscious experience may be conceived as a rather distinct entity built into brain organization and expressly designed for specific functional effects, as opposed to viewing it as a general pervasive property of complex neural integration. There is reason to believe it is present in the higher brain centers but not in the spinal cord, for example, or lower brain stem, and probably not in the cerebellum either. The commissurotomy evidence indicates that the system for inner conscious representations in primates and cats, at least, is confined mainly to the cerebral hemispheres proper and the upper brain stem. We assume it to be rather diffusely represented within the forebrain but by no means extending throughout all neural activity at forebrain levels. On the input side of the conscious system, a great deal of the sensory processing is completed automatically and unconsciously. The integrations required for constancy effects like those for perceived position in space during head, eye, and body movements, or for the union of monocular two-dimensional patterns into novel three-dimensional percepts, or the processing of elemental auditory sounds into perceived speech, etc., are extremely complex neural functions but appear to be processed without conscious mediation. Similarly, on the output side, most or all of the complicated processing required to translate conscious aims, percepts, and volitional intent into appropriate motor-behavior patterns also takes place automatically and unconsciously. The intricate arrays of requisite muscle-contraction patterns involve a complexity that goes far beyond the ability of the conscious mind to understand and direct. This is another reason to identify the conscious properties with the relatively simple holistic features rather than with the whole intricate inframechanism of brain processing.

Though representing a rather small fraction of the total brain activity in physiological terms, the conscious properties are of prime importance from the organizational standpoint. For example, the laying down, storage cataloging, and retrieval of memories seems to proceed very largely on the basis of their holistic conscious properties rather than those of the neuronal inframechanisms. Most higher brain processing in many can be viewed as being designed for, and directed toward, the generation, maintenance, or expression of aspects of conscious awareness. Older stimulus-response and central-switchboard concepts of brain organization that arose out of spinal cord physiology and were congenial to behaviorist interpretation may be replaced by a model in which the brain is seen to be organized as a decision-making control system monitored with value priorities, and in which conscious phenomena confer certain operational advantages over and above those obtainable in systems that lack consciousness.

REFERENCES

Akelaitis, A. J. "Studies on the Corpus Callosum. VII. Study of Language Functions (Tactile and Visual Lexia and Graphia) Unilaterally Following Section of Corpus Callosum." *Journal of Neuropathology and Experimental Neurology* 2 (1943): 226–62.

Anderson, S. L. "On the Problem of Personal Identity." Ph.D. dissertation, University of California, Los Angeles, 1974.

Bogen, J. E. "The Other Side of the Brain. II. An Appositional Mind." *Bulletin of the Los Angeles Neurological Societies* 34 (1969): 135–62.

Bogen, J. E., and Vogel, P. J. "Neurological Status in the Long Term Following Complete Cerebral Commissurotomy." In *Les Syndromes de disconnexion calleuse chez l'homme*, edited by F. Michel and B. Schott. Lyon: Hôpital Neurologique, 1976.

Boring, E. G. *Sensation and Perception in the History of Psychology*. New York: Appleton-Century, 1942.

Bremer, F. "Physiology of the Corpus Callosum." *The Brain and Human Behaviour: Research Proceedings of the Association of Nervous and Mental Disease* 36 (1958): 424–48.

Bremer, F.; Brihaye J.; and André-Balisaux G. "Physiologie et pathologie du corps calleux." *Schweizer Archiv fuer Neurologie, Neurochirurgie und Psychiatrie* 78 (1956): 31–87.

Denny-Brown, D. "Discussion." In *Interhemispheric Relations and Cerebral Dominance*, edited by V. B. Mountcastle. Baltimore: Johns Hopkins Press, 1962.

DeWitt, L. "Consciousness, Mind and Self: The Implications of the Split-Brain Studies." *British Journal for the Philosophy of Science* 26 (1975): 41–47.

Dimond, S. J. "Depletion of Attention Capacity after Total Commissurotomy in Man." *Brain* 99 (1976): 347–56.

Doty, R. W. "Consciousness from Neurons." *Acta Neurobiologiae Experimentalis*, vol. 35 (1975).

Downer, J. L. "Interhemispheric Integration in the Visual System." In *Interhemispheric Relations and Cerebral Dominance*, edited by V. B. Mountcastle. Baltimore: Johns Hopkins Press, 1962.

Eccles, John C. *The Understanding of the Brain*. New York: McGraw-Hill Book Co., 1973.

Franco, L. "Hemispheric Interaction in the Processing of Concurrent Tasks" (in press).

Franco, L., and Sperry, R. W. "Hemispheric Lateralization for Cognitive Processing of Geometry." *Neuropsychologia* 15 (1977): 107–14.

Gazzaniga, M. S. *The Bisected Brain*. New York: Appleton-Century-Crofts, 1970.

Gazzaniga, M. S., and Sperry, R. W. "Language after Section of the Cerebral Commissures." *Brain* 90 (1967): 131–48.

Geschwind, N. "Discussion." In *Les Syndromes de disconnexion calleuse chez l'homme*, edited by F. Michel and B. Schott. Lyon: Hôpital Neurologique, 1976.

Geschwind, N., and Kaplan, E. "A Human Cerebral Deconnection Syndrome." *Neurology* 12 (1962): 675–85.

Hecaen, H. "Clinical Symptomatology in Right and Left Hemispheric Lesions." In *Interhemispheric Relations and Cerebral Dominance*, edited by V. B. Mountcastle. Baltimore: Johns Hopkins Press, 1962.

Koffka, K. *Principles of Gestalt Psychology*. New York: Harcourt Brace, 1935.

Kohler, W. *Gestalt Psychology*. New York: Liveright, 1929.

Kohler, W., and Held, R. "The Cortical Correlate of Pattern Vision." *Science* 110 (1949): 414–19.

Levy, J. "Lateral Specialization of the Brain." In *Annual Colloquium on Biology of Behavior*, edited by J. A. Kiger, Jr. Corvallis: Oregon State University Press, 1972.

Levy, J.; Trevarthen, C.; and Sperry, R. W. "Perception of Bilateral Chimeric Figures Following Hemisphere Deconnection." *Brain* 95 (1972): 61–78.

Levy-Agresti, J., and Sperry, R. W. "Differential Perceptual Capacities in Major and Minor Hemispheres." *Proceedings of the National Academy of Sciences* (USA) 61 (1968): 1151.

MacKay, D. "Discussion." In *Brain and Conscious Experience*, edited by J. C. Eccles. New York: Springer-Verlag, Inc., 1966.

Milner, B. "Hemispheric Specialization: Scope and Limits." In *The Neurosciences Third Study Program*, edited by F. O. Schmitt and F. G. Worden. Cambridge, Mass.: M.I.T. Press, 1974.

Milner, B., and Taylor, L. "Right Hemisphere Superiority in Tactile Pattern-Recognition after Cerebral Commissurotomy: Evidence for Non-verbal Memory." *Neuropsychologia* 10 (1972): 1–15.

Milner, B.; Taylor, L.; and Sperry, R. W. "Lateralized Suppression of Dichotically Presented Digits after Commissural Section in Man." *Science* 161 (1968): 184–85.

Myers, R. E. "Transmission of Visual Information within and between the Hemispheres." In *Interhemispheric Relations and Cerebral Dominance*, edited by V. B. Mountcastle. Baltimore: Johns Hopkins Press, 1962.

Myers, R. E., and Sperry, R. W. "Interocular Transfer of a Visual Form Discrimination Habit in Cats after Section of the Optic Chiasm and Corpus Callosum." *Anatomical Record* 115 (1953): 351.

Nagel, T. "Brain Bisection and the Unity of Consciousness." *Synthese* 22 (1971): 396–413.

Nebes, R. "Hemispheric Specialization in Commissurotomized Man." *Psychological Bulletin* 18 (1974): 1–14.

Penfield, W. "Speech, Perception and the Cortex." In *Brain and Conscious Experience*, edited by J. C. Eccles. New York: Springer-Verlag, 1966.

Puccetti, R. "Brain Bisection and Personal Identity." *British Journal for the Philosophy of Science* 24 (1973): 339–55.

Puccetti, R. (1976). "The Mute Self: A Reaction to DeWitt's Alternative Account of the Split-Brain Data." *British Journal for the Philosophy of Science* 27 (1976): 65–73.

Sperry, R. W. "Neurology and the Mind-Brain Problem." *American Scientist* 40 (1952): 291–312.

Sperry, R. W. "Cerebral Organization and Behavior." *Science* 133 (1961): 1749–57.

Sperry, R. W. "Problems Outstanding in the Evolution of Brain Function." James Arthur Lecture, American Museum of Natural History, New York, 1964.

Sperry, R. W. "Mind, Brain, and Humanist Values." In *New Views on the Nature of Man*, edited by J. R. Platt. Chicago: University of Chicago Press, 1965. Reprinted in the *Bulletin of the Atomic Scientists* 22 (1966): 2–6.

Sperry, R. W. "Brain Bisection and Mechanisms of Consciousness." In *Brain and Conscious Experience*, edited by J. C. Eccles. Heidelberg: Springer-Verlag, 1966.

Sperry, R. W. "Mental Unity Following Surgical Disconnection of the Cerebral Hemispheres." *Harvey Lectures*. New York: Academic Press, 1968.

Sperry, R. W. "Toward a Theory of Mind." *Proceedings of the National Academy of Sciences* (USA) 63: (1969): 230–31. (*a*)

Sperry, R. W. "A Modified Concept of Consciousness." *Psychological Review* 76 (1969): 532–36. (*b*)

Sperry, R. W. "Perception in the Absence of the Neocortical Commissures." *Association for Research in Nervous and Mental Diseases* 48 (1970): 123–38. (*a*)

Sperry, R. W. "An Objective Approach to Subjective Experience: Further Explanation of a Hypothesis." *Psychological Review* 77 (1970): 585–590. (*b*)

Sperry, R. W. "Science and the Problem of Values." *Perspectives in Biology and Medicine* 16 (Autumn 1972): 115–30. Reprinted in *Zygon* 9 (March 1974): 7–21.

Sperry, R. W. "Lateral Specialization in the Surgically Separated Hemisphere." In *The Neurosciences: Third Study Program*, edited by F. O. Schmitt and F. G. Worden. Cambridge, Mass.: M.I.T. Press, 1974. (*a*)

Sperry, R. W. "Messages from the Laboratory." *Engineering and Science* 37, no. 3 (1974): 29–32. (*b*)

Sperry, R. W. "Left-Brain, Right-Brain." *Saturday Review* (August 9, 1976), pp. 30–33. (*a*)

Sperry, R. W. "Mental Phenomena as Causal Determinants in Brain Function." In *Consciousness and the Brain*, edited by G. Globus, G. Maxwell, and I. Savodnik. New York: Plenum Publishing Corp., 1976. Reprinted in *Process Studies* 5 (1976): 247–56. (*b*)

Sperry, R. W. "A Unifying Approach to Mind and Brain: Ten Year Perspective." *Progress in Brain Research*, vol. 43 (1976). (*c*)

Sperry, R. W. "Changing Concepts of Consciousness and Free Will."' *Perspectives in Biology and Medicine* 20 (1976): 9–19. (*d*)

Sperry, R. W. "Bridging Science and Values: A Unifying View of Mind and Brain." *American Psychologist* (1977).

Sperry, R. W., and Gazzaniga, M. S. "Language Following Surgical Disconnection of the Hemispheres." In *Brain Mechanisms Underlying Speech and Language,* edited by C. H. Milikan. New York: Grune & Stratton, 1967.

Sperry, R. W.; Gazzaniga, M. S.; and Bogen, J. E. "Interhemispheric Relationships: The Neocortical Commissures; Syndromes of Hemisphere Disconnection." In *Handbook of Clinical Neurology,* vol. 4, edited by P. J. Vinken and G. W. Bruyn. New York: North-Holland Publishing Co., 1969.

Sperry, R. W., and Green, S. M. "Corpus Callosum and Perceptual Integration of Visual Half Fields." *Anatomical Record* 148 (1964): 237.

Sperry, R. W.; Stamm, J.; and Miner, N. "Relearning Tests for Interocular Transfer Following Division of Optic Chiasma and Corpus Callosum in Cats." *Journal of Comparative and Physiological Psychology* 49 (1956): 529–33.

Sperry, R. W., and Zaidel, E. "Level of Consciousness in the Surgically Disconnected Minor Hemisphere." *Proceedings of the 14th Annual Meeting of the Psychonomic Society* (Abstr.), 1973.

Tieman, S., and Hamilton, C. "Interhemispheric Communication between Extraoccipital Visual Areas in the Monkey." *Brain Research* 67 (1974): 279–87.

Trevarthen, C. B. "Double Visual Learning in Split Brain Monkeys." *Science* 136 (1962): 258–59.

Trevarthen, C. "Psychological Activities after Forebrain Commissurotomy in Man." In *Les Syndromes de disconnexion calleuse chez l'homme,* edited by F. Michel and B. Schott. Lyon: Hôpital Neurologique, 1976.

Wigan, A. L. *The Duality of the Mind.* London: Longman, 1844.

Zaidel, E., and Sperry, R. W. "Performance on Raven's Colored Progressive Matrices Test by Subjects with Cerebral Commissurotomy." *Cortex* 9 (1973): 34–39.

Zaidel, E. "Linguistic Competence and Related Functions in the Right Cerebral Hemisphere Following Commissurotomy and Hemispherectomy." Doctoral dissertation, California Institute of Technology, 1973. *Dissertation Abstracts International* 34 (1973): 2350B. University Microfilms no. 73-26, 481.

Zaidel, E. "A Technique for Presenting Lateralized Visual Input with Prolonged Exposure." *Vision Research* 15 (1975): 283–89.

Zangwill, O. L. "Consciousness and the Cerebral Hemispheres." In *Hemisphere Function in the Human Brain,* edited by S. Dimond and J. Beaumont. London: Paul Elek, 1974.

Author Index

Numbers in *italics* denote pages with complete bibliographic information.

C

E

F

G

N

R

S

T

U

V

W

X, Y, Z

Subject Index

For Product Safety Concerns and Information please contact our EU representative GPSR@taylorandfrancis.com
Taylor & Francis Verlag GmbH, Kaufingerstraße 24, 80331 München, Germany

www.ingramcontent.com/pod-product-compliance
Lightning Source LLC
LaVergne TN
LVHW021003300926
849160LV00007B/234

9781138593329